A TEXT BOOK OF
MEDICAL INSTRUMENTS

A TEXT BOOK OF
MEDICAL INSTRUMENTS

S. Ananthi

B.E., M.Tech. (I.I.Sc.), Ph.D.,
M.I.E.E.E., M.I.E.T.E., M.I.S.O.(I)
Instrumentation Dept., A.C. Tech. Campus
University of Madras, Chennai-600 025

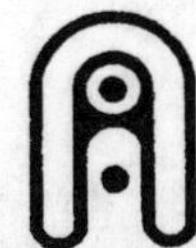

PUBLISHING FOR ONE WORLD

NEW AGE INTERNATIONAL (P) LIMITED, PUBLISHERS

New Delhi • Bangalore • Chennai • Cochin • Guwahati • Hyderabad
Jalandhar • Kolkata • Lucknow • Mumbai • Ranchi
Visit us at **www.newagepublishers.com**

Published by New Age International (P) Ltd., Publishers
First Edition: 2005
Reprint: 2010

Branches:

- 36, Malikarjuna Temple Street, Opp. ICWA, Basavanagudi, **Bangalore**. © (080) 26677815
- 26, Damodaran Street, T. Nagar, **Chennai**. © (044) 24353401
- CC–39/1016, Carrier Station Road, Ernakulam South, **Cochin.** © (0484) 4051303
- Hemsen Complex, Mohd. Shah Road, Paltan Bazar, Near Starline Hotel, **Guwahati**. © (0361) 2543669
- No. 105, 1st Floor, Madhiray Kaveri Tower, 3-2-19, Azam Jahi Road, Nimboliadda, **Hyderabad**. © (040) 24652456
- RDB Chambers (Formerly Lotus Cinema) 106A, Ist Floor, S.N. Banerjee Road, **Kolkata**. © (033) 22275247
- 16-A, Jopling Road, **Lucknow**. © (0522) 2209578
- 142C, Victor House, Ground Floor, N.M. Joshi Marg, Lower Parel, **Mumbai**. © (022) 24927869
- 22, Golden House, Daryaganj, **New Delhi**. © (011) 23262370, 23262368

ISBN (10): 81-224-1572-5
ISBN (13): 978-81-224-1572-8

Rs. 275.00

C-09-10-4143

Printed in India at Ramprintograph, Delhi.
Typeset at Goswami Associates, Delhi.

PUBLISHING FOR ONE WORLD
NEW AGE INTERNATIONAL (P) LIMITED, PUBLISHERS
4835/24, Ansari Road, Daryaganj, New Delhi-110002
Visit us at **www.newagepublishers.com**

PREFACE

The field of medical diagnostic instruments has developed very well during the past 25 years with the impact the Electronics Engineering has provided to it. Today, more and more of Electronic & Instrumentation Engineering students have taken to work on the development of either better Instruments using the Technology or of new instrumental techniques for better and non-invasive diagnostics. In the U.S.A., graduate students from India are now being taken to work in this area for research projects in the Universities and hospitals. Side by side, medical graduates also are now taking interest in learning about the develpments in Electronics so that they can use its components and circuits for making better use in Medical Technology.

Therefore, today, most Engineering graduate and Science post-graduate courses have included the subject in the curriculum. It is now well understood that for a technology researcher to interact with the hospital surgeons and seniors in projects of medical instrumentation, he or she should have a good knowledge of the principles of early-day medical instruments, physiology basics and medical terminology.

This book has therefore subdivided the realm of medical instruments into the same sections like a text on physiology and introduces the basic early-day methods well, before dealing with the details of present-day instruments currently in use. Some principles of diagnosis are also included in order that a new researcher could understand the requirements of the Physician rather than blindly proceed in his developments using his knowledge of circuity, software and methods of signal processing. Further, medical diagnostic practice has been conservative in preserving the acumen the Physicians have imbided from their seniors. For example, in the ECG, the very same trace occupying just 2 mm–3 mm with a chart paper is the vital (QRS) component in diagnosis, though, at present, the same information can be presented in a much better time-scale with greater detail. Because ECG diagnosis is still based on this standard record, a researcher intending to produce a new algorithm for a detection of typical pathology (automatically) would need to know the principles of pathological detection from the ECG in current use. That is why, the book has spent some pages on such aspects as well.

After covering the several instruments under the different heads of Physiology, the later-day instruments like the CT scanner, the MRI, Ultrasound and lasers are included. These deserve typically separate volumes on their own, but even here, the essentials are covered both from the medical and technical angles.

Particular importance has been given to safety aspects as has been widely made known through several papers in the IEEE magazines, in a separate chapter. A chapter on possible further developments and another on signal processing examples have been included to the advantage of a medical reader intending to exploit the technological developments.

A final chapter on the use of computers for medical data management and the use of the Web at large concludes the book.

In a book of this kind, meant to be of use for the student who gets himself introduced to medical instruments for the first time, a large number of books, journals and manufacturers' material had to be referred to. Today, the subject is growing at a very fast pace and newer methods in surgery and diagnostics are coming up every day. The book could cover only such material as are current and it is up to the reader to keep himself abreast of the developments by looking into the useful journals for example, the IEEE issues. A little work done by the author's own Biomedical and Engineering group has been included in the chapter on New developments.

It is hoped that the book will meet the needs of all these who take to the study of this subject either in a course or for research applications, both in medical and in electronic technology.

I have to express my thanks to my erstwhile Professors. K. Padmanabhan, K. Chandrasekharan and V. Mohan for their guidance. Particularly I wish to express my thanks to my husband Mr. S. Rajendran, to my brother-in-law Mr. S. Udayakumar, to Mr. R. Vijayarajeswaran of VI Microsystems and to Mr. P. Swaminathan for their interaction and help in this preparation. I am to record also the tolerance and appreciation exhibited by my sons R. Pradeep and R. Babu when their mother was found busy spending her time late into the night on her computer for this preparation for quite some months.

Dr. S. Ananthi

CONTENTS

Chapter 1

Electrophysiological Measurements

1. INTRODUCTION

From the biological cell, electrical potentials are generated and it is due to the electrolytes inside and outside of the cell. A bioelectric potential may be defined as the difference in potential between the inside and the outside of a cell; there exists a difference in potential existing across the cell wall or membrane. A cell consists of an ionic conductor separated from the outside environment by a semi permeable or selectively permeable cell membrane. Human cells may vary from 1 micron to 100 microns in diameter, from 1 millimeter to 1 meter in length and have a typical membrane thickness of 100 Angstrom units. Bioelectricity is studied both from the viewpoint of the source of electrical energy within the cell and also from the viewpoint of the laws of electrolytic current flow relative to the remote ionic fields produced currents by the cell. We make measurements external to a group of cells while these cells are supplying electrolytic current flow.

1.1. Cell Potential Genesis

Experimental investigations with microelectrodes have shown that the internal resting potential within a cell is approximately – 90 mV with reference to the outside of the cell.

The equation for resting potential is $e = \dfrac{\mathrm{RT}}{\mathrm{F}} \log_e \left(\dfrac{c_2}{c_1}\right)$

where R = Gas constant = 8.31436 Joule mole^{-1} deg^{-1}

T = Temperature, °kelvin

F = Faraday constant = 96488 coulomb/gm–equivalent.

(c means concentration, 1 for inside and 2 for outside.)

This potential changes to approximately + 20 mV for a short period during cell depolarisation. Cell activity results from some form of stimulation. The Hodgkin – Huxley excitation by stimulus theory was initially postulated (Nobel Prize winners) during the 1950's. This theory is briefly described as follows :

The interior of a cell primarily contains concentrations of sodium and potassium ions. These concentrations within a cell differ markedly from the concentrations of these ions in the space outside the cells (Fig. 1.1). Elementary ionic theory states that, under suitable conditions, any uneven distribution of ionic concentration in an aqueous solution will result in a potential difference between the regions of different concentration. If, for example, solutions containing unequal concentrations of ions are separated by membrane semi permeable to these ions, a potential will be found to exist (Fig. 1.2).

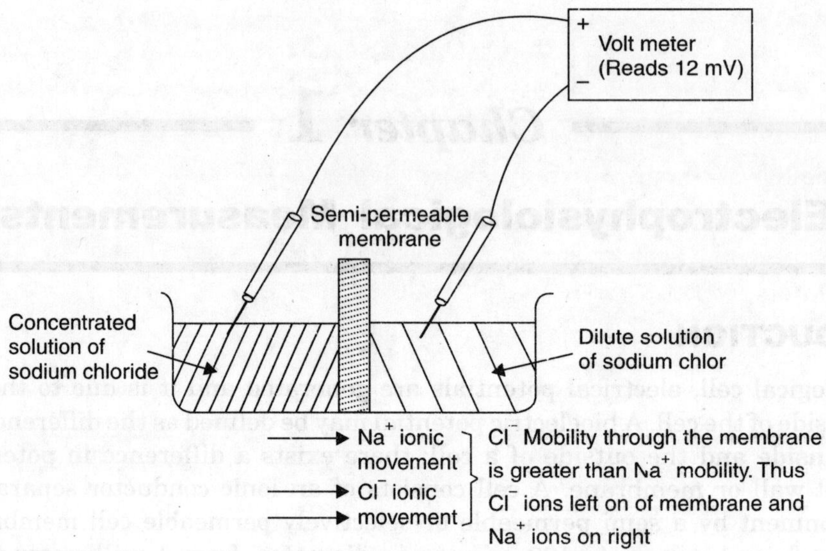

Fig. 1.1 Shows the potential generated ionic concentration difference between two solutions.

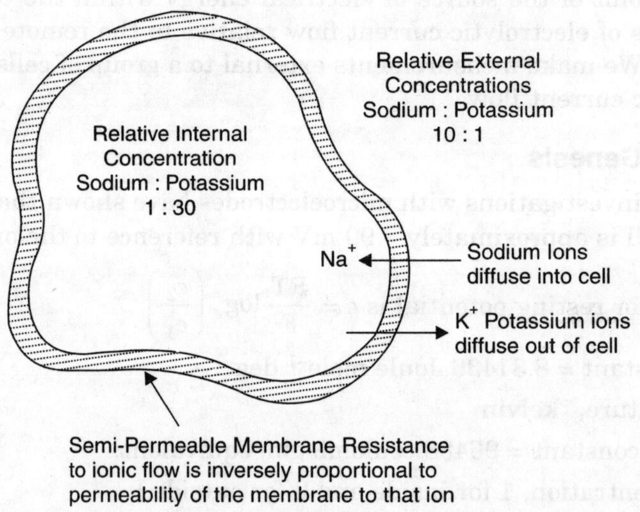

Fig. 1.2 Shows typical concentratioin of sodium and Potassium ions within the cell.

1.2. Chemical Gradient

This potential, which is referred to later as the chemical gradient, is given by the Nernst relations : (T = 293°K)

1.2.1. Nernst Relation

$$\text{Potential (mV)} = 61.6 \log_{10} \frac{\text{concentration one side of membrane}}{\text{concentration, other side of membrane}}$$

or for univalent ionic solutions, the Nernst relation simplifies to :

$$\text{Potential (mV)} = 61.6 \frac{U - V}{U + V}$$

where U = Mobility of the negative ions (anions) through the membrane

V = Mobility of the positive ions (cations) through the membrane

Referring to Fig 1.2, for a 10 : 1 activity (concentration) ratio at 37°C, the relative mobilities of chloride and sodium ions are 65.4 and 43.6 respectively. Applying these values to the Nernst relation gives :

$$\text{Potential (mV)} = \frac{65.4 - 43.6}{61.6 \times 65.4 + 43.6} = 12 \text{ mV}$$

This can be confirmed with a voltmeter as shown in Fig. 1.2. This potential will, of course, run down as diffusion proceeds, unlike that of a living cell.

1.3. Net Gradient

The ionic current produced by ion movement through a semi-permeable membrane depends on the permeability of the membrane and also on the "gradient" that forces the ion through the membrane. This gradient, referred to as the net gradient, consists of both a chemical gradient and an electrical gradient. A chemical gradient is formed due to a difference in concentration producing a potential gradient as given by the Nernst relation. An electrical gradient is formed as a result of a potential that may exist across the membrane due to some other source.

1.4. Cell Concentrations

Experimental investigation have shown that a marked difference in concentrations of both sodium and potassium ions exists across a cell membrane. In mammalian nerve cells as shown in Fig. 1.1. the concentration of potassium ions is in the vicinity fluid external to the cell. On the other hand, sodium ions are approximately 10 times more concentrated in the fluid external to the cell than in the fluid within the cell.

1.5. Cell in Resting State

Consider a cell in its resting or polarized state (Fig 1.3*a*). In this state the membrane is moderately permeable to potassium ions, that is, potassium ions can pass fairly readily through the membrane as the membrane offers medium resistance. This membrane is, however, almost impermeable to sodium ions and, thus, offers a high resistance to the passage of these ions. A large net gradient affects the movement of sodium ions into the cell. This net gradient consists of a chemical gradient produced by the 10 to 1 concentration difference between sodium ions on each side of the membrane and a 90mV electrical gradient produced by the standing potential within cell.

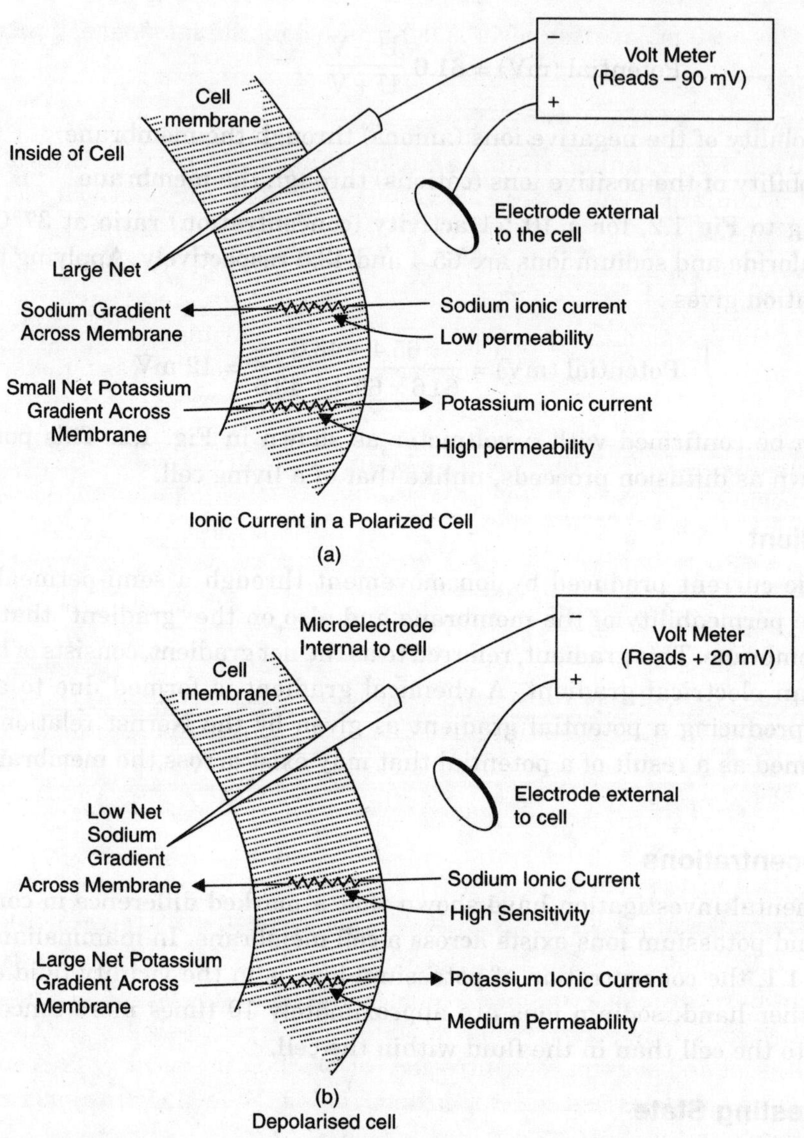

Fig. 1.3

Net Gradient

The net gradient affecting the movement of potassium ions out of the cell is considerably less than the net sodium gradient. This gradient consists of a large chemical gradient due to the 30 to 1 concentration difference across the membrane; however, this chemical gradient is opposed by the electrical gradient produced by the 90 mV standing potential within the cell. Thus, although the membrane is almost impermeable to sodium ions, the net sodium gradient is high. Conversely, although the membrane is moderately permeable to potassium ions, the net potassium gradient is low. The net result is that the sodium and potassium currents are equal; the sodium current balances the potassium current with a resultant current of zero. Since the net current though the membrane is zero, the cell's internal potential will not change and will remain at its – 90 mV resting level.

Indeed, this – 90 mV resting level is determined by the internal cell potential required for sodium and potassium current balance.

Cell Condition after a Stimulus

If the cell receives a stimulus from an outside source, the characteristics of the membrane at the point of stimulation will change and, thus, the ionic currents will also change. After stimulation, the membrane permeability to potassium ions is unaltered but the permeability to sodium ions is increased. A much lower resistance is offered to the flow of sodium ions, thus increasing the sodium ionic current. This increased sodium ionic current causes more positive ions to pass into the cell than are passing out of the cell, causing the internal cell potential to drop from – 90 mV in an attempt to achieve sodium current and potassium current balance.

Cell Depolarization

As this potential decreases, the net sodium gradient across the membrane decreases and the net potassium gradient across the membrane increases, causing the currents to decrease and increase, respectively. This process continues until current balance is again obtained, at which time the internal cell potential is + 20 mV. The cell is then referred to as being in a depolarized state.

Cell Repolarization

By the time the cell has fully depolarized the characteristics of the membrane have begun to revert back to their pre-stimulus state. This causes the sodium ionic current to be considerably lower than the potassium ionic current ; the internal cell potential thus begins to go negative with the process continuing until the – 90 mV resting potential of the cell is once again obtained.

Electrical Analog of the Cell

An electrical analogy to a cell membrane is shown in Fig. 1.4. This circuit cannot strictly be referred to as an equivalent circuit as the electronic current flow in an electrical circuit and the ionic current flow through a cell membrane cannot be said to be equivalent. After assigning resistance values inversely proportional to the relative permeability of the membrane and assuming potassium and sodium concentration ratios, then the intracellular potential for both a polarized cell and a depolarized cell can be determined. The values assumed are analogous to actual values four in a cell.

Assume :

Relative values for R_K R_{Na} and R_D are 1 K, 150 K and 0.35 K respectively.

Potassium ion concentration ratio of 30 : 1 inside to outside.

Sodium ion concentration ratio of 10 : 1 outside to inside.

Then,

$$E_k = 61.6 \log \frac{30}{1} = 91 \text{ mV} - \text{by Nernst relation}$$

$$E_{Na} = 61.6 \log \frac{10}{1} = 62 \text{ mV} - \text{in opposite polarity to } E_k\text{—Nernst}$$

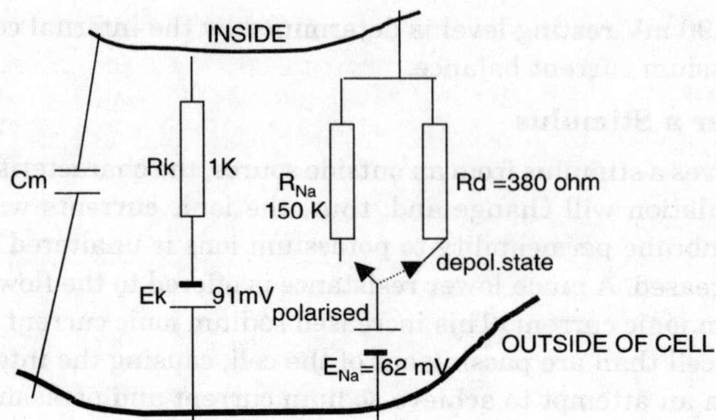

Fig. 1.4. The Electrical analog circuit of the membrane is shown. Cm = membrane capacitance, E_{Na} E_k are the Sodium potassium Nernst potentials, R_K,R_{Na}, the permeability of membrane to K and Na ions flow through membrane, R_d is the permeability of membrane to Na ion flow in depolarizing condition.

For a polarized cell :

$$\text{Net potassium current + net sodium current} = 0$$

$$\frac{\text{Net potassium gradient}}{R_k} + \frac{\text{net sodium gradient}}{R_{Na}} = 0$$

$$\frac{\text{Potassium Chemical gradient + Potassium Electrical gradient}}{R_k}$$

$$+ \frac{\text{Sodium Chemical gradient + Sodium Electrical gradient}}{R_{Na}} = 0$$

$$\frac{E_k + E_c}{R_k} + \frac{-E_{Na} + E_c}{R_{Na}} = 0$$

$$\frac{91 \times 10^{-3} + E_c}{1 \times 10^3} + \frac{-62 \times 10^{-3} + E_c}{150 \times 10^3} = 0$$

Solving

$$E_c = 90 \times 10^{-3} = -90 \text{ mV (polarized)}$$

Similarly, for a depolarized cell, R_{NA} is replaced by R_D (0.35 K)

$$E_c = +20 \text{ mV (Depolarized)}$$

1.6. Action Potential from a Cell

Suppose a microelectrode were inserted into the cell as shown in Figs. 1.3*a* and 1.3*b* and a stimulus were applied to the cell, the output of the microelectrode would appear as shown in Fig. 1.5. this waveform is known as the "Cell action potential". It should be noted that the currents involved in biuelectricity are unlike the currents involved in electronics. Bioelectric currents are due to positive and negative ion movement within a conductive fluid. As these ions possess finite mass and encounter resistance to movement within the fluid their speeds are limited. The cell action potential, thus, shows a finite "rise time" and "fall time".

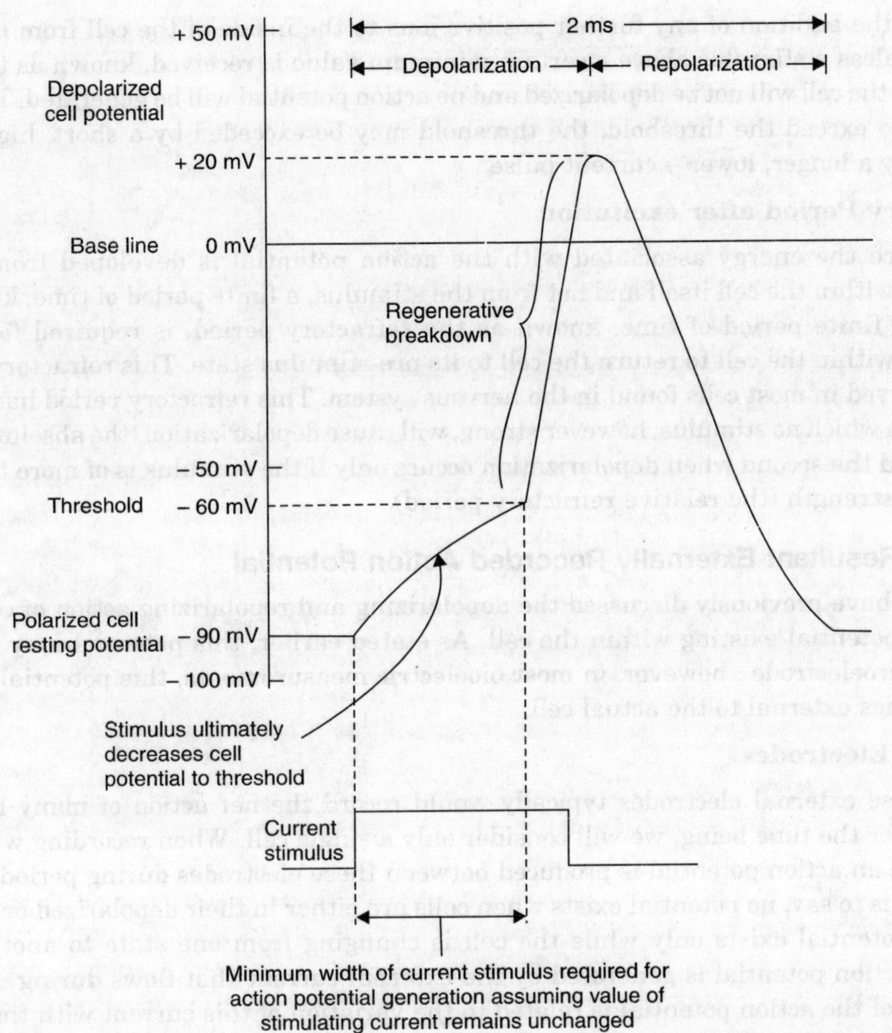

Fig. 1.5. Shows the Cell action Potential (Internally recorded with Micro-electrode).

Sodium Potassium Pump Phenomenon

The ionic concentration gradient across the cell membrane is maintained by virtue of metabolic energy expended by the cell in "Pumping" ions against the ionic gradient formed by the differing ionic concentration between the inside and outside of the cell. This action has been referred to as the "Sodium – potassium pump".

Threshold of Stimulus Causing Action Potential

A cell may be stimulated, or caused to depolarize and then repolarize, by subjecting the cell membrane to an ionic current. This current may be produced by other cells, it may be produced by ionic currents existing as nerve impulses, or it may be artificially produced by some external current stimulus. A cell will be stimulated when sufficient positive ions are added to the inside of the cell to cause its resting potential to be decreased from its – 90 mV level to approximately – 60 mV. Once this threshold level is reached, the cell depolarizes without requiring the addition of any further positive ions to the inside of the cell from the stimulus source. Unless a stimulus above a certain minimum value is received, known as the stimulus threshold, the cell will not be depolarized and no action potential will be generated. The stimulus required to exceed the threshold, the threshold may be exceeded by a short, high – current pulse or by a longer, lower – current pulse .

Refractory Period after excitation

Since the energy associated with the action potential is developed from metabolic processes within the cell itself and not from the stimulus, a finite period of time, known as the refractory finite period of time, known as the refractory period, is required for metabolic processes within the cell to return the cell to its pre-stimulus state. This refractory period has been observed in most cells found in the nervous system. This refractory period has two parts : The first in which no stimulus, however strong, will cause depolarization (the absolute refractory period) and the second when depolarization occurs only if the stimulus is of more than normal threshold strength (the relative refractory period).

1.6. The Resultant Externally Recorded Action Potential

We have previously discussed the depolarizing and repolarizing action of cells and the resulting potential existing within the cell. As stated earlier, this potential may be recorded with a microelectrode ; however, in most bioelectric measurements, this potential is recorded by electrodes external to the actual cell.

External Electrodes

These external electrodes typically would record the net action of many hundreds of cells, but for the time being, we will consider only a single cell. When recording with external electrodes, an action potential is produced between these electrodes during periods of current flow ; that is to say, no potential exists when cells are either in their depolarized or repolarized state. A potential exists only while the cell is changing from one state to another. As the external action potential is generated by the external current that flows during cell activity, the shape of the action potential is related to the variation of this current with time.

External Action Potential

The external potential field rises to its maximum value sometime during the regenerative breakdown phase of the membrane. The external action potential that is recorded from the cell is somewhat similar to a mathematical time derivative of the trans-membrane potential. This potential is detected with maximum amplitude when one electrode is placed as near as possible to the active area and the other electrode is located in a completely inactive or remote area. It is detected with reduced amplitude as the electrodes are placed closer to each other so they intercept smaller elements of potential difference.

Depolarization Current

In a single polarized cell, the inside of the cell is negative with respect to the outside environment, which may be regarded as a reference. As stated previously, the net ionic current flow across the membrane is zero; thus, ionic current flow to and from the cell is zero. If these conditions are altered due to the presence of a stimulating current through the cell membrane, then regenerative membrane breakdown will occur and the cell will depolarize. During the depolarization process the net current through the membrane is not zero; there is a net positive ionic current into the cell through the cell membrane. This current may be detected as a potential difference between two electrodes placed in the vicinity of the cell with the potential difference being produced across the finite resistance of the fluids external to the cell.

This current continues until the cell is fully depolarized, thus, the potential will appear between the two electrodes while the cell is undergoing depolarization. For the short time that the cell exists in a depolarized state, the net current through the membrane is once again zero, thus, no potential will appear between the electrodes.

Repolarization Current

Almost immediately after depolarization, the cell begins to repolarize again. During repolarization, positive ionic current flows from the cell membrane, that is, in the opposite direction to ionic current flow during depolarization. During this period of current flow, a potential will be detected between the electrodes and, since this current is in the opposite direction to the depolarization current, the potential produced between the electrodes during repolarization will be of the opposite polarity to the potential produced during depolarization. The area included by the depolarization and the repolarization potential waveforms is the same since the quantity of current involved in each process is the same. It should be noted that the process described above is somewhat theoretical as it describes the external action potential generated by single cell. In the following discussion we show that single cell depolarization invariably results in depolarization of the adjacent cells and, hence, this externally recorded action potential will be the net summation of the results obtained from these cells.

1.7. Externally Recorded Action Potential from a Group of Cells, the Travelling Wave of Depolarization

Synchronous Depolarization

The preceding discussion must be modified to allow for many cells in close proximity to one another and to allow for the appreciable length of many of these cells. Consider a group of cells in close proximity to one another, under certain conditions of stimulation, these cells may all depolarize at the same time (synchronous depolarization) ; however, the repolarization process is random. Repolarization of the individual cells will occur at different times. The resultant externally recorded action potential is shown in Fig 1.6. Once again the area included under each wave is the same since the quantity of current involved in each process is the same.

Asynchronous Depolarization

Under other conditions of stimulation, the group of cells described previously will not all depolarize at the same time (asynchronous depolarization). The stimulation may result in one cell depolarizing; the action of this cell depolarizing will then act as a stimulus on its adjacent cell causing it to depolarize also. This chain reaction would proceed until all cells in a particular area have depolarized. The resultant externally recorded action potential would appear as shown in Fig 1.6. In practice, combinations of synchronous and asynchronous depolarization occur in a group of cells.

Travelling wave within cells

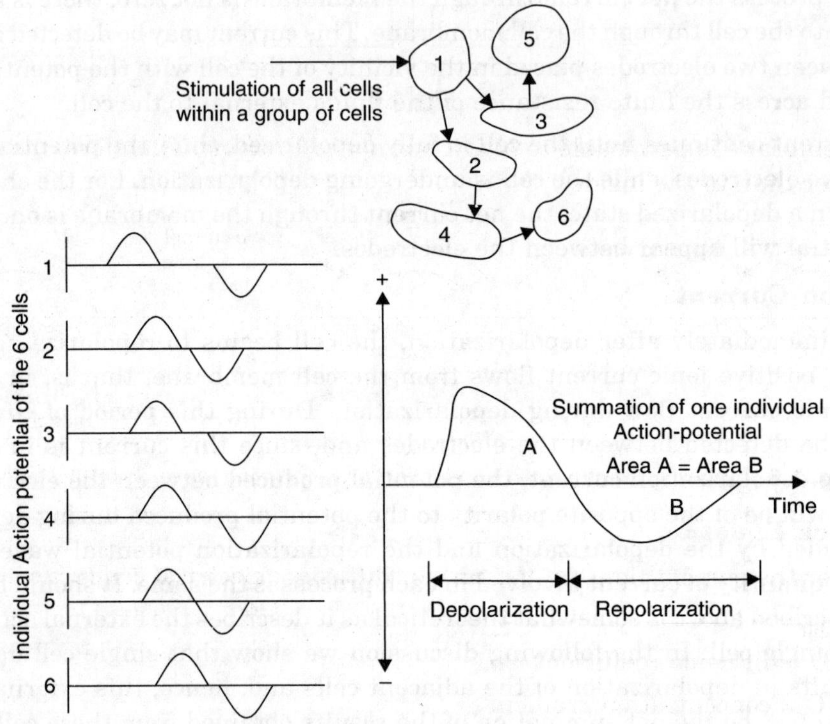

Fig. 1.6. Shows the stimulation is not synchronous and the potential externally seen.

In the same way as the depolarization of one cell causes adjacent cells to depolarize, depolarization of a localized area of an individual cell will cause depolarization of other parts of the same cell. Thus, the depolarization process will appear to travel along the length of the cell causing a travelling wave of depolarization as shown in Fig. 1.8.

As most bioelectric potentials are recorded as external cell action potentials, the results obtained are a summation of the action of many cells. The action potential wave form may be modified by the number of cells, the shape of these cells, and the type of stimulation applied.

The cell already passing a wave cannot respond to a second stimulus – it has become refractory. But there is a variation in excitability, as at point 3 units in time, a smaller response can depolarise once again, while at a point in time t_4, a greater stimulus is required.

The experiments on action potential measurement are usually done on the Squid's axon, which is a large nerve fiber. It is originally called a 100 micron axon. Its action potential varies from – 45 to + 40 mV.

For the Frog's skeletal muscle fiber, it is from – 92 to 30 mV. A contraction follows the wave.

Caridac muscle of frog has a – 55 mV to + 25 mV change, and recovery is prolonged in any cardiac muscle. The top is flat almost.

Inside to outside, the concentration of Na^+,K^+ and Cl^- ions vary in a nerve cell.

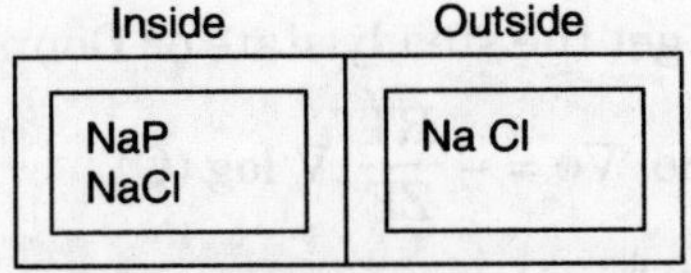

Fig. 1.7

The membrane is permeable to Na,Cl but not to Proteins. Therefore, the concentration of Na is greater than in the inside.

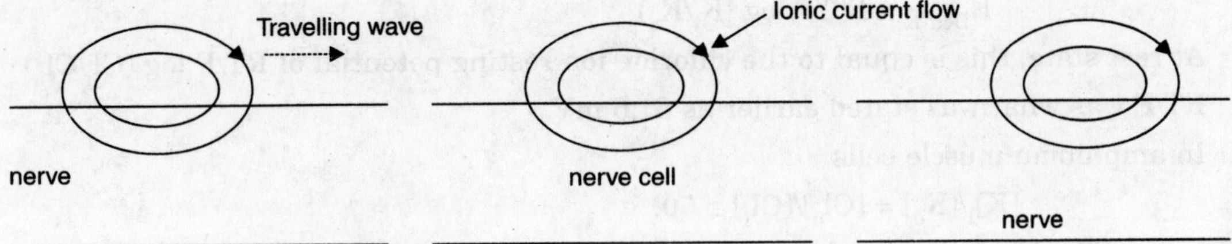

Fig. 1.8 Showing Electro-tonic conduction as a traveling wave down the nerve.

Nernst Planck Equation

Consider the current flow (in A/s. cm) for diffusion, electrical conduction one by one.

$$J_{diff} = -D\nabla C$$

D = diffusion coefficient,

∇C = concentration gradient

$$J_{elec} = -uze\,C\,\nabla\phi$$

u = elec. Field mobility of ion

$= v/\nabla\phi$ = velocity/elec. field

z = valency of ion,

$\nabla\phi$ = field Electric.

The ionic current totally is

So, $$J_{ion} = -D\{\nabla C + (uze\,C/D)\,\nabla\phi\}$$

Using Einstein relation

$D = ukT$ k being Boltzmann's constant,

$$J_{ion} = -D\left\{\nabla C + \frac{zeC}{kT}\nabla\phi\right\}$$

$$J_{ion} = -D\left\{\nabla C + \frac{zFC}{RT}\nabla\phi\right\} \text{(F is Faraday constant)}$$

$R = kL$ where L is Avogadro no.

Faraday is defined as $F = eL$.

e is electronic charge and F is in Coulombs.

The above equation is known Nernst Planck Equation. Using this only, the equation of the wave of action potential can be obtained.

Donnan Equilibrium. We get the steady state or Donnan Potential. When current J = 0.

$$J = 0 \text{ So, } \nabla\phi = -\frac{RT}{ZF} \nabla \log (C)$$

Integrating, $E_{Don} = \phi_I - \phi_{II}$

where the I and II denote the inside and outside of the cell.

This is nothing but the potential difference across the cell membrane.

Thus, for Pottassium ions,

$$E_{Don\ K} = RT/F \log \{K_i/K_o\}$$

At rest state, this is equal to the chloride ion resting potential of RT/F log (Cl_i/Cl_o)

RT/F was what was stated earlier as 61.6 mV.

In amphibian muscle cells,

$$[K]_I/[K_o] = [Cl_o]/[Cl_i] \cong 50.$$

E_{rest} – 99 mV, while actual measurement gave 80 to 100 mV.,

But, if for Na+ ion, E_{Don} is calculated, it is not in agreement. So, the Sodium pump is a metabolic action of push out.

As per $[Na_o]/[Na_i] = 10$, we get

$E_{Don\ Na}$ – 60 log 10 = + 58 mV, which is not true.

Permeabilities of ions

From measured values of V for varying outside concentrations, Hodgkin and Katz found

$$P_K : P_{Na} : P_{Cl} = 1 : 0.04 : 0.45$$

Keynes found $P_K : P_{Na}$ = 1:0.013 using influx and efflux measurements.

$$V = \{RT/F\} \log \frac{P_K C_{Ko} + P_{Na} C_{Nao}}{P_K C_{K\ in} + P_{Na} N_{Nain}}$$

= – 90 mV which agrees with the value of measurements.

It is noted that in the above, Keynes [1951] assumes Cl^- is in equilibrium and does not enter calculations.

Electrotonus–Longitudinal Spread of Current in Nerve Fibres

The resting nerve cell membrane resistance is 1000 ohm/cm², while the capacitance is around 1 μF/cm².

If r_1 and r_2 are external and internal fluid resistances per unit length,

$$\frac{\partial V_1}{\partial x} = -r_1 i_1$$

$$\frac{\partial V_2}{\partial x} = -r_2 i_2$$

$$V_1 - V_2 = -Z_m i_m$$

If there is no current flow in this system,

$$i_1 + i_2 = 0$$

$$\partial i_1/\partial x = -\partial i_2/\partial x = i_m \text{, the trans-membrane current.}$$

And $$\partial^2 V/\partial x^2 = -(r_1 + r_2)\, i_m$$

Also $$V = V_1 - V_2$$

$$i_3 = -C_m\, \partial V/\partial t$$

$$i_4 = (E - V)/r_4$$

$$i_3 + i_4 = i_m$$

$$= -C\, \partial V/\partial t + (E - V)/r_4$$

$$\partial^2 V/\partial x^2 = -\frac{(r_1 + r_2)}{r_4}\{E - V - r_4 C_m\, \partial V/\partial t\}$$

The characteristic length is defined by $\lambda = \sqrt{r_4/(r_1 + r_2)}$

And $\tau_{memb} = r_4 C_m$ which is a time constant.

Therefore we get

$$\lambda^2 \partial^2 V/\partial x^2 - \tau_m\, \partial V/\partial t - V = -E$$

If the above is expressed in a moving co-ordinate system, $y = x - vt$, we get

$$\lambda^2\, d^2V/d y^2 + v\tau_m\, \partial V/\partial y - V = -E$$

$$E - V = e \text{ or } v = E - e$$

e = voltage spread from the active area

$$\lambda^2 \partial^2 e/\partial y^2 - \tau_m\, \partial e/\partial y - e = 0$$

Except at $y = 0$, λ is a constant.

So, $$e = e_0 \exp(-y/\lambda_a)$$

Here, λ_a is a space constant and τ is a time constant for the wave.

Current of conduction in the nerve falls off exponentially with distance from the edge of the (stimulated) active region.

For $\tau^2 v^2/\lambda^2 >> 4$, (nerve and muscle fibres)

$$e = e_0 \exp[-t/\lambda_a]$$

$$\lambda_a = \lambda^2/\tau^2 v^2 = 1/v^2\, C_m (r_1 + r_2)$$

The critical period is the period of latent addition, which is maximum interval between successive sub-threshold stimuli to cause excitation.

EXERCISE

1. Assuming that the net flow of ionic change in an action potential goes up only to charge the membrane capacitance ($C = 1\mu F/cm^2$) calculate the net micro moles transferred per unit action potential rising from – 50 mV to + 65 mV.

The change transferred $Q = CV = 1 \times 10^{-6} \times (115*10^{-3})$

$= 115 \times 10^{-9}$ C/cm^2

The no. of. Coul. per mole $= 9.65 \times 10^4$

Micromoles transferred $= ((115 \times 10^{-9}$ C/cm$^2)/(9.65\ (10^4$ C/cm$^2))$

$= 1.2$ Moles

2. Calculate the change in concentration due to the entry of 3μM/cm^2 of Na into an axon 500 microns as a fraction of the initial concentration, which is 50μM/cc.

$$\Delta C_{Na} = (3 \times 10^{-12} \times d)/(d^2/4)$$

$$= 12*10^{-12}/d \quad (d \text{ is in cm}).$$

$$d = 500\mu = 500 *10^{-4} \text{ cm}.$$

therefore $\Delta C_{Na} = 1.4 \times 10^{-10}$ moles/cc

$$\Delta C_{Na}/C_{Na} = 1.4 \times 10^{-10}/50 \times 10^{-6} = 3 \times 10^5$$

Note that is why a huge number of action potentials can be elicited.

Chapter 2

Electrocardiography

INTRODUCTION

This chapter covers some of the more common measurement techniques used in the medical diagnostics. It is intended to give both Medical and Engineering oriented basis for developing measuring techniques in physiological field. But this covers more of the Engineering aspects that have been employed in most of the medical equipment. The Electrocardiogram and electrocardiograph will be dealt in this chapter.

Generation of electrical activity within the heart is discussed in this chapter. Electrocardiography (ECG) is the art of analyzing this electrical activity by measuring potentials at the surface of the body resulting form this electrical activity within the heart. This is achieved by applying electrodes to certain positions on the body and recording the potentials generated between various combinations of these electrodes with an amplifier and CRT display or strip chart recorder.

ELECTROCARDIOGRAPHIC PLANES

The heart can be regarded as an electrical generator enclosed in a volume conductor, the torso. As this electrical generator is completely enclosed by the torso, a direct measurement of the generator output is impossible without resorting to surgery. The electrocardiographer measures the potential existing between various points on the surface of the volume conductor and uses the information obtained to determine the clinical condition of the heart. The measurement can be carried out in three different planes as discussed below.

1. The Frontal plane
2. The transverse plane and
3. Sagittal plane

These various planes are shown in Fig. 2.1.

The projection of the cardiac potential is referred to as electrocardiogram (abbreviated as ECG). Various techniques are used to measure the projection of the cardiac potential along axes existing on each of the three planes.

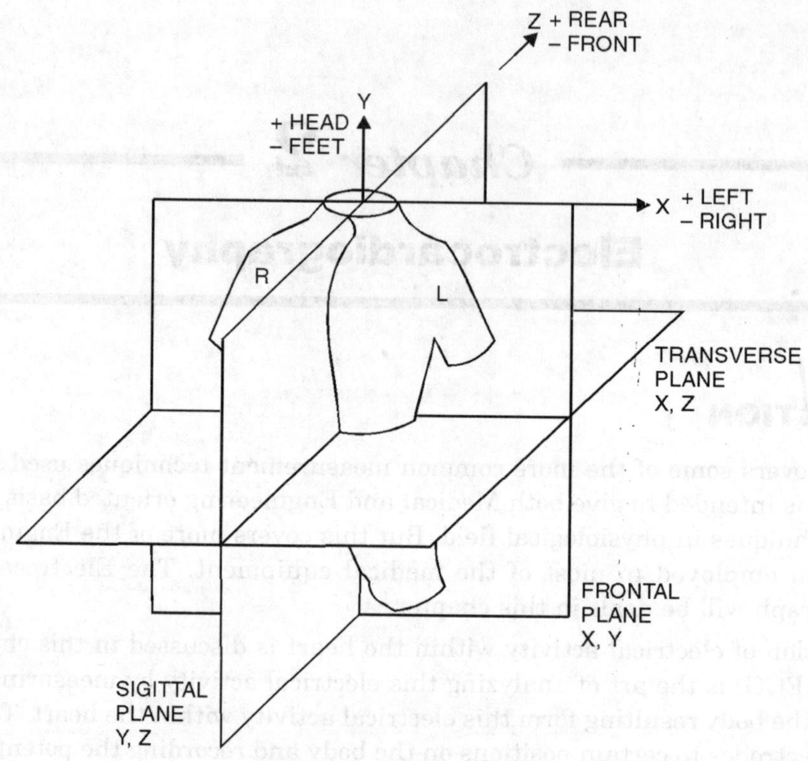

Fig. 2.1. Shows various planes.

FRONTAL PLANE ECG MEASUREMENTS

The electrical potential generated within the heart as projected along axes existing on the frontal plane of the body is known as the frontal - plane cardiac vector as shown in figure. As with vector measurements in the physical sciences, the relative amplitude and angular position of this vector at any instant can not be measured with a single measurement. Two separate measurements are required and the results of these measurement are plotted on vector diagram to determine the relative amplitude and angular position of the vector. In the area of Physical sciences, the two measurements usually determine the projection of the vector along two axes at 90° to one another. In electrocardiography, the projection of this vector is recorded along two axes at 60° to one another as it allows the limbs to be used for the attachment of electrodes; the results obtained are relatively independent of where on the limbs the leads are placed.

EINTHOVEN TRIANGLE

Although only two measurements are theoretically necessary to determine the relative amplitude and angular position of the frontal plane vector, it is common electrocardiographic practice to record at least three projections of the frontal plane vector along three axes, which forms what is known as the Einthoven triangle as shown in figure. William Einthoven, a dutch cardiologist, pioneered many of the Electrocardiography techniques in use today. He has discovered this during the first quarter of this century. His approach to Electrocardiography stated that the vector sum of the projections of the frontal plane cardiac vector at any instant onto the three exes of the Einthoven triangle will be zero (Fig. 2.2*a*). This is well known physical law; Einthoven realized that it did in fact also apply to cardiology. Although the above supplies to the cardiac vector at any instant, cardiologists are usually only interested in the cardiac vector at the peak of the R wave. Thus when the term cardiac vector is used, it implies that "cardiac vector at the peak of the R wave".

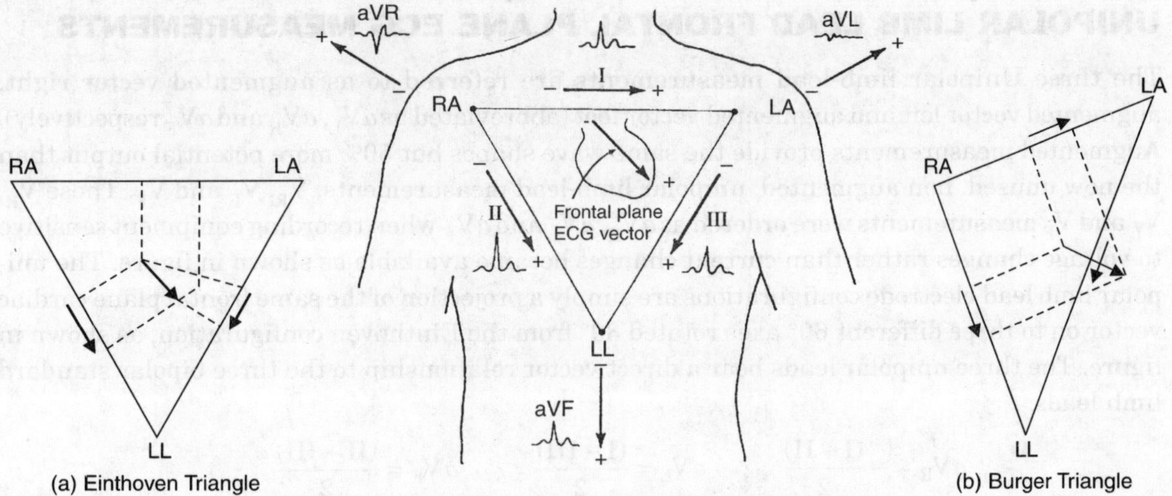

Fig. 2.2. Shows the Einthoven triangle and Burger triangle.

BURGER'S DISTORTED TRIANGLE

More recent advances in electrocardiography have pointed out the well kncwn fact that the human torso is neither homogenous nor triangular and that this leads to a distortion of the electrical field. Thus the angle of the vector deduced from Einthoven's triangle would be in error. Burger attempted to allow for the non-homogeneity of the torso by introduction of the distorted triangle shown in Fig. 2.2*b*, which compensates for the effect of the lungs and the spine. Although Burger's triangle is a more accurate representation of the frontal plane cardiac vector, it is not widely used and cardiologists still prefer to use the Einthoven's approach only. Though we realize that Einthoven's vectors are only approximation, we still use them largely for convenience. The clinical interpretation of ECG's is quite empirical in practice, being done by reference to the enormous number of records which have been correlated with known cardiac disorders, usually at autopsy.

BIPOLAR LIMB LEAD FRONTAL–PLANE ECG MEASUREMENTS

The three potential measurements commonly used to determine the frontal plane ECG vector in conjunction with the Einthoven triangle are :

1. Potential between the right arm and left arm
2. Potential between the right arm and left leg
3. Potential between the left arm and left leg.

These three ECG measurements are known as the standard frontal-plane or bipolar limb lead measurements and these are more commonly referred to as lead I ECG, Lead II ECG and Lead III ECG as shown in the figure.

UNIPOLAR LIMB LEAD FRONTAL PLANE ECG MEASUREMENTS

The three Unipolar limb-lead measurements are referred to as augmented vector right, augmented vector left and augmented vector foot (abbreviated as aV_L, aV_R and aV_F respectively). Augmented measurements provide the same wave shapes but 50% more potential output than the now unused. non augmented, unipolar limb-lead measurements, V_R, V_L and V_F. These V_R, V_L and V_F measurements were ordered as aV_R, aV_L and aV_F when recording equipment sensitive to voltage changes rather than current changes became available as shown in figure. The unipolar limb lead electrode configurations are simply a projection of the same frontal plane cardiac vector on to three different 60° axes rotated 30° from the Einthoven configuration, as shown in figure. The three unipolar leads bear a direct vector relationship to the three bipolar standard limb leads.

$$aV_R = -\frac{(I + II)}{2} \quad ; \quad aV_L = \frac{(I - III)}{2} \quad ; \quad aV_F = \frac{(II + III)}{2}$$

The aV_R unipolar measurement refers to the potential at the right arm using the left arm and left leg to form the indifferent electrode. The aVL measurement refers to the potential at the left arm using the right arm and left leg to form the indifferent electrodes. And aVF refers to the potential at the left leg using both arms to form the indifferent electrode. It should be noted that in these three measurements the indifferent electrode is formed at the negative input of the amplifier in all cases. The ECG waveform will thus be positive for aV_L, positive to aV_F but negative for aV_R.

The science of electrocardiography is based on a physiological phenomenon, first noted in 1856 by Kollikar and Muller that, the heart contraction is accompanied by the production of an electrical current. This current travels through the fluids and tissues of the body to the shoulders and hips and form there runs down the extremities. If the limbs are connected to a galvanometer, the current can be recorded. The limbs must include the heart between them.

Einthoven was the first to put this physiological fact to clinical use. In 1901, he introduced his "string galvanometer". With this instrument he recorded the heart beats. Between 1906 and 1910, he published his clinical studies. Further advance in the knowledge of electrocardiography, especially in the field of arrhythmias, was due to Sir. Thomas Lewis who in 1913 and 1930, by his experimental and clinical studies, has put electrocardiography on a firmer footing. Finally, it was Frank N.Wilson who has brought order and logic into this science. In 1933, he introduced his unipolar system, which is universally accepted today.

ELECTROCARDIOGRAPHIC LEADS

The term lead has two meanings,

1. It is used to indicate the area of the body from which the tracing is taken, for example, lead I, lead aV_R, and lead V_5 etc.
2. The term lead is used for the paper record made by connections from different parts of the body.

It is customary to take twelve different leads. The twelve leads are divided into three groups.

1. Bipolar leads–I, II and III
2. Unipolar limb leads–aV_R, aV_L and aV_F
3. Precordial leads V_1 and V_6.

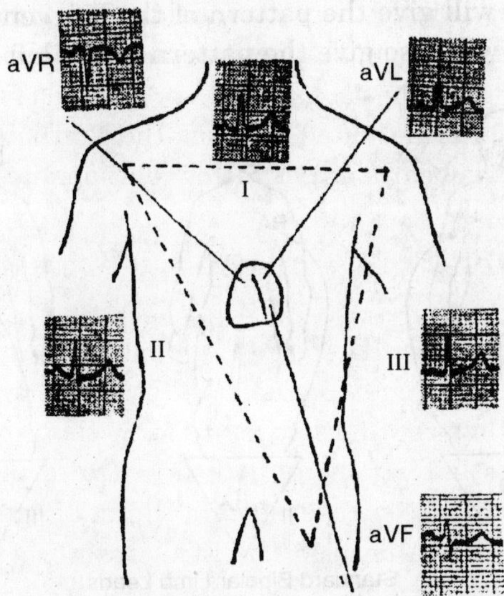

Fig. 2.3. Shows the Unipolar and Bipolar limb leads.

BIPOLAR LIMP LEADS

Bipolar limb leads are the **STANDARD LIMB LEADS.**

The three leads are numbered as given below.

1. Lead-I—this lead connects the right arm and left arm.
2. Lead-II—this lead connects the right arm and left leg.
3. Lead-III—this connects the left arm and left leg.

These leads are bipolar leads because the electrical pattern of leads I, and III are actually patterns from two different portions of the body. Thus lead I pattern is from right and left shoulders. Lead II pattern is from right shoulder and left hip, while lead III pattern is from left shoulder and left hip.

UNIPOLAR LIMB LEADS

These leads are also called " Augmented Unipolar limb leads". The letter **'a'** is used to indicate augmented, 'V' unipolar lead and last letter *R*, *L* or *F* to indicate the portion of the body from which lead is taken. If the lead comes form the right shoulder, the letter 'R' is used and 'L' if the lead is from left shoulder and 'F' if the lead is from the left hip.

There are three augmented uni-polar limb leads.

Lead a VR — from the right shoulder

Lead a VL — from the left shoulder

Lead a VF — from the left hip.

These leads are called unipolar leads because the electrical patterns of leads *aVR*, *aVL* and *aVF* are patterns from one portion of the heart only. Normally, the right shoulder faces the right ventricle. Lead *aVR* will give the pattern of the right ventricle. The left shoulder face the left ventricle. Lead *aVL* will give the pattern of the left ventricle. Similarly left hip faces the left ventricle. Lead *aVF* will also give the pattern of the left ventricle (Fig. 2.4).

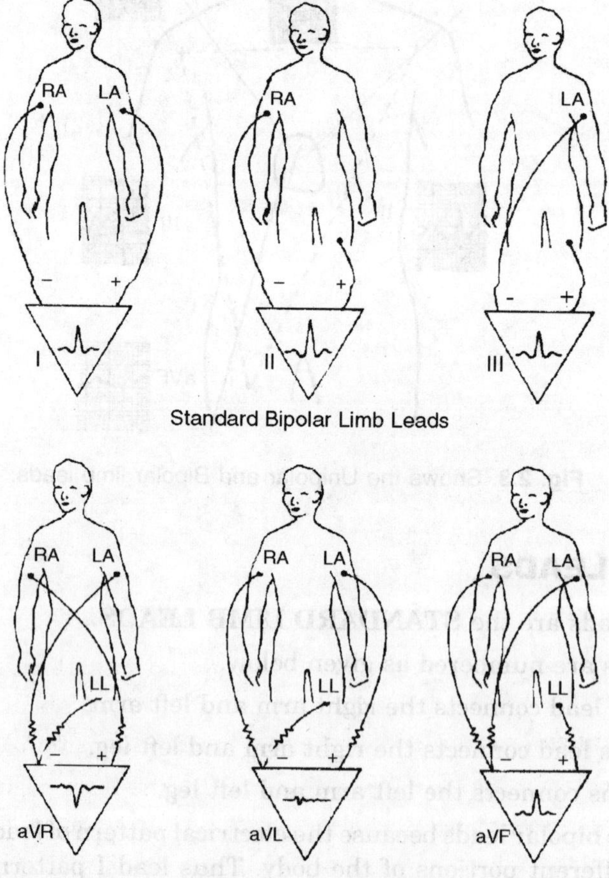

Fig. 2.4. Shows a Electrode position—frontal plane ECG.

PRECORDIAL LEADS

The precordial leads are also unipolar leads and hence they are designated "V" leads. Fixed position on the chest are used.

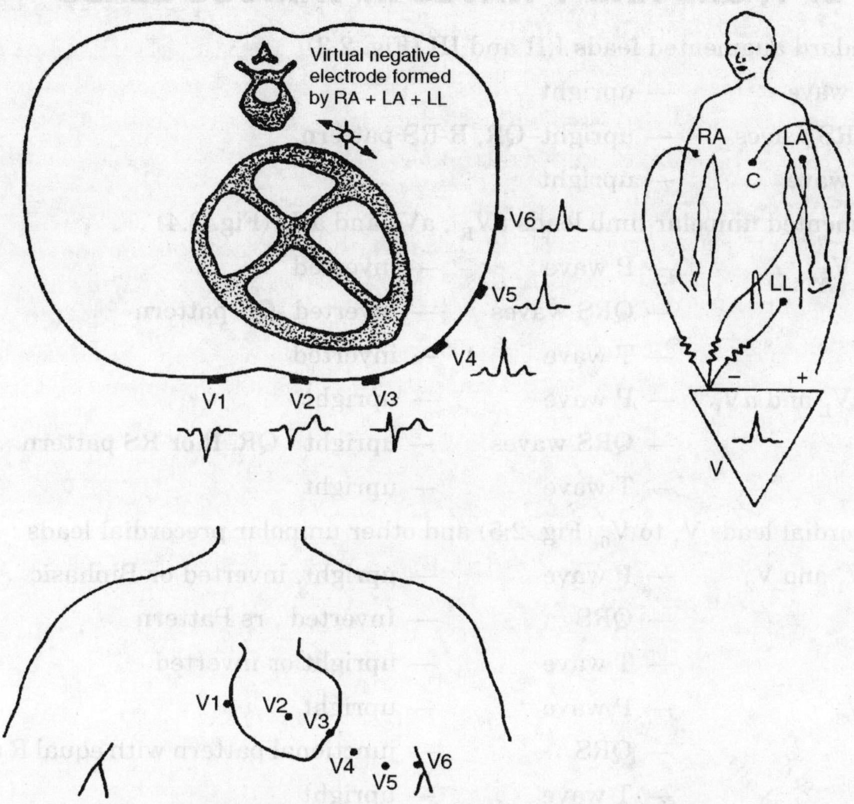

Fig. 2.5a. Shows the Transverse plane ECG.

Fig. 2.5*b* shows the Precordial Leads.

V_1 — 4th intercostal space at the right margin of the sternum

V_2 — 4th intercostal space at the left margin of the sternum

V_3 — 5th Rib in left parasternal line

V_4 — 5th intercostal space in the left midclavicular line.

V_5 — 5th and 6th intercostal space in the left anterior axillary line in a straight-line from position V4.

V_6 — in left mid axillary line, in a straight line from position V_4 and V_5.

V_7 — in left posterior axillary line, in a straight line from positions V_4, V_5 and V_6.

V_8 — in left side at the level of the inferior angle of the scapula.

V_E — at the inferior angle of the sternum to the left on the ensiform cartilage.

V_{3R} — on the right side of the same position as V_3.

V_{4R} — on the right side of the same position as V_4.

PATTERN OF P, QRS AND T WAVES IN VARIOUS LEADS

1. Standard augmented leads I,II and III (Fig. 2.3)

1. P wave — upright
2. QRS waves — upright–QR, R-RS pattern.
3. T wave — upright

2. Augmented unipolar limb leads aV_R , aV_L and aV_F (Fig. 2.4)

aV_R	— P wave	— inverted
	— QRS waves	— inverted -QS pattern
	— T wave	— inverted
aV_L and aV_F	— P wave	— upright
	— QRS waves	— upright - QR, R or RS pattern.
	— T wave	— upright

3. Precordial leads V_1 to V_6 (Fig. 2.5) and other unipolar precordial leads :

V_1 and V_2	— P wave	— upright, inverted or Biphasic
	— QRS	— Inverted , rs Pattern
	— T wave	— upright or inverted
V_3	— P wave	— upright
	— QRS	— junctional pattern with equal R and S waves
	— T wave	— upright
V_4, V_5 and V_6	— P wave	— upright
	— QRS waves	— upright -qr, R or Rs pattern
	— T wave	— upright
V_7 and V_8	— P wave	— upright
	— QRS waves	— upright -qr pattern
	— T wave	— upright
V_{3R}, V_{4R} & V_E	— P wave	— upright, inverted or biphasic
	— QRS waves	— inverted RS or QS pattern
	— T wave	— upright or inverted

Fig. 2.5*b*. showing the Precordial leads. As the electrode is moved from the right ventricle to the left ventricle the R wave increase in size and S wave diminishes in size.

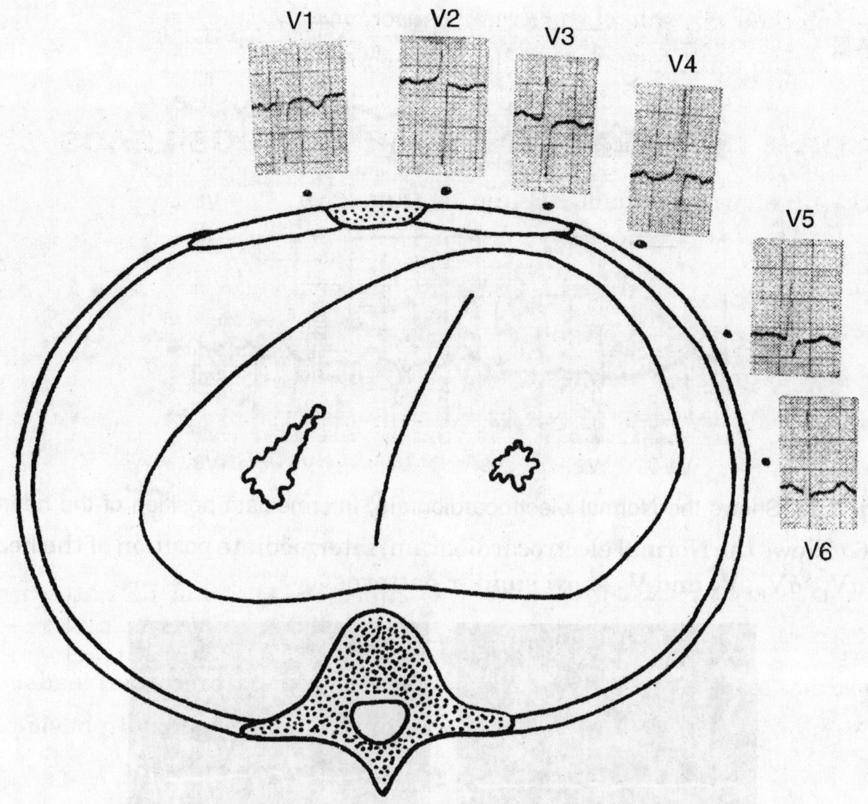

Fig. 2.5b. Shows Precordial Leads. As the electrode is moved from the right ventrical to the left ventrical the R wave increases in size and the S wave diminishes in size.

RELATIONSHIP BETWEEN THE VARIOUS LEADS

The various leads of the ECG electrode are interrelated. Left shoulder and left hip face the left ventricle. Leads aV_L and aV_F show the left ventricular surface pattern. Similarly, leads V_4 and V_5 and V_6 show left ventricular surface pattern, as they are from positions over the left ventricle. Lead I resembles aV_L, while leads II and III resemble aV_F. As lead aV_L and aV_F give left ventricular surface pattern, similar patterns will also be seen in leads I, II and III.

As seen in Fig. 2.5*b*, the precordial leads, as the electrode is moved from the right ventricle to the left ventricle the R wave increase in size and S wave diminishes in size.

Right shoulder faces the right ventricle. Similarly positions V_1 and V_2 are over the right ventricle. Leads aV_R, V_1 and V_2 show similar patterns of right ventricle.

Thus in a normal electrocardiogram, leads I, II and III, aV_L, aV_F, V_5 and V_6 show similar patterns. All these leads show *q*R, R or R*s* patterns of the left ventricle. Leads aV_R, V_1 and V_2 show similar patterns. These leads show *r*S or Q*s* patterns of the right ventricle (Fig. 2.6*b*).

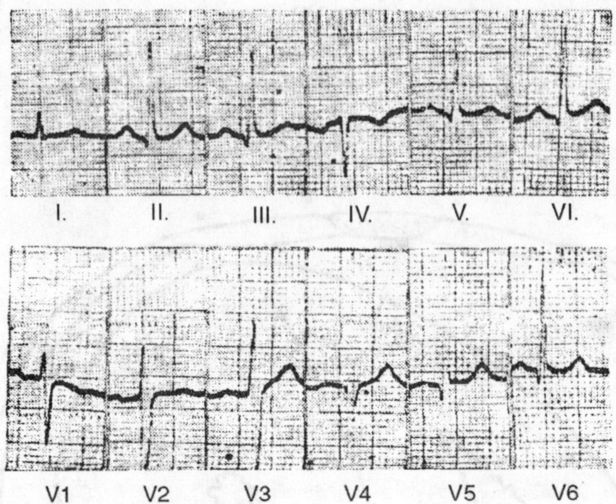

Fig. 2.6a. Shows the Normal electrocardiogram, Intermediate position of the heart.

Fig. 2.6*a* shows the Normal electrocardiogram, intermediate position of the heart. Leads—I, II and III, aV_L, aV_F, V_5 and V_6 show similar patterns.

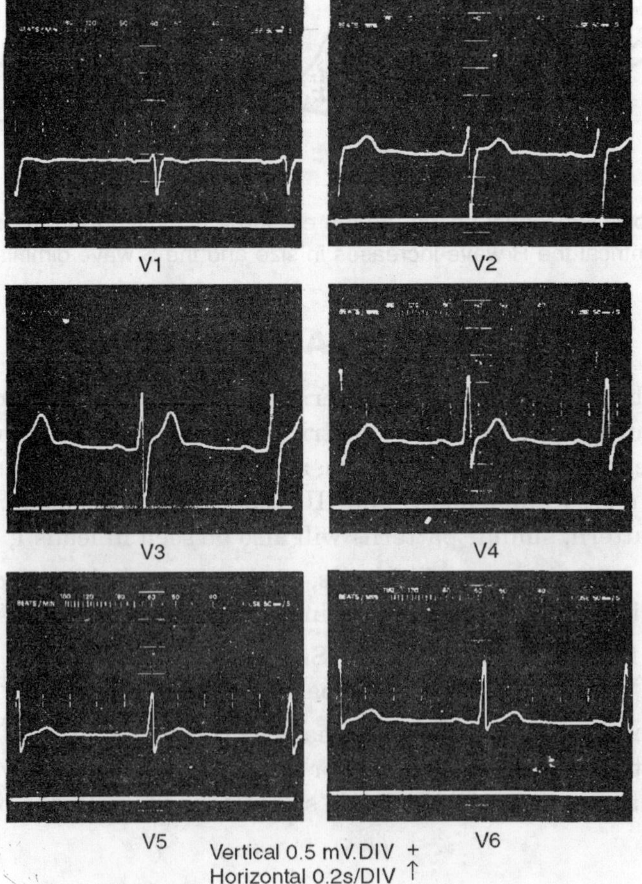

Fig. 2.6b. Shows the typical transverse plane ECG's (recorded with Tek. Type 410 Physiological Monitor).

ALTERNATIONS IN THE NORMAL VENTRICULAR PATTERNS

Variations in the ventricular patterns in the twelve leads are frequently observed in the normal electrocardiograms. Such alternations are physiological and no abnormality. These variations depend on the following three factors.

1. Electrical axis
2. Positions of the heart
3. Rotations of the heart.

These changes are observed in different groups of leads. They are noted as:

(*a*) Changes due to electrical axis are observed in standard limb leads I, II and III.

(*b*) Changes in the positions of the heart are best observed in augmented unipolar limb leads aV_R, aV_L and aV_F.

(*c*) Changes due to rotations of the heart are observed in precordial leads V_1.

ELECTRICAL AXIS

The term electrical axis refers to a pattern form the spread of the electrical process of excitation. It produces changes in the electrical pattern of the leads I, II and III. These changes are called axis deviation. Axis deviation does not depend on the anatomical position of the heart.

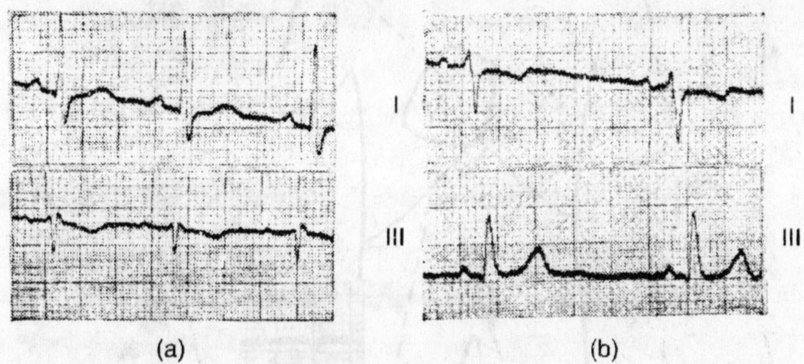

Fig. 2.7. Shows the axis deviation (*a*) Shows left axis deviation, R wave is prominent in lead I and S wave in lead III, (*b*). Shows the right axis deviation. S wave is prominent in lead I, & R wave in lead III.

1. Normally the prominent waves of the **QRS** complex in leads-I and III point upwards. R wave is prominent in both leads (Fig. 2.7). There is no axis deviation.
2. If the prominent wave is R in lead I and S in lead III, there is left axis deviation. R and S in Lead I and Lead III point in opposite direction.
3. If the prominent wave is S and lead I and R in lead III, there is a right axis deviation (Fig. 2.7*b*). S and R waves in leads I and III, point towards each other.

POSITIONS OF THE HEART

The heart is fixed above by the big blood vessels, but it is relatively free at its diaphragmatic surface. It can move in the chest form side to the left or to the right—like the pendulum of a clock. Different positions of the heart will thus lie opposite the shoulders and left hip in different positions. Whatever the position of the heart, the right shoulder will always face the right ventricle. So no change will occur in lead aV_R. Change will only occur in leads aV_L and aV_F. Thus to study the positions of the heart, look at leads aV_L and aV_F. There are important positions of the heart.

1. Normally or immediate position of the heart–left shoulder and the left hip face ventricle (Fig. 2.3). Leads aV_L and aV_F both show left ventricular surface pattern. R wave is prominent in leads aV_L and aV_F.
2. Horizontal position of the heart–the heart has shifted to the left side. Left shoulder faces the left ventricle (Fig. 2.8). Lead aV_L shows the pattern of the left ventricle while aV_F shows the pattern of the right ventricle. In the horizontal position of the heart, R wave is prominent in a aV_L and S wave is prominent in aV_F.

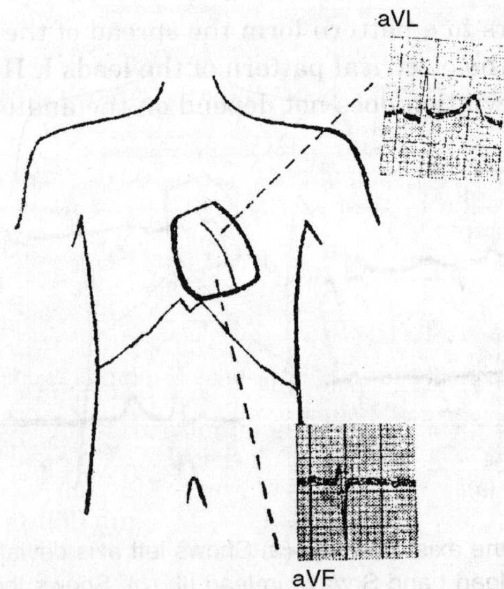

Fig. 2.8. Shows the horizontal position of the heart. R wave is prominent in aV_L and S wave is prominent in aV_F.

3. **Vertical position of the heart.** The heart has shifted to the right side. The left shoulder faces the right ventricle and left hip faces the left ventricle (Fig. 2.9). As in Fig. 2.9, lead aV_L shows the pattern of the right ventricle and aV_F that of left ventricle. In the vertical position of the heart, S wave is prominent in aV_L and R wave is prominent in aV_F.

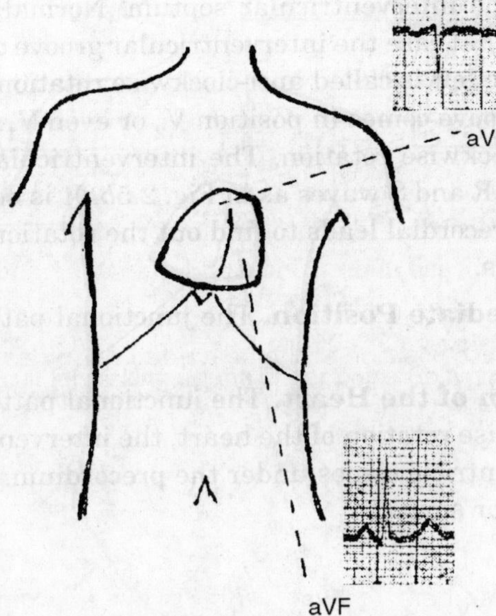

Fig. 2.9a. Shows the vertical position of the heart. S wave is prominent in aVL and R wave in aVF.

There are intermediate positions, *e.g.*, semi-horizontal and semi-vertical positions, but they are not so important.

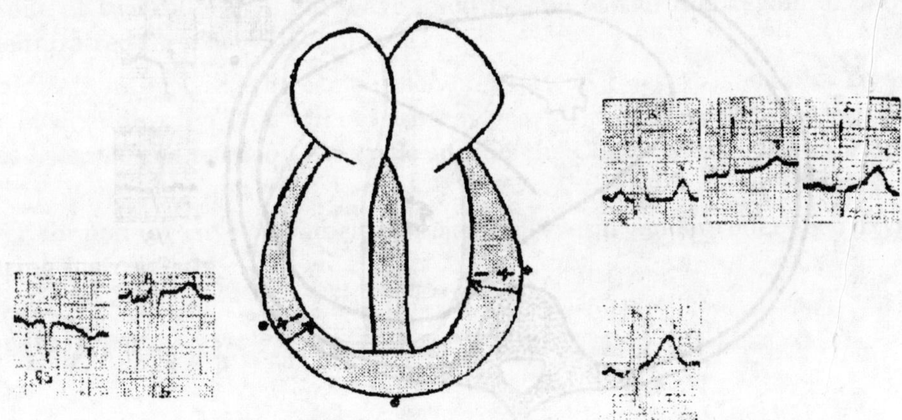

Fig. 2.9b. Shows the pattern of the ventricular waves. In the ventricles, repolarisation spreads from the epicardium to the endocardium.

ROTATIONS OF THE HEART

The heart is a round structure. Above, it is fixed by the great vessels but its diaphragmatic surface is free. It can spin or rotate at its free surface from right to left or vice versa like the balance of a watch. On the anterior surface of the heart is the anterior interventricular groove.

It indicates the position of the interventricular septum. Normally, it is in position V_3. The heart may spin to the left. In that case the interventricular groove comes to V_4 or V_5 or even V_6. This rotation movement to the left is called anti-clockwise rotation. The heart may spin to the right. The interventricular groove comes in position V_2 or even V_1. This rotation movement to the right is called the anticlockwise rotation. The interventricular septum always gives the junctional pattern with equal R and S waves as in Fig. 2.5*b*. It is necessary to find the position of the junctional pattern in precordial leads to find out the rotations of the heart. Rotations of the heart gives three positions.

1. **Normal or Intermediate Position.** The junctional pattern is in position V_3 (Figs. 2.2, 2.3 and 2.4).
2. **Clockwise Rotation of the Heart.** The junctional pattern in position V_4, V_5 or V_6 (Fig. 2.10). In clockwise rotation of the heart, the interventricular groove shifts to the left. More of right ventricle comes under the precordium. Left ventricle becomes less visible on the anterior surface.

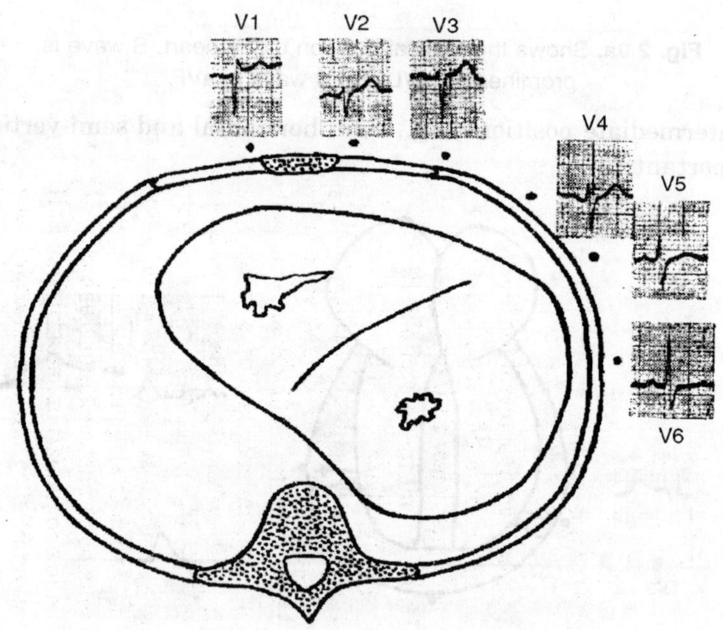

Fig. 2.10a. Shows the clockwise rotation of the heart. The junctional pattern is in position V5.

Anticlockwise Rotation of the Heart. The-junctional pattern is in position V_2 or V_1 (Fig. 2.10*b*). In anticlockwise rotation, the interventricular groove shifts to the right. More of the left ventricle lies under the precordium. Right ventricle becomes less visible on the anterior surface.

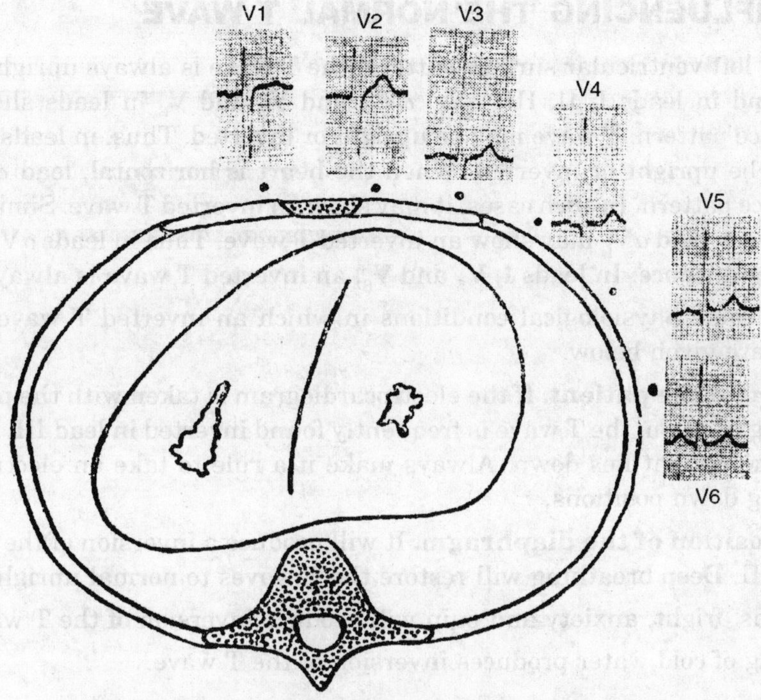

Fig. 2.10b. Shows the Anticlockwise rotation of the heart. The junctional pattern is in position V_2.

FACTORS INFLUENCING THE NORMAL ELECTROCARDIOGRAM

The pattern of the normal electrocardiogram may be affected as a whole by a number of factors. Such factors are listed as follows :

1. Muscle tremors
2. Loose attachment of the electrodes
3. Instrumental errors
4. Electrical interferences
5. Sudden movement on the part of the patient

The above factors produce wavy or fuzzy waves. In severe cases it is impossible to identify the waves. They may also produce shifting of the base line. The electrocardiogram does not remain steady, but runs up and down as if going up or down a hill.

6. **Wrong lead connections.** If the lead wires of lead-I, II and III are wrongly attached, they will alter the pattern of the waves.
7. **Deep breathing.** In some electrocardiograms, a deep Q wave is seen in leads II and III, or in lead III alone. This is due to high position of the diaphragm. This disappears on deep breathing.

FACTORS INFLUENCING THE NORMAL T WAVE

In leads showing left ventricular surface pattern, the T wave is always upright. Thus upright T waves are found in leads I, II, III, aV_L, aV_F, and V_5 and V_6 in leads showing the right ventricular surface pattern, T wave may be upright or inverted. Thus, in leads aV_R, V_1 and V_2, the T wave may be upright or inverted. When the heart is horizontal, lead aV_F shows right ventricular surface pattern. In such cases, it may show an inverted T wave. Similarly, in vertical position of the heart, lead aV_L may show an inverted T wave. Thus in leads aV_L and aV_F of the T wave has no significance. In leads I, V_5 and V_6, an inverted T wave is always abnormal.

There are some physiological conditions in which an inverted T wave may be found. Such conditions are given below.

1. **Position of the patient.** If the electrocardiogram is taken with the patient sitting or standing position, the T wave is frequently found inverted in lead III. This disappears when the patient lies down. Always make it a rule to take an electrocardiogram in the lying down positions.
2. **High position of the diaphragm.** It will produce a inversion of the T wave in leads II and III. Deep breathing will restore the T waves to normal upright position.
3. Emotions, fright, anxiety and pain will produce inversion of the T wave.
4. Drinking of cold water produces inversion of the T wave.

RECORDING OF ECG WAVES

In each cardiac cycle, a series of waves are observed in the electrocardiogram (Fig. 2.11). Einthoven names these waves P, Q, R, S and T waves. These letters are arbitrary as he did not know at that time this significance of these waves.

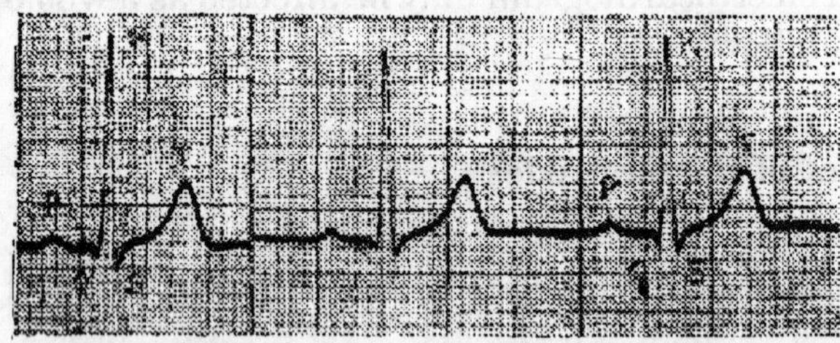

Fig. 2.11. Shows the Nomenclature of the waves.

P-wave. It is the wave auricular depolarization. It denotes auricular activity. It is usually an upright rounded wave. An inverted or biphasic P wave is frequently obtained over the right ventricle.

R-wave. It is the first upright wave after the P wave.

Q-wave. It is the negative wave that precedes the R wave.

S-wave. It is the negative wave that follows the R wave.

QRS wave. The QRS wave is always taken as single unit. It denotes ventricular activity. It is the polarization wave of the ventricle. It is most prominent wave in the whole cardiac cycle. It shows a variety of shapes—QS pattern, *r*S pattern, RS pattern, R pattern, R*s* pattern and *q*R pattern. Of these the QS and *r*S patterns are obtained over the right ventricle, RS is a junction pattern, while R, Rs and qR patterns are obtained over the left ventricle.

As the electrode is moved from the right ventricle to the left ventricle the R wave increases in size and the S wave diminishes in size.

T wave. It is also a wave of ventricular activity. It is the repolarisation wave of the ventricles. It is upright and rounded wave. Over the right ventricle T wave may be inverted.

QRS-T. Waves are designated as the QRS–T complex. They represent complete ventricular activity. The P, QRS and T waves represent the electrical activity of the whole heart with each cardiac cycle.

PR interval-from the beginning of the P wave to the beginning of the QRS complex. PR interval is the measure of the atrioventricular conduction time- the time taken by the excitation process to travel from S.A. node to the ventricular muscle fibers (Fig. 2.12).

QT-interval. From the beginning of the Q wave to the end of the T wave. It represents the total systolic time of the ventricles–the total time of the depolarization and repolarization of the ventricular muscles.

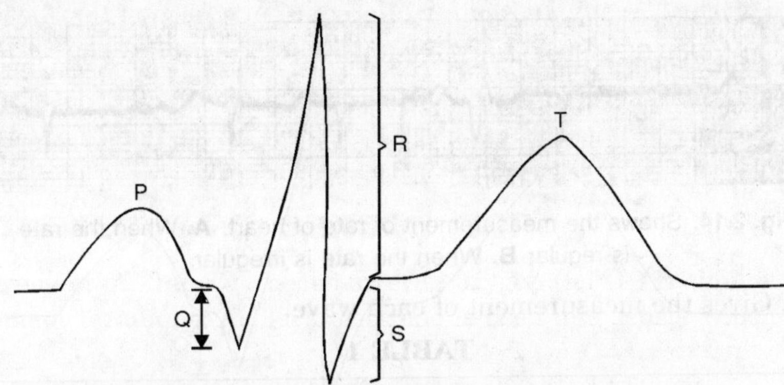

Fig. 2.12. Shows the measurement of waves and base line.

DEFINITIONS

Electrocardiograph. It is the instrument which records the electrical currents generated in the heart.

Electrocardiogram. It is record of the heart's action on a special electrocardiograph paper.

ELECTROCARDIOGRAPH PAPER

It is usually, six centimeter wide (6 cm). The paper is black and it is covered with white wax. When the heated stylus of the electrocardiograph moves over the paper, the wax melts exposing the black paper. The paper moves at the rate of 25 mm per second.

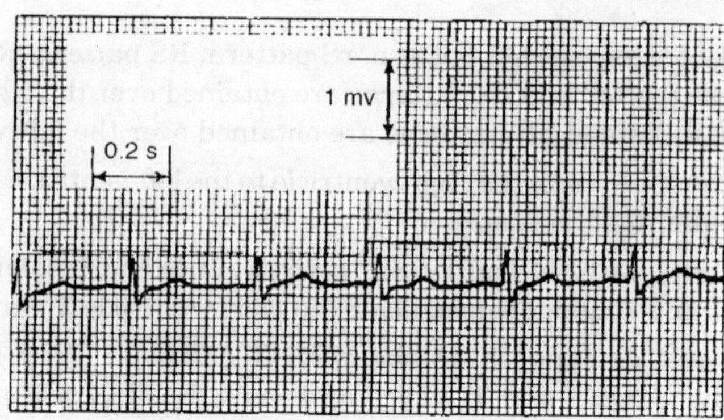

Fig. 2.13. Shows a typical electrocardiograph tracing.

Fig. 2.13. Shows the Electrocardiograph paper.

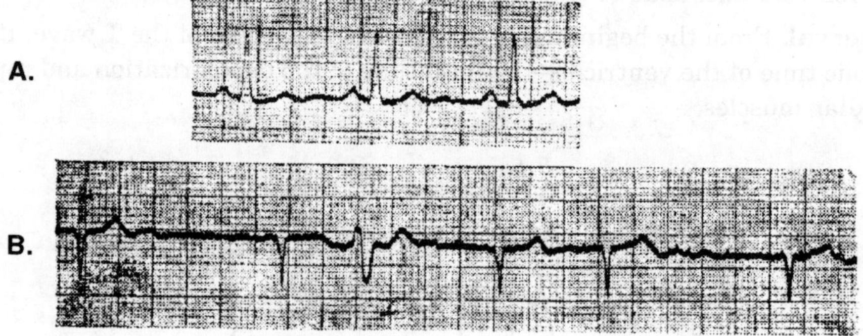

Fig. 2.14. Shows the measurement of rate of heart. **A.** When the rate is regular **B.** When the rate is irregular.

Table. 2.1. Gives the measurement of each wave.

TABLE 1

Wave	Voltage (mm)	Duration (Seconds)
P	Minimun – 0.2	0.02
	Average – 0.5	0.08
	Maximum – 1.5	0.1
QRS	Minimun – 5	0.04
	Average – 8	0.06
	Maximum – 17	0.1
T	Minimun – 0.5	0.1
	Average – 5	0.16
	Maximum – 11	0.22

Intervals		Min. – 0.1
PR		Ave. – 0.16
		Max. – 0.22
QT		Min. – 0.3
		Ave. – 0.34
		Max. – 0.42

Measurement of rate of the heart

Table 2 Rate of heart ready reference. Count the number of small squares between two R waves.

No. of small squares	Rate per minute	No. of small squares	Rate per minute	No. of small squares	Rate per minute
8	187	20	75	32	47
9	166	21	71	33	45
10	150	22	68	34	44
11	136	23	65	35	43
12	125	24	62	36	42
13	115	25	60	37	40
14	107	26	58	38	39
15	100	27	56	39	38
16	94	28	54	40	37
17	88	29	52	41	36
18	83	30	50	42	35
19	79	31	48	43	34

The electrocardiograph paper has horizontal and vertical lines (Fig. 2.12). The vertical and horizontal lines have at intervals accentuated lines. Vertical lines indicate time. Each small division represents 0.04 seconds. Between each accentuated line the time interval between ten such lines is one cm. To deflects the stylus of the electrocardiograph 1cm, a current of one millivolt is needed. The heart produces a current of one millivolt each time in contracts. Thus horizontal lines indicate voltage.

This is the standard type of paper used universally.

NORMAL MEASUREMENTS OF THE WAVES AND THE BASE LINES

An ECG record consists of two parts, wave and base lines. Each wave has a height (voltage), a time interval (duration) and a shape. Each base line has a time interval (duration) and shape. Normally the base lines are flat and remain at the isoelectric line. The important normal measurements are given (Fig. 2.13).

MEASUREMENT OF THE RATE OF THE HEART

The rate of the heart is counted from the number of QRS complexes that occur in one minute. The time interval between two small lines of the electrocardiograph paper is 0.04 seconds.

There will therefore be 1500 small squares in one minute. Similarly there will be 300 big square in one minute, as the time interval between two accentuated lines is 0.2 seconds.

There are two methods of counting the rate of the heart.

1. When the rate of the heart is regular–count the number of small squares between any two R waves (R-R intervals). Divide 1500 by that figure. In Fig. 2.14, the number of small squares between two R waves is 19. The rate of the heart is 155/19 = 79 per minute.
2. Use table. In table 2, it is given the rate of the heart from the number of small squares, for ready reference.

PRESENT DAY ECG INSTRUMENTS AND SPECS

Presently, ECG machines are available with the latest of technological developments. Fig.2.15 shows some excerpts from present day models in use in hospitals. These are seen to reflect the computer based hardware in each of them, though, the standard format of a recorder output is also made available. The first machine seen is using a front panel LCD display of colour, similar to what we find in laptop computers. This has a membrane keyboard and a built in recorder, which is not seen from the top view, but produces a paper output on the left side. The second machine shown right in fig. has full fledged PC like keyboard and a colour LCD display. There is a possibility to view all ECG signals simultaneously on the screen. There might be other features such as the ones listed below in this section. The third machine shows below in the figure is again a typical portable instrument, but one might note the use of a keyboard instead of the earlier control potentiometer. The chart output is coming out on the left.

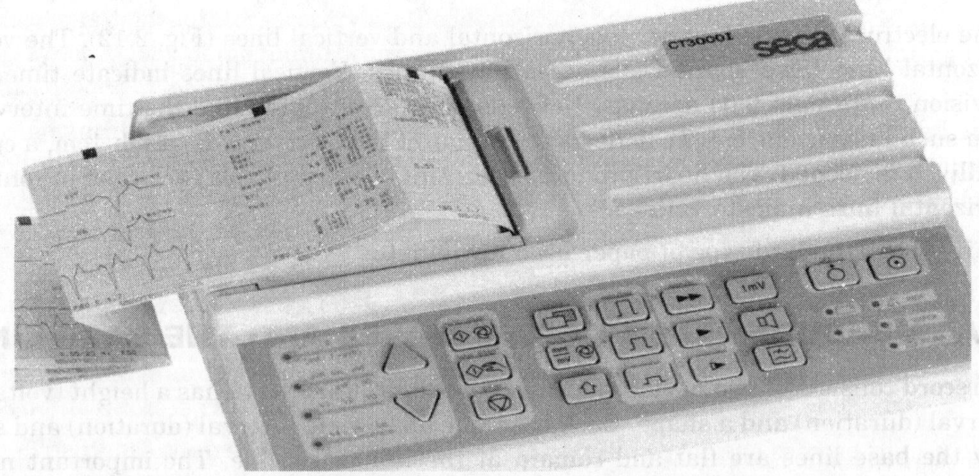

Fig. 2.15. Shows photographs of typical today' latest ECG machines.

The typical specs for these units are that they have:

Thermal paper 4.25″ × 75″ roll

Computer calculated digital detection of arrhythmias

12 μV resolution at standard gain

Auto or manual lead switching

Frequency response 0.01 to 109 Hz at 5 mm recorded signal

Input impedance of 100 MΩ

Defibrillation protection

Patient leakage current less than 10 μA

Common mode rejection ratio (CMRR) 130 dB

Analog to digital converter used – 20 mV, 12 bits

The instrument has RS 232 output links which can use up to 19200 baud rate

Protocol is X modem, 8 second

Uncompressed *e.c.g.* is transmitted in 90 seconds.

Special Functions Provided

1. Arm lead reversal detection
2. Optional trace position
3. Lead off and artifacts detection
4. Sensitivity detection
5. Drift detection
6. A.C. interference detection

From the above, it is clear that the advent of the computer hardware into the ECG machine is already very much into technology, but the retention of the paper records is still considered necessary. Completely virtualisation of the ECG. is not yet considered advisable, because, it is difficult to detract the doctors from the usual small trace short wave pattern ECG that they have been all along trained for diagnosis. The present acumen in ECG is that they have been on the accumulated knowledge which is based on reading just 0.06 second QRS in a very short 2mm trace width for finding any abnormal Q-wave. The trend to use better waveform displays available in the virtual instrument should be developed by the doctors, which would prove to be more accurate in their judgment and diagnosis.

CASE STUDIES OF ELECTRO-CARDIOGRAMS ON THE NORMAL AND COMPUTER BASED INSTRUMENTS

Electrocardiography is broadly divided into two main groups :

1. Ventricular complex abnormalities and
2. Arrhythmias.

The ventricular complex abnormalities involve the QRS–T waves and RS–T segment. Arrhythmias result from disturbance of the cardiac rhythm mechanism. They are disorders of the heart beat.

VENTRICULAR COMPLEX ABNORMALITIES

1. Ventricular hypertrophy
2. Bundle branch block

3. Myocardial infarction
4. Other conditions, like certain cardiovascular diseases-angina pectoris ; certain systemic diseases–diptheria, hyper–thyroidism ; effect of certain drugs–digitalis and changes in the electrolyte balance–hyperkalemia.

Ventricular hypertrophy is a very common condition. In it the ventricular muscle mass is increased in thickness. It occurs in a variety of diseases of the heart.

Diagnostic electrocardiographic signs of ventricular hypertrophy: There are five characteristic signs of ventricular hypertrophy.

1. Increased voltage of the QRS waves.
2. Widening of the QRS complex
3. RS-T segment is depressed.
4. T wave is inverted.
5. Q wave is frequently present.

The ventricular hypertrophy of the heart pattern is easy to spot.

In **marked hypertrophy** of the heart, the voltage of the QRS is increased. There is widening of the QRS complex up to 0.10seconds. The RS-T segment is depressed. The depression may be slight or marked. The taller the R wave, the more marked is the RS-T depression. The RS-T segment gradually runs downwards from the iso-electric line. It is convex upwards and blends with the apex of the T waves. The inverted T wave has apex close to its end (Fig. 2.16*b*).

In mild hypertrophy, all the characteristics of hypertrophy pattern may not be present. The R wave may not be tall. There is no widening of the QRS complex. But there is a characteristic depression of the RS-T segment. It may not be marked but the depression is present. The T-wave is inverted (Fig. 2.16*c*).

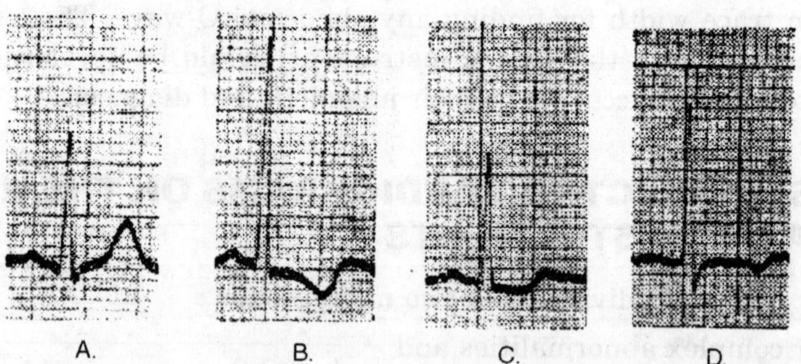

Fig. 2.16. Shows the Pattern of the QRS-T waves. (*a*) Normal (*b*) Marked ventricular hypertrophy (*c*) Mild ventricular hypertrophy (*d*) Ventricular Strain

The change of the ventricular hypertrophy are best seen in precardial leads V1 to V6. Similar changes will also be found in standard limb leads I, II and III and in unipolar limb leads aV_R, aV_L and aV_F. But they are not constant. They depend on the position of the heart. To diagnose ventricle hypertrophy, look for the hypertrophy pattern.

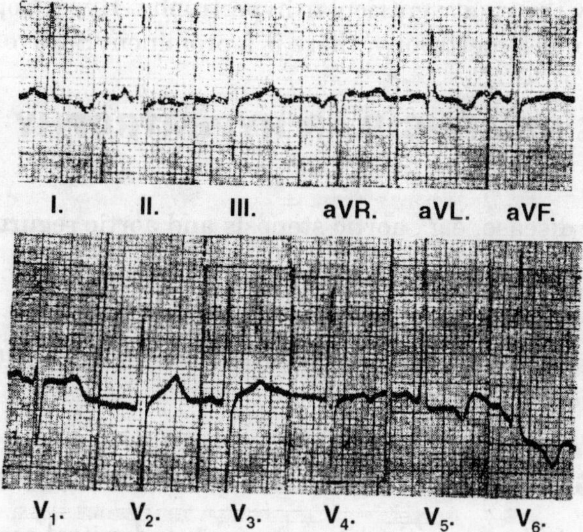

Fig. 2.17. Shows the Left ventricular Hypertrophy. Note the hypertrophy pattern in leads V5 and V6.

Fig. 2.17 shows the left ventricular hypertrophy. (Hypertrophy pattern in leads V_5 and V_6).

1. If the hypertrophy pattern is seen in leads V_5 and V_6 there is left ventricular hypertrophy. If the hypertrophy pattern is seen in leads V_1 and V_2, there is right ventricular hypertrophy. (Fig. 2.18).

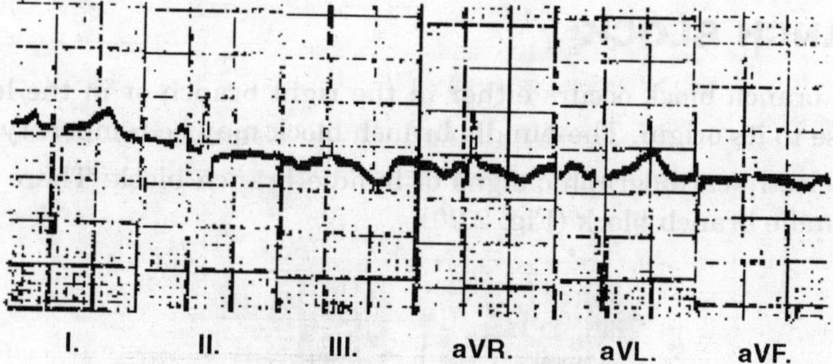

Fig. 2.18. Right ventricular hypertrophy in main ECG leads.

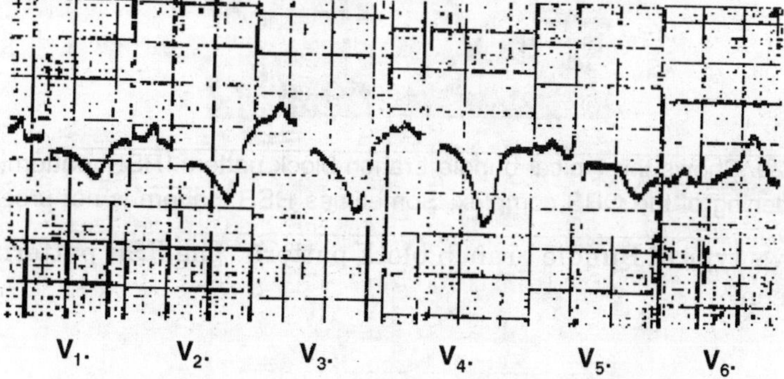

Fig. 2.19. Shows the same in pre cordial leads.

Figs 2.18, 19 show the right ventricular hypertrophy. Hypertrophy pattern in leads V1 and V2. In right ventricular hypertrophy, there is a prominent S wave in left precordial leads.

CAUSES OF LEFT VENTRICULAR HYPERTROPHY

1. Hypertension
2. Aortic valvular disease, e.g., aortic stenosis and aortic regurgitation.
3. Angina Pectoris
4. Chronic nephritis.
5. Some congenital heart diseases–patent ducts arteriosus, coarctation of the aorta.
6. Mitral insufficiency.

CAUSES FOR RIGHT VENTRICULAR HYPERTROPHY

1. Rheumatic heart disease with mitral stenosis and mitral regurgitation
2. Chronic cor pulmonale.
3. Pulmonary Emphysema.
4. Certain congenital heart diseases of the cyanotic type ECG, Tetrology of Fallot, congential pulmonary stenosis, etc.

Reversibility of ventricular hypertrophy: The changes of ventricular hypertrophy are reversible and the ECG can become normal again.

BUNDLE BRANCH BLOCK

The bundle branch block occurs either in the right branch or in the left branch of the bundle of His, clcse to its origin. The bundle branch block may be temporary or permanent.

Diagnostic electro-cardiographic signs of bundle branch block: There are four characteristic signs of bundle branch block (Fig. 2.20)

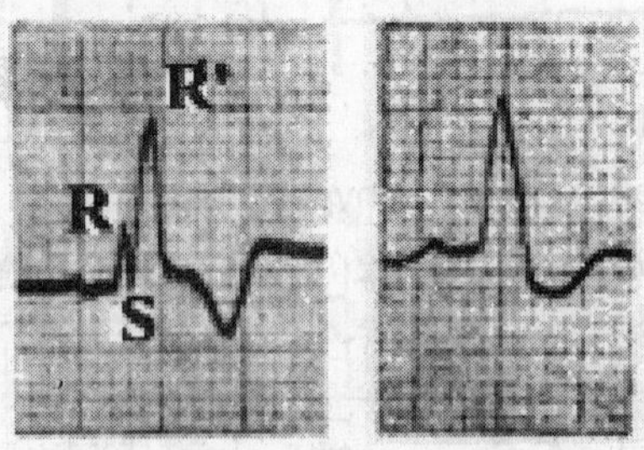

Fig. 2.20. Shows the typical bundle branch biock pattern. RSR' pattern, and 2. Widening of the QRS complex. Sometimes RSR' pattern is not present.

Fig. 2.20 shows typical Bundle branch block pattern. The RSR pattern, Widening of the QRS complex are seen.

Widening of the QRS complex, Notching of the QRS complex. Depression of the RS-T segment and inversion of the T-wave will be there if the bundle branch block occurs.

The pattern of bundle branch block is easy to spot.

In bundle branch block, the QRS complex is widened more than 0.10 seconds. If the QRS complex is widened more than 0.12 seconds, the bundle branch block is complete. If the widening of the QRS complex is between 0.10 and 0.12 seconds, the bundle branch block is incomplete.

The QRS complex is notched. There are two R waves. They are called R and R' waves. R' wave is taller than the R wave. The two R waves are separated by a big or small S wave. This pattern of the QRS complex is called RSR' pattern and it is characteristic of bundle branch block (Fig. 2.20*b*).

WOLF-PARKINSON-WHITE SYNDROME

This is a condition in which the cardiac impulse reaches the ventricles straight from the auricles, via accessory conduction bundles called the Bundles of Kent. The cardiac impulse does not pass down via the Bundle of His. Electrocardiographically, it has two characteristics:

1. PR interval is less than 0.10 seconds and
2. The QRS complex is wide, more than 0.1 seconds (Fig. 2.21).

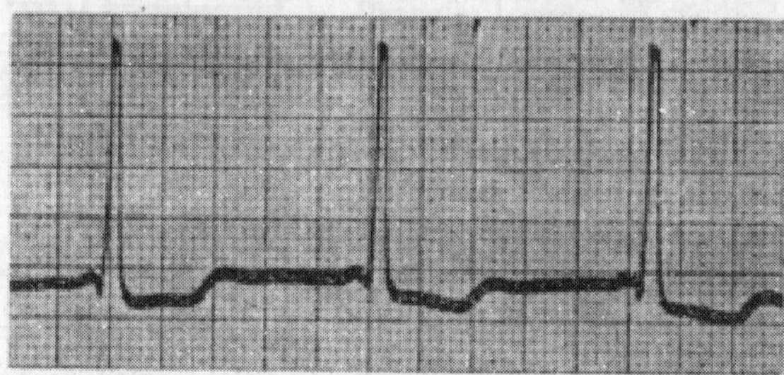

Fig. 2.21. Shows the Wolf-Parkinson-White syndrome.

Fig. 2.21 shows the Wolf-Parkinson-White Syndrome. PR interval is short and QRS wider.

MYOCARDIAL INFARCTION

Occlusion of the coronary artery produces three grades of muscle injury. Each grade produces characteristic electrical effects.

1. **Ischemia effect.** The T wave is inverted. The inverted T wave has a characteristic appearance. The forward limb is upwardly convex and passes downwards into a sharp pointed apex. The hind limb of the T wave is also convex and has the same general outline as the former but oppositely oriented. The T wave has a bilaterally symmetrical form. (Fig. 2.22*a*).
2. **Injury Effect.** This effect manifests itself by displacement of the RS-T segment above the isoelectric level. The displacement is always upwards over the infarct area (Fig 2.22*b*). It also shows an upward convexity. Injury shortens the amplitude of the

R-wave. The higher the RS-T displacement, the shorter the R wave. When the displacement is not marked the R wave is tall. Changes also occur in the T wave. When the RS-T is upwardly displaced, the T wave is inverted and if the displacement of the RS-T is marked, the T-wave disappears.

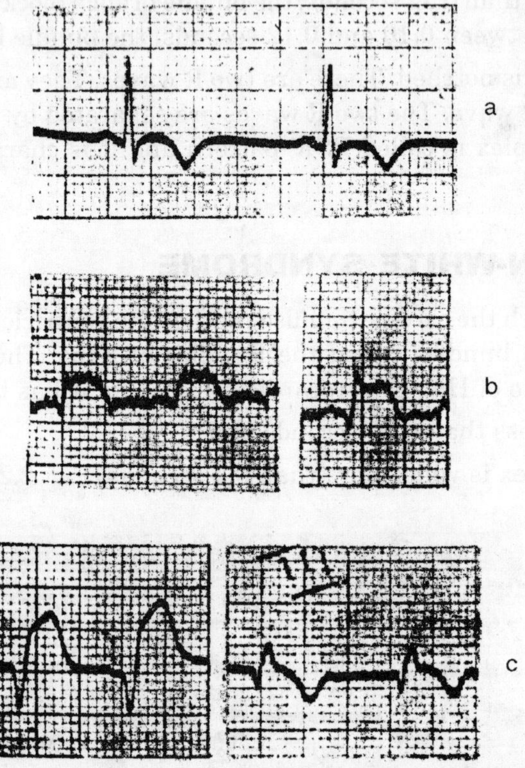

Fig. 2.22. Shows the electrical effects of myocardial infarction. (a) Ischaemia (b) Injury effect (c) Necrosis effect.

3. **Necrosis effect.** If the injury is more severe it causes death of the muscle. The dead muscle produces a Q wave (Fig. 2.22*c*).

ARRHYTHMIAS

Arrhythmias are disorders of rhythm and conduction of the heart beats. Many arrhythmias occur in normal healthy individuals. They are due to the effect of normal vagotonia. Such Arrhythmias are:

Sinus tachycardia

Sinus bradycardia

Sinus Arrhythmias

Electrical alternans.

These Arrhythmias soon disappear and are not of clinical importance.

1. Normal Cardiac impulse

The cardiac impulse: originates in the S.A. node. The S.A. node is named 'cardai pace maker'. The impulse passes over the auricles and reaches the A.V. node. It then passes down the Bundle of His, its right and left branches and their terminal ramifications, to the Purkinji fibres. The Purkinji fibres are in intimate contact with the ventricular muscles. They transmit the impulse to the ventricular muscles.

2. S.A. Block

S.A. block is a more severe condition than sinus arrest. Sinus arrest is due to temporary failure of the S.A. node to initiate the cardiac impulse. In S.A. block the impulse is formed in the S.A node, but it is blocked and does not reach the auricular musculature. In S.A block there is interference in the transmission of the impulse leaving the S.A. node. In both conditions there is auricular standstill. P, Q, R, S and T waves are absent in one or more cardiac cycles. There is a prolonged pause. The duration of the pause varies. If one cardiac cycle is missing, the next cycle appears at practically double the normal interval, *i.e.,* the prolonged P-P interval is twice the size of the normal P-P interval.

When the S.A. node fails as a pace maker to initiate the cardiac impulse, either from sinus arrest or S.A. block, the function of the "cardiac pace maker" is taken over by the A.V. node. The P wave is absent but the QRS and T waves are present and they are of normal shape. If the nodal beat occurs once and is followed by other sinus beats, it is called NODAL ESCAPE (Fig. 4.7*a*). In nodal escape, nodal beats—QRS-T waves occur at intervals. Other beats are sinus because the S.A. node resumes its function again, the block being temporary. If the S.A. block is complete, then no sinus beats will occur at all. In its place nodal beats will occur regularly. This is called nodal Rhythm (Fig. 2.23*b*).

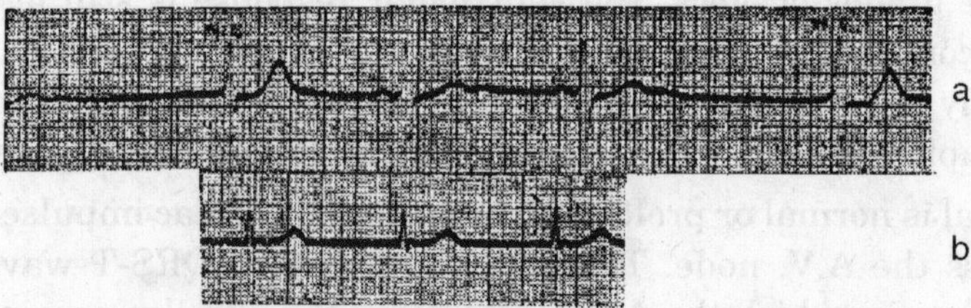

Fig. 2.23. Shows the (a) Nodal escape (b) Nodal rhythm.

Rarely even the A.V. node is in block. In such case the ventricular muscle itself acts as a "pace maker". If the S.A. and A.V. blocks are temporary, it will produce ventricular escape. If the S.A. and A.V. block is complete there will be ventricular rhythm.

Atrio-ventricular Block

A.V Blocks are classified into **three degrees :**

1. First degree heart block or incomplete heart block
2. Second degree heart block or partial heart block
3. Third degree heart block or complete heart block.

First Degree Heart Block

The first degree heart block or incomplete heart block is a condition in which the cardiac impulse originating in the S.A. node takes longer time to reach the ventricular muscles. The delay is in the A.V.node. The PR interval is increased beyond 0.2 seconds. All the P waves are followed by the QRS-T waves. The shape of the P and QRS-T waves are normal. The only abnormality is the prolonged PR interval (Fig. 2.24).

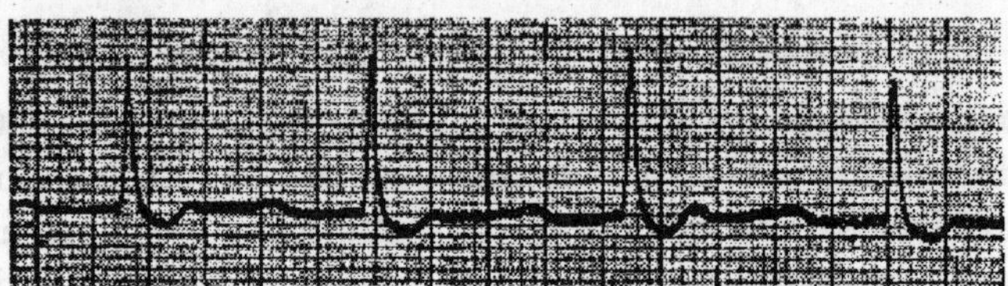

Fig. 2.24. Shows the first degree heart block. PR interval 0.40 seconds. All the P waves are followed by the QRS-T waves.

Second Degree Heart Block

The second degree heart block or partial heart block is a more severe condition than the first degree block. In this condition, some of the S.A. node impulses do not reach the ventricles. They are completely blocked at the A.V. node. The P waves are present, and they are normal in shape and occur regularly. Most of the P waves are followed by the normal QRS-T waves. A few of the P waves are not followed by the QRS-T waves. The block may occur at any interval. There may be 4 : 3 or 6 : 5 or any other interval. 6 : 5 block means that after 5 sinus beats the 6th atrial beat is not followed by QRS-T waves. The 7th atrial impulse again initiates the ventricular response.

In most severe grades of block, the ventricular response is still less. The block occurs regularly at every second, third or more P waves so that there is 2 : 1, 3 : 1 or 4 : 1 heart block. It means that so many P waves are not followed by the QRS-T waves. After two, three, four or five P waves one complete P-QRS-wave is seen. This is normal sinus wave.

The PR interval is normal or prolonged. Some of the cardiac impulses arising in the S.A. node are able to pass the A.V. node. The produce normal P-QRS-T waves with normal PR interval. There are cases in which the A.V. node delays the impulse passing down and in such cases the PR interval is prolonged.

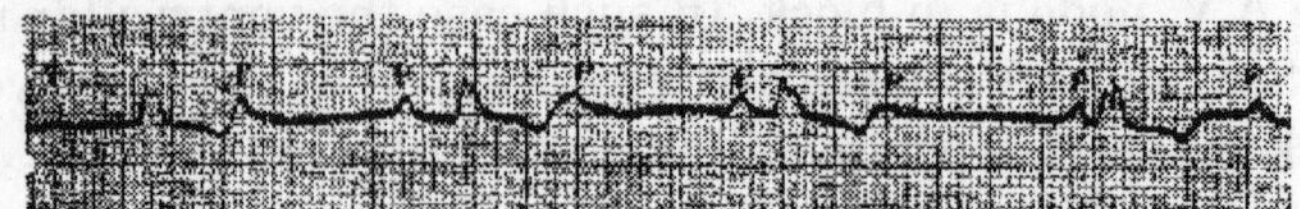

Fig. 2.25. Shows the second degree heart block. All the P waves are not followed by the QRS-T waves.

Fig. 2.25 shows the second degree heart block. All the P waves are not followed by the QRS-T waves. This is 2 : 1 ventricular response *i.e.*, for every two P waves, there is one QRS-T response. Auricular rate is about 100 per minute, while the ventricular rate is 50 per minute.

Third degree heart Block is also called complete heart block. The cardiac impulse originating at the S.A. node can not pass down the A.V. node. The P waves are normal and occur at regular intervals. The rate of the auricular waves is about 80 per minute. At intervals QRS-T waves occur. The QRS-T waves are of normal shape and they occur at irregular intervals. The time relations between the P and QRS-T waves is completely lost. P wave may be in front of QRS, in the notching the QRS complex, in between the QRS and T waves, embedded in the T wave-producing a notching of the T wave, or producing a T wave of different shape, or in the TP interval. The rate of the QRS-T waves is from 20 to 40 per minute (Fig. 2.26).

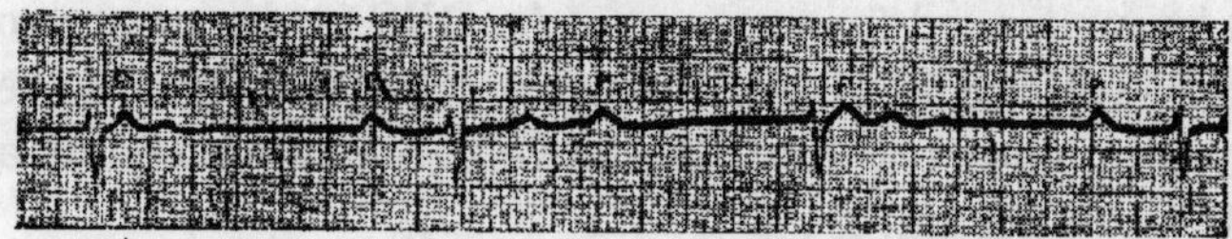

Fig. 2.26. Shows the third degree or complete heart block. Auricular rate is 60 per minute, while the verticular rate is 40 per minute.

Fig. 2.26 shows the third degree heart block. Auricular rate is 60 per minute while the ventricular rate is 40 per minute. The P waves occur at regular intervals. The QRS-T waves are of the nodal type and their rhythm is completely independent of the S.A node rhythm.

Reading of Electrocardiogram

Interpretation of an electrocardiogram requires a careful study of all the waves and base lines in all the leads. Before commencing the study of the record, look at the **standardisation.** Note the calibration. It must be exactly ten mm in height (Fig. 2.27).

The ECG instrument is so standardised that one millivolt current produces a deflection of one cm. Next, glance over the whole record to find any glaring abnormality. If it is found make a note of it. A number of factors influence the normal electrocardiogram. Next one proceeds as follows:

Rate

Rhythm

Voltage

Axis deviation

Extra-systole

P wave

PR interval

QRS complex

RS-T segment

T wave

QT interval

Summary

ECG diagnosis

Rate of the heart.

Rhythm

The cardiac impulse originates at the S.A node and spreads down to the ventricular muscles. It produces normal P, QRS and T waves at regular intervals. This is called normal **SINUS RHYTHM.** Thus rhythm means regularity. Find out whether the Rhythm is regular or irregular. Irregular rhythms constitute arrhythmias.

To find out rhythm, measure P-P, and R-R intervals. Also measure PR and QT intervals.

Voltage

The voltage can be measured for any wave. As QRS is the most prominent wave in the whole electrocardiogram, voltage is always measured for the QRS wave only. Measure the voltage of the QRS waves in leads I, II and III.The voltage can also be measured in pre-cordial leads V_1 to V_6. The voltage is normal if :

1. QRS complex is 5 mm. In standard limb leads I, II and III.
2. Sum of the QRS complexes of leads I, II and III is 10 mm or more.
3. If the QRS complex is 8mm or more in any one of the precordial leads V_1 to V_6.

The voltage may be

1. **Normal.**
2. **High.** A high voltage means a normal healthy myocardium. High voltage is obtained in normal healthy muscular person, ventricular hypertrophy and ventricular extra-systole.
3. **Low.** Low voltage means a poor myocardium. It is common in old age, wasted and emaciated persons, pericardial effusion, myocardial infarction, myxoedema and other conditions of failing heart.

Axis Deviation

Normally there is no axis deviation.

1. Right axis deviation is found in–right ventricular hypertrophy an congenital heart disease *e.g.*, congenital pulmunory stenosis. Tetralogy of fallot, Eisenmenger's syndrome etc.
2. Left axis deviation is found in left ventricular hypertrophy, horizontal heart and congenital heart diseases *e.g.* patent ducts arteriosis, coarctation of the aorta, congenital tricuspid atrasia etc.

Extra systoles. Extra systoles have one important characteristic. The R-R interval between extra systole and the normal beat that precedes it is less than the normal R-R interval, while the R-R interval between the extra-systole and the next normal beat that follows it is longer than the normal R-R interval. There is always a pause following the extra systole.

The extra systole may be

1. Auricular
2. Nodal or
3. Ventricular.

Ventricular systoles are easily made out. Nodal extra-systole has no P wave. The auricular extra systole may need to be differentiated from-a) S.A block or S.A. arrest.

P Wave

Examine all the P waves in all the leads–their shape, voltage and duration. Prominent P waves are found in left and right auricular hypertrophy. P waves are absent or poorly defined in auricular flutter and fibrillation, S.A arrest and block, nodal extra-systoles and nodal rhythm and paroxysmal supra-ventricular tachycardia.

In lead I, P wave is always upright. It is inverted in lead aV_R, dextrocardia, wrong lead attachments of leads I and II, auricular extra-systole and A.V. nodal rhythm.

PR interval. Measure the PR interval in a lead where it is the longest. Normal PR interval is 0.12 to 0.20 seconds. The PR interval is increased more than 0.20 seconds–in first and second degree heart block and in Weinkebach phenomenon. PR interval is less than 0.12 seconds in Wolff-Parkinson-white syndrome and the upper and Lower A.V. nodal rhythm.

QRS Complex is the most important wave of the electrocardiogram. The following points to be noted are :

Normal pattern is altered by :

1. Axis deviation—leads I, II and III.
2. Positions of the heart—leads *a*VR, *a*VL and *a*VF.
3. Rotations of the heart—leads V1 to V6.
4. Other factors like Muscle tremors and loose attachment of the electrodes

Now look for the abnormal QRS patterns

1. Ventricular hypertrophy pattern
2. Ventricular strain pattern
3. Bundle branch block pattern
4. Myocardial infarction patterns

Abnormal QRS complexes are also observed in Ventricular extra-systole, supra-ventricular paroxymal and paroxysmal ventricular tachycardia.

Notching or slurring of the QRS should also be noted. If it occurs near the base of the waves or the apex of the waves when the QRS is tall, then it has no significance. But if notching or slurring occurs in QRS which are short, then it is definitely abnormal.

Notching and slurring occurs in bundle branch block, ventricular extra-systole and paroxysmal ventricular tachycardia.

Q-wave is important in electrocardiography. Normally a Q wave is seen in leads III, V5 and V6. A normal Q wave is never more than 3mm or more than 20% the size of the R wave that follows it. A Q wave ¼th the size of the R wave is always pathological. A prominent Q wave is frequent in myocardial infarctions. In myocardial infarctions Q wave is also wide, 0.03 seconds or more.

II. Duration of the QRS complex-QRS complex must not measure more than 0.10 seconds. A duration greater than 0.10 seconds is always abnormal. Wide QRS occur in–Bundle branch block, intra-ventricular block, Wolff Parkinson-white syndrome, myocardial infarction, ventricular extra-systole, paroxysmal ventricular tachycardia and sometimes in ventricular hypertrophy.

RS-T Segment

The RS-T segment is always iso-electric. An elevation or depression of the RS-T segment by one mm is not abnormal. Beyond one mm, the elevation or depression of the RS-T segment is pathological. Elevation above the base line is called LOW take off. For purpose of high or low take off the RS-T segment must be compared with the TP segment that follows it, and not with the PR segment which precedes it.

Elevations of the RS-T segment occurs in

1. Myocardial infarction
2. Acute pericarditis
3. Ventricular extra-systole
4. Paroxysmal ventricular tachycardia

Depression of the RS-T segment occurs in

1. Myocardial infarction–opposite to the site of infarction
2. Myocardial anoxaemia
3. Ventricular hypertrophy
4. Ventricular strain
5. Bundle branch block
6. Digitalis
7. ventricular extra-systole

In ventricular hypertrophy and bundle branch block, the RS_T deviation is in the same direction as the T wave. In myocardial infarction, the RS-T deviation is in opposite direction to the T wave. In digitalis saturation, the RS-T segment is cup shaped or of the straight line type.

T Wave

Like Q wave, T wave is important in electrocardiography. Normal T wave characters must always be remembered.

Note the shape of the T waves. T wave has the special characteristics in-

1. Ventricular hypertrophy
2. Ventricular strain
3. Bundle branch block
4. Myocardial infarction
5. Myocardial ischaemia
6. Digitalis saturation
7. Ventricular extra-systole

In ventricular hypertrophy, bundle branch block, and ventricular strain, the T wave is asymmetrical. The hind limb of the T wave is short and nearer the apex of the wave. In myocardial infarction, the T wave is symmetrical, the two limbs being the mirror images of each other.

The T wave is inverted in many physiological conditions. Important pathological conditions I which the T wave inversions are:

1. Ventricular hypertrophy
2. Ventricular strain
3. Bundle branch block
4. Myocardial infarction
5. Myocardial ischaemia
6. Digitalis saturation
7. Ventricular extra-systole

Low voltage of the T wave is found in the same conditions described above.

High voltage T waves are obtained in

1. Marked ventricular hypertrophy
2. Bundle branch block
3. Hyperkalemia

Q-T Interval

Q-T interval is the total time of ventricular activation. It is prolonged in:

1. Myocardial infarction
2. Bundle branch block
3. Quinidine
4. Hypokalemia

QT-interval is shortened in

1. Digitalis
2. Hypercalcemia

Summary

Then the summary is made for the abnormal features detected. This gives the important points to concentrate on.

Diagnosis

After considering all the points, one has to try to give the possible the ECG diagnosis of the record. It may be possible to state definitely the underlying pathological diagnosis of the disease. But for this the ECG findings must always be considered in conjunction with the history of the patient, the clinical findings, pathological and other investigation reports and the clinical diagnosis whenever available. Never venture a diagnosis from the ECG alone.

Use of Virtual ECG Instrument

Having considered some of the important areas of diagnosis with a view to understand the waveform patterns which lead to a diagnosis, the virtual display with an ICU ward's Computer monitor enables the features to be noted continuously rather than from a hard copy. To this purpose, the comparison of the past records of the same or any other known patient with the particular waveform pattern can be made. The recognition has not been possible, as yet, to be made automatic, because such an expert system is not presently available. The display of the waveform has been proceeding only on the basis of the same Einthoven's recording even today. That is, we still use the same length of time period for the display (with only 3mm length allotted for the entire QRS complex). At the time recorders existed in those days, perhaps it was not possible to increase the speed of recording. On a virtual instrument, it is possible to view the QRS complex itself on one full frame, with more samples per second during that 0.06-0.08 second interval. In that case, it may not fit in with the experience of the observing diagnostic Physician to find an abnormal ST depression or an S wave convexity, since he has been all along trained to look at a small kink in a 1 mm space of the chart record. However, with the feasibility of providing a clear view of the signal in the region of interest, the virtual instrument definitely provides much more information, though it would be somewhat long before its use is clinically recognised.

A modern Electrocardiographic instrument is based on a software module packaged to have the look and feel of a physical instrument. The computer display can be a stand alone instrument like an oscilloscope with its familiar knobs, switches, and scope display, or it can represent the controls of an ATE setup or of a set of monitoring devices. A user interface can be created regardless of the hardware involved; the software becomes the instrument. The implementation of the Electrocardiograph (ECG machine) on the personal computer is a Virtual Instrument. The only external hardware is the E.C.G. preamplifier board along with the data acquisition board which is interfaced via the printer port. All controls are via keyboard and the display is similar to the normal E.C.G. recorder. The instantaneous heart rate is also displayed. Alarm provision is also made feasible in this unit when any abnormalities are found for a particular patient when E.C.G. recording is carried out. This paves the way for an intelligent E.C.G. diagnosis using a PC.

ECG CIRCUITS

1. A Typical Recorder type analog ECG machine

Circuits of standard earlier version machines use only analog components. They may or may not have opto isolation between the preamplifier and the further circuits. This is not essential because the further thing to preamplification is only to drive the recorder, which is the hot stylus wax paper recorder, built into the machine. There are no interfaces for computer connection in these units.

The circuit diagram of a typical machine of this category, (which is important because these are the machines found today with many Doctors), is shown in Fig. 2.27. These also need servicing now a days and a description of the pre-amplifier circuit is well in order.

Preamplifier for Analog ECG Machine

A circuit of the typical "Cambridge" ECG recorder is given in figure. This is a differential amplifier whose input stage is a matched pair of n-channel silicon field effect transistors 2N2935. The output is single ended.

Diathermy filter. R1, C1, R2, C2 form a filter to eliminate interference from 27 MHz diathermy radiation possibly used in the same environment. R1, R2, MR1, MR2, MR3, MR4 protect the amplifier from damage due to surges, such as from an defibrillation equipment, likely to be used along with this.

VT3, a BC108 small signal transistor, is wired as a constant current source for the field effect transistors. RV2 is for balancing the two FET currents.

Transistors VT4-5, 6, 7 form a differential *Beneteau pair*. (2N4126, BC108) Their output is feedback by R15,16. The gain up to this stage is about 30.

VT8, 10 are a differential pair with a single ended output. (2N1306).

There is provision for varying the gain using emitter resistors in steps.

VT8 and VT10 must be carefully matched to avoid D.C. shifts when the gain is changed. The fine control RV4 varies the resistance between pins 9 and 10. This is called as the Sensitivity control.

VT9 provides constant current for VT8 and VT10. RV3 changes the current through VT8 and VT10, and hence the voltage across R30 and the DC output level.

VT11 and VT12 are a current output stage with temperature compensation from MR5. The output current is 4.5 mA and the amplifier voltage gain into a 1Kohm load is now greater than 700.

Drive Amplifier

General. The frequency response of the amplifier is flat from DC to 2KHz. A bridge system is employed. The input signal is amplified by VT2 and drives one end of the gavonometer (hot stylus recorder's). This is via the VT3 and VT5 emitter followers. The other end of the coil is driven by an "error" amplifier. This is by VT13 and emitter followers VT11,12. This keeps the coil centre at a fixed potential determined by Zener diode Z3. A phase splitting action is produced, causing the ends of the gavo coil to "see-saw" about the centre point. This system provides a good stability against temperature variations.

The emitter follower VT5 uses another transistor VT4 as the emitter load resistor to give high efficiency and at the same time, to prevent VT5 from cutting off due to transients from the back e.m.f. of the galvo coil.

The transistor VT5 acts as a simple emitter follower for driving the load. For deflection one way, its base potential goes negative and thus the load current rises, allowing a larger voltage to develop across R7. This cuts off VT6 which in turn cuts off VT4. Further increases in load current would cause a larger voltage drop across R7, which cannot have a lower value without upsetting the whole sequence of events. This large voltage rise is prevented by VT7 which clamps the maximum voltage to a value determined by base bias.

For deflection in the opposite direction, the galvo coil current passes via VT4, but to ensure that VT5 can control the voltage across the coil, a small amount of this current is allowed to flow through VT5- this current must not be too high or efficiency will be reduced..This minimum current through VT5 is defined or clamped by R7 and the bias on the base of VT6. If the current tries to fall below the clamping value, VT6 conducts more and provides additional current through VT4. If VT5 passes too high a current, the conduction in VT6 and VT4 decreases in proportion. The current in VT5 is clamped to a minimum value of 8 mA.

The other half of the galvo coil is driven in the same manner by the voltage at the base of VT11, which is derived from the reference amplifier VT13 and is in anti-phase.

Error amplifier

If the voltages across the galvo coil are not equal and opposite, an error voltage occurs at the center tap of this coil. . This error voltage is coupled through Z3 into VT13 base, which amplifies this error and applies feedback through VT12 and VT11 to reduce the error.

If the position control is rotated in such a direction as to drive the base of VT5 negative, then once VT13 has "bottomed", further rotation causes a rapid rise in base current of VT13 through Z3 and half the galvo coil. It is prevented from becoming excessive by the limiting action of Z2.

Drive amplifer

The input signal from the preamp is applied to VT2 base, amplified and then coupled to the coil through VT3 and VT5. The linearity is improved to the desired value by feedback R4 and choice of VT2 current.

Position control

This is located in the circuit containing VT1 and Z1. This provides a variable current drain for the 4.5 mA current flowing out of the preamplifier. The difference between the output current of the preamp and the collector current of VT1 is seen by the drive amplifier VT2 and is amplified.

Recording unit

The recording uses the pen heat oscillator, the drive motro, the galvo and the stylus. 25KHz is the pen heat frequency.

The stylus deflector is a highly damped moving coil galvanometer. High dampling is achieved by a shorted turn, which is the former itself. A strong return spring gives the galvanometer a good frequency response.. The galvanometer takes about 10 V for full deflection to one side. It can withstand some amount of overload current as well.

Chart drive is single speed operation, as per ECG standard. A mechanical governor is used for adjusting the speed variations, (as in tape recorders).

A TYPICAL LABORATORY ECG PRE-AMPLIFIER CIRCUIT

Fig. 2.28 shows a typical circuit showing the various parts of the ECG pre-amplifier.

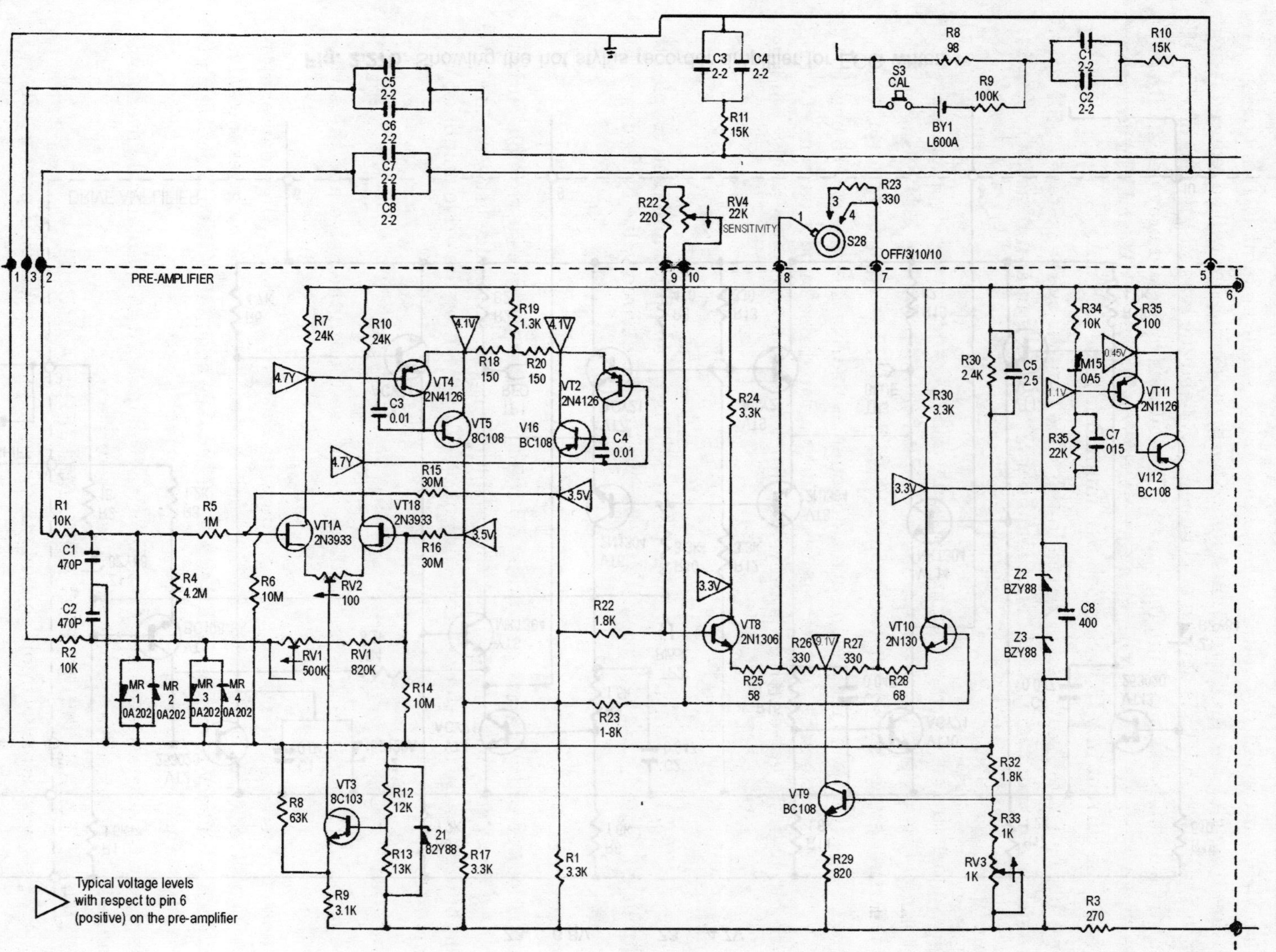

Fig. 2.27a. Shows the pre amplifier of the ECG writer.

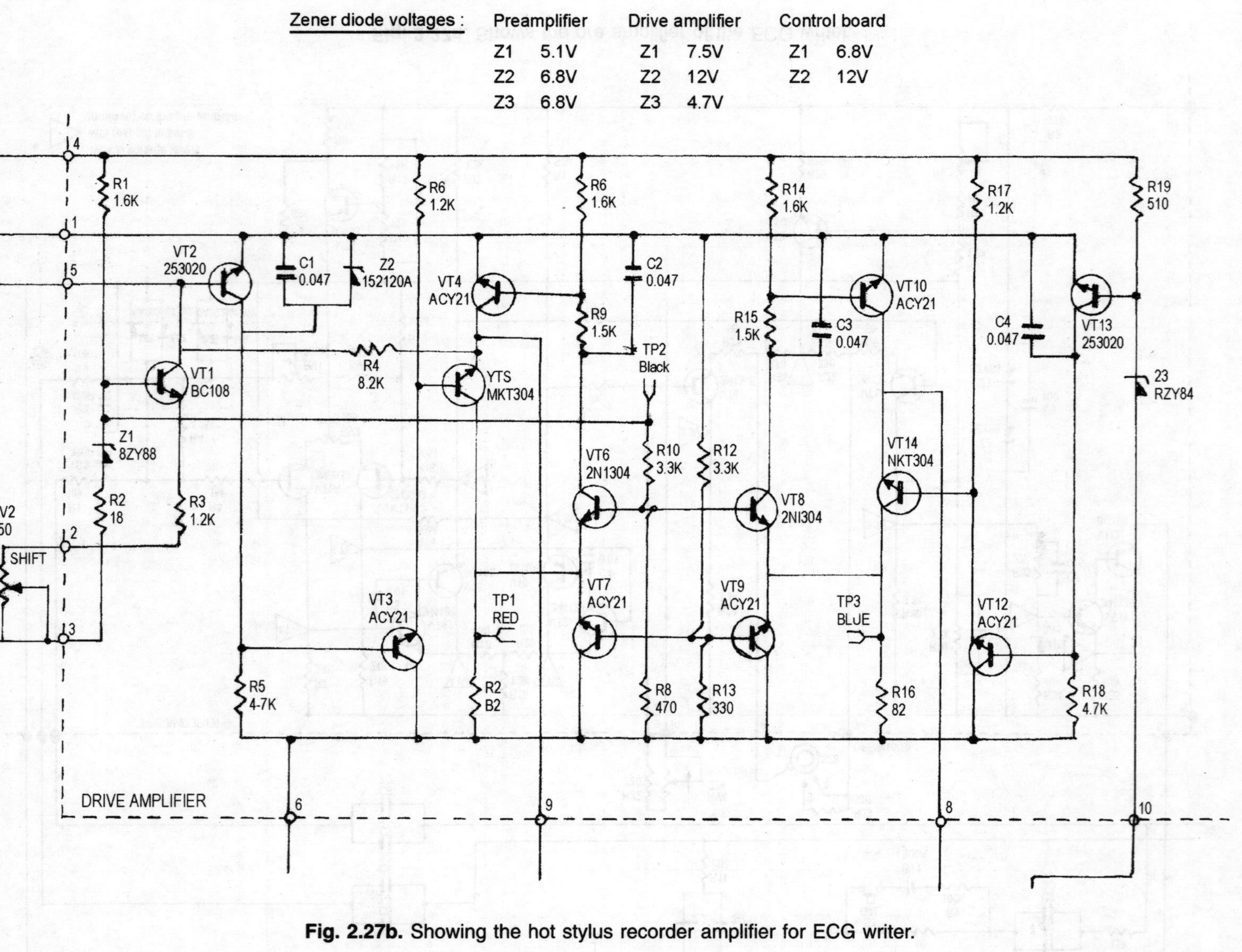

Fig. 2.27b. Showing the hot stylus recorder amplifier for ECG writer.

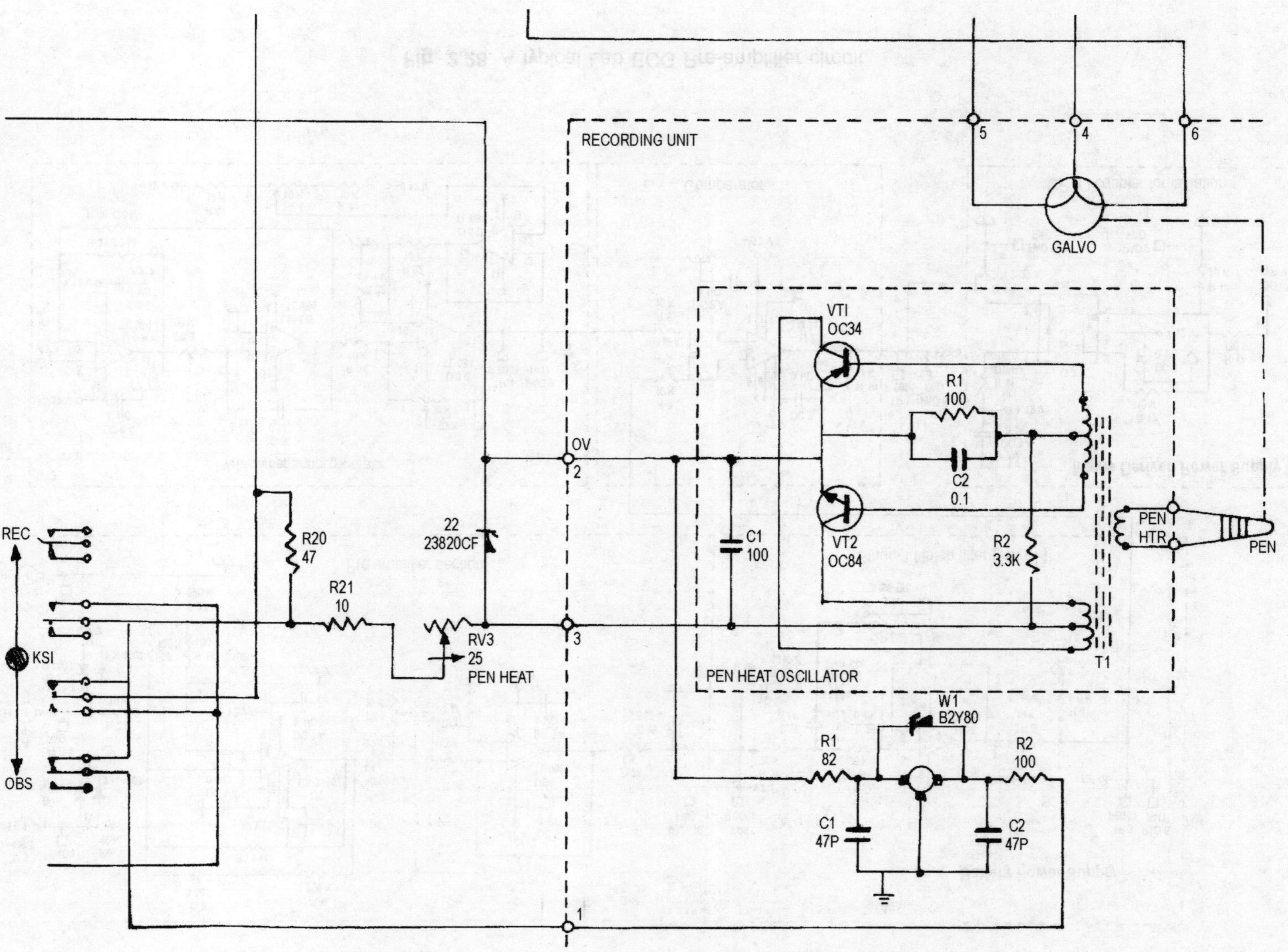

Fig. 2.27c. Shows the pen heat oscillator and chart drive motor circuit for the ECG writer.

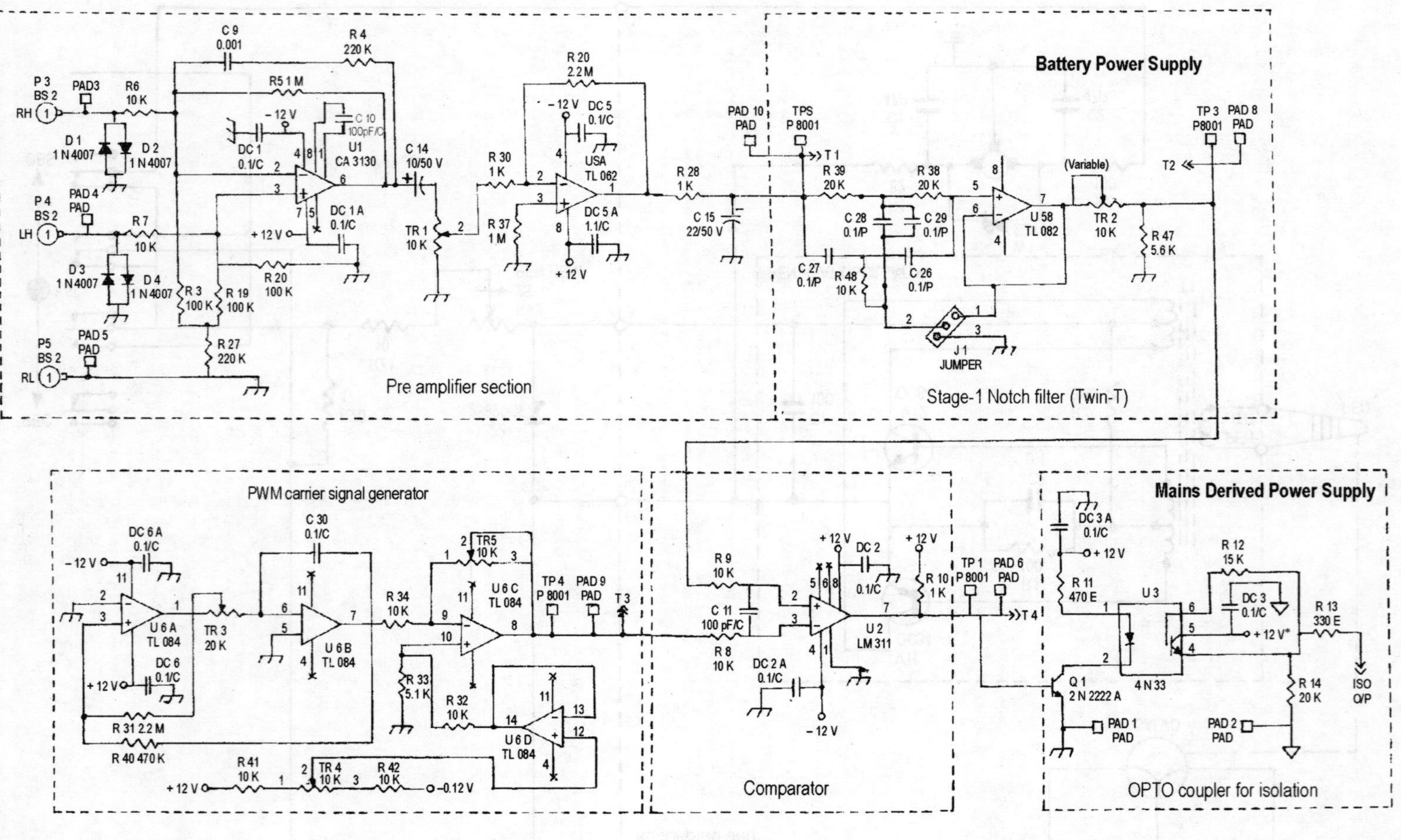

Fig. 2.28. A typical Lab ECG Pre-amplifier circuit.

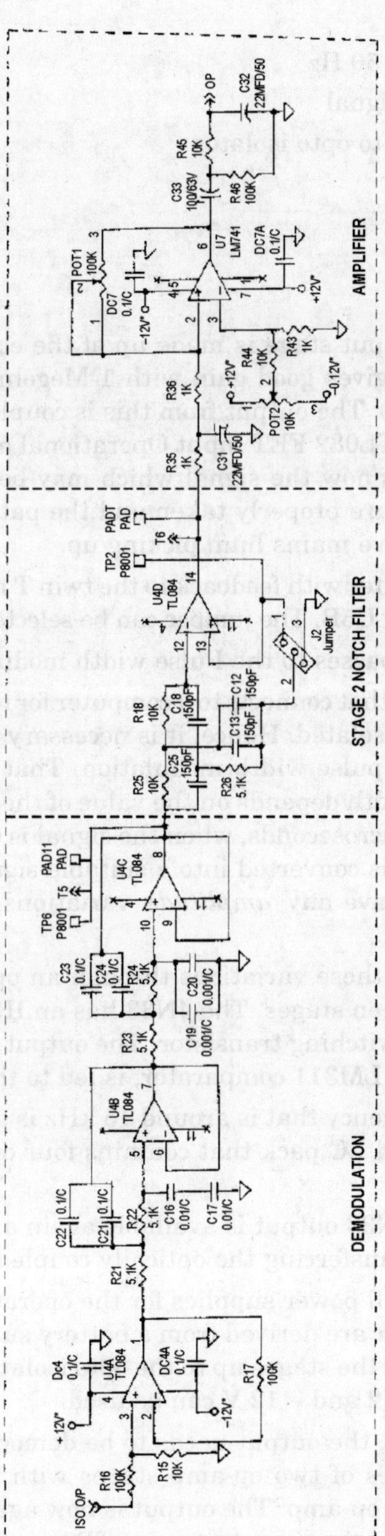

Fig. 2.28 (Contd.)

1. The input stage
2. The active notch filter for 50 Hz
3. The conversion to PWM signal
4. The comparator for input to opto isolator
5. The opto isolator
6. The demodulator
7. Stage 2 filter
8. Final amplifier

In this circuit shown, the input stage is made up of the economical but high performance CMOS RCA3130 Chip. This gives good gain with 1 Megohm in the feedback path and series input resistors of 10K (R6, 7). The output from this is coupled capacitively through C14 and TR1 to the next stage using a TL082 FET input Operational amplifier. This works at very high, typically 1000. The output is now the signal which may be having considerable mains from component, unless the leads are properly taken and the patient is kept on an insulated table, with no possibility of excessive mains hum picking up.

The notch filter is an active filter with feedback to the twin T network found via the jumper J1, which uses operational amplifier U5B. The jumper can be selected with no feedback also.

The output from this stage passes to the Pulse width modulation circuit.

Every typical e.c.g. amplifier that connects to a computer for further processing or analysis or whatever, needs to be optically isolated. Hence, it is necessary to convert the analog signal into a digital pulsed signal, using pulse width modulation. That means the analog signal is replaced by a pulse train, whose width depends on the value of the signal. For e.g., if the signal is 1 V and the pulse width is 100 microseconds, when the signal is 0.5V, the width 50 microseconds and so on. In other words, it is converted into a suitable signal for digital transmission, since the PWM output does not have any *amplitude* variations, but merely varies in time width as per the signal.

So, it is possible to transfer these variations through an opto-coupler, which is typical component used for isolation between stages. The 4N33 has an IR diode at the input which is driven by a transistor 2N2222, a switching transistor. The output from the comparator, which gets the PWM signal from the fast LM311 comparator, is fed to the opto isolator.

The PWM signal of the frequency that is around 15 kHz is generated by a pair of operational amplifiers using TL084 quad LC pack that contains four operational amplifiers in one 14 pin chip.

The optical isolation from 4N33 output is available again a PWM signal, with the right hand side transitor of the 4N33 transferring the optically coupled signal information.

It is necessary to note that all power supplies for the operational amplifiers, right from the front–end up to the opto isolator are derived from a battery supply. This ensures low noise and hum. The currents required for the stages up to the opto isolator is around 50 mA only and suitable chargeable batteries of + 12 and – 12 V can be used.

Then, after the opto-isolator, the output needs to be demodulated. After a buffer stage in U4A, the demodulator comprises of two op-amp stages with filtering using fourth order filter, using R-C twin stage in each op-amp. The output is now again an analog signal, similar to what was present in the previous circuit at test point TP2.

Now, a second Notch filter stage is used to eliminate all mains hum, which is also a twin T notch with active feedback. The selection is by jumper J2 in the bottm figure part.

Thereafter, a final amplification stage is added with again of about 100, to raise the signal nominally above 1 V at the output. The signal is capacitive coupled using a large capacitor C33 of 100 μF.

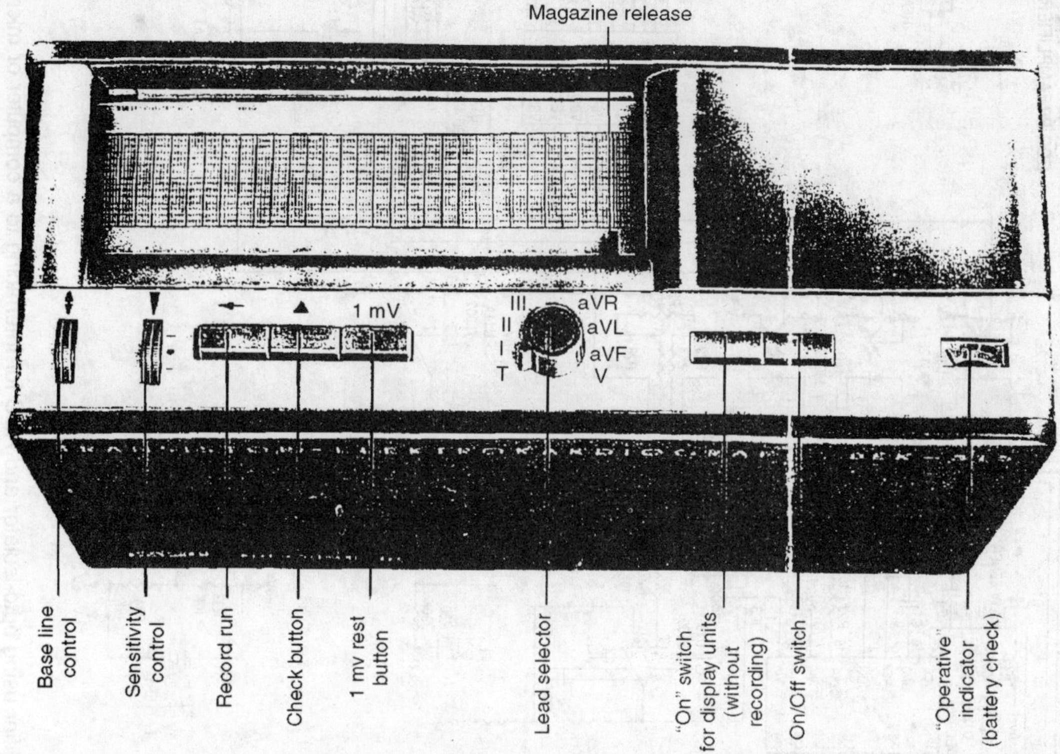

Fig. 2.28a. Photograph of portable ECG Unit.

2. A modern ECG PRE AMPLIFIER BOARD

In contrast with the earlier models which even exist today both for sale and from earlier hospitals, the modern machine approach the problem with certain features not previously possible.

1. Use of stepper motor for chart drive (of course, with a gear train)
2. Use of opto isolator at the preamp to drive amp
3. provision for RS232 or similar computer interface
4. Display like LCD or LED in addition to the chart recorder
5. User friendliness in lead selection through analog switch Ics

Let us now consider a modern ECG preamplifer.

Fig. 2.28 gives a description of the E.C.G. pre-amplifier and interface circuit. At the extreme left is shown the twin row header for connecting to the Computer's Printer port through a flat ribbon cable. This connects the data bits of the ADC to the ports on the printer port. Opto-isolators U1 to U8 (IC 4N27) connect the ADC's 8 bit data signal from pins 18 to 11 for isolating the patient data acquisition circuits from the Computer's signal lines.

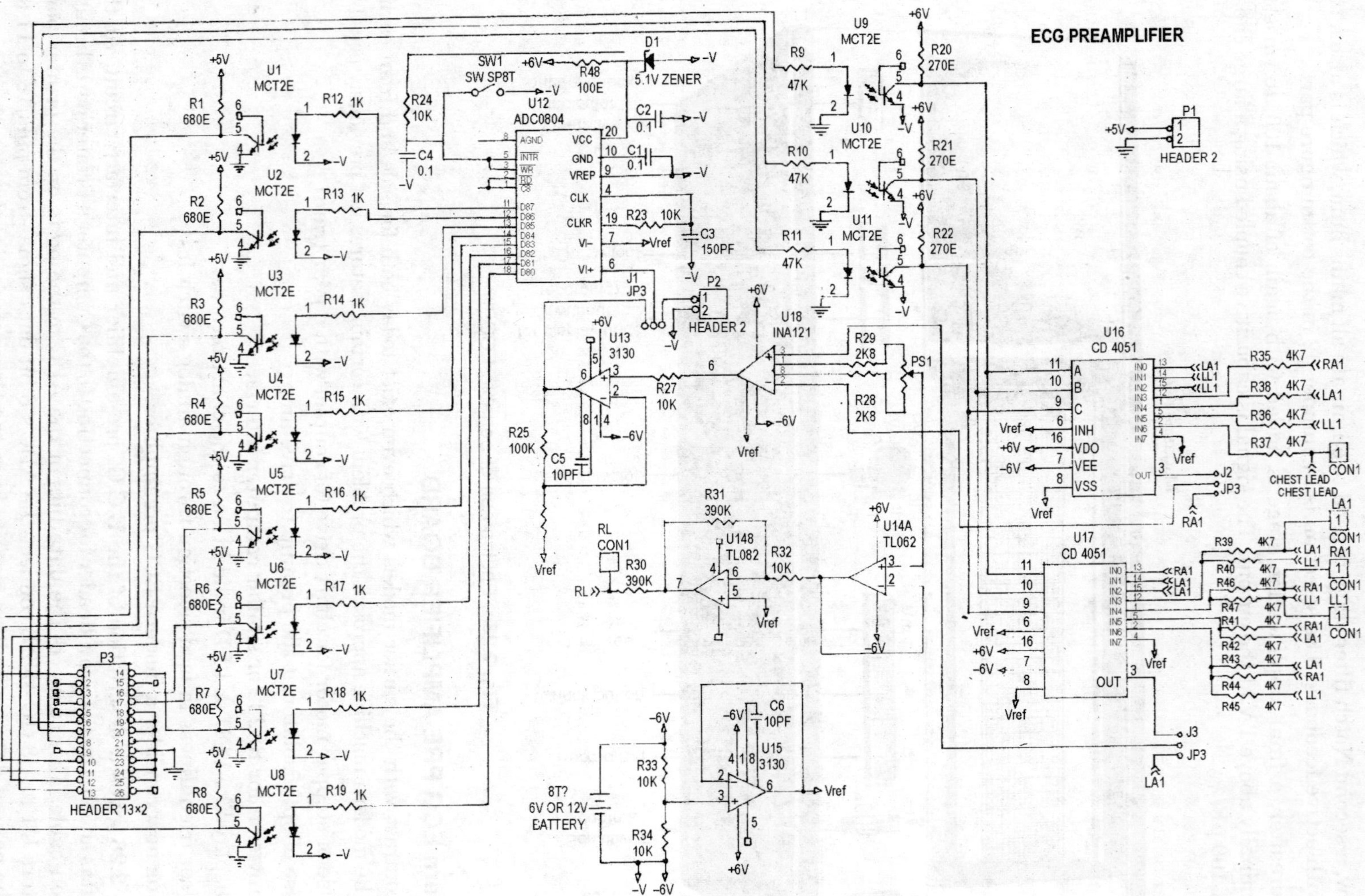

Fig. 2.29 (a). Shows a modern ECG pre amplifier using opto-isolator and ADC for Interfacing to a computer or microcontroller.

The I.C. U12 is just an 8 bit ADC, the National's 0804, presently employed, and has a sampling time of 100ms. The eight bits output from the ADC are logic signals, which are to be read by the port bits of the printer port. Hence, eight opto-isolators are used for the purpose. The ADC clock is set by resistor R23 and Capacitor C3. The ADC 0804 operates on a 5V supply, which is provided by the Zener diode D1 from the circuit's battery supply. The ADC is made to continuously converting, by wiring the INTR\ and WR\ pins together. A switch SW1 is used for momentarily grounding these pins to start off the continuous ADC action. Pin 6 of U12, the ADC, receives the pre-amplified E.C.G. signal from the Instrumentation amplifiers U18 and U13. Because distortion is produced at lower input impedance values, we use instrumentation amplifiers. (Fig. 2.29*a*)

U13 is a CMOS hi-input impedance Operational amplifier which can work from a low voltage supply of 6V. The U18 is an instrumentation amplifier INA 121 from Burr-Brown. It has FET inputs, uses low power and works from 3V supply also. Its offset voltage and drift are 200 μV-2 μV, while it has a common mode rejection of over 100 dB. It is a simple 8 pin plastic package and is not expensive. Its FET- input circuitry provides a low power instrumentation

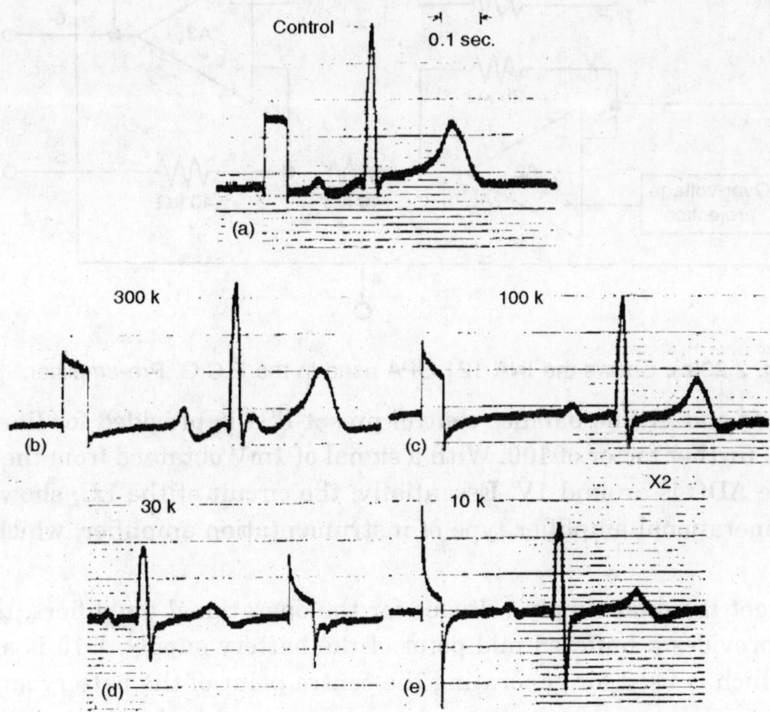

Fig. 2.29 (b). Distortion of e.c.g. at lower input impedance values.

amplifier offering excellent accuracy. Its versatile three- op amp design and very small size makes it ideal for battery operation purpose. Particularly noteworthy is its low bias current of (4pA which permits the use of high impedance on input leads. Using a single external resistor it provides a high gain and a CMRR of 100 dB. Hence it is very useful for the E.C.G. application where the signals are usually very weak. Circuits with battery operation with as low as 3V is possible with this device. Hence the ECG preamplifier makes use of this for the front end circuitry. It is always advisable to avoid 220V AC based power supplies for these circuitry to avoid risk of dangerous leakage currents. Thus, the E.C.G. preamplifier circuit using INA121 has been experimented and found to be satisfactory.

A resistor between the pins 1 and 8 does the gain adjustment. This controls the gain because the ratio of the internal 25 K (Fig. 2.29) to this resistor value governs the feedback ratio for the two input operational amplifier stages. The resistors R29 and R28 control the gain

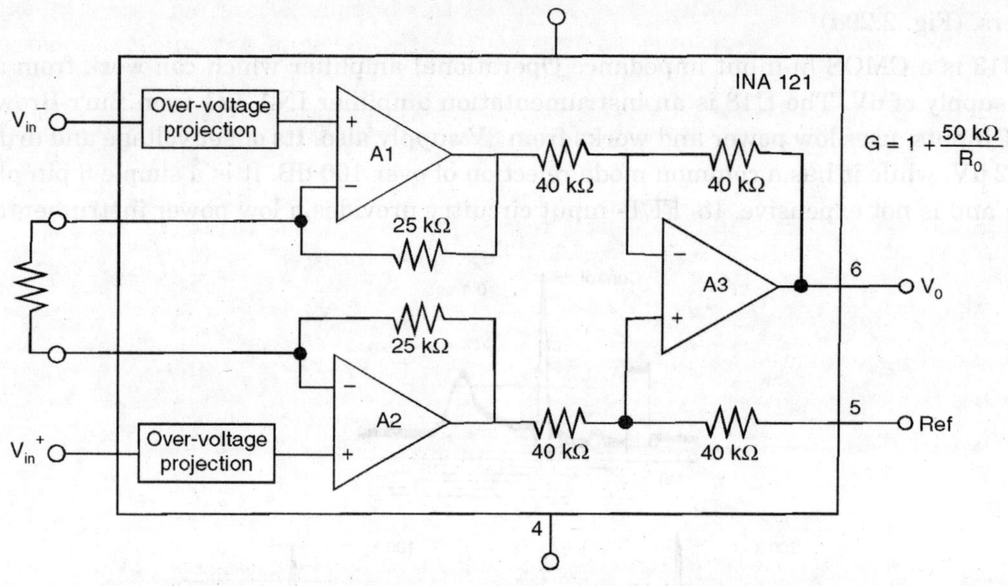

Fig. 2.29(c). Shows the INA 121 OPA used in the E.C.G. Pre-amplifier.

to be 10 in the front end. A fine balance control preset PS1 is provided for fine balance. The U13 amplifies by a further factor of 100. With a signal of 1mV obtained from the leads, the net signal given to the ADC is around 1V. Essentially, the circuit of the I.C, shown in Fig. 2.29 below, is a three operational amplifier type of instrumentation amplifier, which is quite well known.

In order to get the dual supply voltages for the operational amplifiers, the I.C. U15 is employed, which provides a buffered mid-point of the battery supply. U15 is a buffer operational amplifier which is used for generating the centre point of the battery supply, which is the effective common point of the operational amplifiers, and is denoted as VREF. R33 and R34 are equal value resistors that divide the battery supply to create the buffered centre voltage, V_{REF}.

THE CONNECTION TO THE RHYTHM STRIP

While working as an E.C.G. monitor in an intensive care bed, it is usual to connect a pair of chest electrodes and a right leg electrode. This is known as the Marriott lead or modified chest lead. This simulates the V1 position with the electrode placement as follows:

Positive Electrode. Fourth Intercoastal space, right sternal border;

Negative Electrode. Just below the outer position of the Left Clavicle;

Ground electrode. Below the right clavicle.

For this lead, the monitor is set as Lead I for this bi-polar recording. This is known also as the rhythm strip, which gives the main pattern of the E.C.G. signal for continuous observation during monitoring. The leads from the electrodes are then directly connected to the input pins of the INA 121. There is no choice of the several E.C.G. leads in this application. Berg strip jumpers J2, J3 are used for this direct connection.

ECG LEAD SELECTION CIRCUIT

The ECG signals are picked off through electrodes on the limbs and chest of the body. The following lead configurations are used.

Lead-1: Right arm-left arm electrodes

Lead-II : Right arm-left leg electrodes

Lead-III : left arm-left leg electrodes

AUXILIARY LEADS

Lead aV_R : Right arm-junction of left arm and left leg via resistor network.

Lead aV_L : Right arm-junction of right arm and left leg via resistor network.

Lead aV_L : Left leg-junction of right arm and left arm via resistor network.

CHEST LEADS

V-Lead. These leads are between the common right leg electrode and the chest-placed Lead in one of the six positions, using a cup electrode. The places of these V1-V6 leads are anatomically located by the physician during the examination.

There are two important aspects of the E.C.G. pre-amplifier hardware.

The selection of a pair of signal wires corresponding to the choice of the lead is unique. For *e.g.*, if LEAD 1 is chosen, then the connections to the amplifier will be made from the right and left arm wires..

Figure also shows the circuit for lead selection using CMOS switches (CD 4051) for making the choice of connections to the patient leads. (4.4)

The CD 4051 is a FET based switch, which has 8 contacts in one package. The selection is based on a one out of eight. The inputs A,B, C to its pins 11,10 and 9 have a range of 0 to 7, so that the choice of one among eight is made. The switch control is through the Inhibit pin 6, which is made low. The IC uses the battery supply, and has a range between its positive and negative rail voltages for the conduction of the signal. The signal input is given to pins IN0 to IN7, of which IN0 is connected to LA1 in U16 and RA1 in U17, so that the choice of input A = 0,B = 0 and C = 0 connects the leads LA1 and RA1 to the output pins (no. 3) of the ICs. Thus, the output pins are connected to the input of the IC U18, the instrumentation OPA through J2, J3.

It may be noted that by selecting the signals to the input pins A,B,C of the pair of CMOS switch ICs U16 and U17, it is possible to choose the various lead configurations for the E.C.G. Further, in order to generate the signals for the auxiliary electrodes, resistors R35 to R45 are employed. e.g., to get the lead aVR, LA1 and LL1 are noted to be connected to the junction of U17 at its pin 12 (IN3). RA1 is connected to the corresponding pin 12 of U16. Thus, the differential signal required for the right auxiliary lead aVr is obtained from the CMOS switches.

Likewise, the other auxiliary electrode connections are made by the selection of the switches through inputs 4 and 5. The chest lead input is given to pin 2 of U16, while the common signal obtained by R42-45 is given to the same pin in U17. The chest lead obtains the difference between the voltage directly picked off the chest lead and the junction point of the arm and leg electrodes.

OPTO ISOLATOR FOR LEAD SELECTION

The three inputs for the CMOS switches for lead selection are opto-isolated again, because they are got from the printer port signals from pins 6 – 8. Opto isolators U9 to U11 are used to input a bit signal to the selection of the leads. The outputs are connected to the CD 4051 (U16 and U17) to the select input pins A,B,C. The printer port ground has connection to the computer ground, but this is isolated from the battery supply. By outputting the bits 000 to 110, the leads I,II,III, aVr, aVL, and aVF are selected through the CMOS switches within the U16 and U17.

The common electrode is right leg electrode .The sum of the lead signals is fed back to the right leg, so as to maintain the right potentials at the common (earth) point. This method minimises hum in the circuit and enhances the common mode rejection.

ISOLATION FOR SAFETY

Isolation of patient leads from any mains derived power supply is mandatory for E.C.G. monitors. In this design, this point has been properly taken care of.

The INA121 FET-input, low power Instrumentation amplifier is used here for pre amplification of the E.C.G. signal. The IC has input protection for excessive voltages which are likely to arise from the patient leads, over – 40 to + 40V.

The signal at the output of this circuit is between 1-2V for a change of 1 mV-2 mV of the physiological E.C.G. signal.

The signal is passed through the opto couplers, U1 to U8, which provide high isolation resistance, all parts being IC 4N27.

ECG PRE AMPLIFIER CIRCUITS

There are two important aspects in the ECG pre-amplifier circuit design.

1. To select the signal pair of wires corresponding to the choice of the lead. For example, if lead-I is chosen, then the connections to the amplifier will be made from the right and left arm wires.
2. To amplify the signal which is just a mV or so, to a level of 2V.
3. To provide isolation for the patient.

Fig. 2.28 shows the typical circuit commonly employed in present day ECG pre-amplifiers. This uses CMOS switches namely CD4051 for making the lead selection. Instead of INA12, the CMOS OPAMP TL061, TL081 also provide good differential amplification of the selected lead. Front end buffers are made up using the low noise, high gain IC LM 348. The common electrode is right leg electrode. The sum of the three lead signals is fed back to the right leg, so as to maintain the right leg potentials at the common (earth) point. This method minimizes hum in the circuit and enhances the common mode rejection.

The signal is passes through an opto coupler circuit, comprising of IC1023. Additionally, an active 50 Hz notch filter is employed to filter out 50 Hz noise signals. The signal at the output of this circuit is between 1 V to 2 V for a change of 1 mV of the physiological signals.

A DIGITAL E.C.G. RECORDER SYSTEM WITH RIGHT LEG DRIVE

A standard ECG consist of 12 channels; each channel "looks" at the heart from a different electrical axis. The different "views" allow us to interpret the activity of different parts of the heart. The timing relationship between different components of the heart will identify defects in the conduction pathways.

In patients with high blood pressure, the left ventricle will become quite large due to its increased load. This is seen as significant increase in the amplitude of the QRS complex. Treatment of the high blood pressure will allow the left ventricle to return normal size which significantly decreases the chance of a heart attack.

Since the amplitude of the electrical signals in the heart are a function of chemicals in the body, it is possible to predict abnormalities. For example, an elevated potassium level will produce a tall peaked T wave.

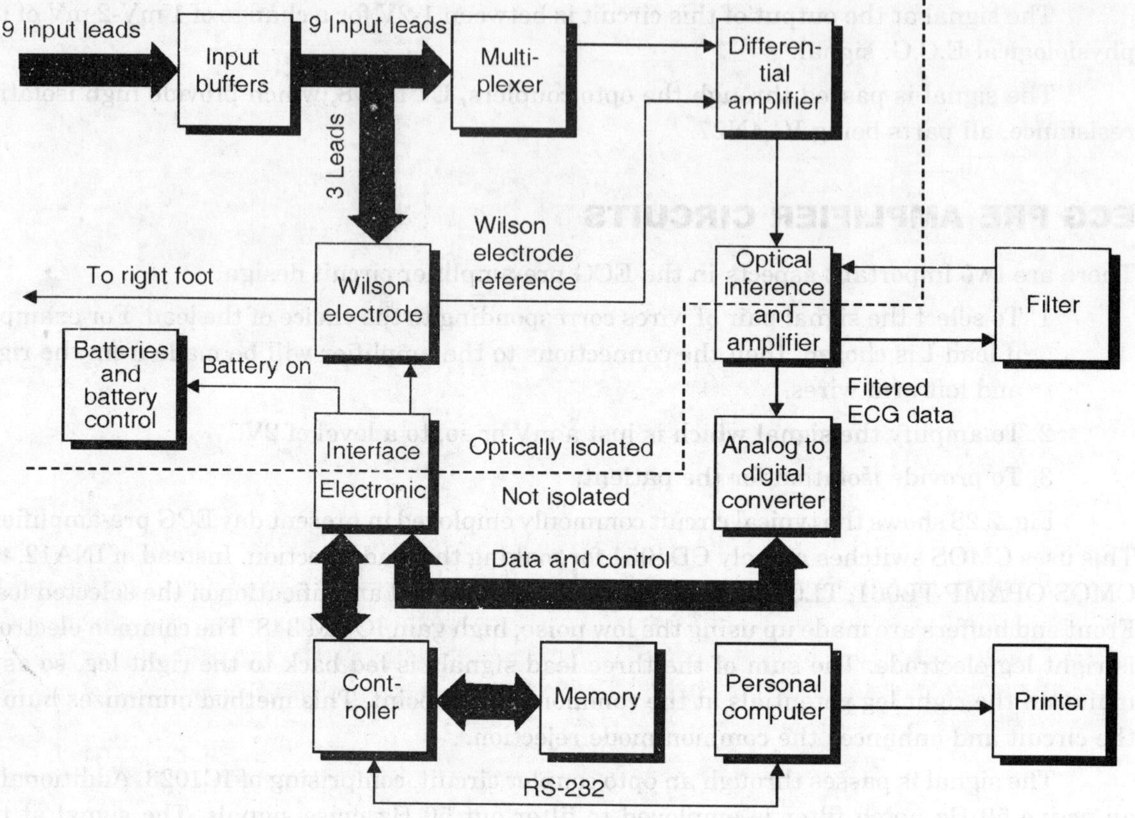

Fig. 2.30. Shows the block diagram of the complete ECG system. The system logically divides into the front-end electronics and the controller, Data communication between the analog and digital portion of the ecg is accomplished through optical isolators, which helps keep the patient isolated.

E.C.G. PRE-AMPLIFIER CIRCUITS

Before proceeding with the modern circuit using single input amplifiers and right leg drive, let us give some simple circuits for use and trial for the students learning to make such amplifiers, in this section.

A simple pre-amplifier based on general purpose op-Amp for lab testing in training students is given below. This uses the differential amplifier configuration with a large input resistance of 1 M across each lead to ground which is wired through a 10 M resistor as a maximum. It is to be emphasized that the two 1 M resistors are to be matched equal for proper Common mode hum signal rejection. The lead wires to the electrodes are to be made via a shielded cable and the shield should be grounded. The gain is such that the two OP-Amp. Configuration gives an ECG signal of 1Vt typically. The second stage is only capacitive coupled. The frequency response is limited by the feedback capacitor on the first Op-Amp.

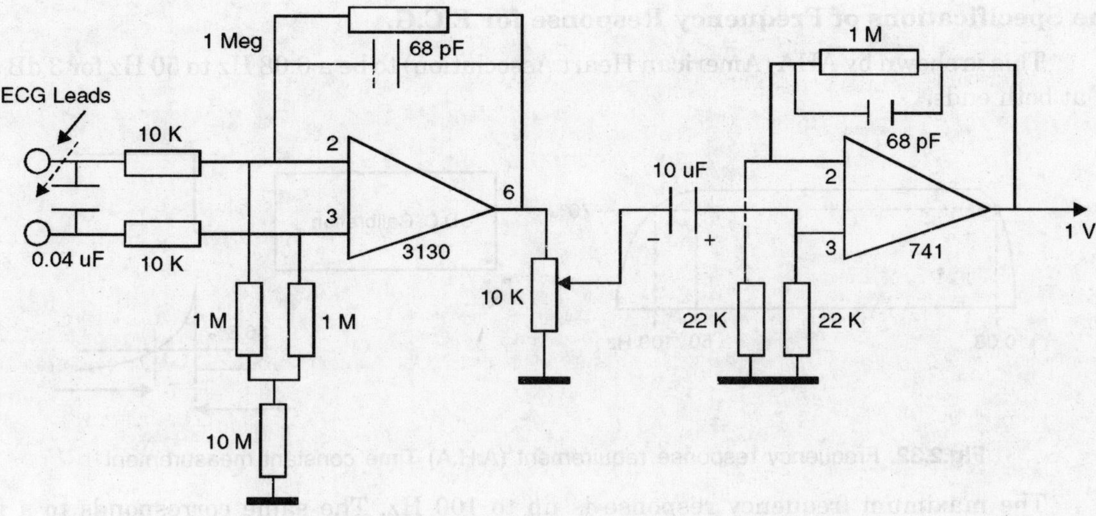

Fig. 2.31. Showing a simple lab ECG pre amplifier Circuit.

Further, in order to reject mains based hum ordinarily picked up in these circuits, as well as in commercial circuits, resort is made to a notch filter of the analog type. Rather than using a simple bridged-T filter configuration which has a low Q factor, an active stage using an OP-Amp. Improves the notch very much. The following is one such lab. Type circuit of the hum filter for 50 Hz.

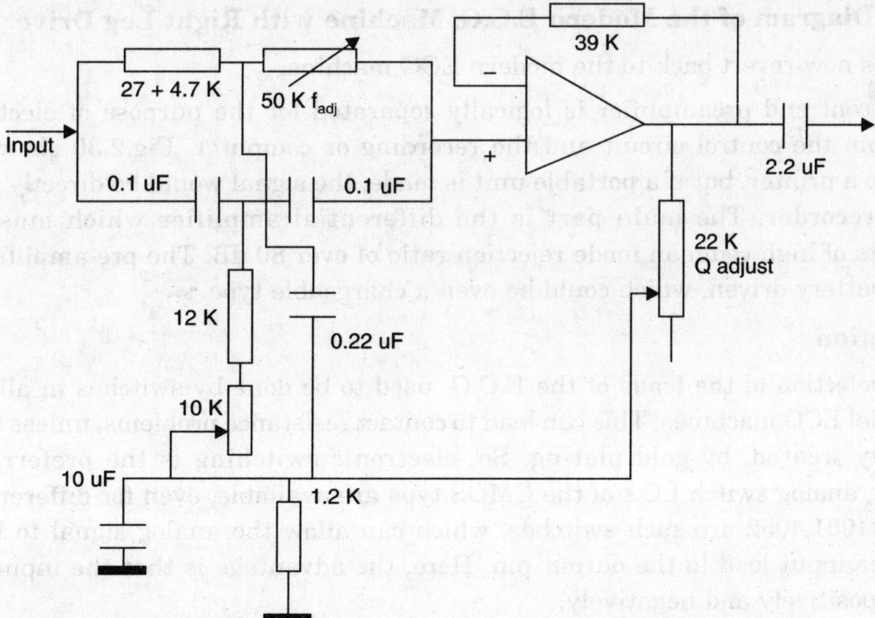

The frequency is adjusted by the 50 K variabie resistor on the bridge arm and the 22 K on the earthed arm. The Q factor is adjusted by the feedback from the Op-Amp.

The Specifications of Frequency Response for E.C.G.

This is shown by AHA (American Heart Association) to be a 0.08 Hz to 50 Hz for 3 dB cut off at both ends.

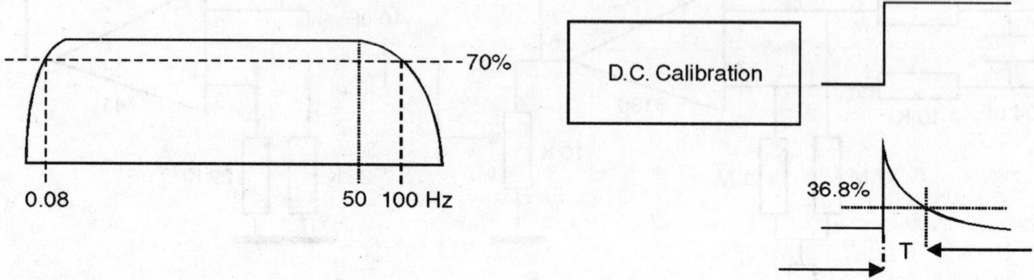

Fig.2.32. Frequency response requirement (A.H.A) Time constant measurement

The maximum frequency response is up to 100 Hz. The same corresponds to a flat response from 0.14 to 50 Hz, wherein the drop may be within ±6% or 0.5 dB. This is equivalent to a time constant of 3.2 s.(0.14 Hz).

Secondly, with a 5 mm (on chart) peak to peak response at 50 Hz, the same must not fall at 100 Hz below 3.5 mm.

The D.C. low frequency response by calibration signal as a step input should be used to determine the T.

The block Diagram of the Modern E.C.G. Machine with Right Leg Drive

Let us now revert back to the modern ECG machine.

The front end preamplifier is logically separated for the purpose of electrical safety isolation from the control circuit and the recording or computer. Fig.2.30 shows the block interfaced to a printer, but if a portable unit is made, the signal would be directly given to the hot stylus recorder. The main part is the differential amplifier which must meet the requirements of high common mode rejection ratio of over 80 dB. The pre-amplifier circuit is preferably battery driven, which could be even a chargeable type.

Lead Selection

The selection of the leads of the E.C.G. used to be done by switches in all the earlier simpler model ECG machines. This can lead to contact resistance problems, unless the contacts are specially treated, by gold plating. So, electronic switching is the preferred method. Fortunately, analog switch I.C.s of the CMOS type are available, even for differential inputs, *e.g.*, the CD4051,4052 are such switches, which can allow the analog signal to be switched from any one input lead to the output pin. Here, the advantage is that the input signal can swing both positively and negatively.

The 12 leads of the ECG including the V leads are all selected from out of the three limb leads, the six chest leads, the right leg being considered to be at earth potential.

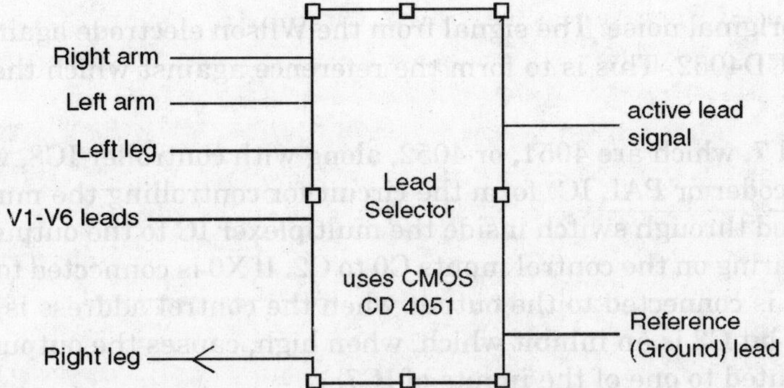

Fig. 2.33 (a). Shows the block diagram of the ECG lead selector unit.

The lead selector can select either directly from the leads of the patient or can be given from the output of an input low noise buffer amplifier.

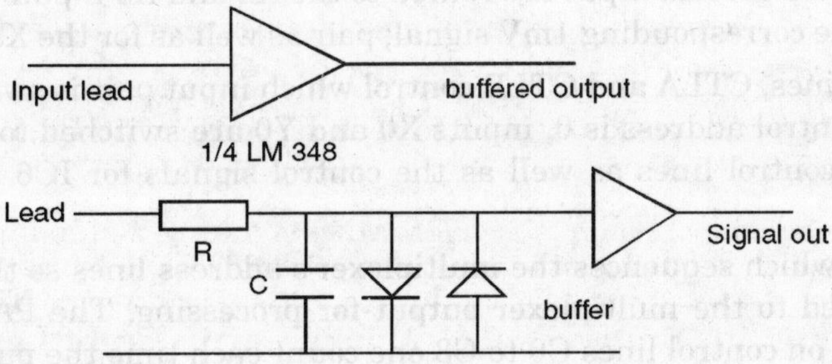

Fig. 2.33 (b). Use of buffer at input lead. Shows protection diodes and capacitor.

The use of the CA 3048, or LM 348 is preferred because these are suitable low noise buffers. So, all the leads are independently buffered from the patient leads. Since the possibility of higher value common mode voltages are eliminated by the use of diode shunts on the input leads, which are always required in ECG machines, due to the possibility of such high voltage transients entering in from the patient electrodes (in surgical theatres, where additional equipment are used for surgical work on the patient).

So, the use of input end diodes with limiting series resistor is able to take care of such high voltages. A shunt capacitor of 220 pF is also required. (Fig. 2.33 (*b*)) The actual e.c.g. signal from the patient leads would ordinarily be just about 0.8 to 1.4 milli volts and the buffer should be able to transmit this without any loss of signal or distortion.

So, the buffered leads from the patient are taken to the analog multiplexer I.C. CD4051 and also to the differential I.C. which is 4052. The first I.C. gives the X output which is taken from one of the leads shown. The second output is the night leg drive.

Right Leg Drive

The output from the three limb leads from IC1 a to c are summed into op-amp IC 3b, inverted and fed back to the patient through the tenth lead, which is attached to the patient's right leg. The composite signal from the three limb leads is called the Wilson Electrode. The Wilson Electrode signal significantly reduces the common mode noise in the system, since unwanted signals common to the of phase with the original noise. The signal from the Wilson electrode again is inverted in IC3c and routed to the CD4052. This is to form the reference against which the nine input signals are compared.

The IC6 and 7, which are 4051, or 4052, along with controller IC8, which is a controller (a programmed decoder or PAL IC) form the circuit for controlling the multiplexer. The eight inputs are connected through switch inside the multiplexer IC to the output X according to the 3-bit address appearing on the control inputs C0 to C2. If X0 is connected to X when the control address is 000, X1 is connected to the output when the control address is 001 and so on. The additional address bit C3 is an inhibit which, when high, causes the output to be floating. The output of IC6 is routed to one of the inputs of IC7.

Another analog switch IC7 has two outputs and four X-Y input pairs (X0-X3 and Y0-Y3). The X0 input is the output from IC6. The corresponding input Y0- comes from the Wilson electrode, IC3c. The signal from IC3a (input 9) is the input to X1. The Wilson electrode signal is also combined with the input 9 on Y1. In addition to the nine signal inputs from the patient, a 1mV test signal and a ground input are routed to the X2 and X3 inputs respectively. Ground is the Y2 input for the corresponding 1mV signal; pair as well as for the X3 ground input on Y3.

Two address lines, CTLA and CTLB control which input pair is switched to the outputs. That is, when the control address is 0, inputs X0 and Y0 are switched to the outputs X and Y respectively. These control lines as well as the control signals for IC6 are derived from the outputs of IC8.

IC8 is a PAL which sequences the multiplexer's address lines so that each input signal is sequentially passed to the multiplexer output for processing. The PAL is programmed to advance the address on control lines C0 to C3 one count each time the pulse is received on the clock input. Additionally, a decode function is programmed in the PAL(Altera EP320) to control the state of the control lines CTLA and CTLB and, hence, which signal pairs from the multiplexer are fed to the differential inputs of the instrumentation amplifier.

Address from PAL				Control from PAL		Multiplexor state IC6	Multiplexor state IC7
C3	C2	C1	C0	CTLB	CTLA	In Out	In → out
0	0	0	0	0	0	X0 → X	X0 → X Y0 → Y
0	0	0	1	0	0	X1 → X	X0 → X Y0 → Y
0	0	1	0	0	0	X2 → X	X0 → X Y0 → Y
0	0	1	1	0	0	X3 → X	X0 → X Y0 → Y
0	1	0	0	0	0	X4 → X	X0 → X Y0 → Y
0	1	0	1	0	0	X5 → X	X0 → X Y0 → Y
0	1	1	0	0	0	X6 → X	X0 → X Y0 → Y
1	0	0	0	0	1	X7 → X	X0 → X Y0 → Y
1	0	0	1	1	0	Z	X1 → X Y1 → Y
1	0	1	0	1	1	Z	X2 → X Y2 → Y
						Z	X3 → X Y3 → Y

Fig. 2.35. Table shows how the signals from the PAL are used to control the sequencing of the input signals to the input of the instrumentation amplifier.

The Analog Interface

The instrumentation amplifier (IC4 and IC 9b) is one of the important elements. It is a differential amplifier which is AD625. Gain is about 1000.

An offset adjust pot R12 is also used to adjust for offset voltages. A precision 2.5V reference diode IC5 is used. The output will be 21.5 V when there is no differential signal.

Final stage of the preamplifier circuit comprises of the isolation using opto isolator IC16c driven by IC 9a.

The output from the opto is 180o phase shifted from the input. IC10d corrects the same. IC10d is an active op-amp type low pass filter at a 100 Hz cut off.

A high pass filter is implemented in the final stage by feed back of the signal from the emitter of IC16 c through an active low pass filter using IC10a and its components. The low pass filter is at 0.1Hz cut off. The output is fed back through IC16d where it is sued to cancel frequencies below 0.1 Hz. As a result the frequency components of the ECG signal are limited between 0.1 and 100 Hz nominally.

The signal can be further digitized in the ADC and fed to the computer interface through RS232 on a microcontroller.

The signal can be given to a recorder in a portable instrument.

The Hot Stylus Recorder

The portable commercial common instrument for E.C.G. is shown in the pictures. The same shows the various switches and controls. The strip chart recorder has a paper which is black coated on the back and has a wax white front layer. When the heated strip is passed over the paper by the moving needle of the recorder, the trace appears fine and black. The records are long lasting for future patient reference and for the Doctor.

The strip chart recorder is basically a moving coil meter used for D.C. ammeters. But, the needle is replaced by a stylus. The stylus moves as per the current fed to the coil of the meter. The coil is of course driven by a power amplified version of the pre-amplifier output signal of the previous section. The current causes the needle to move on the circular arc, but this arc movement is converted to a linear movement.

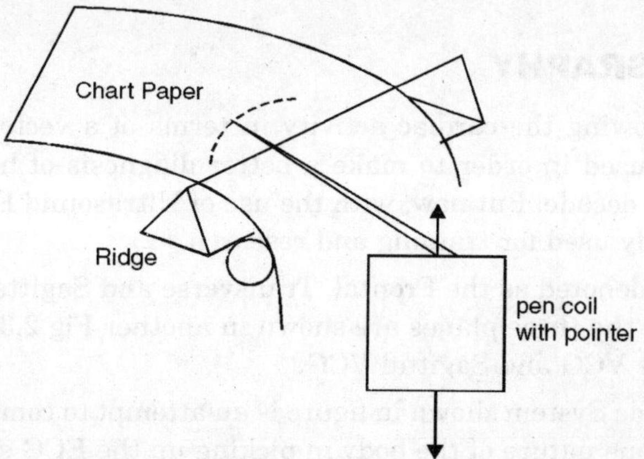

Fig. 2.36. Showing Pen drive for hot stylus Recorder.

The linear movement of the stylus which is hot in this type of recorder is made to be a straight line even though the same moves on an arc, by making the movement to be over a ridge, on which the chart paper is made to pass.

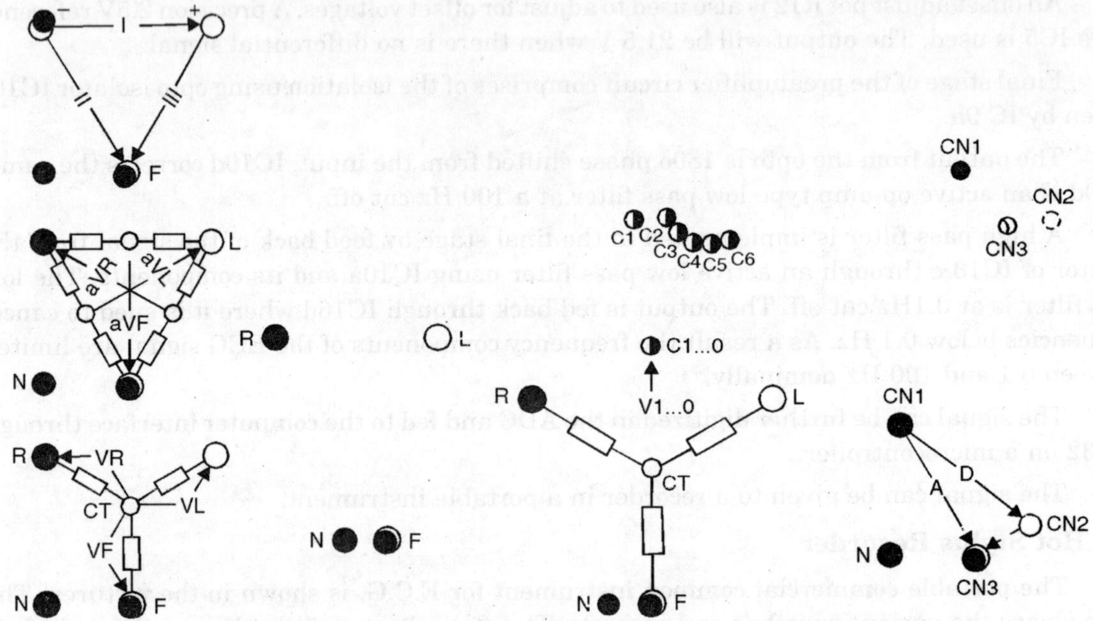

Fig. 2.37. The pattern of the leads and selection for the ECG.

Fig. 2.37 gives the pattern of selections of the leads of the ECG Instrument.

The hot stylus recorder has a good frequency response, enough to display up to 100 Hz signal components in the ECG record.

There are various alternative versions of the basic instrument. For the purpose of monitoring in intensive care units, the pre-amplifier of the ECG is attached to a monitor, which was, in earlier days, a long persistence C.R.O., but today, on raster scan monitors, using graphics display controllers. Such monitoring systems are discussed in a later chapter.

VECTOR CARDIOGRAPHY

The method of showing the cardiac activity in terms of a vector on the three planes shown in Fig. 2.38 was used in order to make a better diagnosis of heart and related lung problems in the previous decade. But now, with the use of Ultrasound Echo Doppler machine, this technique is generally used for training and research.

The three planes, denoted as the Frontal, Transverse and Sagittal are shown in figure. The spatial projection on the three planes are shown in another Fig 2.38*b*. They are called as Frontal VCG, Transverse VCG and Sagittal VCG.

The Frank Electrode System shown in figure is an attempt to compensate for the drop of voltage and inhomogeneous nature of the body in picking up the ECG signals along the three axes. The compensation network shown by resistors was also for the same purpose. The path of the loops indicate the nature of the heart conduction system better than the plain ECG.

The directions of the signals are positive X to the left side and positive Y to the head and positive Z to the back. There are many other electrode system signal tracings such as the axial, cube and tetrahedron arrangements, with the compensating resistors.

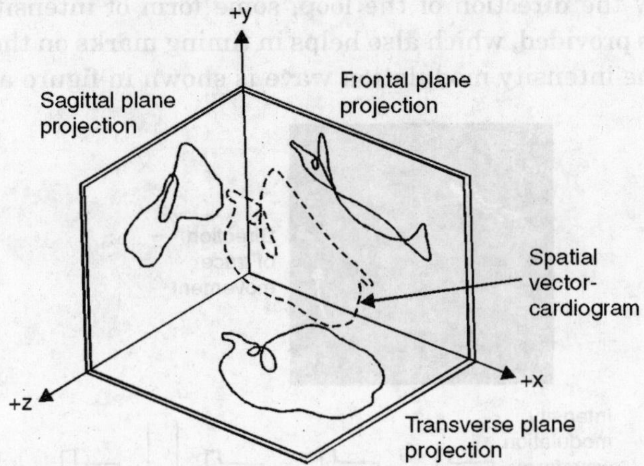

Fig. 2.38a. Shows the electrode positions in Sagittal plane (Frank).

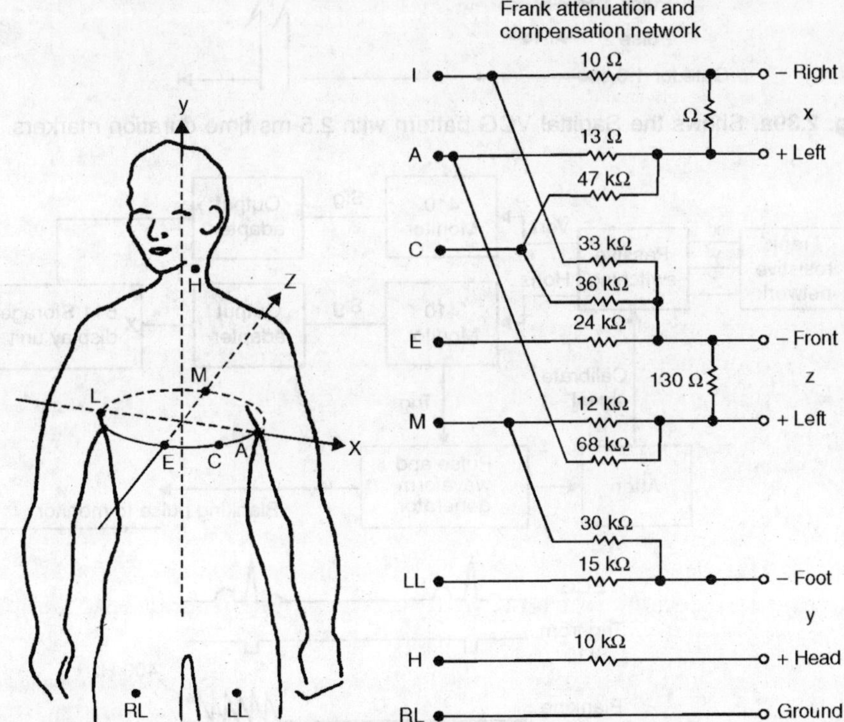

Fig. 2.38b. Shows the Frank electrode positions.

A careful observation of the ECG waveform shown in the record of the VCG pictures indicates that the phases of the QRS wave (shown broader in this picture), are not same; in fact, if they were in phase, the loops will all be just straight lines. The loop of the P-wave is not important and is not shown well because of its lesser amplitude. If the gain of the VCG on the CRO is increased, the P loop and the T wave loop will also appear in closed loops. The phase of the respiratory cycle and the posture of the patient are also involved in the wave patterns.

In order to show the direction of the loop, some form of intensity modulation on the screen at 400 Hz dots is provided, which also helps in timing marks on the loop. An arrow head effect is also shown. The intensity modulation wave is shown in figure along with the loop.

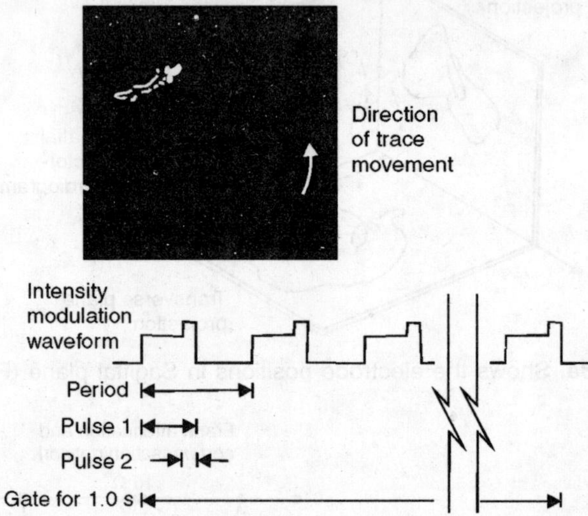

Fig. 2.39a. Shows the Sagittal VCG pattern with 2.5 ms time duration markers.

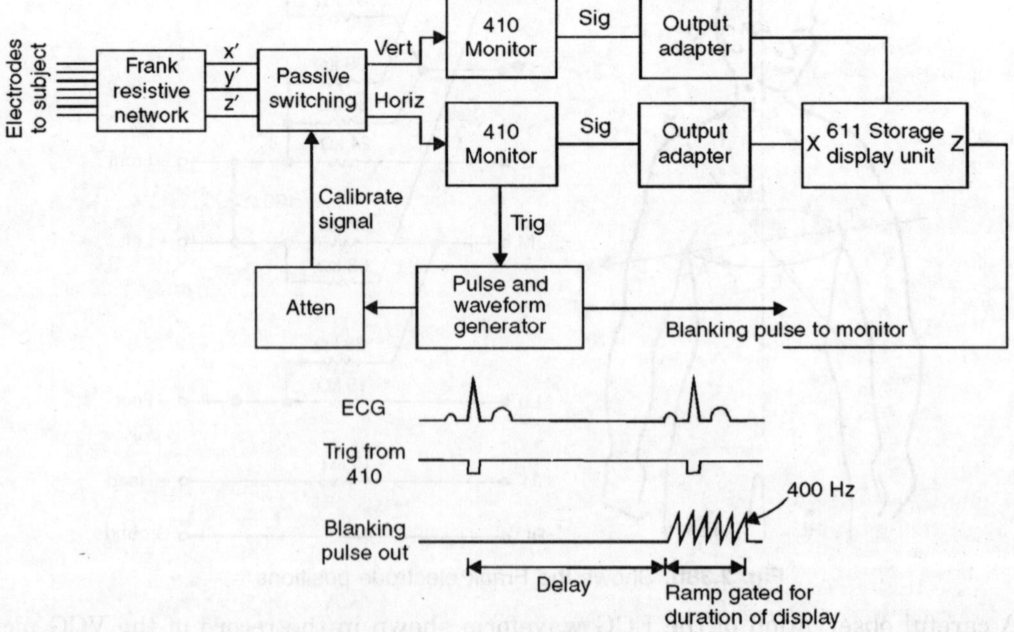

Fig. 2.39b. Shows the VCG system using two monitors and incorporating intensity modulation.

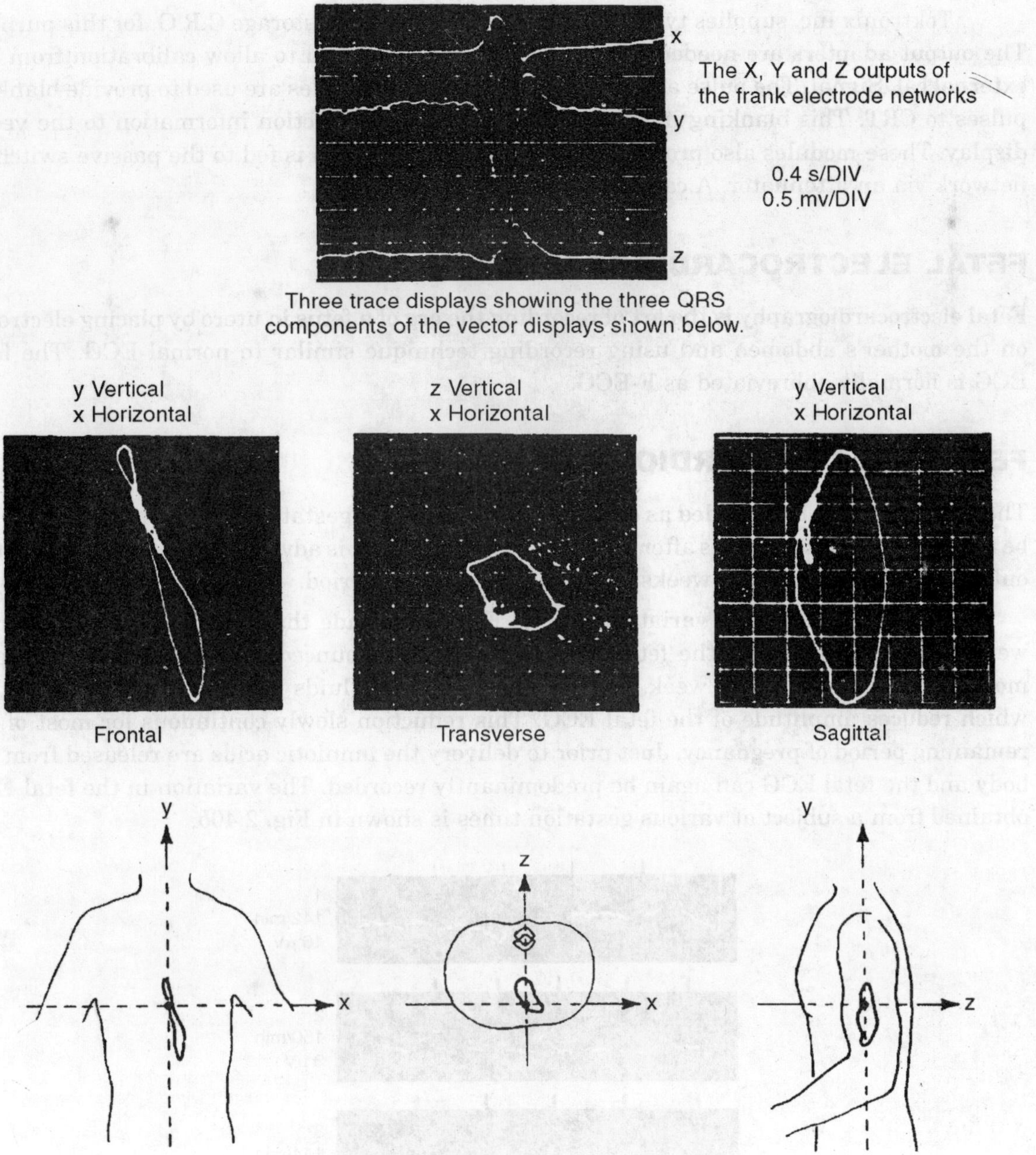

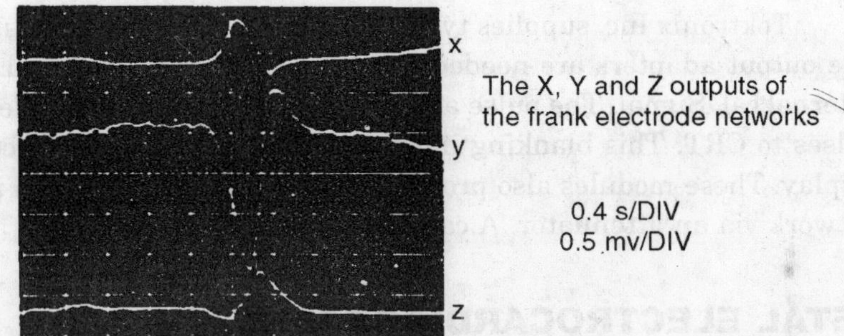

Three trace displays showing the three QRS components of the vector displays shown below.

y Vertical
x Horizontal

z Vertical
x Horizontal

y Vertical
x Horizontal

Frontal

Transverse

Sagittal

y x

z x

y z

Fig. 2.39c. Shows the Frank Vector Cardiogram.

Fig. 2.39*c* showing the VCG system with two monitors and incorporating intensity modulation is also shown below. A VCG measurement system needs:

1. Two separate ECG measurement modules
2. Frank electric resistive network
3. X-Y storage C.R.O.

Tektronix Inc. supplies type 410 monitors and Type 611 storage C.R.O. for this purpose. The output adapters are needed to adjust the signal level and to allow calibration from any external cal. Signal. The pulse and waveform generation modules are used to provide blanking pulses to CRT. This blanking information adds time and direction information to the vector display. These modules also provide a calibration signal which is fed to the passive switching network via an attenuator. A camera is useful for recording.

FETAL ELECTROCARDIOGRAPHY

Fetal electrocardiography is the art of recording the ecg of a fetus in utero by placing electrodes on the mother's abdomen and using recording technique similar to normal ECG. The fetal ECG is normally abbreviated as F-ECG.

FETAL ELECTROCARDIOGRAM

The fetal ECG may be recorded as early as the 11th week of gestation in some subjects and can be recorded in almost all cases after 16 weeks gestation. But it is advisable to get best information out of the record is after 16 weeks to 24 weeks gestation period.

Fig. 2.40*a* shows the variation in fetal ECG amplitude that may be expected after 16 weeks. By the 18th week, the fetal ECG invariably pronounced and continuous to become more evident to about 24th week. At this stage, amniotic fluids begin to form in the mother which reduces amplitude of the fetal ECG. This reduction slowly continuous for most of the remaining period of pregnancy. Just prior to delivery the amniotic acids are released from the body and the fetal ECG can again be predominantly recorded. The variation in the fetal ECG obtained from a subject at various gestation times is shown in Fig. 2.40*b*.

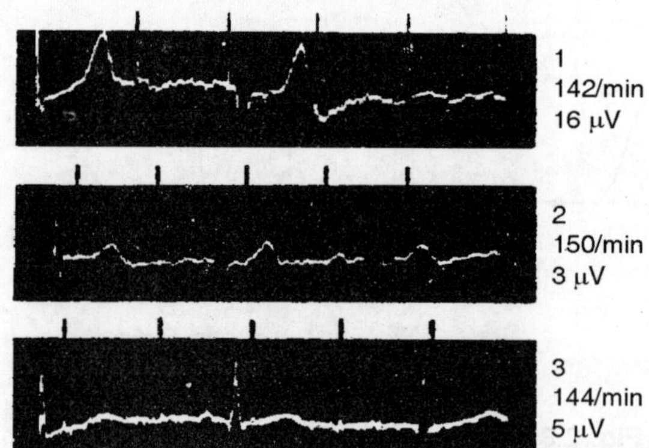

Fig. 2.40a. Shows Fetal ECG's at 16 weeks on several subjects.

Fig. 2.40*a* shows a Fetal ECG at 16 weeks on several subjects and (b) shows a fetal ECG variations with gestation time.

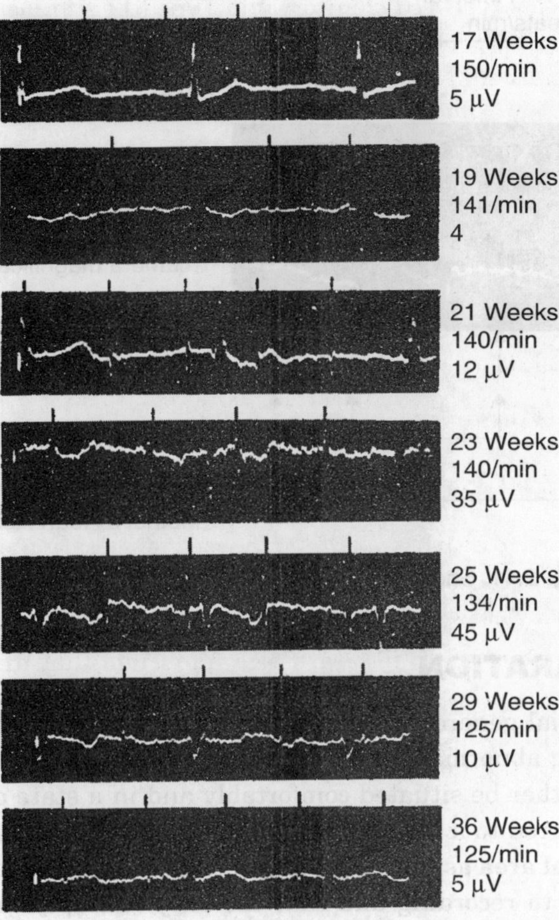

Fig. 2.40b

THE NORMAL FETAL ECG

As discussed in the previous paragraph, the fetal ECG amplitude varies greatly with gestation time and also varies from one subject to another. A typical fetal ECG obtained at 18 weeks is shown in Fig. 2.41.

The mother's ECG is clearly evident and , being many times greater in amplitude than the fetal ECG, may camouflage the fetal ECG. The fetal ECG can clearly be observed during the isoelectric period between the mother's ECG. The technique used to record this fetal ECG will be discussed later in this chapter. From this record, it is evident that the mother's heart rate is 62 beats per minute and the fetal heart rate is 158 beats per minute. In the early stages of pregnancy, the fetal heart rate is normally between 140 to 160 beats per minute. If the mother is relaxed during recording of the fetal ecg, it is expected that her heart rate would be under 80 beats per minute. Due to the low amplitude of the fetal ecg, the fetal R wave is normally the only part of the fetal ECG complex which is more evidently seen.

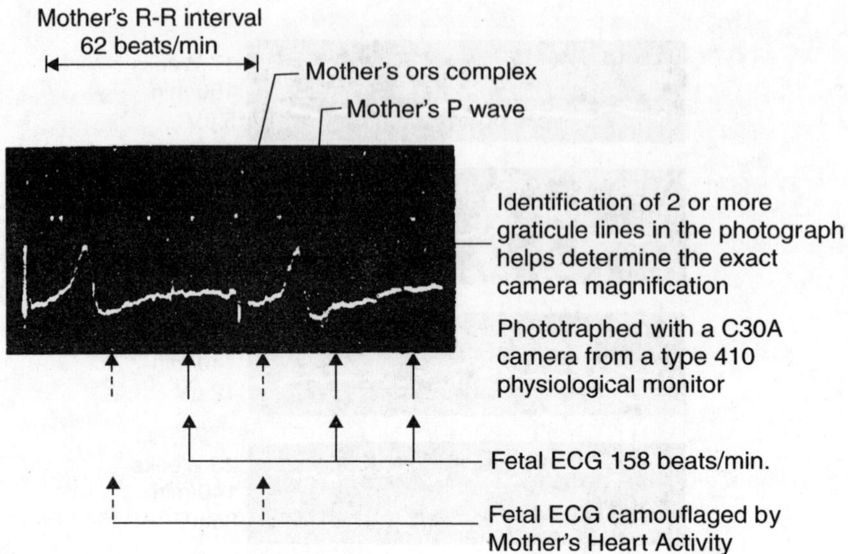

Fig. 2.41. Shows a typical Fetal ECG display at 18 weeks.

SUBJECT PREPARATION

As the electrical potential generated by muscular activity within the mother's abdomen will clearly be present using abnormal electrodes when attempting to record the fetal ECG, it is imperative that the mother be situated comfortably and in a state of complete rest. A bed or couch is normally preferred to a clinical examination table. To reduce the mother's muscular activity in the abdominal area as much as possible, it is desirable that the subject does not eat for several hours prior to recording and that the subject empty her bladder shortly before recording.

ELECTRODE PLACEMENT

Many electrode positions have historically been used to record the fetal ECG. It is now generally acceptable method is the abdominal electrode configuration. Due to the variation expected in the fetal position, many electrodes should be applied to the abdomen and the fetal ECG recorded between various combinations of these electrodes until a positive recording is obtained. The most common fetal ECG lead configuration is the **Blondheim configuration** shown in Fig. 2.42. This configuration consists of three electrodes namely A, D and F placed at the vertices of a 60°triangle and an additional three electrodes namely **B, C** and **E** placed at the vertices of an inverted 60° triangle. Figure 2.42 also shows two more electrodes on the back of the subject **(G** and **H).** It has been found that, during the early stage of pregnancy, a recording from one of these two back electrodes to any abdominal electrodes produces more reliable output. It is important that care must be taken when applying the electrodes.

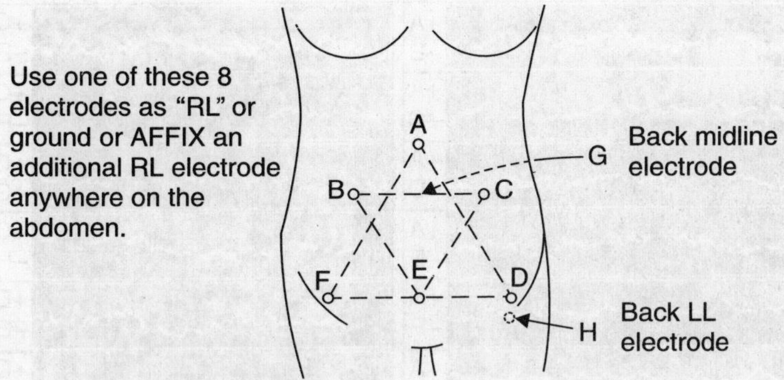

Fig. 2.42. Shows the Fetal electrode positions.

It has been reported that, during early stages of pregnancy, better results may be obtained by exerting considerable pressure onto the electrodes so as to move these electrodes closer to the actual fetus.

ELECTRICAL INTERFERENCES

Particular care must be taken to eliminate line frequency interference from the fetal ECG recordings. Adequate instrumentation can eliminate any line frequency interference if it appears as differential signal using 50 Hz notch filter. The leads connecting the patient to the monitor be as short as possible, preferably no longer than two feet.

Electrodes should be placed on the mother's abdomen as shown in Fig. 2.43. If it is intended that the fetal ECG form many patients be recorded, it is better that some form of custom electrode selection switching unit be built to avoid the necessity of having make separate connections to the recording equipment for each electrode configuration. A typical set of fetal ECG's obtained by recording all combinations of the electrodes shown in Fig. 2.43. Normally, it is not necessary to record all possible combinations of these electrodes and the procedure is usually considered complete when a fetal ECG has clearly been observed in two or three configurations.

In early stages of pregnancy, the following combinations appear to give the greatest possibility of observing the fetal ECG. C-F, B-D, A-F, A-D and if the G and H are present then G-F, G-D and B-H. The later stages of pregnancy when the fetal ECG is pronounced, it is normally only necessary to record from either of the three set of electrodes forming 60° triangles of brodheim configuration, that is electrodes A, F and D or electrodes B, C and E. Ac the amplitude of the fetal ECG is normally between 5 and 50 mVolts, and, as it is preferable to use battery operated equipment to record fetal ECG for reasons discussed earlier most commercial electrocardiographs or physiological monitors are not comparable with fetel ECG recording. It is common practice to use EEG recorder or physiological monitor operated in the EEG position to monitor the fetal ECG.

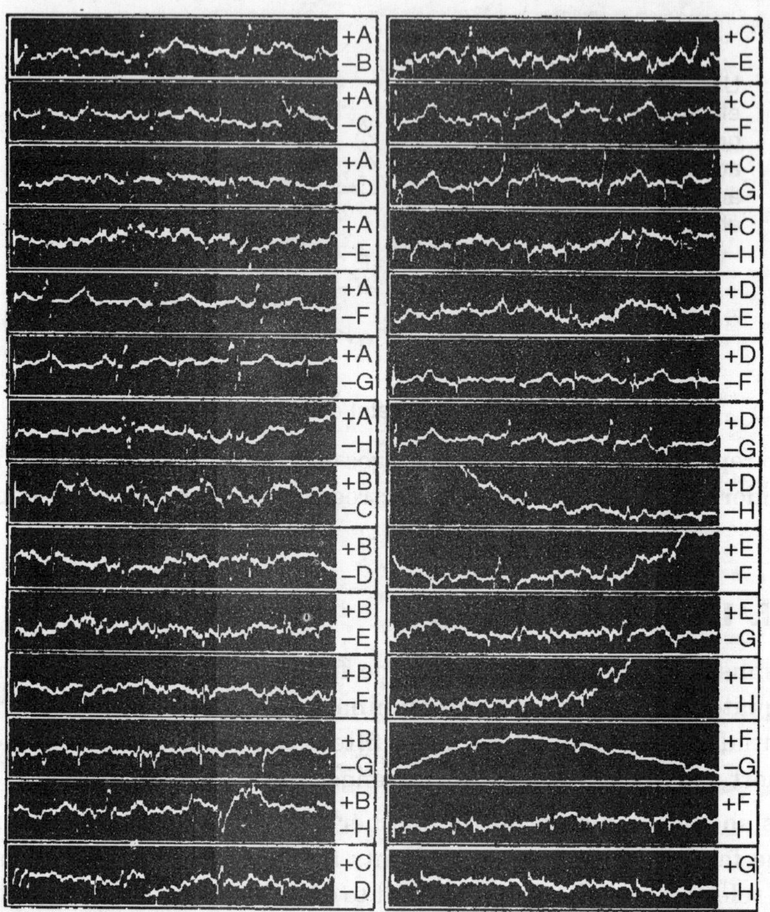

Fig. 2.43. Shows the Fetal ECG variations with various electrode positions (23 weeks gestation).

ALTER LOW FREQUENCY CUTOFF

Using EEG machines to record the fetal ECG is a recommended technique. EEG position is the function selector switch is selected and fetal ECG electrodes are connected to the EEG position of the patient cable. A standard 410, as well as any other commercially available EEG recorder, may give satisfactorily good results. However, the frequency response of EEG recorders have the low frequency response extending below 0.1 Hz. Muscle activity within the mother's abdomen will probably result in severe interference causing the trace to be off screen most of the time. This can be overcome by increasing the frequency response of EEG recorders. A modification that may be added to the monitor to increase the low frequency response in EEG position from below 0.1 Hz to approximately 1 Hz. This modification also reduces the gain in the EEG position form 50 to 100 μV per centimeter. The gain can however, be increased with the variable control by a factor of 3 to give a maximum gain of 33 μV per centimeter. All fetal ECG photograph shown in this chapter will be having a sensitivity of 33 μV per cm and at a sweep speed of 50 mm per second.

PHOTOGRAPHY OF FETAL ECG WAVEFORMS

As detailed analysis is often required to detect the fetal ECG, particularly to the earlier stage of pregnancy, it is desirable to take the photograph of the information appearing on the CRT monitor. All photographs shown in this chapter were recorded in this way. When photographing from the 410 with the C-30A camera, the shuttle should be in the B position and operated manually for 2 seconds. Optimum results are obtained using aperture of f/16 and a magnification factor of 0.9X. Certain nonlinearities exist and the same be overcome by the given formula;

For Fetal ECG spacings measured near the center of the screen using a sweep speed of 50 μV per second :

$$\text{Fetal heart rate Beats per min.} = \frac{300 \times \text{graticule mark spacing}}{\text{Fetal ECG R wave spacing}} \times 0.9$$

For fetal ECG spacings measured near the edge of the screen using a sweep speed of 50 mm per second.

$$\text{Fetal heart rate Beats per min.} = \frac{300 \times \text{graticule mark spacing}}{\text{Fetal ECG R wave spacing}}$$

Due to the nonlinearities mentioned earlier, a correction factor of 0.9 is necessary for information at the edge of the screen.

INTERPRETATION OF THE FETAL ECG

When attempting to record the fetal ECG, positive results give positive indication that the fetal ECG does exist.; however, negative results are non conclusive and give an indication as to the viability of the fetus. Although the fetal ECG can be recorded in almost all cases by the 16th week.

FETAL ECG AND STETHOSCOPE

It is generally accepted that fetal heart activity cannot be detected by a standard stethoscope earlier than approximately the 20th week. Thus the fetal ECG can give a positive indication of the existence of a live fetus several weeks earlier that can be obtained with a stethoscope

Fig. 2.44 shows the orientation of the electrical axis of the fetal heart compared to the orientation of the electrical axis of the mother's heart.

As the electric field generated by the mother's cardiac vector produces " mother's ECG" activity when recording fetal ECG, the axes of this mother's ECG activity will be tangential to this field and not necessarily parallel to the direction of mother's cardiac vector. Within a few weeks after the fetal ECG is first detected, its amplitude is great enough for accurate measurement and the results can be plotted on a vector diagram. An error triangle is obtained by plotting the intersection of all vectors; the head of the fetal ECG vector must be somewhat lie somewhere within the error triangle.

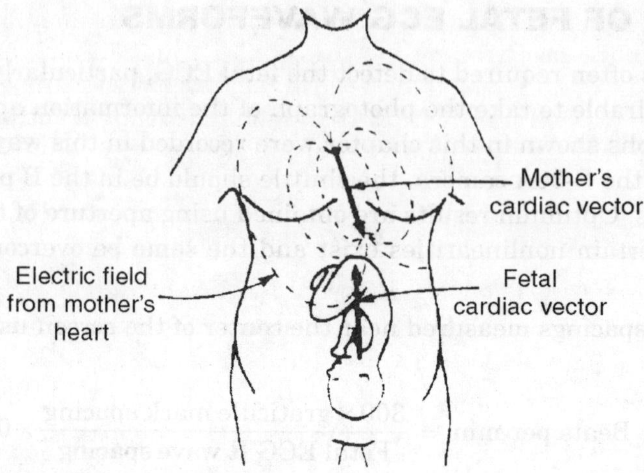

Fig. 2.44. Shows fetal cardiac vector vertex presentation at full term.

MULTIPLE PREGNANCY

Fetal electrocardiography is perhaps most useful when attempting to diagnose multiple pregnancy. X-ray techniques are known to be harmful to the fetus; however, fetal ECG techniques are completely harmless and can detect multiple pregnancy as early as the 16th week. Fig. 2.45 shows a fetal ECG recording of twins at 21 weeks. As the fetal R waves are of opposites, *i.e.*, one twin is breech and the other is cephalic.

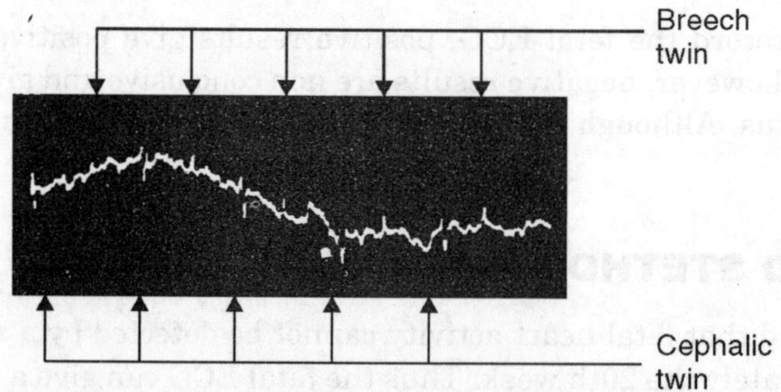

Fig. 2.45. Shows the Twin gestation fetal ECG at 21 weeks.

As the fetal R waves in direction opposite are of opposite polarity, it is obvious that their electrical vectors are in opposite directions, i.e., one twin is breech and the other is cephalic. Fetal R waves in the same direction as the mother's QRS complex represent the breech represent the cephalic twin.

The fetal ECG is often recorded during fetal delivery to indicate the delivery will be from the vertex of the breech position and to give an indication of fetal distress during labor.

SAGITTAL PLANE ECG MEASURMENTS

The measurements of the cardiac vector projection in the sagittal plane are referred to as "the unipolar esophageal lead ECG measurement" or the "E lead ECG measurements". Although the unipolar esophageal lead ECG is rarely recorded these days, it can be recorded by attaching an esophageal lead to the positive input of the amplifier and forming an indifferent negative electrode using both arms and the left leg as with the transverse-plane V leads. Esophageal lead measurements are recorded from within the esophagus using a catheter, or fine rubber tube, threaded with wire with an electrode attached to its tip.

ECG INSTRUMENTATION REQUIREMENTS

Already, we have been discussing about the electrode placement and its various configurations. The potential appearing at these electrodes must be amplified by a differential amplifier and recorded on either a strip chart recorder, a CRT display or occasionally, magnetic tapes are used. Commercial instruments usually include electrode selection, amplification and either a CRT display or a strip chart recorder. These instruments are commonly referred to as ECG monitors or physiological monitors if they utilize a CRT display and as electrocardiographs if they utilize a strip chart recorder display. The commercial electrocardiographs preceded commercial physiological monitors by 70 years or so; thus, many of the features on physiological monitors are carried over from electrocardiographs even though they may not be optimally suited for use with CRT displays.

Electrocardiographs almost all machines invariably use graph paper with horizontal and vertical lines at 1mm intervals and a heavier line at 5 mm intervals as shown in Fig. 2.13. In regular electrocardiography, the recording speed is 25 mm per second; thus 1mm horizontal intervals each represent 0.04 second and 5 mm intervals represent 0.2 seconds. As far as the sensitivity of electrocardiographs is concerned, it is typically 100 microvolts per millimetre. (1 mV/cm)

CRT DISPLAYS IN ECG MACHINES

When referred to CRT displays, it is normal practice in the electronics industry to refer to mV/centimeter vertically and seconds/centimeter horizontally. However, due to the historical influence of electrocardiographs, the reciprocal of these dimensions is used in electrocardiography; that is millimeter/millivolt and millimeter/second. Physiological monitors commonly use twice the vertical sensitivity and twice the sweep speed of electrocardiographs; that is 20 mm/mV and 50 mm/second.

HOLTER ECG MACHINE

The Medilog FDS is the next step in the evolution of digital Holter recorders. With a simple user interface and compact design, it provides all the capabilities required for reliable ECG recording.

The Holter is a standard old E.C.G. recorder with tape for 12 hours in case of patients needing monitoring. The unit shown is a later day version, with magnetic digital recording and a display as seen.

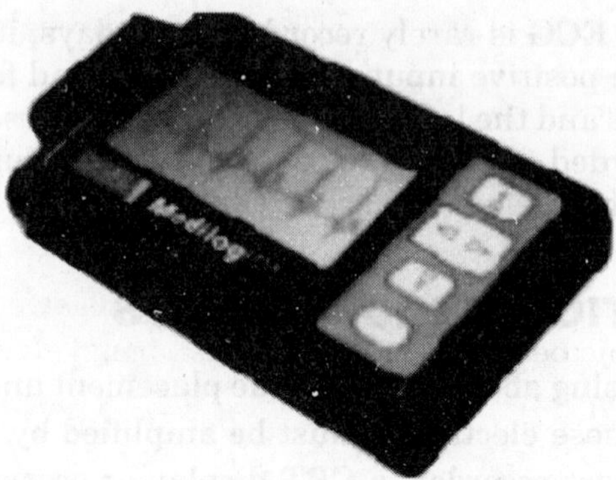

Fig. 2.46. The Holter ECG recorder.

INPUT IMPEDANCE

As high input impedance differential amplifiers are invariably used in modern electrocardiograph machines and physiological monitors, some ground reference must be maintained between the subject and the amplifier. This is usually accomplished by attaching an electrode to the subject's right leg and connecting this electrode to the ground of the amplifier. These amplifiers should have common mode impedance of at least 10M Ω per input and should have a common mode rejection ration of 10000:1. Frequency response within the ECG extend from 0.05 Hz to approximately 80 Hz; most of the commercial amplifiers will exhibit adequate high frequency response of up to 120 Hz but exhibit the low frequency response to 0.05 Hz or better.

PATIENT SAFETY

It is highly desirable that any amplifier used to record ECG's are used to record other potentials from the human bed, should incorporate internal circuitry to protect the subject against electrical shock should the amplifier fail. More of protection circuits and safety measure are covered in a separate chapter.

INSTRUMENTATION OF THE ELECTROCARDIOGRAM

Interpreting the results obtained from various ECG measurements discussed in earlier chapters, it is an art in itself and should only be attempted by suitable trained medical personnel. Although it is not possible to cover all the aspects of interpretation in the medical field, it is desirable that the reader should have some concepts of what is considered normal and what is considered abnormal and appreciate the meanings of the more important terms used by cardiologists when discussing the scope of the ECG waveforms.

The 'normal' ECG has come about by observing the distribution in many thousands of healthy subjects. The ECG presented in Fig. 2.46*b* are normal ECGs for a healthy adult male. Any variation from the normal rhythm is known as an arrhythmia. As arrhythmias may be more evident in certain ECG measurements, a set of frontal-plane and transverse-plane ECG is usually required for a complete analysis of the electrocardiogram.

A fast heart rate in excess of 100 per minute is known as tachycardia. A slow heart rate of less than 60 per minute is known as bradycardia. An excessively large and continuous ECG with no recognized, QRS or T waves is a sign of ventricular fibrillation, a condition where the ventricular muscle goes into local oscillation in a "circus movement", waves of depolarization going round and round the ventricural tissues. A random and changing phase relationship between P and QRS and T indicates adioventricular rhythm, in which a complete bundle block occurs in the bundle of His and the auricles and ventricles slower. Arrhythmias also appear as extra beats, known as ectopic beats, on an otherwise normal electrocardiogram. This has been discussed earlier in this chapter.

Chapter 3

Circulatory System

MYOCARDIAL INFARCTION

Coronary heart disease is the greatest single cause for death in most cases in the Universe. The most frequent cause is the myocardial infarction. So, lots of efforts have been put forth both in research work as well as in clinical fields. Therefore, it is important to understand the cardiovascular system thoroughly, so as to take subsequent prevention against the heart disease.

THE CARDIOVASCULAR CIRCULATORY SYSTEM

In a complex multi cellular animal with a high density of cell population and a relatively small volume of tissue fluid bathing these cells, a continuous and rapid revitalization process must take place.

CELL REVITALIZATION

The revitalization is the fundamental purpose of the cardiovascular circulatory system. In the first chapter, the potential produced within a single cell was discussed. This potential is a result of continuous metabolism within the cell. This metabolism process needs nutrients and excretes waste products; the circulatory system provides these nutrients and removes these waste products.

The major component of the circulatory system is the heart . The heart supplies the power required to circulate blood throughout the body. The heart is two pumps in series; the right hand section, the smaller one, provides the power required to force the blood through the lungs. The larger one, is a more powerful left hand section provides the power required to force the blood through the body.

A simplified block diagram of the circulatory system is shown in Fig. 3.1. The blood flow from the heart to the aorta is shown in Fig. 3.2. The aorta curves in an arch up from the heart, down along the back bone and into the abdomen; from it other large arteries lead to the head, the digestive organs, the arms and the legs. From these arteries branch the smaller arterioles and from these, branch billions of tiny capillaries. By the time blood has reached the capillaries, it is moving slowly along channels. These channels are only about 10 microns in diameter. Here the blood discharges its load of dissolved food and oxygen to the body cells. These cells in turn deposit waste materials such as carbon-di-oxide into the blood stream. In yielding oxygen and taking on the waste, the blood turns colour form bright red to dull red or "blue". The blood now starts back to the heart passing from the capillaries into the venules. The venules converge into larger veins and then into the two largest veins just above and below the heart, known as vena cava. The blood empties into right atrium. It is pumped into the right ventricle and then moves out through the pulmonary artery to the lungs. The lungs then supply the blood with fresh oxygen.

The blood passes form the lungs to the left atrium, then is pumped into the left ventricle and passes via the aorta This is done for repeating the circulation process. This general flow throughout the body is known as the **"systemic circulation"**; the flow to and from the lungs is known as the **"pulmonary circulation".** Local circulations within the systemic system include the renal (to the kidneys), the hepatic portal (to the liver), the cerebral and (to the heart itself). The waste products contained in the blood are removed by the kidneys and liver. The average quantity of blood in man is about five liters. This is completely circulated through the body in approximately one minute.

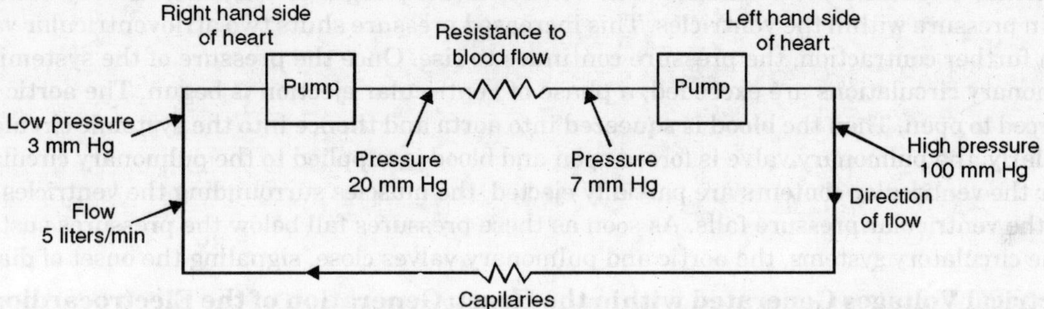

Fig. 3.1. Shows the simplified block diagram of the circulatory system.

THE HEART

In this section, the cardiac cycle is to be described. The heart itself weighs less than half a kilogram, is almost about 15 cm long at its maximum dimension. The heart lies pointed downward to the chest cavity to the left of the mid-center body line. The entire walls of the heart are made of muscle; within these walls are four hollow chambers, a left and right receiving chamber (atrium) and below them a left and right pumping chamber (ventricle).

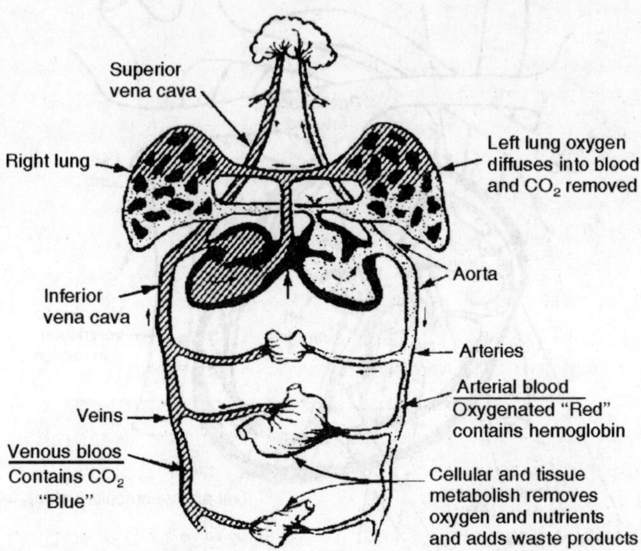

Fig. 3.2. The cardiovascular circulatory system.

CARDIAC CYCLE

The cardiac cycle is characterized by the following mechanical events. Between beats, the heart mechanically rests and this is known as the period of **diastole**. During diastole, the heart assumes its maximum size and fills with oxygenated blood returning from the lungs and venous blood returning from the body. The heart's period of mechanical activity is known as **systole.** The onset of systole is initiated by contraction of the muscles surrounding the atria. This propels additional blood into the ventricles. The ventricles then begin to contract, thereby causing a rise in pressure within the ventricles. This increased pressure shuts two atrioventricular valves. With further contraction, the pressure continues to rise. Once the pressure of the systemic and pulmonary circulations are exceeded, a phase of ventricular ejection is begun. The aortic valve is forced to open. Then the blood is squeezed into aorta and thence into the systemic circulation. Similarly, the pulmonary valve is forced open and blood is supplied to the pulmonary circulation. After the ventricular contents are partially ejected, the muscles surrounding the ventricles relax and the ventricular pressure falls. As soon as these pressures fall below the pressures sustained in the circulatory systems, the aortic and pulmonary valves close, signaling the onset of diastole.

Electrical Voltages Generated within the Heart: Generation of the Electrocardiogram Waveform (ECG)

In the preceding section, we studied about the mechanical activity of the heart. It is well known that the mechanical activity is initiated by contraction of the muscle surrounding the atria. The detailed relationships between cells, nerve and muscle is complex. This is sufficient at this stage to state that muscle contraction is initiated by stimulation.

Sino-artrial node. The right atrium consists of a bundle of nerves known as the sino-artrial node (**A** node). This type of nerve system is found nowhere else in the body. Its function

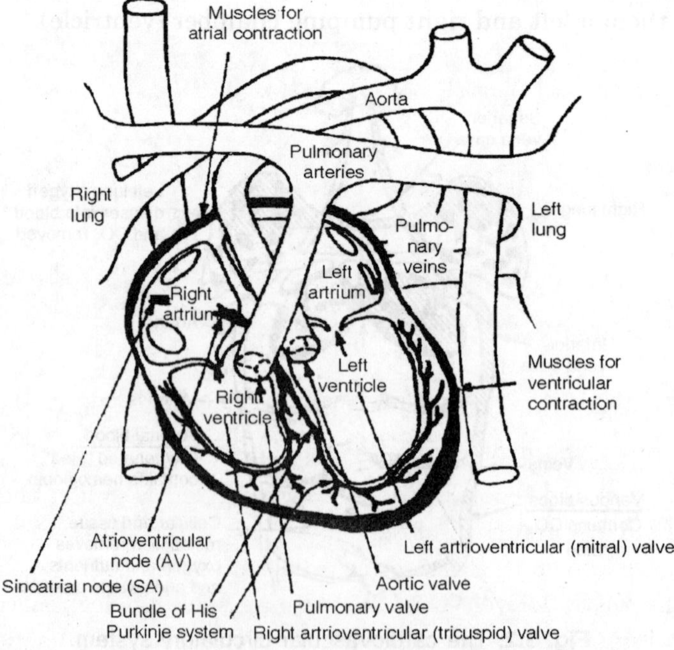

Fig. 3.3. Shows the Heart.

is to start the heart beat and set its rhythm of pace. The electrical and mechanical output from the heart is initiated. This results in contraction of the various heart muscles. The basic rhythm of the heart is self-sustaining through synchronization from the *SA* node within the heart. This rhythm is modified by certain nerve fibers external to the heart that affect the *SA* node. These nerves have a function in the normal control to the heart rate to respond to increased or decreased demand for blood by the body.

Atrioventricular node. Impulses are generated by the *SA* node stimulate contraction of the muscles comprising of atria. These impulses also travel along the conducting fibers in the atrium to the ventricular node or *AV* node, stimulating depolarization of this node as shown in the Fig. 3.3. Stimulation of atrioventricular node causes impulses to be sent to the myocardium or muscles comprising the ventricles via the *'bundle of His'* and the Purkinje conducting system resulting in contraction of this muscle. Thus, the muscular contractions necessary to maintain the heart's pumping action, are initiated by depolarization and repolarization of the *SA* node and then depolarization and subsequent repolarization of the *AV* node.

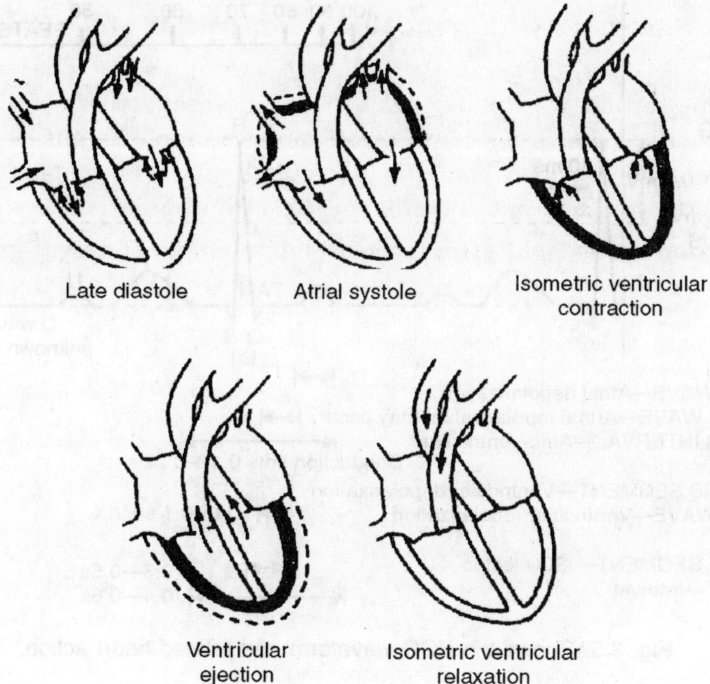

Fig. 3.4. Shows the mechanical cycle of the heart.

Fig. 3.4 shows the mechanical activity of the heart.

These depolarization and repolarization generate external action potentials. The action potentials can be recorded at the surface of the body. These external action potentials generated from within the heart are known as the electrocardiogram or ECG. It is common, also, to refer to this waveform as the EKG, derived form the German spelling electrocardiogram. The ECG waveform as shown in Fig. 3.5, gives the relationship to the mechanical action of the heart and the resultant arterial pressure.

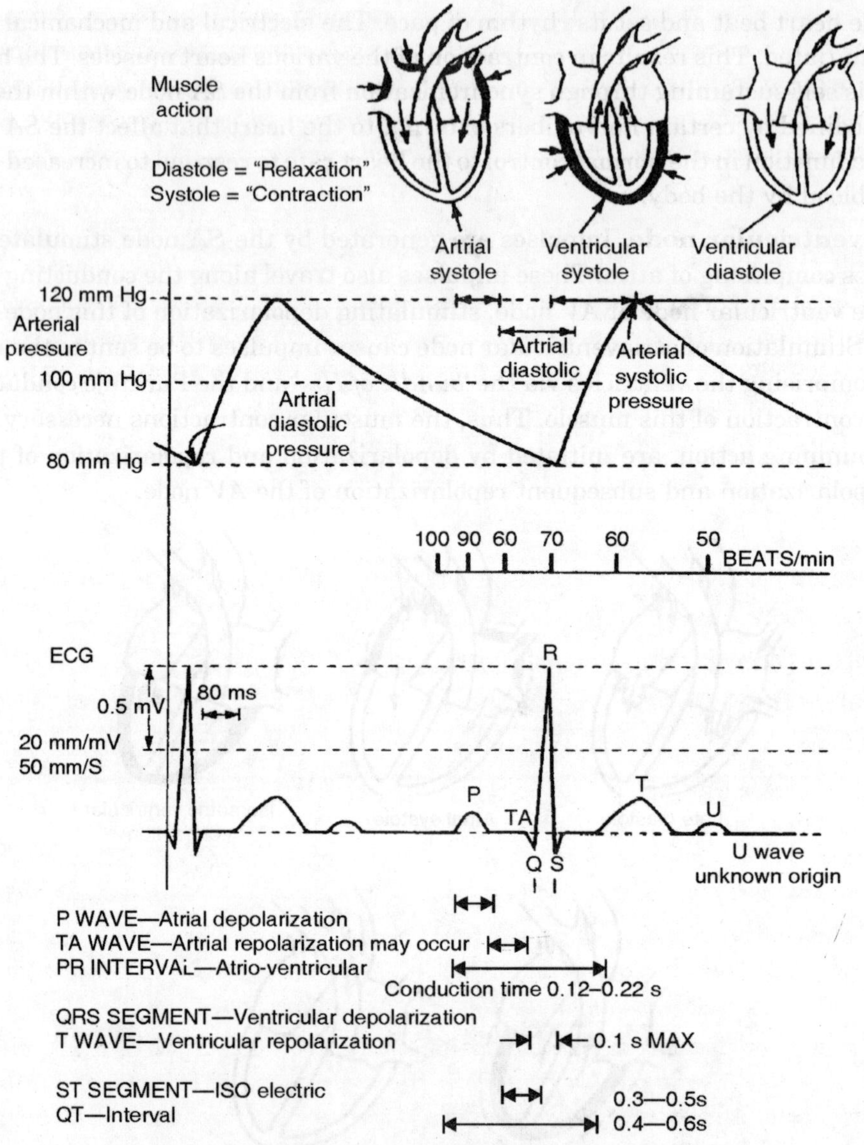

Fig. 3.5. Shows the ECG waveform and related heart action.

HEART ELECTRICAL ACTIVITY (ECG)

Electrical activity of the heart is, as discussed earlier, initiated by depolarization of the *SA* node and a resulting contraction of the muscles surrounding the atria. This results in external action potential known as *P* wave. Immediately following this depolarization, repolarization of the atria occurs. However, for some reason, this does not generate a pronounced action potential. This potential is known as the *TA* wave and is rarely observed in practice. Electrical activity produced by depolarization of the *SA* node travels through fibers within the atrium to the *AV* node. The time taken for this electrical stimulation to travel form the *SA* node to the *AV* node is known as the atrioventricular conduction time and is typically between 120ms and 220ms. When this stimulation reaches the *AV* node, this node depolarizes and the depolarization is conducted down through the *'bundle of His'* to the myocardium muscle causing ventricular depolarization. The external action potential is referred to as *QRS* complex. Immediately following this depolarization, the cells concerned repolarize. This results in ventricular repolarization or the **T** wave. Many ECG waveforms also show an additional wave occurring after the **T** wave. This is designated the **U** wave and its origin is unknown. The ECG Waveform and related heart action is shown in Fig. 3.5.

The ECG waveform is recorded at maximum potential when one electrode is placed slightly above the heart and to the right and the other electrode is placed slightly below the heart and to the left; thus, the potential output of the heart can be said to be generated along this axis. In the chapter on **Electrocardiography,** variations in the ECG waveform with different electrode positions are described.

BLOOD PRESSURE MEASUREMENT

Blood pressure measurement can be classified into three groups. They are :

1. Direct Blood Pressure measurement
2. Indirect Blood Pressure measurement and
3. Relative Blood Pressure measurement

Direct blood pressure measurement involves gaining access to the circulatory system and measuring the pressure in the system directly by using some form of pressure transducer.

Indirect blood pressure measurement involves application of pressure external to the circulatory system. The blood pressure is observed due to the effect of this external pressure on the circulatory system.

And finally a third group of measurement, *i.e.*, the relative blood pressure measurements is nothing but the uncalibrated indirect measurement which is usually performed in a simpler way, and inherently more convenient , instrumentation.

Blood flow is derived from the measurement of blood velocity which necessitates access to one or more of the primary arteries within the body using surgical techniques. The blood pressure information and blood flow information is enough for analysis of the circulatory system. However, a complete hydrodynamic analysis of the circulatory system can only be accomplished by also measuring blood volume.

DIRECT BLOOD PRESSURE MEASUREMENT

Direct Blood Pressure measurement is done by inserting a pressure transducer somewhere within the circulatory system. Figs. 3.1, 3.2 and 3.3 refers to this circulatory system. The transducers can be designed in such a way that one can insert them directly into the circulatory system. However, it is more common to connect the circulatory system with either a catheter or a hypodermic needle and to record the pressure with a pressure transducer attached to the catheter or needle.

Cardiac catheter consists of a rubber, Teflon or polyethylene tube with one end formed to a smooth bullet like shape so as to allow to introduce the same into vein and arteries easily. A small opening is provided about 1cm at the end as shown in Fig. 3.6. The catheter as shown is approximately 40 cm long and 5mm in diameter. Catheters are generally available form 1mm to 10 mm in diameter with various lengths. Cardiac catheters are described by their circumference also.

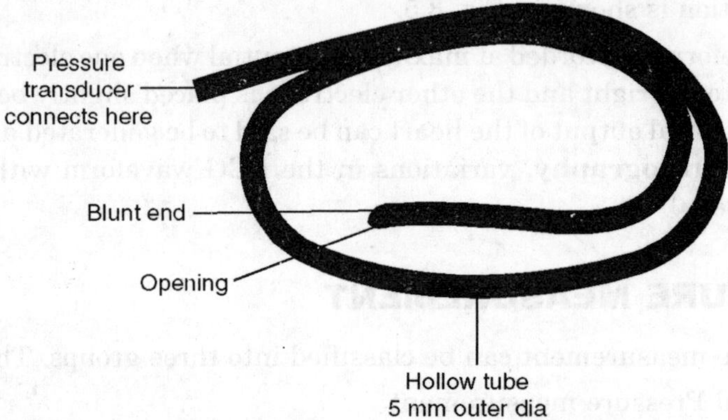

Fig. 3.6. Shows a 5 mm cardiac catheter.

As shown in Fig. 3.7*a*, the pressure transducer is configured. The pressures can be measured in almost any portion of the circulatory system. The entry to the circulatory system may be at either at the arms or legs; a catheter may be manipulated throughout the circulatory system as shown. It should be noted that the pressure measured will be the pressure at the blunt end of catheter and not the pressure at the point where the catheter enters the circulatory system.

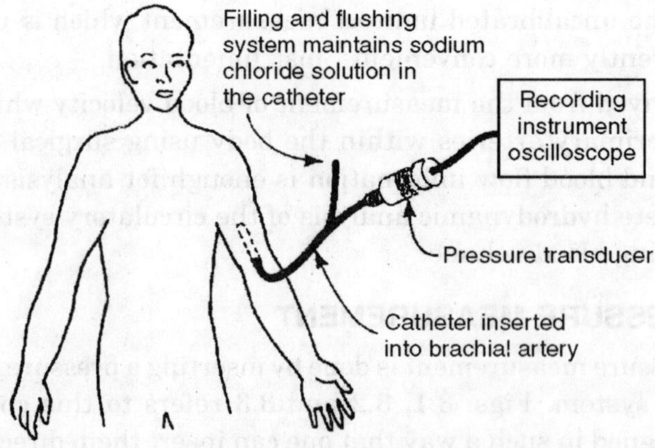

Fig. 3.7. Shows the direct blood pressure measurement.

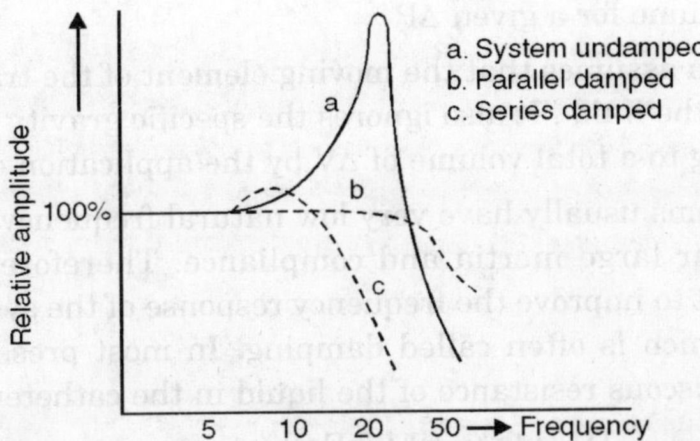

Fig. 3.7a. Shows the frequency response of fluid-filled catheter system.

It is also possible, to actually introduce the smooth end of the catheter into the right atrium via the inferior vena cava with careful manipulation. Cardiac defects, such as holes in the heart, were explored. This method or the procedure is referred to as **cardiac catheterization.** The investigations can be obtained at left ventricle by catheterization via the aorta and is referred as **arterial catheterization,** which almost always causes trouble with arterial damage and leakage into the tissues.

ARTERIAL PRESSURE MEASUREMENT

The most common pressure measurement is arterial pressure since this is usually measured by introducing the catheter into the brachial artery at the elbow of either arm.

Frequency Response and Damping Adjustment of the Fluid Filled Catheters

The frequency components of a normal pressure pulse consists of a DC (zero frequency) component, a fundamental component at the heart rate and the harmonics of the fundamental rate frequency. For recording the pressure pulse without any distortion, the measuring system should be capable of recording all frequency components with equal amplification and phase shift. The range of frequency response starts from the DC and is determined from an estimation of the highest heart rate expected and the number of harmonics to be taken into account. Generally, the blood pressure contains 6 to 20 significant harmonics, but it is accepted that the frequencies up to 10th harmonics produce sufficient components in the pressure pulse. Suppose if the heart pulse is 99 (beats per second), the same will be rate of the arterial pressure waves. This means that the upper frequency response should be at least 15Hz for a heart rate of 90 per minute.

A special consideration requires in relation to a fluid column pressure measuring system which is 'the natural frequency or the resonant frequency of the system'. The measuring system can respond accurately only up to frequencies well below the natural frequency. A simplified equation (1) which defines the natural frequency of the system is given by

$$f = (D/4)\ \sqrt{1/\pi L \times \Delta P/\Delta V} \qquad \ldots(1)$$

where D = diameter of the fluid column

L = length of the fluid column

ΔP = change in pressure

ΔV = change in volume for a given ΔP

The above equation assumes that the moving element of the transducer is very small as compared to the mass of the fluid . It also ignores the specific gravity of the fluid. ΔP is change in pressure corresponding to a total volume of ΔV by the application of the assumed pressure.

Fluid column systems usually have very low natural frequency to be measured with the requirement, due to their large inertia and compliance. Therefore, to record the pressure accurately, it is important to improve the frequency response of the system. This may be one by compensation method which is often called damping. In most pressure measuring systems, damping is provided by viscous resistance of the liquid in the catheter and is given by

$$D = [4\eta/(r_c)^3][l_c/\pi E\rho]^{1/2} \qquad \text{...(2)}$$

where η = viscosity (liquid)

D = damping coefficient

ρ = liquid viscosity

r_c = radius of the catheter bore in cm

l_c = length of the catheter bore in cm

E = volume elasticity of the sensing element in dynes/cm^3.

The above eqn.(2) shows that the damping increases inversely as the cube of the catheter diameter. Eqns. (1) and (2) become contradictory because natural frequency decreases directly with the diameter of the fluid column while the damping ratio increases. A compromise must be reached to obtain a maximum flat frequency response. To obtain a uniform flat response, the system has to be suitably damped. This can be done by two ways; they are as given below :

1. A series damper which makes the use of the capillary introduced between the catheter and the manometer. With this series damper, it is possible to effect a considerable decrease in the height on the resonance peak. But, the resonance peak is shifted to a lower value which makes the frequency response worse than without damping.
2. Another method is by using a parallel damper consisting of a variable needle resistance parallel to the manometer and in series with the distensible plastic tube connected to a syringe. The parallel damper is able to flatten the resonance peak and a flat response curve is achieved almost up to the original peak.

Catheter Pressure Transducers

A typical pressure transducer for use with a catheter is shown in the Fig. 3.8*a*. Since a very little pressure difference is encountered throughout the arterial system, it is unnecessary to introduce the catheter to any great distance into the circulatory system. The catheter/ transducer combination may be replaced by a needle transducer as shown in Fig. 3.8*b*. The needle/ transducer combination which is also available in a syringe configuration as shown in Fig. 3.8*c*. These combinations using needles rather than a flexible catheters are obviously much easier to introduce it into the subject's circulatory system and are thus preferable for direct blood pressure measurement. They are introduced into the femoral artery near the groin as this artery is close to the surface at this point. The syringe configuration allows administration of an arterial injection while recording arterial pressure.

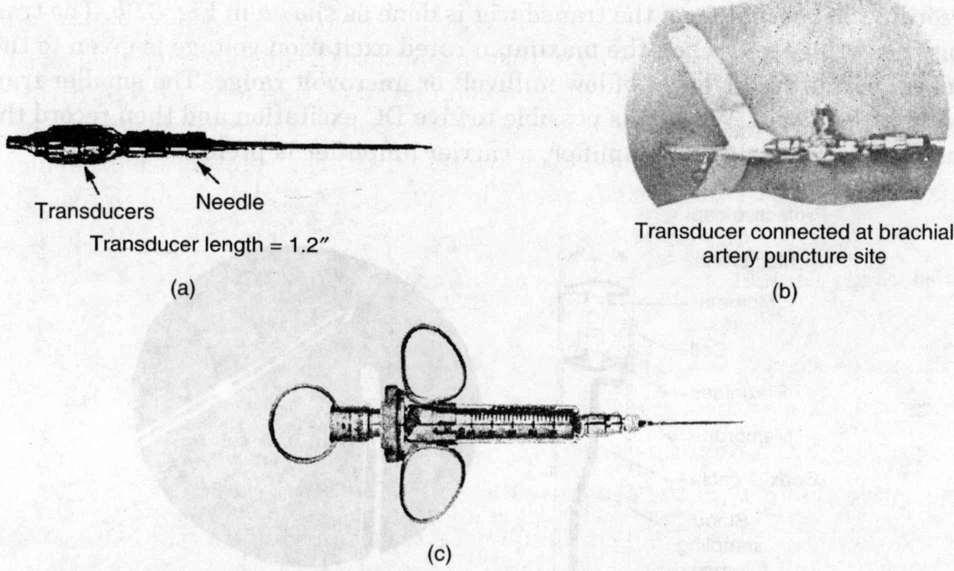

Fig. 3.8. (a) Shows the needle transducer, (*b*) Shows a needle blood transducer, (c) Shows a syringe blood pressure transducer.

For measurement of blood pressure within the heart, very small catheters typically in the order of 1millimeter diameter are required. These are known as drift catheters. The small diameter catheters are used so as not to interfere with the normal operation of the heart. These small catheters are inserted into the venous system and "drift" with the blood flow, eventually reaching the heart. Actually, they may be passed through the heart into the pulmonary circulatory system. The main disadvantage of these small catheters is the damping effect they have on the pressure pulse waveform of the system which limits the high frequency response of the system and gives erroneous readings. To avoid this problem, the catheter tip transducer as shown in Fig. 3.9*a* is preferable which incorporates a small pressure transducer built into the end of the catheter, the combination being less than 2mm in diameter. This allows introduction of the actual transducer into the heart and thus avoids the damping problem inherent with very small catheters.

Fig. 3.9a. Shows a catheter tip pressure transducer.

Bridge Type Transducers

Recording the output from the transducer is done as shown in Fig. 3.9*b*. The transducers are arranged as bridge and when the maximum rated excitation voltage is given to the bridge, it produces an output in the order of low millivolt or microvolt range. The smaller transducers produce very little output. While it is possible to give DC excitation and then record the output directly using a high sensitivity amplifier, a carrier amplifier is preferable.

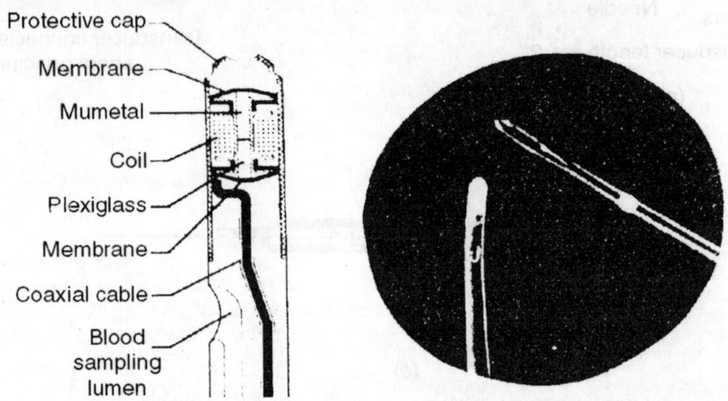

Fig. 3.9b. Shows the Catheter tip inductance pressure transducer. (Courtesy Carolina Medical Electronics, Winston-Salem, N.C.)

There are Catheter-tip transducers also. These have a catheter at whose tiny tip, an LVDT type transducer is built. Pressure applied to the membrane alters core position of the inductor which is part of an oscillator. A frequency modulated signal, is thus obtained. Fig. 3.9*b* shows the one by Carolina Medical Inc.

Very small direct blood pressure transducers are available presently, and they have been developed for research purposes. These transducers have an effective diameter of 10 microns. The transducer consists of a 10 micron micro electrode filled with an electrolyte having a different resistivity than that of a blood or body fluids. A pressure system is connected to the microelectrode and the impedance between the center of this electrode and the body is monitored. A servo control system controls the pressure in the microelectrode driving pressure system to keep the impedance between electrode and the body constant by exerting a pressure on the electrolyte in the microelectrode equal to the pressure external to the microelectrode tip. This pressure exerted on the electrolyte is therefore a measure of the blood pressure at the tip of the microelectrode.

Arterial pressures are normally measured as millimeters of mercury, mm/Hg, and venous pressures are usually measured as centimeters of water, cm/H_2O. These units are derived from older pressure measuring techniques using either mercury or water manometers. A typical arterial blood pressure waveform is shown in Fig. 3.10. The peak pressure is referred to as the **systolic** pressure and the minimum pressure is referred to as the **diastolic** pressure. It is common terminology to refer to an arterial blood pressure of, say 120 millimeter systolic and 80 millimeter diastolic as "120" and "80" or 120/80. As discussed earlier in chapter-2, the pressure in the arteries is many times greater than pressure in the veins, typical arterial pressure being 120/80 and typical venous pressure being 9/5 mm/Hg or, in the more common terminology, 12/7 cm/H_2O.

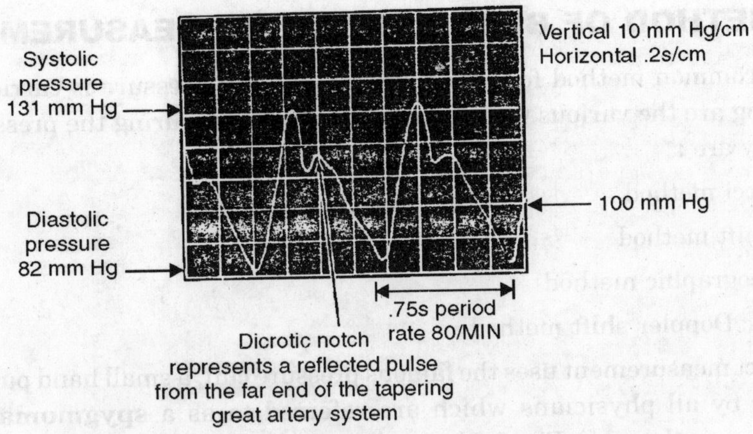

Fig. 3.10. Shows the arterial blood pressure waveform.

The direct blood pressure method is relatively easy to measure, but it requires an incision in an artery for introduction of a catheter or insertion of hypodermic needle. Very often, this results in the permanent loss of the artery used, it is regarded with some disfavor in most countries except USA. But the results obtained by this method are accurate for clinical purposes and are usually obtainable by indirect method also.

ARTERIAL PRESSURE MEASUREMENT BY PUNCTURE

In the area of arterial pressure measurement tests were carried out at desired point of the blood connecting flex tubing of the "artificial kidney", and in the event of "shunt" patients, directly at the arterial shank of the Scribner by-pass. (3.11*b*).

The instrument is linked through a flexible cable to the transducer which is made in the form of a cartridge having a length of approximately 15 cm and a diameter of 3 cm. An optically enlarging pressure dome of "piacryl" allows clear sight into the measuring chamber of the transducer. Connection between the transducer and the point of measurement is made through a thin flexible tube of PVC (1 m). To prevent entering of blood into the measuring chamber it is filled with a sterile physiological salt solution, because there would be improper measurement results if the fluids are separated by an intermediate layer of air. Since the internal components of the transducers are sensitive to temperature, sterilization by hot stream or air is not feasible. For this reason, disinfection by measuring a 2% formalin solution or 1-2% solution of ammonium base (C_4 solution) is essential. To obtain accurate measurements, it is necessary to mount the transducer in a horizontal position to a tripod. Recalibration of the bio-meter is to be carried out before each measurement. This technical procedure is not difficult but presupposes some familiarities.

There is also provision for connection to a display unit, recording instrument; integrated and instantaneous pressure can be measured. (0 to ± 300 torr).

INDIRECT METHOD OF BLOOD PRESSURE MEASUREMENT

The most common method for measurement of blood pressure is carried out indirectly only. The following are the various techniques involved in measuring the pressure by this indirect method. They are :

1. Riva-Rocci method
2. Phase shift method
3. The Rheographic method
4. Ultrsonic Doppler shift method

This indirect measurement uses the famous pressure cuff, a small hand pump and pressure dial device, used by all physicians which are referred to as a **spygmomanometer.** This spygmomanometer, as shown in Fig. 3.11*a* incorporates a pneumatic cuff encircling the upper arm. An inflatable section of this cuff is inflated by a small hand pump and the pressure in the

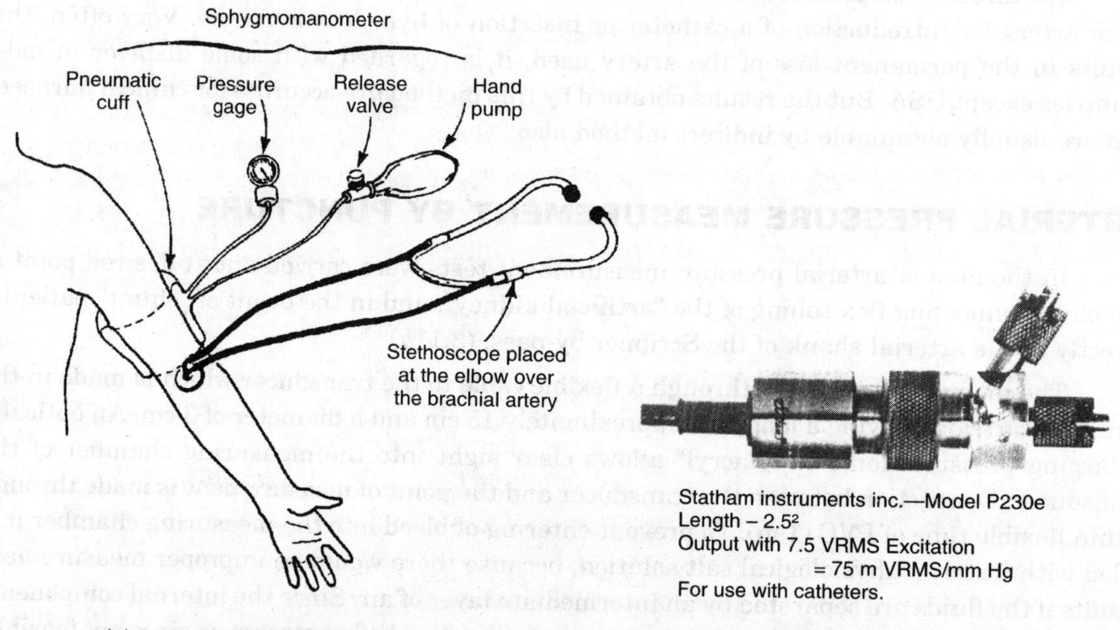

(a) Indirect Pressure Transducer, (b) A conventional blood pressure transducer (direct type)

Fig. 3.11. Shows the indirect blood pressure measurement with a sphygmomanometer.

system is indicated by a mechanical pressure gauge or in some models, a mercury manometer. Now we have LCD digital display based instruments also available. The cuff is inflated to a pressure greater than the blood pressure in the large brachial artery of the arm. The pressure thus collapses the artery and cuts off the blood flow to the arm. As the pressure in the cuff is gradually released using a release valve built into the hand pump, a point is reached where the cuff pressure and the peak or systolic arterial pressure are the same. At a pressure slightly below this level, the peak arterial pressure slightly exceeds the cuff pressure and blood is able to squirt through the compressed segment of the brachial artery. This squirting blood results in turbulence within the artery creating sounds known as **"Korotkoff"** sounds. These sounds are usually detected with a stethoscope placed over the brachial artery. As the pressure in the cuff is further decreased, Korotkoff sounds continue until a point is reached where no further turbulence is produced as no constriction exists in the brachial artery. This point represents the diastolic blood pressure. Actually, Korotkov identified a second sound also, though it is not clinically used for the measurement, but it gives the diastolic end point more accurately, if sensed by a suitable microphone and amplified for hearing.

As it is somewhat difficult to detect the pressure where the Korotkoff sounds begin and cease, this sphgmomanometer techniques cannot be relied upon to produce accuracy of much better than about 10mm of mercury (Hg). While the technique is inaccurate, it is simple to perform and very little discomfort is felt by the patient. In the hands of a skilled operator highly repeatable results are obtained and, since the clinician or the doctors are usually more interested in trends than exact numbers, the technique is entirely appropriate.

It is possible that this sphygmomanometer technique may be automated by replacing a hand pump with an automatic cuff pump. The automatic cuff pump may be operated by pushing a panel-mounted button to produce a single cycle inflation and deflation. Also it may be set for repeat cycles at various intervals for continuous monitoring of blood pressure over longer period of time. The stethoscope may be replaced by Korotkoff - sound microphone as shown in Fig. 3.12. This microphone consists of a piezoelectric transducer specifically designed to produce the Korotkoff sounds clearly and efficiently. Similarly, the pressure indicating dial may also be replaced with a pressure transducer as used for the direct pressure measurement.

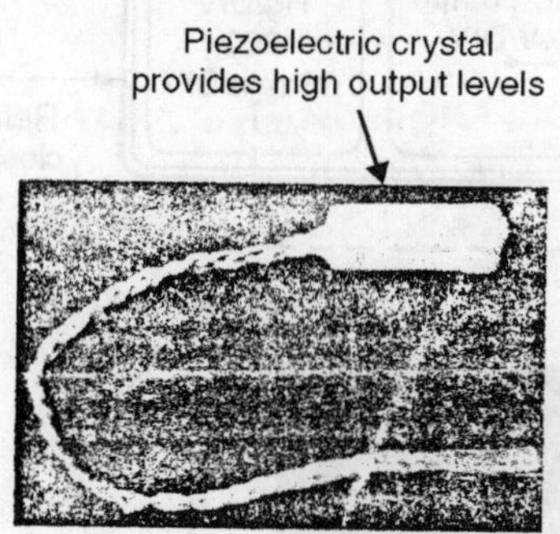

Fig. 3.12a. Shows a korotkoff sounds microphone.

In the indirect blood pressure measurement method, the subject's/the patient's blood pressure can be conveniently recorded. An oscilloscope is used here for displaying the pressure waveform. The vertical channel of the oscilloscope displays the output of the Korotkoff sound microphone signal while the horizontal channel displays the output signal received from the pressure transducer. A typical display produced by this method is shown in Fig. 3.13.

The horizontal axis is calibrated in pressure; the points at which vertical information appears and then disappears are the systolic and diastolic pressures. This system is capable of giving better accuracy than the conventional cuff/stethoscope. This avoids the human judgment in determining the presence of Korotkoff sounds. A high pass filter may be used for rejecting

the information from the microphone below 150Hz so as to get clear display. This high pass filter is employed between the microphone and the oscilloscope vertical channel.

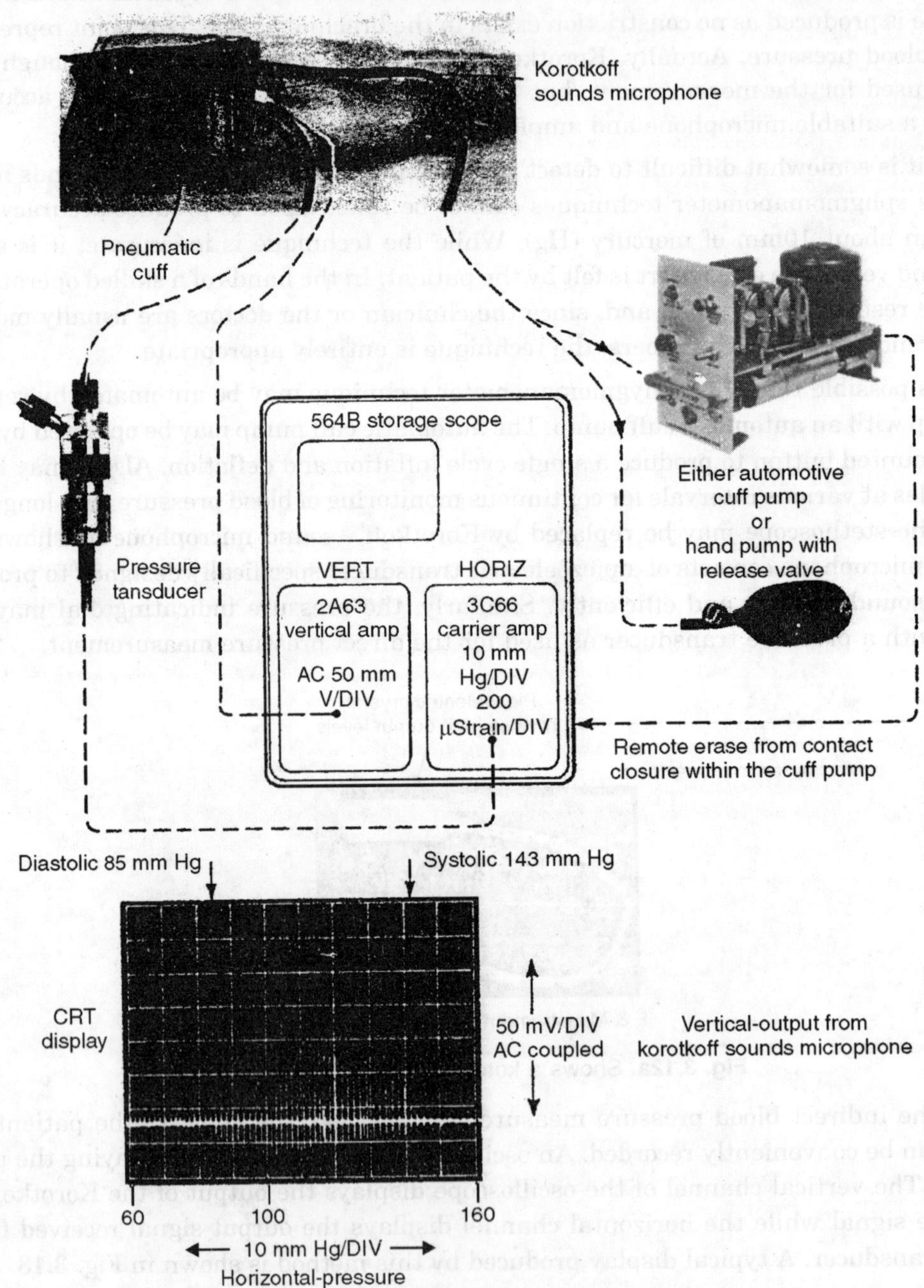

Fig. 3.13. Shows a Automatic indirect blood pressure measurement.

Indirect method of blood pressure is an attempt to measure intra-arterial pressures non-invasively. The most standard manual technique employs either the palpation or the auditory detection of the pulse distal to an occlusive cuff. Fig. 3.11 shows one indirect method of way measuring blood pressure. It employs a sphygmomanometer consisting of an inflatable cuff for occlusion of the blood vessel, a rubber bulb for inflation of the cuff, and either a mercury or an aneroid manometer for detection of pressure.

Procedurally, the blood pressure is measured as given below :

The occlusion cuff is inflated until the pressure is above systolic pressure and then slowly bled off (2 to 3 mmHg/s) or (0.3 to 0.4 kPa/s). When the systolic peaks are higher than the occlusive pressure, the blood spurts under the cuff and causes a palpable pulse in the wrist (***Riva-Rocci method)***. Audible sounds are (***Korotkoff sounds)*** are heard through the stethoscope, held over the brachial artery near the elbow. The manometer pressure at the first detection of the pulse indicates the systolic pressure. As the pressure in the cuff is decreased, the audio Korotkoff sounds pass through five phases (Geddes–1970). The period of transition from muffing (phase IV) to silence (phase V) brackets the diastolic pressure.

This technique may not be suitable for the infants and hypotensive patients since it requires several measurements and because normal respiration and vasometer waves modulate the normal blood pressure levels.

Using occlusive cuff of the correct size is important if the clinician is to obtain accurate levels. The pressure applied to the artery wall is assumed to be equal to that of the external cuff. However, the cuff pressure is transmitted via interposed tissue. With a cuff of sufficient width and length, the cuff pressure is evenly transmitted to the underlying artery. Generally, this is accepted one that the width of the cuff should be about 0.40 times the circumference of the extremity. However, no general agreement appears to exist about the length of the pneumatic cuff. If a short cuff is used, it is important that it be positioned over the artery of interest. A longer cuff reduces the problem of misalignment. The cuff should be placed at heart level to avoid hydrostatic effects.

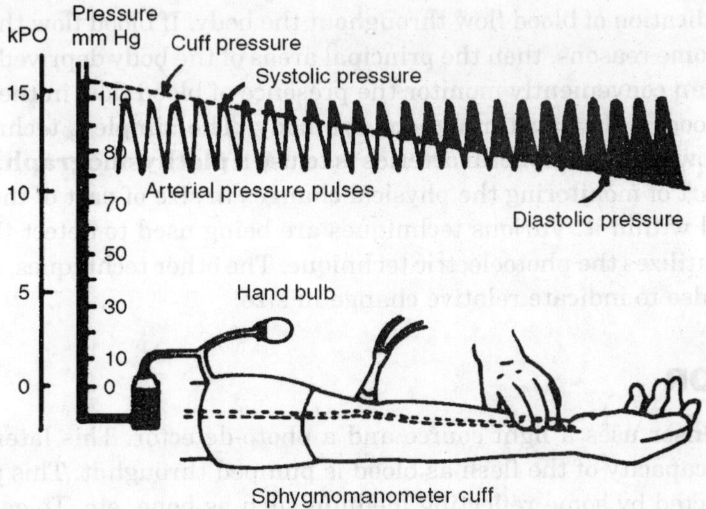

Fig. 3.14. Shows the typical indirect blood-pressure measurement.

Fig. 3.14 shows a typical Blood pressure measurement using indirect method.

The sphygomomanometer cuff is inflated by the hand bulb to pressures above the systolic level. Pressure is then slowly released. Blood flow under the cuff is monitored by a microphone or stethescope placed over a down stream artery. The first Korotkoff sound detected indicates systolic pressure whereas the transition from muffing to silence brackets diastolic pressure.

The auscultatory technique is simple and requires a minimum equipment. However, it cannot be used in a noisy environment, whereas the palpation technique can. The hearing acuity of the user must be good for low frequencies from 20 to 300Hz, the bandwidth required for these measurements.

A number of techniques have been proposed auomatically and indirectly, to find the systolic and diastolic blood pressures in humans. The basic technique involves an automatic sphygomomanometer that inflates and deflates occlusive cuff at a predetermined rate. A sensitive detector is used to measure the diastole pulse or cuff pressure. A number of kinds of detectors have been employed for research. Some of the detectors are given below :

1. Ultrasonic
2. Piezo electric
3. Photoelectric (Shygmo pick up)
4. Electroacoustic
5. Thermometric
6. Electrocardiographic
7. Rheographic and
8. Tissue impedance

PLETHYSMOGRAPHY

In many cases, the absolute values of the blood pressure need not be measured ; all that is required is an indication of blood flow throughout the body. If blood flow throughout the body diminishes due to some reasons, then the principal areas of the body deprived will be the fingers and the toes. One can conveniently monitor the presence of blood flow in these areas. This will ensure that the blood is flowing throughout the body. The simplest technique of recording presence of blood flow in the peripheral arteries is to use a **plethysmograph**. Plethysmography is nothing but the art of monitoring the physical changes in size of part of the body as modified by the flow of blood within it. Various techniques are being used to detect this change in size. The **pulse sensor** utilizes the photoelectric technique. The other techniques, such as impedance measurement are also to indicate relative change in size.

PULSE SENSOR

The pulse sensor uses a light source and a photo-detector. This later device is used to record a change in capacity of the flesh as blood is pumped through it. This pulse sensor relies on light being reflected by some reflecting medium such as bone, etc. To get sufficient output potentials, a fairly high concentration of arteries near the surface is required.

These pulse transducers are suitable for application to the finger. But it is less suitable for toe, ear and nose use.

When the patient is in drugged state, or if he is affected by coldness then vasoconstriction will occur and tends to limit blood flow to the limbs. Under these conditions, it is preferable to tape the pulse sensor to the forehead of the subject. A typical pulse sensor is shown in Fig. 3.15. This is applied to the finger and forehead as shown. A typical Plethysmogram recorded with this pulse sensor and physiological monitor is as shown in Fig. 3.16.

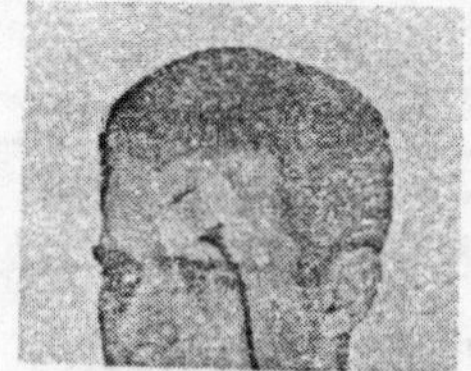

Plethysmograph held in place by tape or by an elastic strap around the head

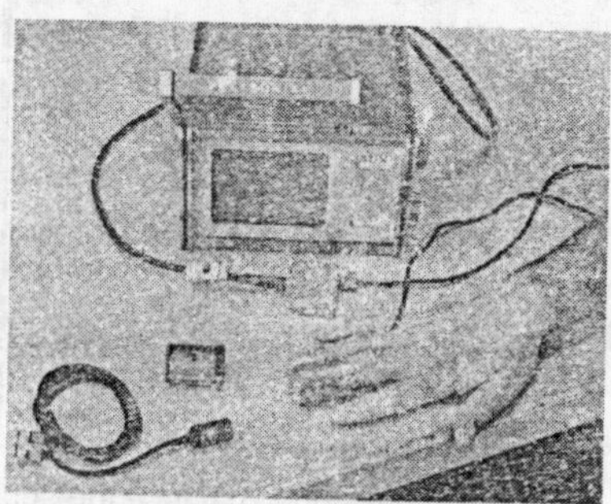

Plethysmograph held in place by the tektronix finger holder

Fig. 3.15. Shows the placement of the tektronix plethysmograph.

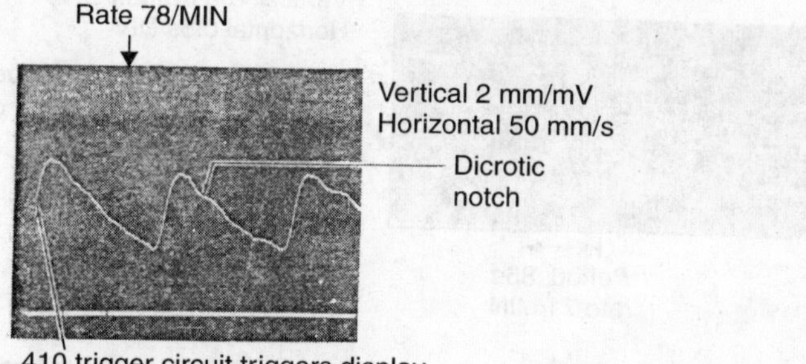

Fig. 3.16. Shows the plethysomgram obtained with tektronix pulse sensor (attached to finger) and 410 monitor.

IMPEDANCE MEASUREMENT

The impedance measurement technique is used to indicate relative changes in size resulting from blood flow. If the impedance between the arms is monitored, it will be found that the impedance change is due to the action of the heart and due to respiration. It is proved that the sensation level of arm to arm electrical current increases with frequency. Some sensation may be felt with 1 mA of DC current. However, at 25 kHz , 10 mA is required to cause sensation. Thus audio frequency currents of at least in the order of 1mA are used to monitor impedance. These frequencies and low currents are also to avoid cell stimulation. It has found that when measuring the impedance between the arms, cardiac action primarily changes the resistive component of the impedance while respiratory action mainly changes the capacitive components. So, for detecting cardiac action, one must use an audio frequency system sensitive only to resistive changes, to avoid respiratory effects.

These system can be incorporated using the Tektronix type 3C66 carrier amplifier with a storage oscilloscope and time base as shown in Fig. 3.17. With this unit, capacitive impedance changes are completely eliminated. This is done by paralleling the impedance to be measured with a large fixed capacitor.

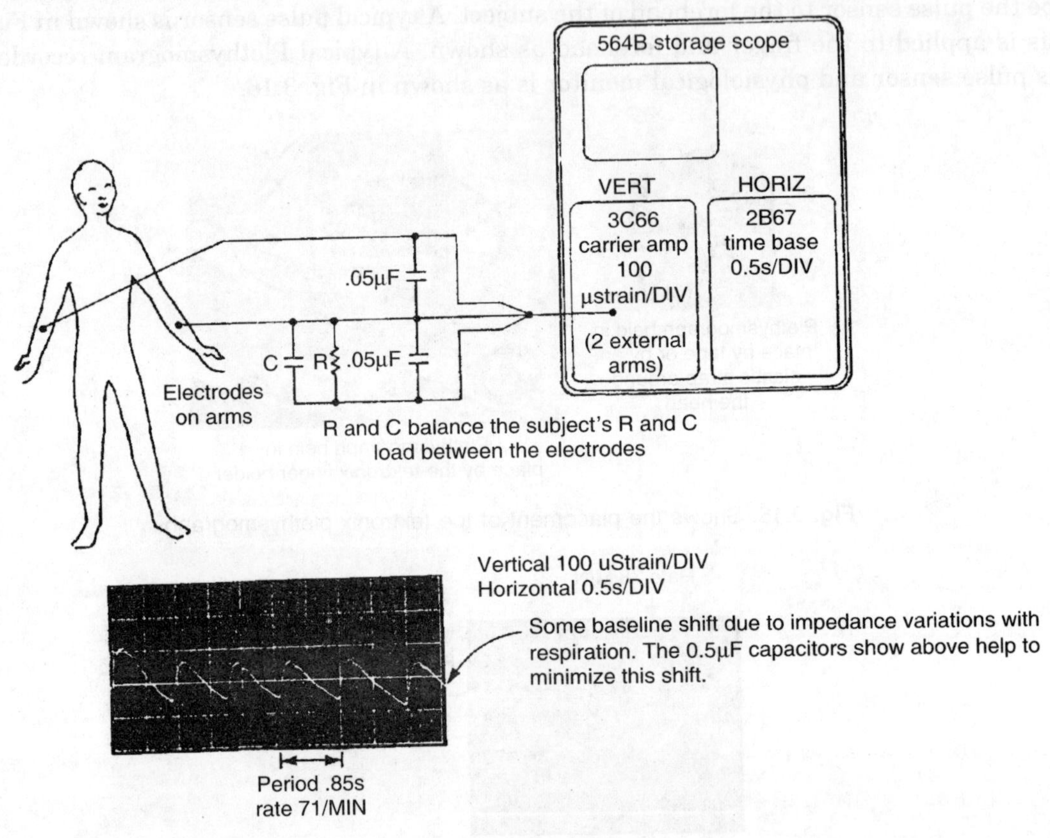

Fig. 3.17. Shows the impedance plethysmography with tektronix 3C66 plug-in.

A similar capacitor is needed to balance the bridge, as also a balancing R and C to simulate the R and C of the subject. The 3C66 is operated with a Wheatstone bridge external to the instrument, the other two arms are internal. A typical impedance plethysmograph recorded with the above technique is shown (Fig. 3.17). The slight change in base line evident in this recording is due to the influence of respiration.

THE ARTERIAL PULSE AND ITS MEASUREMENT

The rhythmic expansion of the arterial wall caused by the systolic rise in pressure is called the Arterial Pulse.

It is easily felt by palpation at the radial and temporal arteries, the dorsal artery of the foot and so on. Feeling the radial pulse was common in our country since the days of Veda, as Ayurveda has taught methods of sensing the lack of six vital elements by just feeling the radial artery pulse with three fingers laid across it near the wrist by the Ayurvedic Physician.

The pulse wave, or pressure increase, arises in the aorta. The wave of such pressure expands the arteries and then passes into the arterioles and then the capillaries at a definite rate. The figure showing the pulse wave as measured on the

1. Carotid Artery,
2. The Radial artery and
3. The finger pulp is given below.

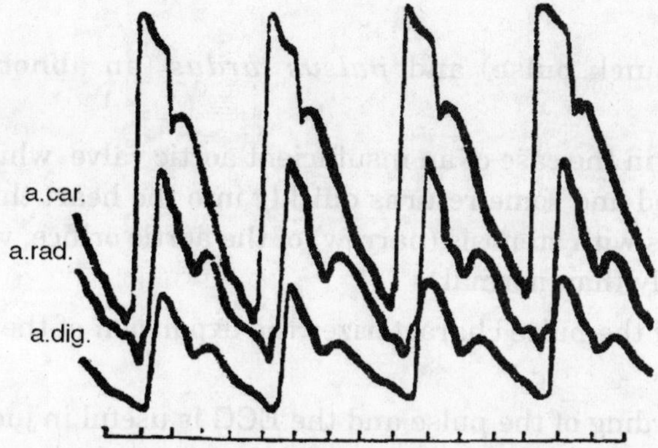

Fig. 3.18. Shows Spygmograme recorded synchronously from the corotid, radial and digital arteries.

Fig. 3.18 showing the Arterial pulse pressure wave as given below.

1.Carotid Artery, 2. The Radial artery and 3. The Finger.

The linear velocity of flow is between 0.3 to 0.5 m/s in the arteries. For detailed analysis of separate pulse waves, the Sphygmograph is used. Pick-ups are used for sensing the signal.

The main parts of the pulse curve which is the sphygmogram or sphygmo signal comprises of

(*a*) an *anacrotic* on the rising edge of the curve

(*b*) a *catacrotic* on the descending part of the curve.

The anacrotic rise results from the increase in arterial pressure and the distension of the artery wall at the beginning of the ejection phase.

The catacrotic descent occurs at the end of systole, as the ventricle pressure begins to fall. At the beginning of ventricular relaxation, when the ventricle chamber pressure is less than in aorta, blood discharged into the artery rushes back toward the ventricle. The pressure drops as a deep notch which shows up on the pulse curve as the "deep incisure" notch. But this happens only momentarily because the semilunar valves are shut by the backward flow. The rise of the wave as a secondary wave of increase of pressure then distends the arterial walls. This is the dicrotic rise on the sphygmogram.

The curve at the finger shows the variations much less than at the major artery.

EXAMINATION OF THE SPHYGMO SIGNAL

It reveals the following important properties :

1. Rate
2. Velocity of flow
3. Amplitude
4. Tone
5. Rhythm

Pulsus celer (a quick pulse) and *pulsus tardus* (an abnormally slow pulse) are distinguished.

The former occurs in the case of an insufficient aortic valve, while the ventricle ejects an increased amount of blood and some returns quickly into the heart through the valve defect if any. *Pulsus tardus* occurs with stenosis (narrow) of the aortic orifice, when the blood is pushed into the aorta more slowly than normal.

The **amplitude** of the pulse characterizes the expansion of the arterial wall during the pulse thrust.

Synchronous recording of the pulse and the ECG is useful in judging cardiac function in certain heart conditions.

Pulse deficit is when an occasional wave of ventricular excitation is not followed by discharge of blood into the vascular system and by a pulse thrust.

If a pulse wave is weak and does not reach the peripheries, then it gives irregular rhythm and is called *allorthymic pulse.*

THE FINGER PULSE PICK UP

A suitable method for easily and non invasively picking up the sphygmo signal at the digit (*i.e.*, finger) is given below.

A lamp of 6V, 60 mA low current is shining light into the finger pulp held inside a slotted tube. On the other side of the finger pulp the light dependant resistor (CdS or CdSe film resistor) is kept so as to face the (reddish) light received through the pulp of flesh on the thumb finger. The transistor circuit shows amplifies it to about 500 times and provides about 100–200 mV of sphygmo signal.

A quick check of the transistor output on a moving coil (multi) meter can show the pulsating signal and a long persistence or storage (Digital Storage scope) can show the variations of the sphygmo signal continuously.

The signal is usually picked up with mains frequency noise and is advisable to use a battery for the power supply shown. The same circuit can also be used for a reflective type pick up, in which the light source is a small thin lamp of the same rating and the LDR is replaced by a phototransistor. The reflective pick up is free from vibrations or movement artifacts since it can be held taped to the finger pulp when used for automatic continuous monitoring.

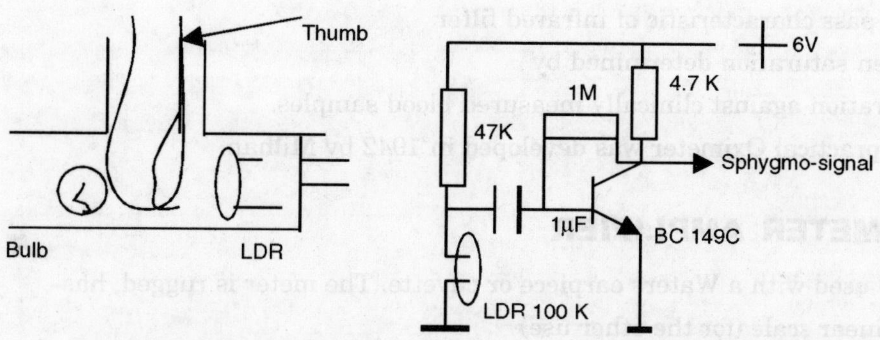

Fig. 3.19. Circuit for picking up the finger pulse Sphygmo signal.

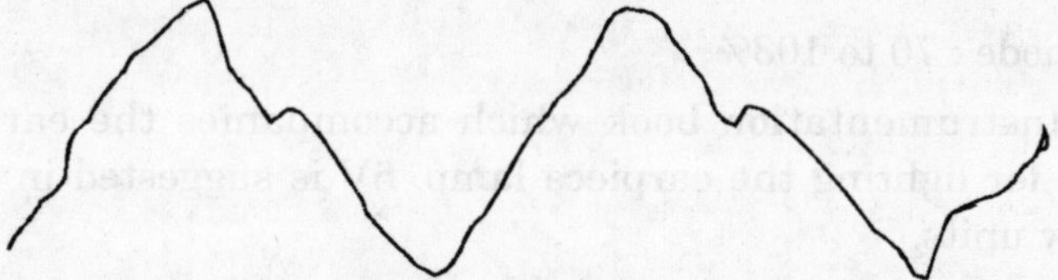

Fig. 3.20. The sphygmo signal picked up from the sensor.

The Principle of the spectrophotometric method of Oxygen Saturation in blood measurement

The saturation of the oxygen in the blood can be measured by observing the sphygmo signal amplitude at two different light wave lengths, one at the Red region of 690 nm and another at the infra red frequency (800 nm).

By a calculation involving the comparison of the two values, it is possible to determine the PO_2 of the blood indirectly. This will not anyway provide a very accurate measurement like taking the blood sample and using an Electrode such as the Clarke Electrode for finding out the PO_2.

However, for non-invasive and quick assessment, several vendors offer such oxygen saturation measuring instruments.

2. DETERMINATION OF OXYGEN SATURATION IN BLOOD

Principle

Detection of colour density change by photoelectric methods "Redness of Blood."

Transluminance of a well of tissue richly endowed with a capillary bed: (lobe, pinna of ear) is the first aspect.

The following two detectors are used for measuring the oxygen saturation in blood.

1. Red–640 mμ–signal is proportional to amount of blood and oxygen saturation

2. Infrared–840 mμ–Signal is independent of oxygen but dependant on amount of blood.

Band pass characteristic of Red filter employing photo voltaic cell.

Band pass characteristic of infrared filter

Oxygen saturation determined by

Calibration against clinically measured blood samples.

First practical Oximeter was developed in 1942 by Milhan.

THE OXIMETER AMPLIFIER

This is to be used with a Waters earpiece or cuvette. The meter is rugged, has

1. A linear scale (for the other use)
2. Marked 'M'mode : 0-105%.
3. Oxygen saturation scale
4. Marked 'N' mode : 70 to 103%

The "Waters" Instrumentation book which accompanies the ear piece indicates the recommended voltage for lighting the earpiece lamp. 5V is suggested in older units; 4V with greater current in new units.

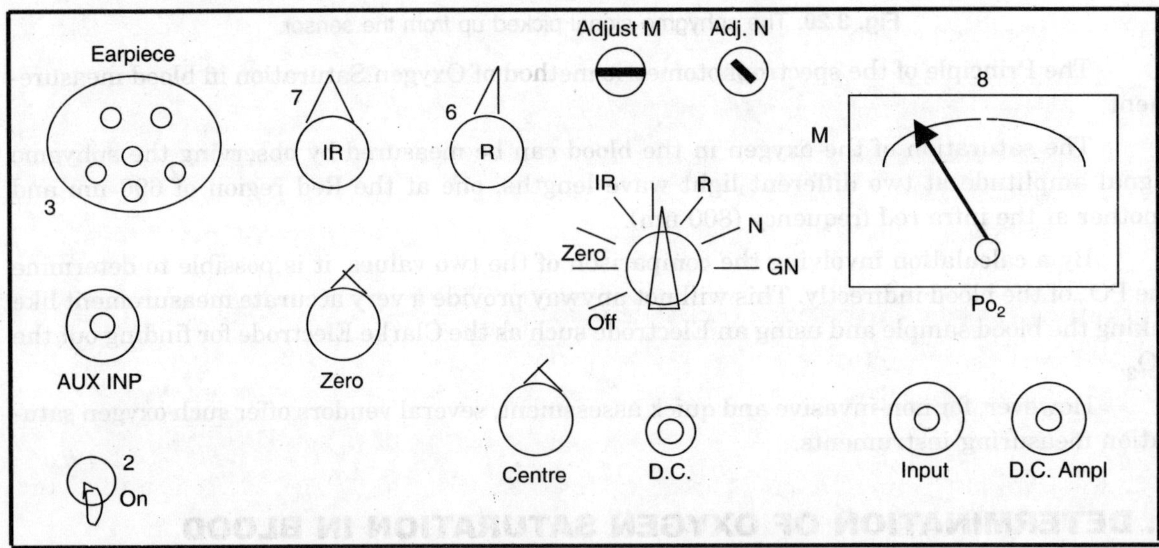

Fig. 3.21a. The Oximeter Amplifier Model Waters make.

Fig. 3.21 shows the front panel picture of the oximeter.

The toggle switch (2) must not be turned on unless the earpiece is plugged into the input socket (3).

Earpiece Calibration with Filter

1. Insert earpiece in socket (3) and turn earpiece switch ON. Insert EW filter -allow 15 minutes warm up.
2. With switch in zero position, adjust electrical zero.

3. Insert E90 earpiece filter; turn switch to TR. Adjust IR control(6) to bring needle to extreme left hand line of meter scale LMN. Adjust 'centre' to position trace on the 'scope' to bottom of screen.
4. Insert EBL filter, turn switch to R-L adjust R control(7) to move needle to arbitrary setting of 98 on M scale, for a first time. More accurate setting on step-9.
5. Insert E35 filter, turn switch to M, adjust M(8) to move needle reading suggested in Waters manual for E35 filter.
6. Insert E90 filter, switch in M position, reading adjusted by R to value indicated in Waters manual.
7. Recheck E35 and E90 settings until both are correct. Repeat steps 5 & 4.
8. With E90 filter in, turn switch to N position, reading should be the same on N-scale as it is for 'M' mode. If not, adjust "N" mode.
9. If R control was adjusted in step-6, reinsert EBL filter, turn switch to R position and note reading. This value should be used as the R-setting in step–4 hence forward and will eliminate the need to repeat step 5,6.

Using Earpiece with Patient after Calibrating with Filter

1. With switch at zero position, set electrical zero.
2. Attach earpiece to patient; allow a 15 minutes warm up. Turn switch to IR; adjust IR to move needle to left hand edge LMN line.
3. Apply pressure to earpiece to make it bloodless and turn switch to R, adjust R to move needle to 98 on M-scale.
4. Remove pressure, read saturation on M or N scales. M for lower range, N for higher range.

With known Bloods, Cuvette for O_2 Determination

1. Insert Cuvette adopter box in earpiece socket.
2. With switch at zero, adjust to red line with zero knob.
3. Insert 100% saturated blood with switch at IR and set IR to left hand LMN line.
4. With 100% saturated sample still in Cuvette, switch to 'R' and adjust R control to return position to red line. Switch to 'M' and adjust R control to read 100%.
5. Flush cuvette and insert unsaturated blood. With switch at M, adjust M control to bring meter to known value of blood.

Not necessary to make repeated adjustment as it will hold as long as photo cells do not deteriorate.

Dye Curves

1. Insert earpiece or cuvette. Allow to warm up.
2. With switch in zero position, adjust electrical zero, adjust to red line with zero control.
3. With earpiece in place or arterial blood in cuvette, turn switch to IR. Turn IR control until needle reaches LMN line. Turn oximeter 'centre' control to set trace at bottom of

screen. Then turn IR control completely clockwise. Then turn N to completely clockwise. Trace will be off screen.

For Evan's Value

4*a*. Turn switch to R, adjust R control until needle is at red line. Trace will return.

5*a*. Turn switch to N. Inject dye , start record, curve will be downloaded.

For Cardiac Green

4*b*. Turn switch to GN, adjust R control to bring needle to 15 on L (linear) scale.

5*b*. Start camera and inject dye. Curve will be upward.

Use smaller amounts of dye if curve is large or turn IR control only part way in (3) above.

While the above procedures indicate the steps of the method, today's instruments have made the same automatic and reading on an LCD display.

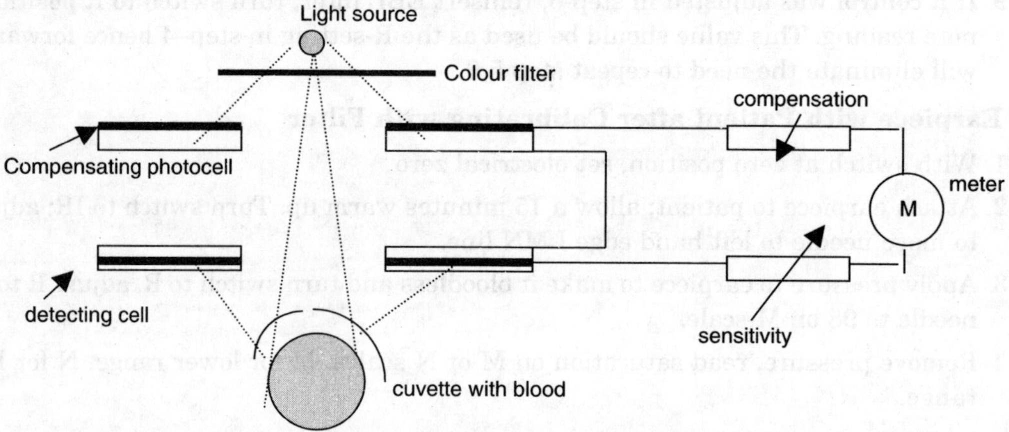

Fig. 3.21b. Shows the basic schematic of a reflection oximeter.

One basic equation for oxygen saturation is given as

$$= 1.13 - 0.28[I_{i\text{-}red}/I_{red}]$$

with $I_{i\text{-}red}$ is at 805nm and I_{red} at 650 nm.

HEMO REFLECTOR

The **Brinkman** Hemo Reflector allows oxygen saturation in blood to be measured, e.g., during cardiac catheterisation. It is used for investigation of small blood samples obtained by puncture or catheterisation. About 3 minutes is the time taken and 1% accurate result is obtained with just half a ml of blood.

1. Diagnosis of cardiac and vascular anomalies
2. Treatment of post operative anoxic conditions
3. Treatment of anoxia due to pulmonary affection.

To specialists of cardiac and pulmonary diseases, anesthetists it is useful. The method is based on the measurement of intensity of light reflected by a blood layer. Light of 600-700

micron which is strongly absorbed by Hemoglobin but lesser by oxy hemoglobin, is used. The reflected light is proportional to oxygen saturation.

The sample is placed in the Hemo-reflector and is turned towards the light path. The galvo shows a deflection, which indicates oxygen saturation. Because of the reflection method blood need not be hemolysed.

Two other cuvettes serve to adjust for sensitivity and compensate for reflections from the glass walls of the cuvette containing the blood.

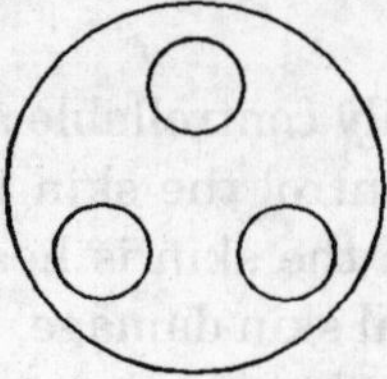

Fig. 3.22. Revolving head with cuvettes in holders.

Detailed instructions for using the instrument is supplied, together with a quantity of reagents sufficient for the measurement of several hundred blood samples. Two syringes are also supplied.

20 bottles 100 gm diluent (2% Nacl, 0.3% Na-Salicylate, 0.05% NaCN)

4 bottles each 100 gm solution (2%$Na_2B_4O_7$ and p.3% Na-Salicylate)

20 ampoules of 200 mg $Na_2S_2O_4$

TRANSCUTANEOUS PO$_2$ SENSOR (TCPO$_2$)

Measurement of Transcutaneous arterial oxygen (tcPO_2) is similar in principle of vitro PO_2 measurement technique. A Clark electrode is used in a sensor which is placed in contact with the skin.

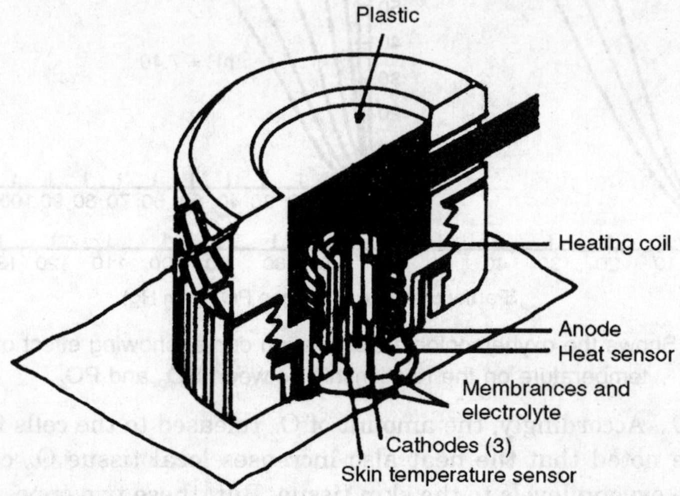

Fig. 3.23. Shows the cross-sectional view of a transcutaneous oxygen sensor.

Fig. 3.23 shows the cross sectional view of a typical Clark electrode-type $tcPO_2$ sensor. This contains three glass sealed pt. Cathodes which are separately connected via current amplifiers to an Ag/AgCl anode ring. A buffered KCl electrolyte, which has low water content to reduce drying of the sensor during storage, is used to provide a medium in which chemical reactions occur. Under normal physiological conditions, the PO_2 at the skin surface is essentially atmospheric regardless of the PO_2 in the underlying tissue.

Hypermia of the skin causes the skin PO_2 to approach arterial PO_2. Hypermia can be induced by the administration of certain drugs, by the heating or abrasion of the skin, or by application of nicotinic acid cream.

Because heating gives most readily controllable and consistent effect, a heating element and a thermistor sensor are used to control the skin temperature beneath the PCO_2 sensor. Sufficient arterioalization results when the skin is heated to temperature between 43°C and 44°C. These temperatures cause nominal skin damage, but with neonates it is still necessary to reposition the sensor frequently to avoid tissue burns. While heating the skin, O_2 diffusion through the stratum corneum increases and vasodilution of the dermal capillaries the blood flow to the skin at the sensor site where the heat is applied. Increased blood flow delivers more O_2 to heated skin region, making the excess O_2 diffuse through the skin more easily. As Fig. 3.24 suggests, heating of blood also causes the ODC to shift to the right, resulting in a decreased

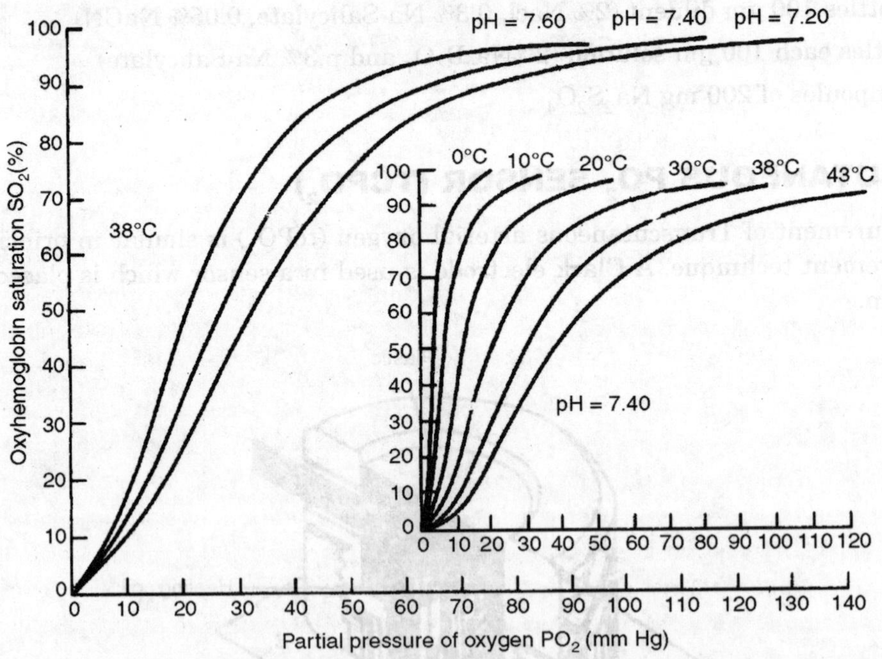

Fig. 3.24. Shows the oxyhemoglobin dissociation curve, showing effect of pH and temperature on the relationship between SO_2 and PO_2.

binding of Hb with O_2. Accordingly, the amount of O_2 released to the cells from a given PO_2 is increased. It may be noted that the heat also increases local tissue O_2 consumption, which tends to decrease the oxygen levels to the skin tissue. But, these two opposing factors approximately cancel each other. Duration of monitoring is a function of the skin's sensitivity to possible burns, as well as to electrode drift. Typically continuous monitoring is recommended for 2-6 hour before moving to a different skin site.

BLOOD FLOW MEASUREMENT

Blood flow is one of the most important physiological parameter. Blood flow is measured by using mean velocity transducer. The transducer is placed in artery having known cross sectional area. Many types of mean velocity (transducers) type of flow meters have been developed and at present these are easily available in the market. But there are various other techniques developed for blood flow measurement also.

This chapter discusses about the various techniques involved in the blood flow measurement. The following are various techniques which are most commonly used for the above purpose, each one having its own merits and demerits.

1. Electromagnetic blood flow meter
2. Ultrasonic Blood flow meter (Presently used)
3. NMR blood flow meter (Presently used)
4. Laser Doppler blood flow meter (Presently used)

ELECTROMAGNETIC BLOOD FLOW METER

The theory of electromagnetic flow meters is based on Faraday's law. When a conductive fluid, such as blood, traverses the lines of force of a magnetic fluid, an electromotive force (emf) is generated in the fluid which is perpendicular to both magnetic lines of force and the direction of motion of the fluid. This electromotive force (emf) is directly proportional to the intensity of the magnetic field, the distance between the sensing electrodes and the fluid velocity. In the blood flow measurement, the sensitivity and the stability requirements are dependant. They are mainly dependent on the magnetic flux in the magnetic flowmeters which are used for blood flow measurement.

The electromagnetic blood flow transducer consists of an electromagnet to generate a magnetic field. Two electrodes are provided to sense the flow signal. These are encapsulated in epoxy in a form to allow them to fit around the blood vessel. The inside diameter fixes the cross sectional area of the vessel, changing the transducer to a flow-rate measuring instrument, although basically this is a velocity transducer. Electrodes make contact with the vessel wall. The flow transducer is connected to a flowmeter. This flowmeter supplies energizing current to the electromagnet, amplifies the flow signal, discriminates it from artifacts and makes it available for display on an oscilloscope.

The above assumes a DC magnetic field which would produce a DC flow signal. Since it would not be possible to differentiate this signal form electrode offset potential, amplifier drift etc., commercial blood flowmeters use AC excitation; either sinewave or square wave can be given as excitation signal ;

The output signal is derived from the transducer is given by

$$e = kBvd \qquad ...(3)$$

where e = the induced voltage

B = Magnetic field strength in tesla

v – velocity of blood flow

d = diameter of the blood vessel.

k = constant of proportionality

If the strength of the magnetic field and the diameter of the blood vessel remain unchanged, the induced voltage will then be a linear function of flow velocity. Therefore $e = k_1$ V where $k_1 = kb\ d$ which is constant.

In general, flow rate Q through a tube is given by

$$Q = vA$$

where A is the area of cross section of the tube. And v is the velocity of blood flow.

$$v = Q/A \qquad ...(4)$$

Hence $e = K_1 \times Q/A = K_2 \times Q$ where $K_2 = K_1/A$ and is a constant . From the above equation, it indicates that the voltage induced is directly proportional to the flow rate through the blood vessel.

The induced voltage picked up by the electrode is amplified and displayed and recorded by using suitable instrumentation setup system.

The instrumentation system is calibrated in terms of volume flow as function of the induced voltage. The diameter of the blood vessel is held constant. The above relation is true only if there exist conditions of a axial symmetry and the blood velocity is independent of the velocity profile. Then only, the induced voltage is directly proportional to the blood volume flow.

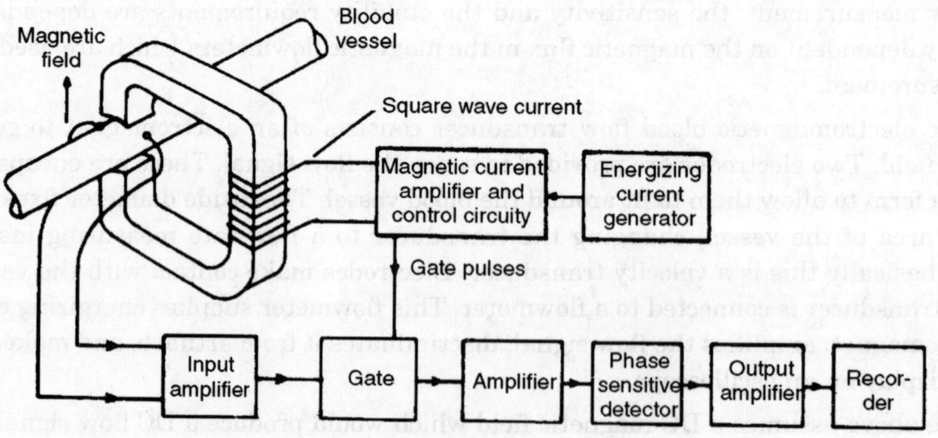

Fig. 3.25. Shows the block diagram of a square wave electromagnetic blood-flow meter.

Fig. 3.25 shows the Electromagnetic flow measurement unit.

Instrumentation requirements

Transducer

Pre-amplifier circuit

Gating circuit

Bandpass amplifier

Detector

Low pass filter and Output

Magnet

As discussed earlier, the standard e.m.f. induced relation due to a velocity of flow v in a magnetic field of B Columbs/s.m is given by

$$e = BLv \qquad ...(5)$$

Limiting factors of this method are

1. Polarization of electrodes
2. Induced (quadrature voltage)—$\partial B/\partial t$
3. Deviation from symmetrically axial flow distribution
4. Externally generated and physico-chemical artifacts.

1. **Polarization of electrodes** results from electro-chemical reactions at the electrode-fluid interface. This produces DC potentials ranging from several millivolts to several volts. To avoid this effect, the field is energized with 400 Hz AC and the emf is amplified by an AC amplifier which rejects the DC components.
2. **Quadrature emf** results from inductive interaction between electrode circuit and the AC magnetic field. This quadrature emf is 90° out of phase with the field and the flow signal. To provide a means of determining this quadrature voltage and minimising its effect, a phase adjustment is provided which positions the demodulator gating intervals. By correctly setting this adjustment, the composite signal may be read at a time when the flow component is maximum and the quadrature component is minimum.
3. **Disturbances in the flow symmetry** caused by side branches kinks or flow obstruction may affect total flow calibration calibration. Experience has indicated that a long smooth section of vessel is best, but where branching vessels cannot be avoided, to probe should be located on the high pressure side.

Other potential limitations of the principles of e.m. flow measurement come from artificial environment. Disturbances caused by surgical tools are also there.

Flow range : 2.5 cc/min–20000 cc/min

Output : 600mV full scale (10 kΩ single ended).

Signal to Noise ratio. This is proportional to the peak to peak to value of the excitation voltage. For sine wave and square wave excitation of the same peak to peak to voltage, the power required for sine wave excitation is only 50% of the power required by the square wave excitation.

Excitation Frequencies

In both sine and square wave excitation systems require excitation frequencies high enough to permit effective sampling, typically form 200 Hz to 1000 Hz.

With a sine wave excitation, to avoid the $\partial \mathbf{B}/\partial \mathbf{t}$ component in the induced Blv signal, the signal is sampled at the peak of the sine wave applied ($\partial \mathbf{B}/\partial t \to 0$).

With a square wave excitation, the $\partial \mathbf{B}/\partial \mathbf{t}$ component is absent except at the transitions and hence the sampling gate is easy to implement at any point in its flat parts.

COMMERCIAL FLOW PROBES

Some commercial blood flow meters are shown in figure given below (Fig. 3.25). The flowmeters are of the intracorporeal type which have a opening to allow placement around the blood vessel. These openings are usually fitted with a cover to maintain a constant blood vessel size. Extracorporeal transducers have tubular sleeve or cannula extensions and are applied by cutting the blood vessel and inserting the tubular sleeve in series with this vessel. Blood is in direct contact with the sleeve lumen in extracorporeal units.

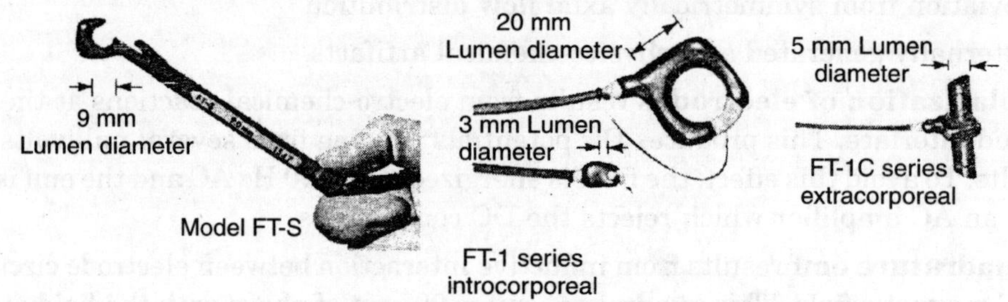

Fig. 3.25b. Shows the commercial blood flow meters.
(In Vivo Metric Systems, Los Angles, Calif)

COMMERCIAL FLOW METERS

Blood flow meters along with suitable flow transducers for use are produced by several manufacturers. In general, these instruments provide either sine wave excitation or square wave excitation in the range of 0.1 A to 1 Ampere and provide an output in the range of 0.1 volt to 1 volt . These outputs are used with an oscilloscope or with a recording device. The recording device should have a response of DC to 100 Hz. The instruments are calibrated to read in cubic centimeters per minute. Usually it covers a wide range from 1 to 100,000 cubic centimeters per minute. Blood velocity in the pulmonary artery may reach 100 centimeters per second. Since the artery has a cross sectional area of about 1.8 square centimeters, the velocity results in a peak flow of 100,000 cubic centimeter per minute. Blood flow systems may be calibrated by allowing blood to escape into a graduated flask for a known small period or by using an external calibration system providing known flow. A typical blood waveform is shown in figure given below (Fig. 3.26).

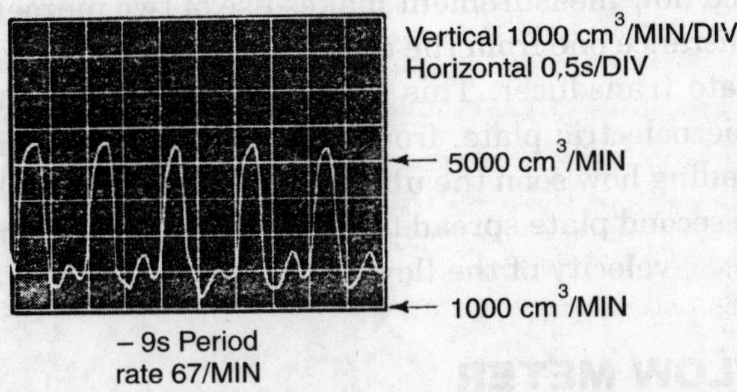

Fig. 3.26. Shows a typical blood flow record from an electromagnetic flowmeter.

The complete measuring system is shown in the Fig. 3.27. These are mostly used on animals now-a-days.

OTHER FLOW MEASURING DEVICES

Other forms of blood flow measuring devices are very rarely used. The isothermal flowmeter places a thermistor within the blood flow. The flow in blood tends to cool the thermistor and a measurement is obtained by recording the increase in thermistor excitation required to maintain the thermistor at a constant temperature, *i.e.*, the constant resistance. The electroturbinometer inserts a minute rotational generator into the blood flow system; this generator is driven by a small propeller driven by the blood flow. Ultrasonic blood flow measuring techniques are popular; these techniques involve the detecting the small phase difference in the direction of flow and in the opposite direction. The actual block diagram of these types are will be explained later in another chapter.

THE BLOOD FLOW IN THE VARIOUS ORGANS

The blood vessels dilate in a good working organ and their resistance therefore decreases. Since this local vascular dilation has little effect on the pressure of the blood, its volume in these vessels increases.

Organ	Blood flow In ml per 100g of organ wt.
Thyroid	560
Kidneys	420
Liver	150
Heart (coronary)	85
intestine	50
Brain	65
Spleen	70
Stomach	35
Muscles of arms	2 to 3 at rest
Muscles of leg	3 to 3.5 at rest

The ultrasonic blood flow measurement makes use of two piezoelectric transducer plates on the artery at a small distance one from the other. The high frequency voltage (about 2 MHz) is applied to the first plate transducer. This causes the sonic oscillations to spread and are received by the second piezoelectric plate, from which the signal is picked up, amplified and seen on the CRO. After finding how soon the ultrasound wave reaches the second plate and how soon oscillations from the second plate spread to the first against the direction of the blood flow, it is possible to calculate the velocity of the flow.

TYPE 4001 E.M. FLOW METER

Carrier suppressed modulation is employed in the M-4001 system so that in the absence of input signal voltage,(no blood flow), the carrier voltage is also zero. When blood is flowing through the Lumen, a 400 Hz carrier modulated by a signal proportional to the rate and flow direction, is sensed by the FLO-PROBE electrodes.

As previously explained, most probes develop an unwanted unmodulated quadrature component due to coupling between magnet and electrode circuit. The signal presented to the differential amplifier therefore includes this component.

The differential amplifier raises the input signal to the level required by the synchronous demodulation and aids in canceling common mode noise due to mains hum pickup or from other electronic instruments. The synchronous demodulator serves a dual function by demodulating the flow signal voltage for presentation and by eliminating the quadrature components (unwanted signal) generated by transformer action in the flow-probe.

A reference voltage from the phase control circuit gates the circuit elements within the synchronous demodulator, preserving the identity of the modulating voltage polarity. The output of the synchronous demodulator therefore corresponds to the original modulating (blood flow) signal.

Quadrature voltage is eliminated in the synchronous demodulator by a method of voltage cancellation. The phase control circuit is adjusted so that one of the two gates in the synchronous demodulator is switched on precisely at the start of each cycle of the 400 Hz carrier while the other is switched off. After a period of time corresponding to half cycle, the action is reversed with the alternate gate conducting and the initially conducting gate switched off. Since the quadrature voltage is exactly 90 degrees out of phase with the 400 Hz carrier frequency, the synchronous demodulator is conducting during a period of time in which the quadrature voltage is equally positive and negative. The summation or the average values of this voltage is therefore zero and its effect is cancelled.

The phase control circuit supplies 400 Hz reference voltage to time the gating action of the demodulator. Circuit times are adjusted so that the reference voltage is exactly 90° out of phase with the quadrature voltage.

The output circuit is essentially a low pass filter (LPF) designed to roll off the response at approximate 100 Hz to eliminate the 400 Hz carrier and reduce any extraneous noise components.

During calibration 10 mV signal is applied to the input by a calibrator, a standard accessory. The sensitivity is then adjusted for full scale output to standardize the gain through the amplifier, so that the individual calibration figures given with each flow probe can be used to determine the flow rate accurately.

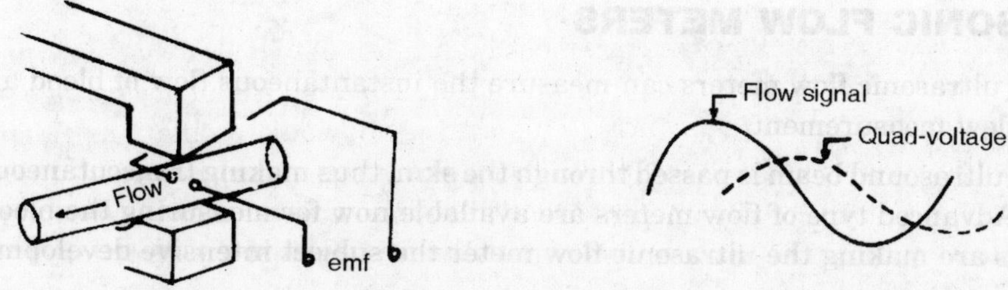

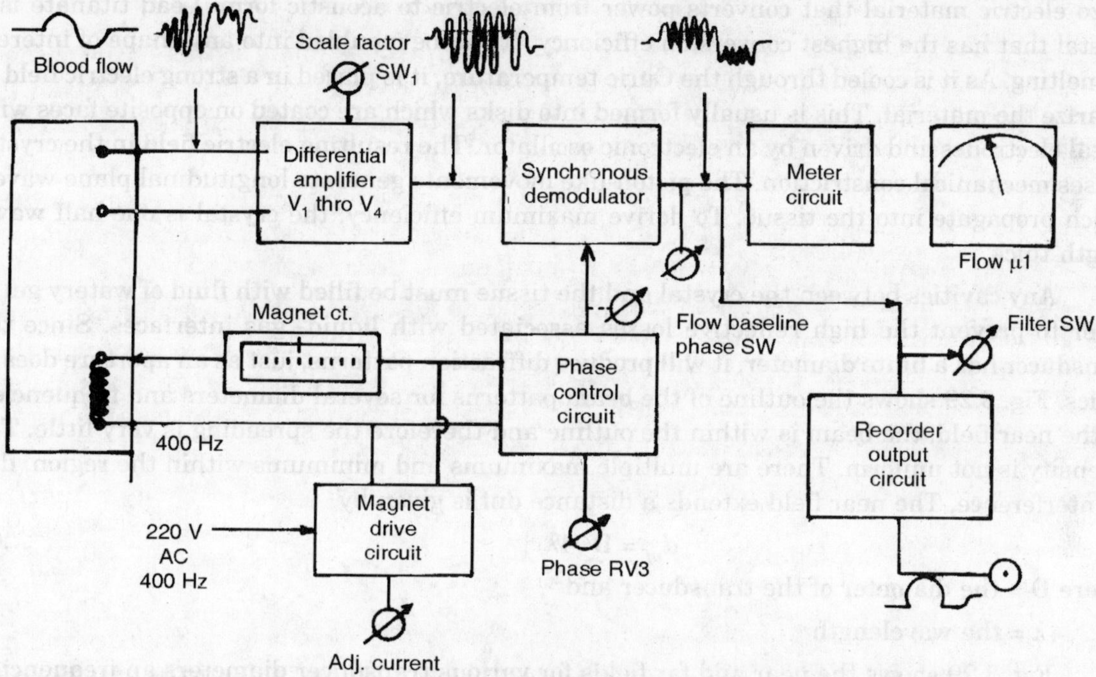

Fig. 3.28. (a) The blood flow measurement unit, (b) Shows the phase changes in the flow signal and the output signal c). Shows the functional Block diagram of the Blood Flow measurement.

LASER DOPPLER FLOW METER

In laser Doppler blood flow meter, a 5 mW He-Ne laser beams (632.8 nm) light through fiber optics into the skin is used. Moving Red blood cells in the skin frequency shift the light and cause spectral broadening. Reflected light is carried by fiber optics to a photodiode. Signal processing of the output is done as given below

1. Filtering
2. Weighting
3. Squaring and
4. Dividing

are necessary for processing the signal of interest.

ULTRASONIC FLOW METERS

The ultrasonic flow meters can measure the instantaneous flow of blood as like electromagnetic flow measurement.

The ultrasound beam is passed through the skin, thus making transcutaneous flow meters practical. Advanced type of flow meters are available now for measuring the blood flow. These advantages are making the ultrasonic flow meter the subject intensive development.

Transducers

Piezo electric type of transducer is employed for the measurement of blood flow. This piezo electric material that converts power from electric to acoustic form. Lead titanate is a crystal that has the highest conversion efficiency. It can be moulded into any shape of interest by melting. As it is cooled through the Curie temperature, it is placed in a strong electric field to polarize the material. This is usually formed into disks which are coated on opposite faces with metal electrodes and driven by an electronic oscillator. The resulting electric field in the crystal causes mechanical constriction. The piston-like movements generate longitudinal plane waves, which propagate into the tissue. To derive maximum efficiency, the crystal is one-half wavelength thick.

Any cavities between the crystal and the tissue must be filled with fluid of watery gel in order to prevent the high reflective losses associated with liquid- gas interfaces. Since the transducer has a finite diameter, it will produce diffraction patterns, just as an aperture does in optics. Fig. 3.29 shows the outline of the beam patterns for several diameters and frequencies. In the near field, the beam is within the outline and therefore the spreading is very little. The intensity is not uniform. There are multiple maximums and minimums within the region, due to interference, The near field extends a distance dnf is given by

$$d_{nf} = D^2/4\lambda \qquad \text{...(6)}$$

where D = the diameter of the transducer and

λ = the wavelength

Fig. 3.29 shows the near and far fields for various transducer diameters an frequencies.

In the far field the beam diverges. The intensity is inversely proportional to the square of the distance from the transducer. The angle of beam diverges by θ as shown (Fig. 3.29) and is given by,

$$\sin\theta = 1.2\lambda/D \qquad \text{...(7)}$$

As seen in the Fig. 3.29, the spatial resolution is very poor in the far field region and it is better to avoid this region.

To achieve near field operation, it is advisable to use higher frequencies with larger transducers.

To select the optimum operating frequency, it is necessary to consider the following factors.

- For a beam of constant cross section, the beam decays exponentially because of absorption of heat in the tissue. This absorption coefficient is approximately proportional to the frequency. Therefore choose low operating frequency

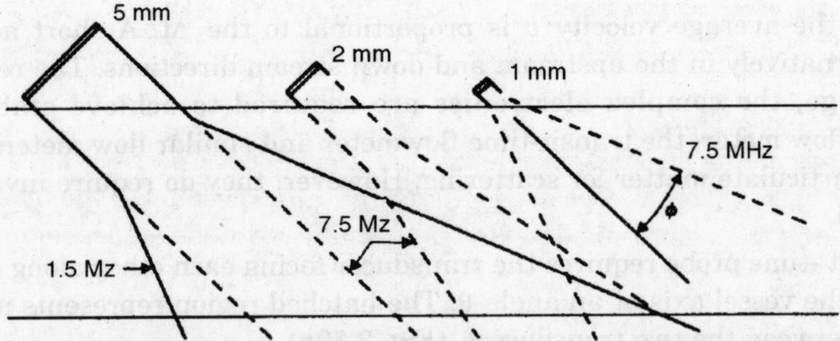

Fig. 3.29. Near and far fields for various transducer diameters and frequencies. Beams are drawn to scale, passing through a 100-mm-diameter vessel. Transducer diameters are 5, 2 and 1 mm. Solid lines are for 1.5 MHz, dashed lines for 7.5 MHz.

- **Regarding power, most ultrasonic flowmeters depend on the power scattered back from the moving blood cells. The back scattered power is proportional to f^4, which suggests to have to higher operating frequency.**

Therefore, after considering the above parameters, the operating frequency is the range of 2 to 4MHz for this application.

TRANSIT–TIME FLOWMETERS

The configuration of the ultrasonic transit- time flow meter is shown in Fig. 3.30.

The transducer arrangement is shown in Fig. 3.30*a* used of transit- time ultrasonic flow mete. The effective velocity of sound in the vessel is equal to the velocity of sound, *c* and the component due to the velocity of blood flow along the path of the ultrasound, v. For laminar flow, $v = 1.33u$ and turbulent flow $v = 1.07u$ where u is the velocity of flow of blood averaged over the cross sectional area.

Because the ultrasonic path is along a single line rather than averaged over the cross sectional area, *v* differs from *u*. The transit time in the down stream (+) and upstream (–) direction is given by

$$\begin{aligned} T &= \text{distance/conduction velocity} \\ &= D/(c \pm u \cos \theta) \end{aligned} \quad \ldots(8)$$

The difference between upstream and downstream (transit - time) is given as follows:

$$\begin{aligned} \Delta t &= 2Du \cos \theta/(c^2 - u^2 \cos^2 \theta) \\ &\simeq 2Du \cos \theta/c^2 \end{aligned} \quad \ldots(9)$$

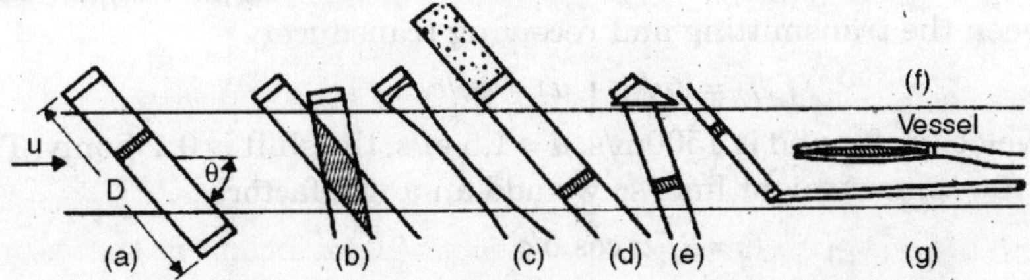

Fig. 3.30. Shows the different ultrasonic transducer configurations used for blood flow measurement.

And thus the average velocity v is proportional to the Δt. A short acoustic pulse is transmitted alternatively in the upstream and down stream directions. The resulting – t is in nanosecond range, the complex electronics are required to achieve stability. Like the electromagnetic flow meter, the transit-time flowmeter and similar flow meters use invariably a not required particulate matter for scattering. However, they do require invasive surgery to expose the vessel.

The transit -time probe requires the transducer facing each other along a path of length D inclined from the vessel axis at an angle θ. The hatched region represents a single acoustic pulse traveling between the two transducers. (Fig. 3.30*a*)

In a transcutaneous probe, both transducers are placed on the same side of the vessel so the probe can be placed on the skin. Beam interaction is shown as hatched (Fig. 3.30*b*).

Any transducer may contain a plastic lens that focuses and narrows the beam (Fig. 3.30*c*).

For pulsed mode of operation, the transducer is loaded by backing it with a mixture of tungsten powder in epoxy. This increases losses and lowers Q. Shaded region is shown for a single time of range gating (Fig. 3.30*d*).

A shaped piece of Luctite on the front loads the transducer and also refracts the beam. (Fig. 3.30*e*).

A transducer placed on the end of a catheter beams ultrasound down the vessel. (Fig. 3.30*f*).

For pulse operations, the transducer is placed at an angle as shown in Fig. 3.30*g*.

CONTINUOUS DOPPLER (CW) FLOWMETER

When a target recedes from a fixed source that transmits sound, the frequency of the received sound is lowered because of the Doppler effect. For small changes, the fractional change in frequency equals the fractional change in velocity.

$$f_d/f_o = u/c \qquad \text{...(10)}$$

where f_d = Doppler frequency shift

f_o = source frequency

u = target velocity

c = velocity of sound

The Doppler ultrasonic flowmeter is shown in Fig. 3.31. This requires particulate matter such as the blood cells to form reflecting targets. The frequency is lowered twice. One shift occurs between the transmitting source and the moving cell that receive the signal. The other shift occurs between the transmitting and receiving transducer.

$$f_d/f_o = 2u/(c + u) \approx 2u/c \qquad \text{...(11)}$$

Since the velocity of sound is 1500m/s. u = 1.5 m/s, the shift is 0.1% only. The velocities do not all act along the same straight line, so we add an angle factor

$$f_d = 2f_o u \cos \theta/c \qquad \text{...(12)}$$

Where θ is the angle between the beam of sound and the axis of the blood vessel as shown in Fig. 3.31. If the flow is not axial, or the transducers do not lie at the same angle, as in Fig. 3.30*b*, it is necessary to add trigonometric factor.

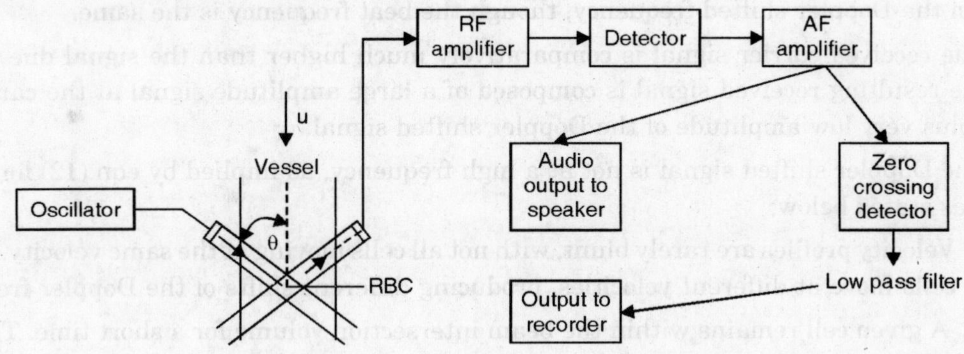

Fig. 3.31

Fig. 3.31 shows the block diagram of a simple continuous wave (CW) Doppler flowmeter. It is required to have a low output impedance for the oscillator so as to drive the low impedance crystal. As a known phenomenon that the crystals are operated at mechanical resonance, where the impedance drops to about 100 Ω. The ultrasonic waves are transmitted to the moving cells, which reflects the Doppler-shifted waves to the receiving transducer. The receiving transducer is identical to the transmitting transducer. The amplified RF (radio frequency) signal at a frequency is given in eqn.(12).

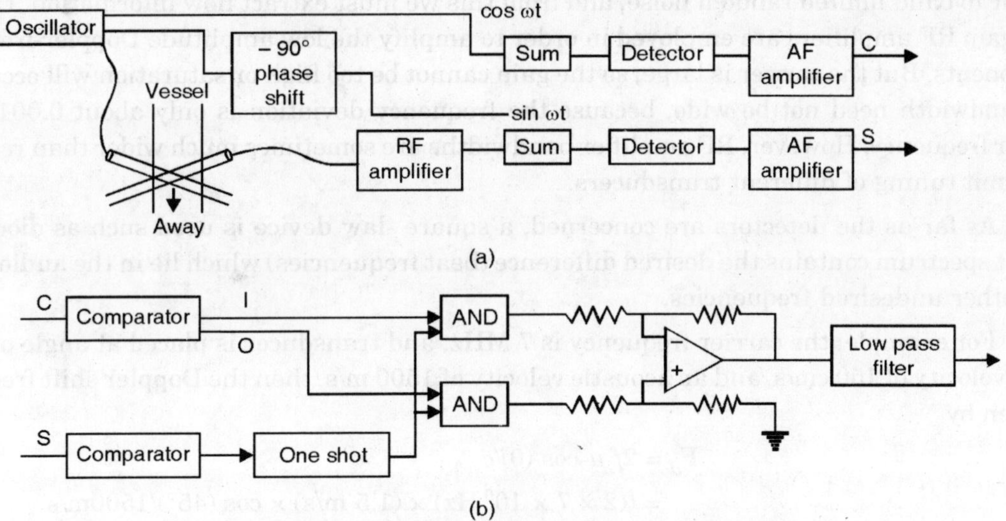

Fig. 3.32. Shows the Directional Doppler Block Diagram.

By hearing the audio output by the use of a speaker, we get much useful qualitative information. A simple frequency to voltage converter circuit is employed to get this qualitative output to a recorder. The zero crossing detector emits a fixed area of pulse each time the audio signal crosses the zero axis. These pulses are low- pass filtered to produce an output proportional to the velocity of the blood cells.

In the case of electro magnetic flowmeter, it is capable of measuring both forward and reverse flow, the simple ultrasonic type flow meter full-wave rectifies the output, and the sense of direction flow is lost. This results because for either an increase or a decrease there is a change in the Doppler shifted frequency, though the beat frequency is the same.

The received carrier signal is comparatively much higher than the signal due Doppler shift. The resulting received signal is composed of a large amplitude signal at the carrier frequency plus very low amplitude of the Doppler shifted signal.

The Doppler shifted signal is not at a high frequency, as implied by eqn.(12) for several reasons as stated below:

1. Velocity profiles are rarely blunt, with not all cells moving at the same velocity. Rather, cells move at different velocities, producing different shifts of the Doppler frequency.
2. A given cell remains within the beam intersection volume for a short time. Thus, the signal received from one cell is a pure frequency multiplied due to time-gate function, resulting in a band of frequencies.
3. Acoustic energy traveling not within the main beam, but at angles to the beam axis, plus energy in the side lobes, causes different Doppler frequency shift due to an effective change in θ.
4. Tumbling of cells and local velocities resulting from turbulence cause different Doppler-frequency shifts.

All these factors combine to produce a band of frequencies. The resulting spectrum is similar to band limited random noise, and from this we must extract flow information. Usually, high gain RF amplifiers are employed in order to amplify the low amplitude Doppler-frequency components. But the carrier is large, so the gain cannot be too high or saturation will occur. The RF bandwidth need not be wide, because the frequency deviation is only about 0.001 of the carrier frequency. However, RF amplifier bandwidths are sometimes much wider than required, to permit tuning of different transducers.

As far as the detectors are concerned, a square -law device is used such as diode. The output spectrum contains the desired difference (beat frequencies) which lie in the audio range, plus other undesired frequencies.

For example, the carrier frequency is 7 MHz, and transducer is placed at angle of 45°, a blood velocity of 150 cm/s, and an acoustic velocity of 1500 m/s, then the Doppler shift frequency is given by

$$F_d = 2f_o u \cos(\theta)/c \qquad \ldots(13)$$

$$= ((2 \times 7 \times 10^6 \text{ Hz}) \times (1.5 \text{ m/s}) \times \cos(45°)/1500\text{m/s}$$

$$= 10 \text{ kHz}.$$

The DC component can be removed by using high pass filter .

In the simple instruments, the AF output drives a power amplifier and speaker earphone. For getting the directional information of the blood flow, directional Doppler block diagram is employed as shown in Fig. 3.32.

(*a*) Quadrature phase sensitive detector is used. Sine and cosine signals at the carrier frequency are summed with a RF output before detection. The output C from the cosine channel then leads (lags) the output S from the sine channel if the flow is away from (or towards) the transducer.

(*b*) The logic circuits in the above figure-32b, route one shot pulses through the top (or bottom) AND gate when the flow is away from or (toward) the transducer. The differential amplifier provides bi-directional output pulses which are then filtered.

This may be understood by much better example:

A better approach is to borrow a technique from a Radar technology, which is used to detect the speed of the aircraft is flying but also its direction. This is the quadrature detection.

As in Fig. 3.32*a*, the analog portion of the qaudrature phase sensitive detector in which the phase shift network splits the carrier into two components that are in quadrature, which means that they are 90° phase shifted signal. These reference cosine and sine waves must be several times larger than the RF amplifier output, as shown in Fig. 3.32*a*. The reference wave and the RF amplifier output are linearly summed to produce the RF envelope shown in figure-33b. We assume that the RF amplifier output contains no carrier.

If the blood flow is in the same direction as the ultrasonic beam, we consider the blood to be flowing away from the transducer as shown in Fig. 3.32*a*. For this direction, the Doppler shift frequency is lower than that of the carrier. The phase of the Doppler wave lags behind that of the reference carrier and the Doppler vector rotates clockwise. In Fig. 3.33*b*, for time 1, the carrier and the Doppler add, producing a larger sum in the cosine channel. The sine channel is unchanged. For time-2, the carrier and the Doppler add, producing a larger sum in the sine channel. Similar reasoning produces the rest of the signals as shown in Fig. 3.33.

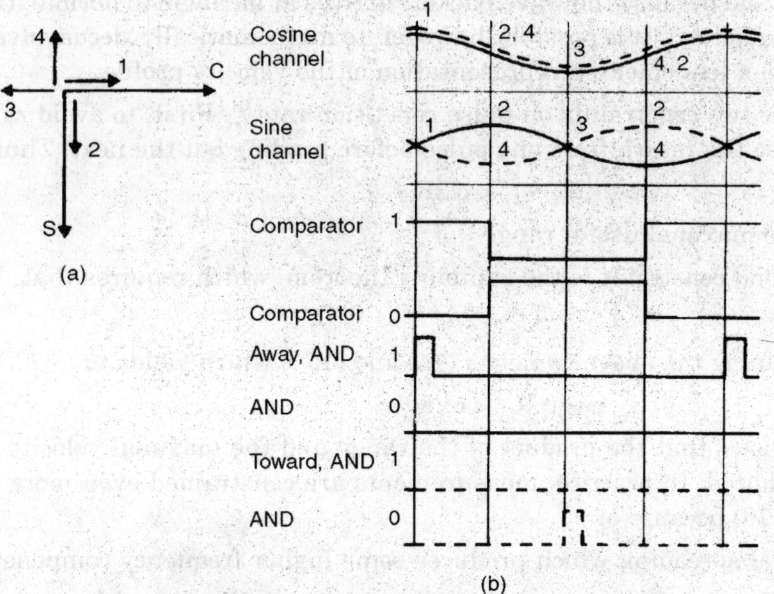

Fig. 3.33. Shows directional doppler signal waveforms.

If the blood flow is towards the transducer, the Doppler frequency is higher than the carrier frequency, and the Doppler vector rotates counterclockwise. This produces the dashed waves shown in Fig. 3.33*b* and phase relation between cosine and channels is reversed. Thus, by examining the sign of the phase, we measure direction of flow. The detector produces AF waves that have the same shape as the RF envelope.

Fig. 3.32*b* shows the logic that detects the signal of the phase. The cosine channel drives a comparator , the digital output of which shown in Fig. 3.33*b*, is used for gating and does not change with the direction of the blood flow. The sine channel triggers a one shot the width of which must be short. Depending on the direction of flow, this one - shot is triggered either at the beginning of or halfway through the period (Fig. 3.33*b*). The AND gates then gate it into the top or bottom input of the differential amplifier, thus producing a bi-directional output.

It is also possible to add another one-shot and several logic blocks to obtain pulse outputs on both positive and negative zero crossings. This doubles the frequency of the pulse train and reduces the fluctuations in the output to 0.707 of their former value.

PULSED DOPPLER

To achieve good range, resolution, it is preferable to use pulsed Doppler than the Continuous wave (CW) Doppler method of flow measurement. The pulse duration should ideally be very short and narrow pulses. To achieve a good Signal to Noise ratio (SNR) and good velocity discrimination, the pulse width should be more. The usual compromise is an 8MHz pulse of 1ms duration, it produces a traveling packet 1.5mm long as shown in Fig. 3.30*d*. The intensity of this packet is convolved with a local velocity profile to produce the received signal. Thus the velocity profile of the blood vessel is smeared to a larger - than - actual value. Because of this problem and because the wave packets arrives at an angle to normal, the location of the vessel valve is indistinct. It is possible, however, to mathematically 'deconvolve' the instrument output to obtain a less smeared representation of the velocity profile.

There are two constraints on pulse repetition rate f_r. First, to avoid range ambiguities, we must analyse the return from one pulse before sending out the next. Thus

$$f_r < c/2R_m \qquad ...(14)$$

where R_m is the maximal useful range.

The second constraint is the sampling theorem, which requires that

$$f_r < 2f_d \qquad ...(15)$$

By combining the above two eqns (14) and (15), which yields to

$$U_m \cos\theta\, R_m < c^2/8f_o \qquad ...(16)$$

Which shows that the product of the range and the maximal velocity along the transducer axis is limited. In practice, measurements are constrained even more than indicted by the above eqn.(16) because of

1. spectral spreading which produces some higher frequency components
2. imperfect cutoff characteristics of the low-pass filters used to prevent aliasing.

Since it is not possible to start and stop the oscillator in 1μs, first stage of the oscillator produces continuous wave. The transmitter and the receiver both uses piezo-electric transducers.

So a gate circuit is provided to turn off the signal from the transmitter during reception. The optimal transmitted signal is a pulse modulated sine wave carrier.

Although it is easy to generate the burst signal at this frequency, it is difficult to transduce this electric burst to a similar acoustic burst. Crystal transducers are suitable since it has got a high Q. The above parameters should be taken care to get accurate measurement.

CARDIAC OUPUT MEASUREMEN|T

Blood flow may be measured in almost any part of the circulatory system by using the blood flow measurement techniques discussed previously. The cardiac output is the quantity of blood delivered by the heart to the aorta per minute. This is a major determinant factor for the quantity of oxygen delivered to the tissue. It is certain that when problems occur in the case of insufficient supply of blood from the heart or unable to meet the demand of the system, then a depression in the cardiac output may result in low blood pressure, reduced tissue oxygenation, acidosis, poor renal function and shock. This is nothing but the reflection of myocardial function and when the measurements in the blood pressure and the central volume pressure is taken, the rationale treatment of cardiac disorders becomes clear. Stroke volume of the blood pumped frcm the heart with each cardiac cycle at rest varies among adults between 70 to 100 ml, while the cardiac output is 40 to 61 per minute.

When blood flow is measured in pulmonary artery or the aorta, this blood flow, integrated over a cardiac cycle, represents the total amount of blood flowing through the heart, This is referred to as the *cardiac output*. The cardiac output may be determined by integrating the results obtained form conventional blood flow measurement at the pulmonary artery or aorta. As this involves critical surgical procedures, cardiac output is more commonly determined using dilution techniques. This dilution technique gives total cardiac output whereas the flow measurement shows the discrete changes in cardiac output over one complete cardiac cycle.

DYE SOLUTION TECHNIQUE

The most commonly used indicator substance is a dye. The use of indocyanine green dye, suggested by Fox and Wood, is usually employed for recording dilution curve, The dilution curve is shown in figure given below. (Fig. 3.34). This dye is preferred since this dye has the property of absorbing light at 800nm. This 800nm region of the spectrum where the reduced and oxygenated haemoglobin have the same optical absorption. Some other dyes such as blue dye can also be used for this purpose. The concentration of cardiogreen can be measured with the help of infra-red photocell transducer. The size of the dye cuvettes is of small volume as 0.01ml.

The injection of dye into the right atrium is by means of venous catheter. Initially, 5 mg cardiogreen dye is injected in a 1ml volume. For children, the quantity may be 2.5 mg. A motor driven syringe draws blood constantly form the radial artery thorugh a cuvette. The curve is traced by a recorder attached to the densitometer. Once the curve is drawn, the dye is flushed out from the circulating blood by injecting saline into the system.

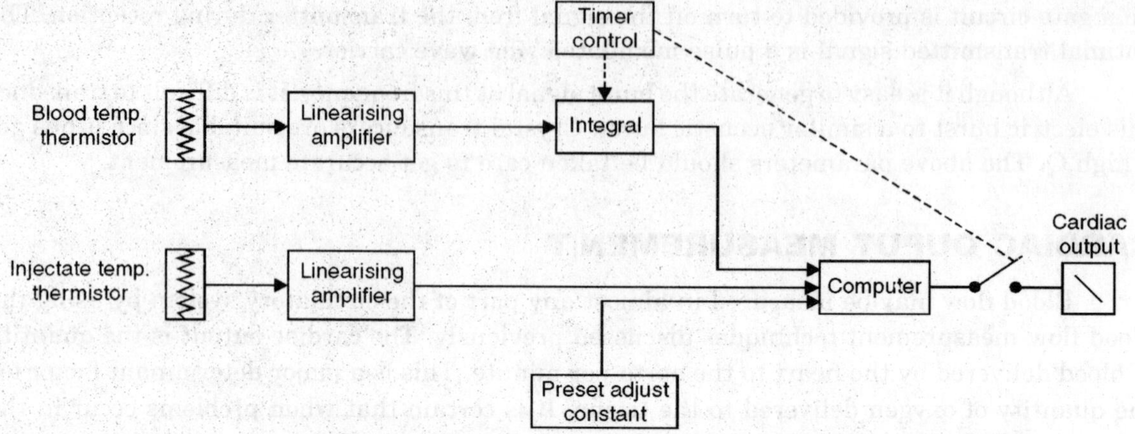

Fig. 3.34. Shows the block diagram of the processing and computing circuit of thermal dilution method.

The photometric part consists of a radiation source and a photocell and an arrangement for holding the disposable polyethylene tube constituting the cuvette. An interference filter is employed here. Its peak transmission capacity is 805 nm, so as to permit only infrared radiation which is the range of interest of transmitting region. This wavelength is isobestic wavelength for hemoglobin at various levels of oxygen saturation. The formation of bubbles may be avoided, by flushing out the cuvette tubing with a solution of silicone in ether initially.

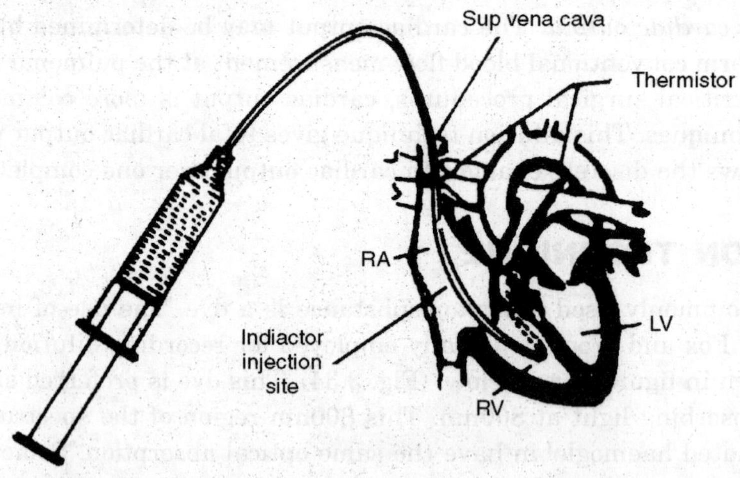

Fig. 3.34a. Shows the cardiac output thermal-dilution set-up.

A flow rate of 40 ml/min is preferred in order to get as short a response time as possible for the sampling catheter. The sampling syringe has the volume of 50ml/min. The output of the photocell is connected to a low drift amplifier. This amplifier has got a high input impedance and low output impedance. The amplification factor is directly proportional to the resistance value of the potentiometer **R.** A potentiometric recorder records the amplifier signal on 200 mm wide recording paper, and a paper speed of 10mm.sec.

The Stewart-Hamilton dye solution technique involves introduction of a known volume of dye into the superior vena cava vessels via the arms. Withdrawals of samples of the blood/

dye mixture are from the aorta via the catheter. The dilution of dye contained in these samples is determined with a densitometer. This is shown in figure given in Figure 3.35. Modern dye solution techniques use radioisotopes instead of dye. Counters are used instead of densitometers. The output from the densitometer or counter is coupled to an analog computer which computes cardiac output directly. Cardiac output in an adult male is approximately 500 cubic centimeters per minute.

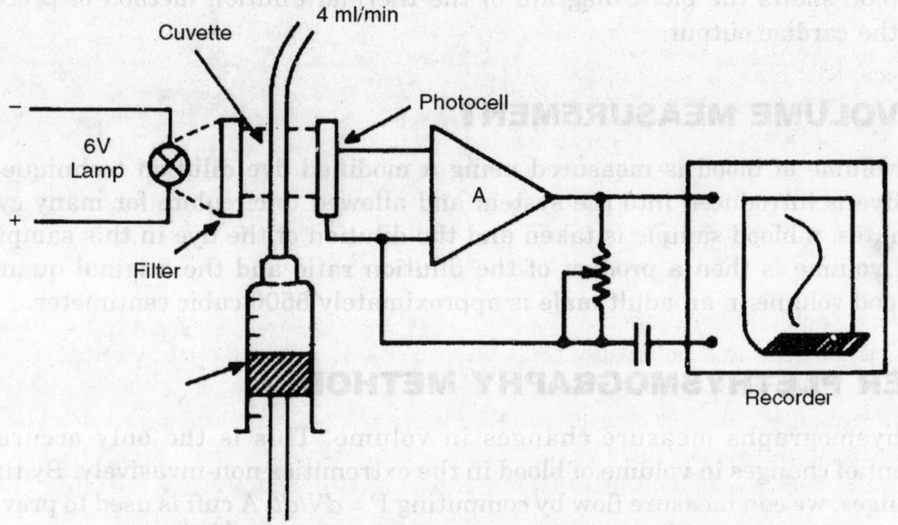

Fig. 3.35a. Shows the Diagrammatic representation of a densitometer for quantitative measurement of dye concentration.

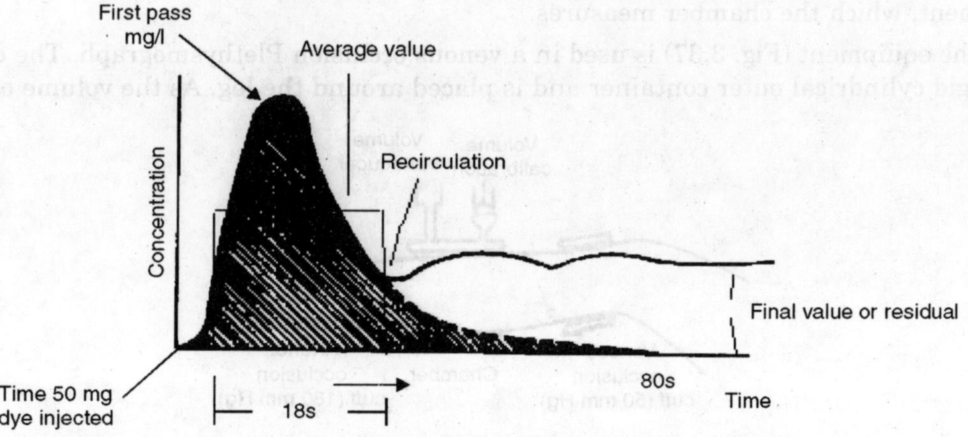

Fig. 3.35b. Shows the dye dilution curve.

Fig. 3.35 shows the densitometer for quantitative measurement of dye concentration for measuring the cardiac output.

Example. The mean concentration of dye in blood was 36.2 mg/litre during the I pass of 18 seconds. The dye injected at $t = 0$ was 50 mg. The final value of dye after (> 80 s) was 15.5 mg/l, Find the blood volume and the cardiac output.

Ans. The Ist pass is 18 seconds.

Mean concentration for 18 s = 36.2 mg/l

Mean concentration per min = 36.2 × 18/60 = 11.4

Cardiac output per min = 50./11.4 = 4.38 lit.

End tail is 15.5 mg/l. So, blood volume = 50/15.5 = 3.2 lit.

Fig. 3.36 shows the block diagram of the thermal dilution method of processing and computing the cardiac output.

BLOOD VOLUME MEASUREMENT

The volume of blood is measured using a modified dye dilution technique. A known amount of dye is introduced into the system and allowed to circulate for many cycles. After several minutes, a blood sample is taken and the dilution of the dye in this sample is noted. Total blood volume is then a product of the dilution ratio and the original quantity of dye injected. Blood volume in an adult male is approximately 5500 cubic centimeter.

CHAMBER PLETHYSMOGRAPHY METHOD

Plethysmographs measure changes in volume. This is the only accurate way of measurement of changes in volume of blood in the extremities non-invasively. By timing these volume changes, we can measure flow by computing $F = dV/dt$. A cuff is used to prevent venous blood from leaving the limb. Hence the name venous occlusion plethysmography.

Fig. 3.37*a* shows the Chamber Plethysmograph, Here, the venous occlusion cuff is inflated to 50mm Hg, stopping venous return. Arterial flow causes the flow to increase in volume of the leg segment, which the chamber measures.

The equipment (Fig. 3.37) is used in a venous occlusion Plethysmograph. The chamber has a rigid cylindrical outer container and is placed around the leg. As the volume of the leg

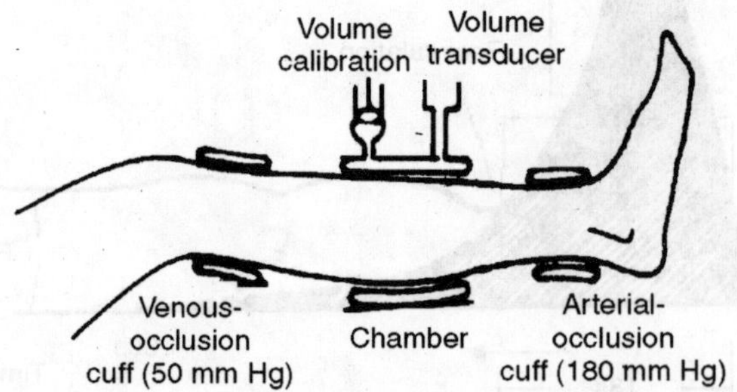

Fig. 3.37a

increases, the leg squeezes some type of bladder and decreases its volume. If the bladder is filled with water, the changes in the volume may be observed by measuring the rise in the water level. For recording purposes, some air may be introduced above the water level and the change in air pressure measured. Water-filled Plethysmographs are temperature controlled to prevent thermal drifts. Because of the hydrostatic pressure, they may constrict the vessels in the limb and cause undesirable physiological changes. Fig. 3.37*b* shows the sequences of operation of the plethysmograph equipment in measuring the blood flow.

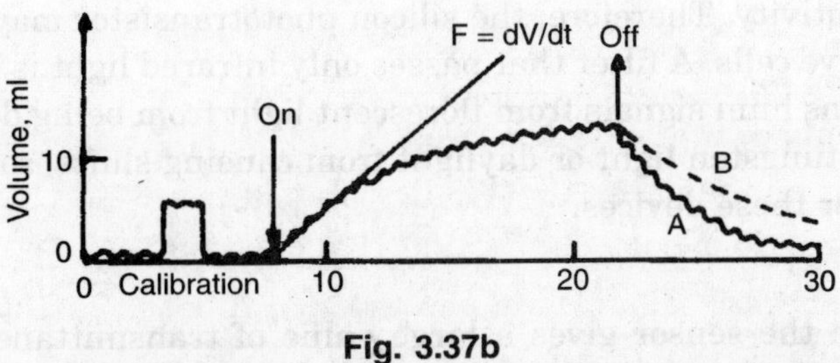

Fig. 3.37b

Air may be used in the bladder and the resulting changes in pressure measured directly. Some systems do not use bladder. They seal the ends of a rigid chamber to the limb, but then leaks may be a problem. One device uses a pneumatic -tachometer to measure the fow of air into and out of the chamber. This flow is then integrated to yield changes in volume.

PHOTOPLETHYSMOGRAPHY

This is another and advanced technique for measuring the blood volume seen in Fig. 3.9. Light can be transmitted enough through the capillary bed, the changes in volume of vessels modify the absorption, reflection, and scattering of light. Although photoplethysmogrphy is simple and indicates the timing of event such as heart rate, it provides a poor measure of changes in volume. Also, it is sensitive to motion artifact.

LIGHT SOURCES

Fig. 3.38 shows the photoplethysmogrphic method of measuring the blood volume. Here, the sources generate light that is transmitted through the tissue. A miniature tungsten lamp may be used as the light source, but the heat generated causes vasodilation, which alters the system being measured. Alternatively, a GaAsLed may be used which produces a narrow band source with a peak spectral emission at a wavelength of 940 nm.

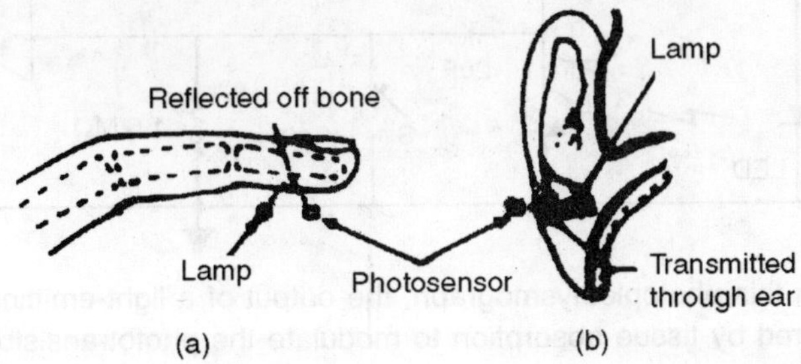

Fig. 3.38. (a) Light transmitted into the finger pad is relfected off bone and detected by a photosensor. (b) Light transmitted through the aural pinna is detected by a photosensor.

Photosensors

Photoconductive sensor cells have been used as sensors, but this is bulky and it is necessary to use a filter to restrict the sensitivity of the sensor to the near infra red region so that changes in blood O_2 content that are of prominence in the visible light region will not causes changes in sensitivity. Therefore, the silicon phototransistor may be used which is not bulky as photoconductive cells. A filter that passes only infrared light is helpful for all types of sensors to prevent mains hum signals from florescent light from being detected, This does not prevent DC light from tungsten light or daylight from causing shifts, so lightproof enclosures are usually provided for these devices.

Circuits

The output form the sensor gives a large value of transmittance modulated by very small changes due to pulsations of blood. To avoid the large baseline value, frequencies above 0.05Hz are passed through a high-pass filter. The resulting signal is greatly amplified to give sufficiently large waveform. Any movement of the photoplethysmograph relative to the tissue causes a change in the baseline transmittance that is many times larger than the pulsation signal. These large artifacts due to motion saturate the amplifier; thus it is necessary to save the output faster.

The design of complete circuit for a solid state photoplethysmogrph is given below.

A typical LED requires a forward current of 15 mA. Using a 15V supply, it would require a series resistor of

$$R_i = V/I = 15/0.015 = 1\ K\Omega$$

A typical phototransistor passes a maximum of 150 μA.

To avoid saturation, $R_p = V/I = 15/0.15 = 100\ K\ \Omega$.

The paper capacitor of 2 μF is used. To get 0.05 Hz low pass response,

The output resistor $R_o = 1/2\pi f_o C = 1/(2\pi\ (0.05)(2 \times 10^{-6})) = 1.6\ M\Omega$.

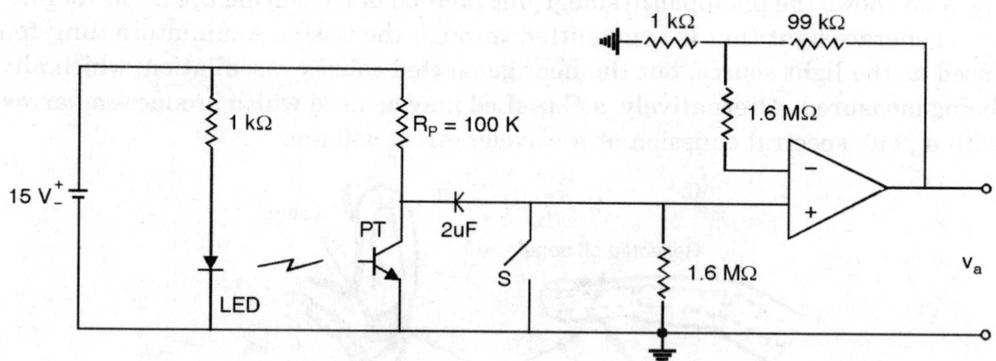

Fig. 3.39. In this photoplethysmograph, the output of a light-emitting diode is altered by tissue absorption to modulate the phototransistor.

Fig. 3.39 shows the circuit diagram of the photoplethysmographic instrument.

APPLICATIONS

When a patient is at rest, the photo-plethyysmograpgh can measure the heart rate. It offers an advantage in that it responds to the pumping action of the heart. When it is properly shielded it is unaffected by the use of electrosurgery, which usually disables the ECG.

Chapter 4

Electroencephalogram

THE BRAIN AND THE CENTRAL NERVOUS SYSTEM

In other chapters, we have discussed about the muscle action and the potential associated with the peripheral and motor, and sensory nervous system. In this chapter, the sensory nerves in connection with the brain are going to be the main cause of our Encephalography. Strictly speaking, most of these nerves connect to spinal nerves in the spinal cord and these spinal nerves carry information to and from the brain.

As we know, all the nerve cells are located throughout the body. These nerves carry information between all body locations. Most of the nerve cells are located in the brain and in the spinal cord. The cell comprising the spinal cord and the brain are similar; the cell body is known as *soma* and surrounding a region is called nucleus.

The cell body has an extension known as *axon*. This axon may comprise part of the spinal cord and interconnect with sensory and motor nerves or may branch into many small fibers known as the terminal arborizations of the axon. Brain cells consist also of projections of the cell

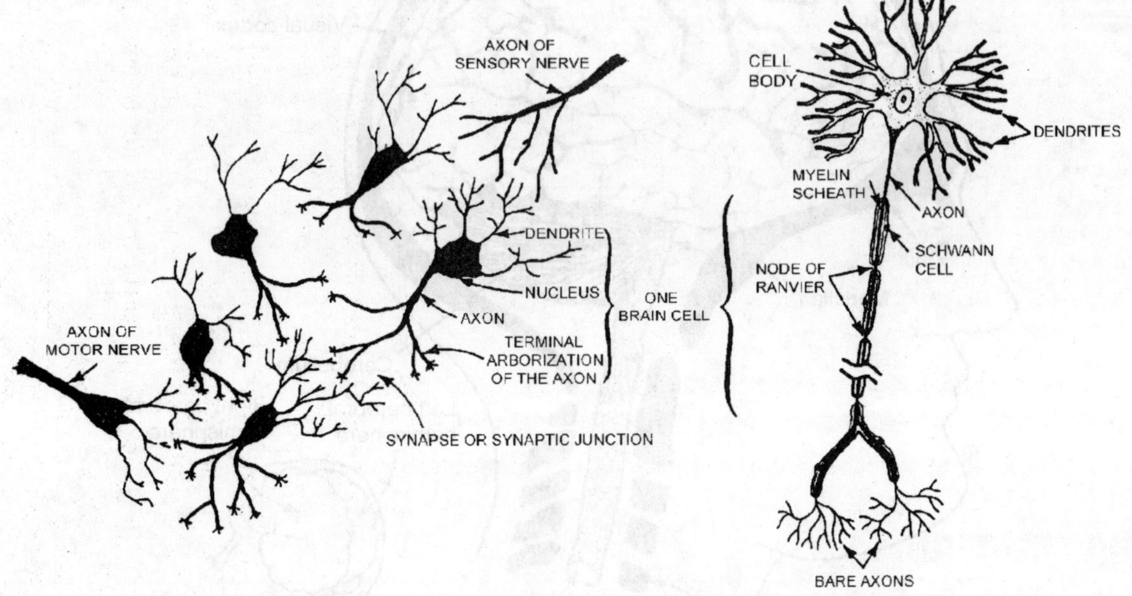

Fig. 4.1. Shows the simplified Brain cell-interconnection.

body known as the dendrite which sense the information from adjoining cells. The terminal arborizations transmit information to adjoining cells either directly in spinal cells or via the dendrite in brain cells. These cell interconnections called Synaptic junctions or simply as the synapse, allow electrical impulses to flow throughout the brain and the central nerve system; one cell acting as a trigger to influence the neighboring cells. Fig. 4.1 shows the brain cell interconnection.

The mechanism by which the information is carried is extremely a complex mechanism. As discussed in Chapter 1, the migration of potassium and sodium ions is a primary factor. However, there are many other chemical interchanges involved, but as far as our aim is concerned, we will discuss only the electrical phenomena of the nervous system. It must be emphasized, that we measure the electrical activity only because of its convenience; it is not the fundamental form of nervous activity.

THE BRAIN AND ITS PARTS

It is true that the brain is a complex structure. It comprises of a very large number of cells. These cells are interconnected among themselves and which also receive data from the various sensory

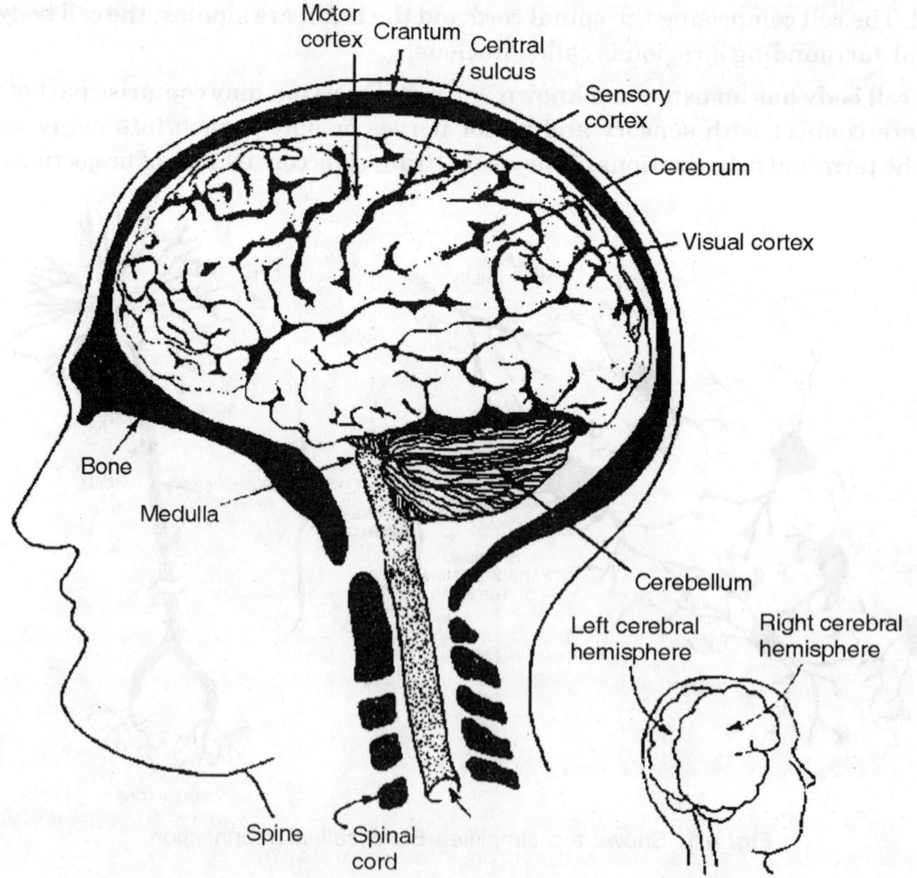

Fig. 4.2. Shows the anatomical sections of the brain.

organs. In one sense, it can be called as supervisory control unit. The brain can override most reflexes and direct the body to act in a coordinated manner. Until recently, it was thought that most of the functions of the brain resulted form the interaction of nervous impulses at the synapse of the cells and many analogies with digital electronic computers were formulated. It is now known that this is only part of the story. For example, the substance in which the cells are embodied, the *neuroglia* (from a Greek word meaning glue), is known to play an important part in brain function and may be vitally concerned with memory. It is thought that oscillatory electrochemical mechanisms are responsible for short term memory but that these impulses gradually modify the chemical structures of parts of the brain, so that the permanent storage of information is chemical rather than electrical.

Anatomically, the brain is divided into several parts as shown in Fig. 4.2. When sectioned along the midline, the appearance is as shown in Fig. 4.3. Generally speaking, the deeper structures of the brain , that is nearest to the spinal cord, are most responsible for the human behavior (anger, fear etc.). These are easily controllable. The cortex (outer structure) is the part of the brain which is highly developed in man and which has enabled him to dominate all other species.

Some areas of the cortex serve specific parts of the body. For example, in Fig. 4.2, the sensory input is handled in the area marked sensory cortex while motor output proceeds from the motor cortex. Likewise, vision is handled at the rear of the brain in the visual cortex. It is less easy to define the areas which serve intellectual functions although the frontal areas are partly responsible. There is a large bundle of fibers which interconnect the left and right hemisphere; this is known as the corpus callosum and its location can be seen in Fig. 4.3.

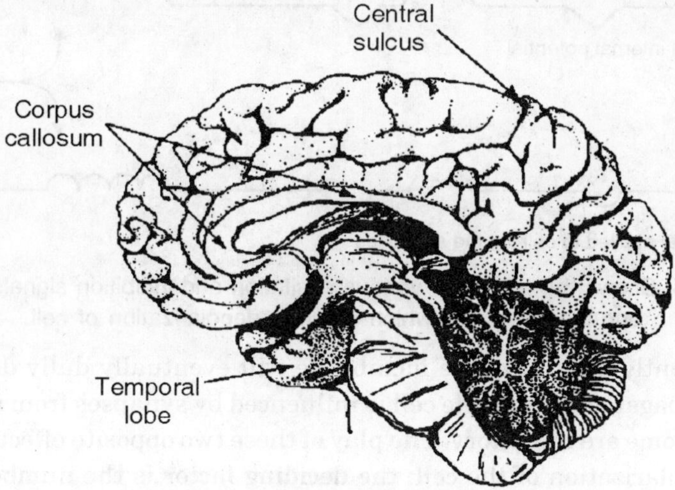

Fig. 4.3. Shows the cross-sectional view of the brain.

CELL POTENTIALS AND ACTION

The properties of excitation and inhibition are however, highly conjectural. These give only part of the story. There is no general scientific agreement on the subject.

As given to chapter 1, the cells were referred to bi-stable devices existing in only two states; a polarized state of – 90 mV and a depolarized state of +20 mV. Intermediate potentials a were regarded as having a little significance. Nerve cells in the central nervous system and the brain exist in a polarized state of between – 70 mV and – 110 mV. The exact cell potential within this range appears to be significant as it determines the cell's vulnerability to a stimulus that would result in regenerative breakdown.

Assume that a group of cells producing zero activity; the cells within this group would rest at the normal polarized level of – 90 millivolts. Assuming that one cell is depolarized from an external stimulus, this depolarization will affect the adjoining cells via synapses, causing a change in the resting potential of these adjoining cells. The effect of these adjoining cells may be either to raise or to lower their resting potential depending on the type of fiber involved in the synaptic junction. If the resting potential is increased, the breakdown of the cell membrane will not occur and the impulses can be thought of as having had an inhibitory effect. If the impulse arriving at this synapse decreases the resting potential, then the cell is more susceptible to depolarization and the impulse can be thought of as having had an excitatory effect. With repeated excitatory

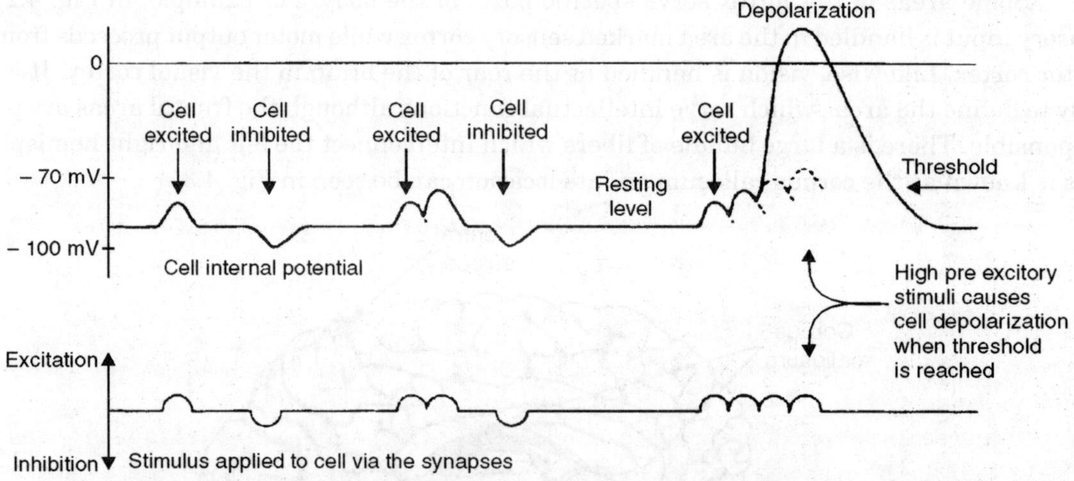

Fig. 4.4. Shows the effects of various excitation and inhibition signals on any one individual cell which result in depolarization of cell.

stimuli at a sufficiently high rate, the membrane will eventually dully depolarize and a new impulse will be propagated. Any single cell is influenced by synapses from any other cells; some are excitatory and some are inhibitory. The play of these two opposite effects on any area may or may not cause depolarization of the cell; the deciding factor is the number of impulses being received per unit time and the balance between excitation and inhibition. Although the effect at a synapse of any sub-threshold impulses dies away rapidly, it does not die away immediately. This allows almost coincident impulses from different sources to build up their effect; thus frequency becomes an important parameter. Fig. 4.4 shows the effects of various excitation and inhibition signals on any one individual cell which result in depolarization of cell once the – 70 mV threshold is obtained.

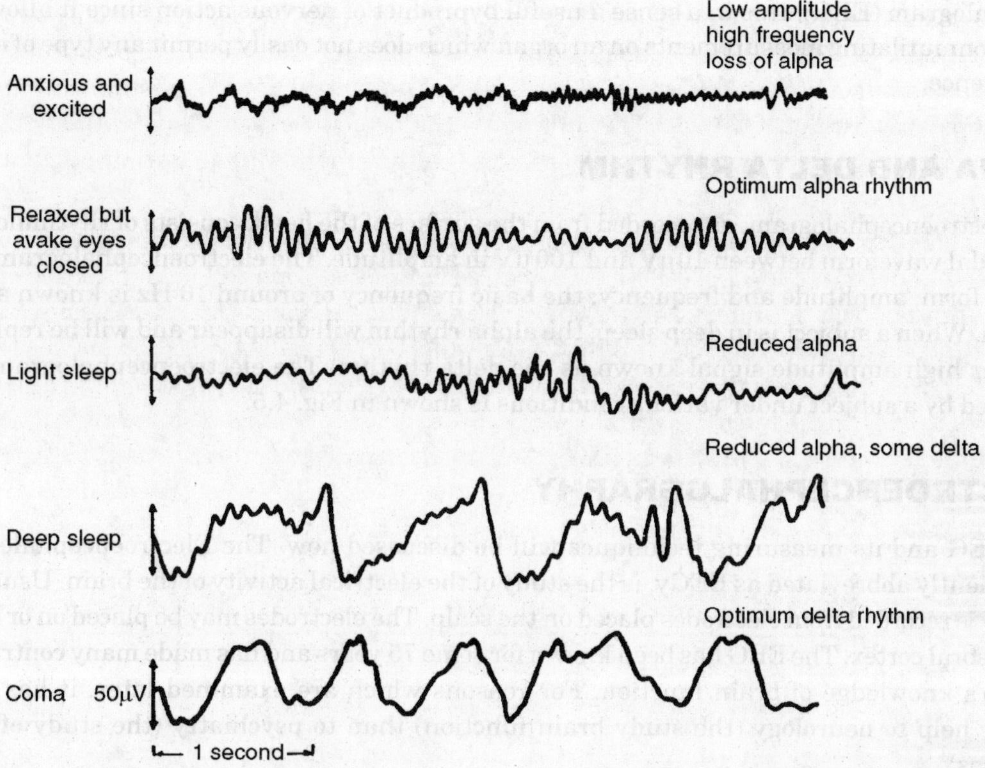

Fig. 4.5. Shows the physiological states and the resultant electroencephalogram (EEG).

PRODUCING EVOKED POTENTIALS

As shown in Fig. 4.2, parts of the surface of the brain have been found to be associated with various sensory systems. When an appropriate stimuli is applied to a sense receptor, the corresponding sensory area of the brain responds by producing an electric potential known as the evoked potential. The evoked potential, as it appears at the surface of the brain, is the integrative result from the action of many cells. When this evoked potential is recorded externally, on the scalp, the output signal will be in the order of 10 μV or so. It is not yet known completely which cortical elements are responsible for these evoked potentials. Often they are camouflaged by the electroencephalogram, thus it may be necessary to remove the electroencephalogram by an averaging technique when attempting to record the evoked potential, which will be discussed later.

THE ELECTROENCEPHALOGRAM (EEG)

As we discussed earlier, the brain can be regarded as a highly developed biochemical factory. The electrical activity which results from so much of chemical change is known as the electroencephalogram (EEG). It is in a sense a useful byproduct of nervous action since it allows us to make nonmutilating measurements on an organ which does not easily permit any type of external interference.

ALPHA AND DELTA RHYTHM

The Electroencephalogram, as recorded from the surface of the head, consists of rhythmical, slow sinusoidal waveform between 10 μV and 100 μV in amplitude. The electroencephalogram, varies in both form, amplitude and frequency; the basic frequency of around 10 Hz is known as alpha rhythm. When a subject is in deep sleep, the alpha rhythm will disappear and will be replaced by a slower high amplitude signal known as the delta rhythm. The electroencephalogram (EEG) produced by a subject under various conditions is shown in Fig. 4.5.

ELECTROENCEPHALOGRAPHY

The EEG and its measuring techniques will be discussed now. The Electroencephalography, conveniently abbreviated as EEGy, is the study of the electrical activity of the brain. Usually this activity is recorded from electrodes placed on the scalp. The electrodes may be placed on or beneath the cerebral cortex. The EEG has been known for some 75 years and has made many contributions to man's knowledge of brain function. For reasons which are examined later, it has been of greater help to neurology (the study brain function) than to psychiatry (the study of mental processes).

THE CHARACTERISTICS OF THE NORMAL EEG

The EEG of a normal adult human, normal being used in the everyday sense of the word, is relatively easily described. When the subject is relaxed, but not drowsy, a relatively smooth oscillation, whose frequency is seldom less than 8 Hz or more than 13Hz can be recorded from the area of scalp immediately over the occipital lobes. Typically this oscillation, the a rhythm, has an amplitude of 50 μV peak to peak, although in rare subjects it may be twice this amplitude and in about 10% of the population it is absent or very small. This rhythm is responsive to mental activity; in most subjects attempting a task such as mental arithmetic will attenuate or abolish it.

Most EEGs are recorded using multi-channel ink writing oscillographs, as shown in Fig. 4.6. These are widely available for the physiologists. Some more sophisticated. frequency information is particularly significant since the basic frequency of the EEG varies with different behavioral states. For analyzing the EEG signals, the normal frequency range of EEG has been sub- divided into five bands. These five bands are below.

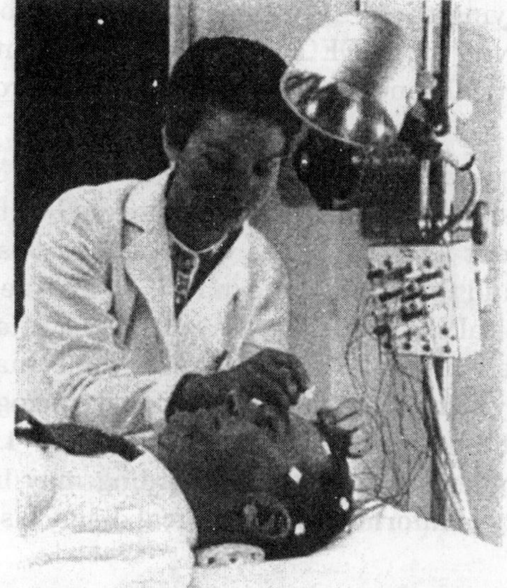

(a) Electrodes are applied to the scalp and plugged into the junction box.

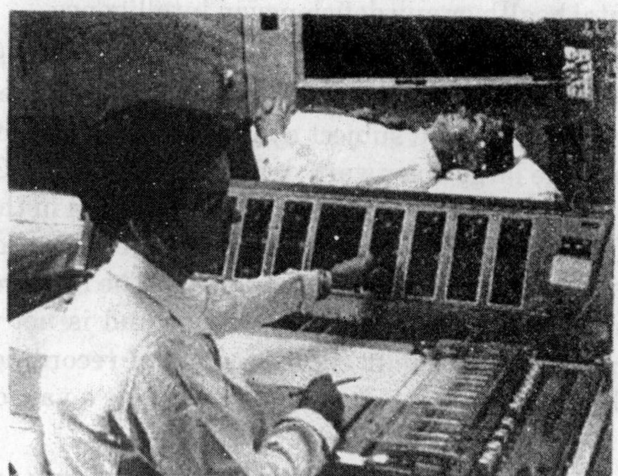

(b) A switch selector allows the desired electrode configuration to be chosen.

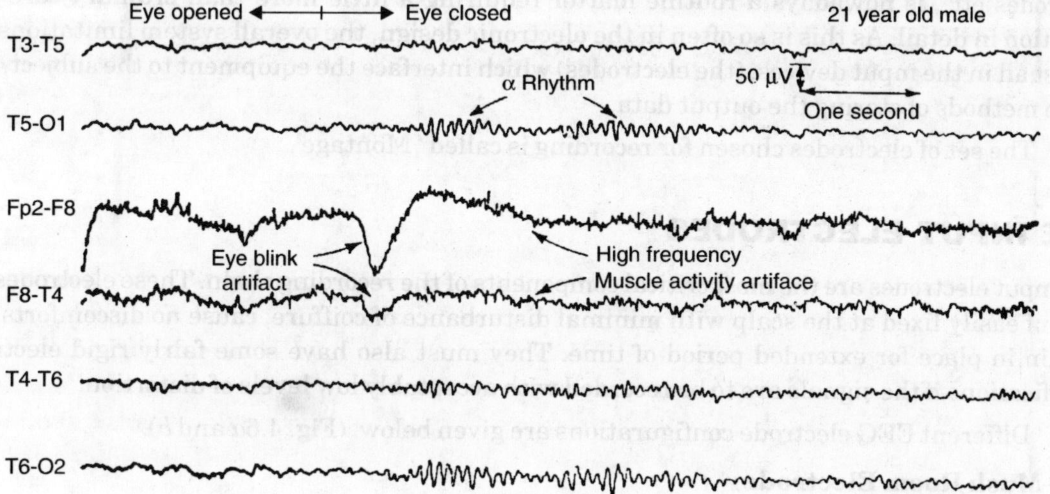

(c) A segment of the record obtained showing six of the sixteen channels recorded.

Fig. 4.6. Shows a typical EEG waveform for a normal adult subject.

Name of the Rhythm	Frequency Range
Delta (δ)	0.5 Hz–4 Hz
Theta (θ)	4 Hz–8 Hz
Alpha (α)	8 Hz–13 Hz
Beta (β)	13 Hz–22 Hz
Gamma (γ)	22Hz–30 Hz

Various techniques have been followed for displaying these EEG signals which will be discussed later. The a rhythm is the most prominent activity in the EEG of healthy adults. But, the a rhythm is not found in very young children and its absence does not indicate a lack of mental health or any deficiency in intelligence.

A segment of an EEG record from a normal subject (adult male) is shown in Fig. 4.6. Six of the 16 channels are commonly used to record the EEG signal. The tracing is read from left to right. Initially, the subject eye's were open but after about 2.5 seconds, he was asked to close them. The large downward deflection in leads FP2 – F8 and the smaller one in F8 – T4 are the " eye blink artifact". The a rhythm can be seen in the occipital channels T5 – 01 and T6 – 02 after the eyes were closed. Although the subject was completely normal, the a rhythm is somewhat smaller and less persistent than usual. The high frequency component in the two middle tracings is an artifact due to muscle activity and is not form the brain. The EEG shown in Fig. 4.6 represents only about eight seconds of recording. However, in practice, a recording may be maintained for an hour or more producing a vast quantity of information for clinical diagnosis.

THE ELECTRODE CONFIGURATION–'MONTAGE'

For an engineering point of view, the design of an EEG instrument and its accessories such as electrodes etc., is nowadays a routine matter requiring a little more than ordinary care and attention in detail. As this is so often in the electronic design, the overall system limitations are almost all in the input devices, (the electrodes) which interface the equipment to the subject, and in the methods of storing the output data.

The set of electrodes chosen for recording is called ' Montage'.

THE INPUT ELECTRODES

The Input electrodes are the most critical components of the recording chain. These electrodes are to be of easily fixed at the scalp with minimal disturbance of coiffure, cause no discomforts and remain in place for extended period of time. They must also have some fairly rigid electrical specifications if the signals are to be recorded with acceptably low levels of distortion.

Different EEG electrode configurations are given below. (Fig. 4.6*a* and *b*).

EEG Mush Room Electrode

- Made of silver alloy.
- They are slipped underneath perforated rubber bands.
- Easy to clean.
- Can be connected with leads by means of small spring contact plugs.
- Z- electrodes is a modification of this and
- Do not require perforations - the rubber band.

EEG Club Shaped Pad Electrode

- fitted with a Perspex or a plastic holder

- the contact surface of the electrode is wrapped in cotton wool or funnel and soaked in saline
- Chloriding the electrodes reduces interfacing polarization effects
- Resistance between electrode and skin must be reduced by conducting medium. R < 5 kΩ or better.
- Use acetone for removing sebum.

EEG Adhesive Electrode

- 5 mm curved silver disc- center perforation admits the point of a glass rod by which it can be sealed to the skin until collodion gets dry. Or it allows spraying through the electrode paste.
- Scrap the skin with needle.

Advantage—Useful for restless patients.

Disadvantage—Position cannot be changed.

Needle

Stainless steel or silver alloy-pushed into scalp . (sterilized and kept in alcohol).

Contact resistance-high

It may give a 'stabling sensation'.

'Suction Electrodes

- fixing and removal is easy

Pharyngeal Electrodes

- S shaped insulated thick silver wire with a bare knob like tip.
- Introduced through the nose 15 cm long, 12 cm curvature.
- Superior to scalp electrodes for recording the basal activity of the temporal lobe.- used
- Pans swallowing movement causes artifacts.
- Breathing disturbances.

Tymponanic Electrode

- Shorter than the above type.
- No curvature
- Tip is covered with soaked pad
- Inserted into external meatus.

Spheriodal Electrodes

- Injection needle 5 cm long varnish insulated has a point bare at end.
- Inserted immediately below zygomatic arch

Cortical electrodes, Depth electrodes and IBM electrodes are some of the electrodes used in EEG measurements.

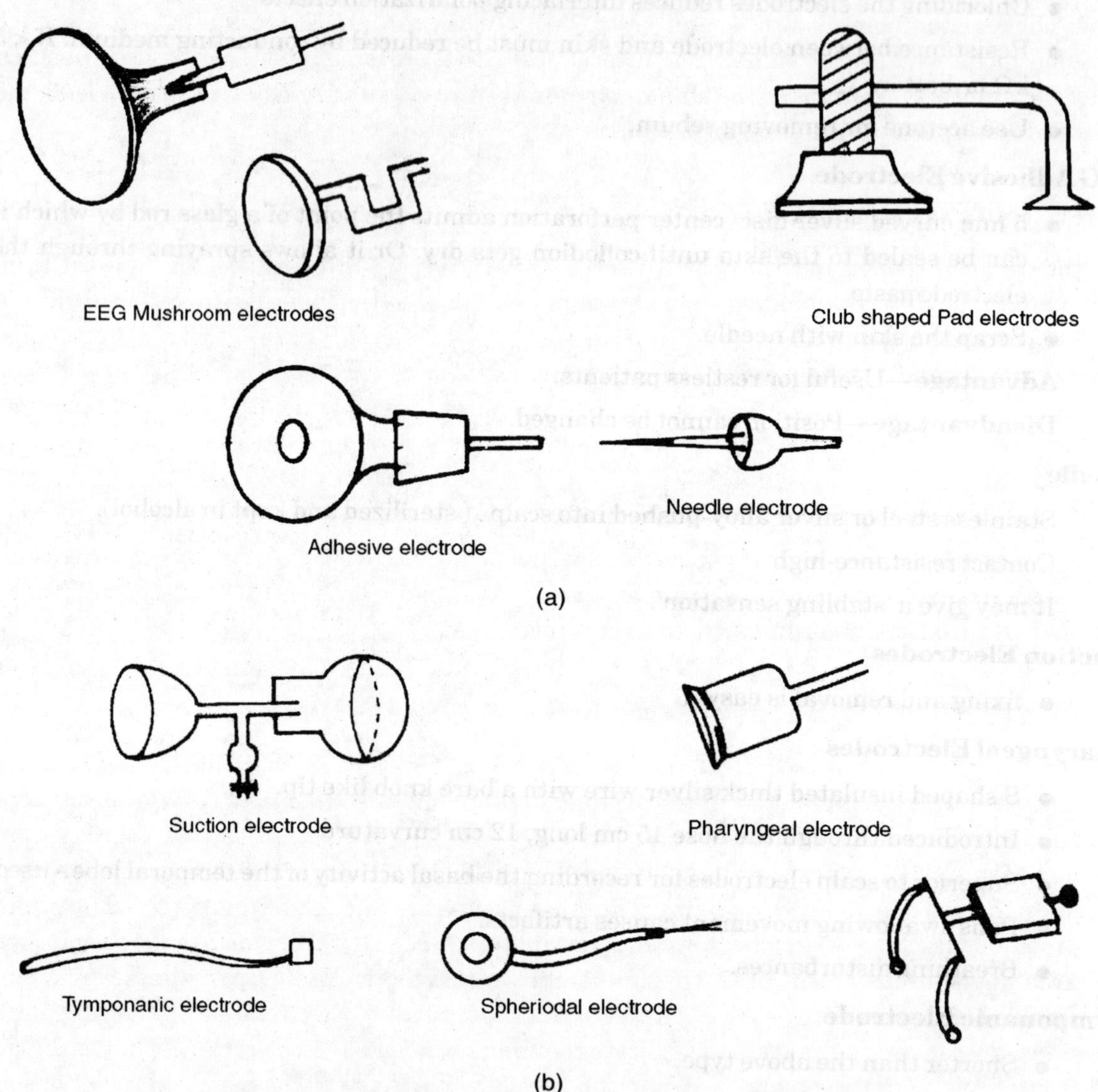

Fig. 4.6a and b. Shows different EEG electrode configurations.

The amplitude of an EEG signal is μVolts level in general. It should be noted that the signal arising is not from the scalp but form the cerebral cortex which is separated from a scalp by the cerebral spinal fluid and by the skull. Parenthetically, we should note that the engineers often suppose the skull to be insulator because they usually see it dried and mounted. The living brain, however, is encased in living bone, which is well permeated with conducting fluid. The amplifying system thus sees signals which arise in generators which have large, complex and variable source impedances. There may be large offset electrode potentials of the order on many millivolts developed between the electrode and the scalp unless a suitable electrode material is used. The high common-mode rejection ratio (CMRR) of the modern EEG amplifier will cancel the common mode part of this signal. But in practice, small movements of the subject's head can cause substantial variations in the standing potential and if these are different in each lead, they will of course appear as differential signals.

LINE INTERFERENCE

Another problem arising in EEG recording is the presence of line interference. This due to the fact that many of the clinical equipments are almost line operated equipments and there are substantial electrical and magnetic fields at the line frequency. The CMRR of the amplifier can, in principle, reduce these signals to insignificance, but only if the entire system, including the electrode impedances, is balanced with respect to ground (common) point of the amplifier. Thus electrode resistance must be reduced as low as possible; with good technique inter-electrode resistance of the order of 1-2 kΩ can be obtained. By using a shielding cage is an alternative technique to reduce the effect of line frequency interference.

Even this technique is not generally satisfactory since the degree of physical isolation it entails can be an emotionally upsetting experience, especially for a child. A relaxed subject is a necessity if good EEG recordings are to be obtained.

ELECTRODE CONSTRUCTION AND CONNECTIONS

The most widely used electrodes are small silver pads electrolytically coated with silver chloride and attached to the scalp with a quick drying adhesive, usually collodion. A harness of rubber straps is also often used to hold the electrodes in place. The scalp area is to be degreased and cleaned with alcohol before the electrodes are placed. Also, the surface resistance should be reduced by the use of a conducting paint. These electrodes are enough for most recordings in the range of 1-60 Hz. If, however, the low frequency limit is to be extended, which is the case in some research applications of the EEG, then electrodes which more closely approximate truly non-polarizable electrodes, such as Ag/AgCl electrodes must be used. Electrodes are generally placed at standard locations on the scalp to facilitate communication between electroencephalographers. These positions, with their usual designations, are shown in Fig. 4.7. The usual abbreviations are as under:

F	—	Frontal
T	—	Temporal
C	—	Central
P	—	Parietal
O	—	Occipital

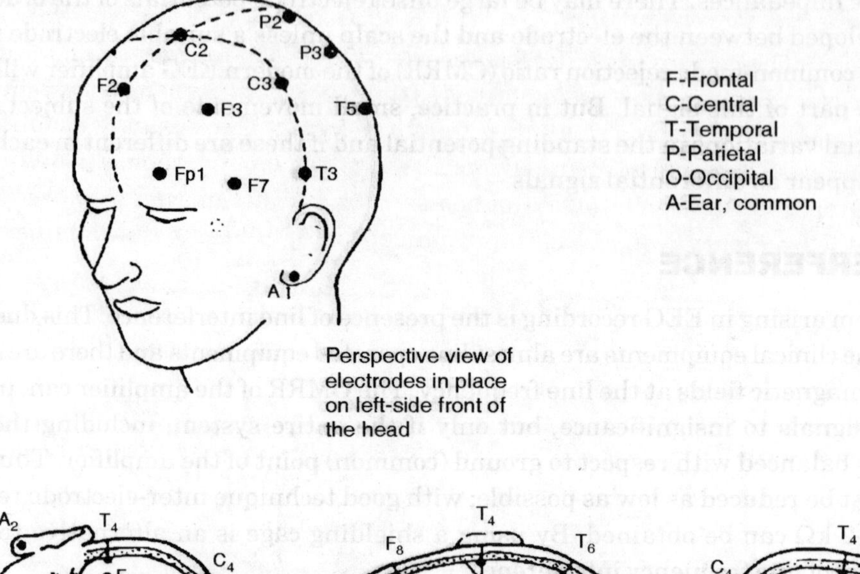

Fig. 4.7. Shows the EEG electrode positions.

EEG RECORDING INSTRUMENTS

Multi-channel, ink-writing oscillographs are generally used for recording of EEG signals. The recording material is relatively cheap. Also, the record is available for inspection as it is being written, the electroencephalographer can quickly flip through a long recording. And it is possible to obtain an "eyeball" impression of its contents. Other media of EEG recording is the use of magnetic tapes, but this is not very popular and it is being used seldom in practice. If visual analysis is to be supplanted by computer or other automated data-processing techniques, then the written record must be supplemented by a magnetic recording or a curve reader (e.g., the multi channel high speed curve reader described by Barlow in 1968) must be used. A graphics tablet or scanner cum software can do the work with some difficulty. The frequency response of most EEG recorders is limited to 60 Hz, but this adequate for most clinical purposes.

MULTI-CHANNEL

EEG recording systems are usually self-contained units consisting of electrode switching networks, high gain differential amplifiers and graphic recorders. Multi-channel recording is almost invariably used, the number of channels ranging between 6 and 32 with 8 or 16 channels being the numbers preferred for routine work.

Multiplicity of electrodes are affixed to the scalp while EEG recording is done as shown in Fig. 4.7, and the recording channels are connected to them via a switching network. The amplifiers are (Fig. 4.7*b*) designed invariably to accept differential inputs. The design is usually optimized for low noise and good common-mode rejection. The low frequency response usually extends to about 0.1 Hz. Of course, the high frequency response is limited to somewhere between 60 Hz and 100 Hz, due to the frequency response of the graphic recorder following the amplifier.

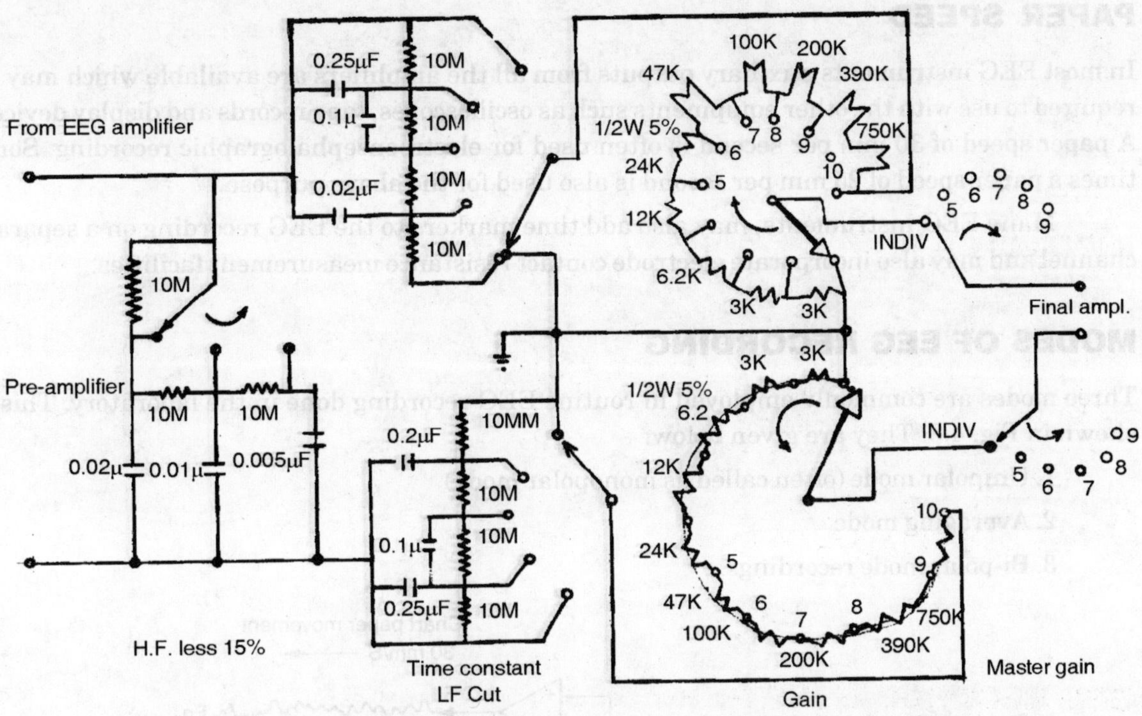

Fig. 4.7b. Shows a typical EEG circuit with lead selector and gain control.

LINE FREQUENCY FILTER

Since the EEG activity occurs below 50 Hz, a notch filter tuned to line frequency is often included in EEG instruments to minimize line frequency interference. But its use is strongly discouraged except as a last resort.

SENSITIVITY OF THE EEG INSTRUMENTS

The gain of the most modern EEG instruments is stable to within a few percent, a 50 µV square-wave calibrator may be included in the instrument. Although the sensitivity of the amplifier may be adjusted to suit particular subjects, the electroencephalographer rarely changes the sensitivity during the recording of an EEG. He usually selects a gain that makes the initial record "look right" and uses the same gain throughout all phases of recording. Since the electro-encephalographer is concerned with relative amplitudes between the channels, it is necessary that each channel has the same sensitivity. It is desirable to standardize on both sensitivity and paper speed to achieve aspect ratio consistency, which allows comparison with other EEGs recorded from other subjects.

Normally, the sensitivity is kept 7 mm per 50 μV for adult subjects, a somewhat lower sensitivity for children and a somewhat higher sensitivity for aged. The range of sensitivities used is usually within the range of 4 mm per 50 μV to 15mm per 50 μV.

PAPER SPEED

In most EEG instruments auxiliary outputs from all the amplifiers are available which may be required to use with the other equipments such as oscilloscopes, tape records and display devices. A paper speed of 30 mm per second is often used for electroencephalographic recording. Some times a paper speed of 25 mm per second is also used for the above purpose.

Many EEG instruments, may also add time markers to the EEG recording on a separate channel and may also incorporate electrode contact resistance measurement facilities.

MODES OF EEG RECORDING

Three modes are commonly employed in routine EEG recording done in the laboratory. This is shown in Fig. 4.8. They are given below:

1. Unipolar mode (often called as monopolar mode)
2. Averaging mode
3. Bi-polar mode recordings.

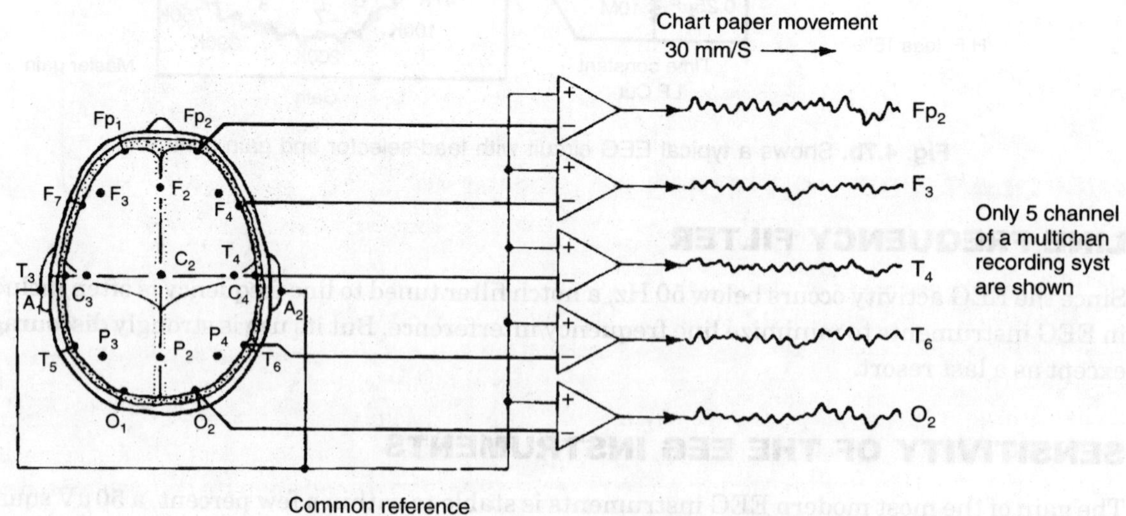

(a) Shows the unipolar mode configuration for recording EEG

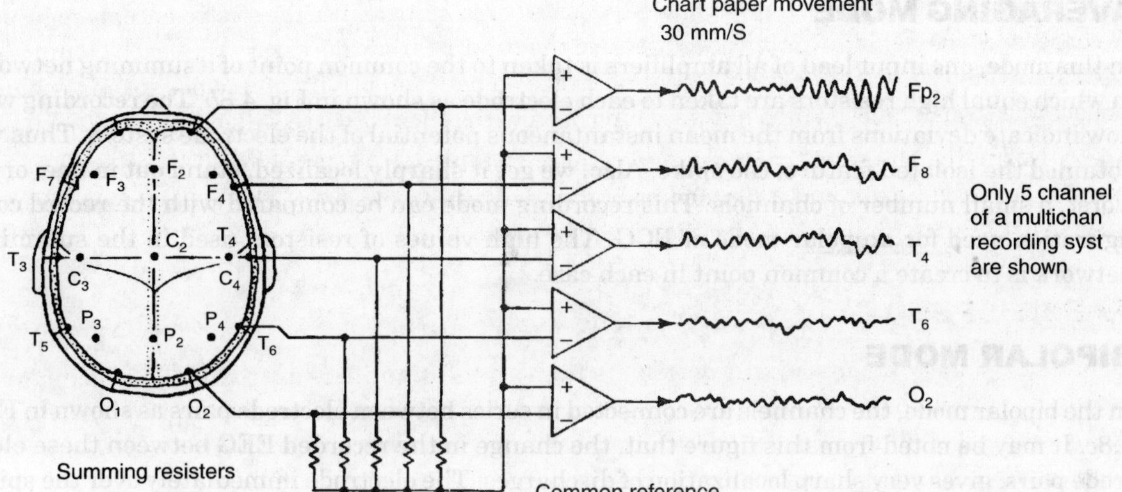

(b) Shows the configuration of Averaging mode technique used for EEG recording.

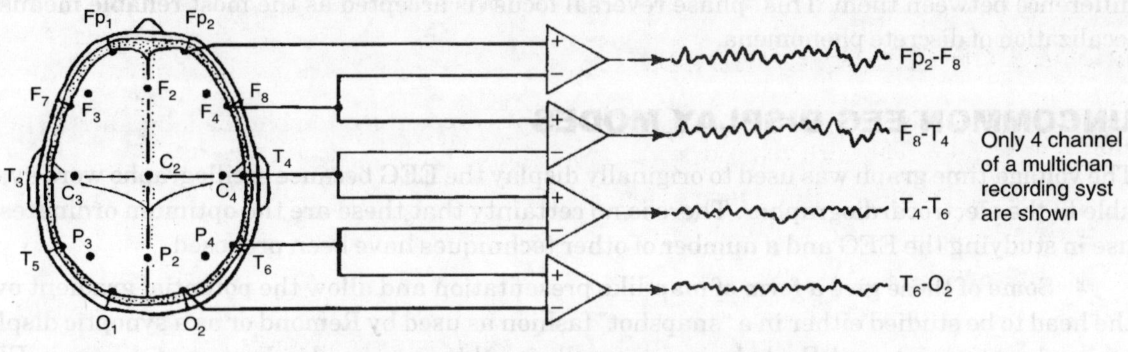

(c) Shows the Bipolar EEG recording configuration

Fig. 4.8. Shows the different modes of EEG recording.

UNI-POLAR MODE OR MONO POLAR MODE

In this unipolar mode, one electrode is common to all channels as in Fig. 4.8*a*. Ideally, this common electrode is regarded as electrically inactive. However, in practice, electrical activity near the electrode will appear in all channels and invariably there are problems in selecting the site for this common electrode. The ear, or both ears connected together, are sometimes used as being generally close to regions of the brain with little on-going electrical activity. If a subject has localized discharge, for simplicity we will assume a spike discharge; then successful localization of the spike will be dependant on its amplitude in the various channels. With some loss of scientific vigor we may say that the amplitude will be greatest in the channel when its active electrode is near the spike focus. In this case, localization is either not possible or very ambiguous. Although one electrode is common to all channels, to reduce interference and artifacts, it is desirable not to ground this common electrode and a separate ground electrode is often connected between the subject and the instrumentation ground.

AVERAGING MODE

In this mode, one input lead of all amplifiers is taken to the common point of a summing network in which equal high resistors are taken to each electrode as shown in Fig. 4.8*b*. The recording will now indicate deviations from the mean instantaneous potential of the electrode system. Thus we obtained the isolated feature, the spike. Also, we get it sharply localized, stand out in one, or at worst, a small number of channels. This recording mode can be compared with the record configuration used for unipolar mode of ECG. The high values of resistors used in the summing network is to create a common point in each case.

BIPOLAR MODE

In the bipolar mode, the channels are connected in series between electrode pairs as shown in Fig. 4.8*c*. It may be noted from this figure that, the change in the recorded EEG between these electrode pairs, gives very sharp localization of discharges. The electrode immediately over the spike generator will cause a positive deflection in one recording channel and a negative deflection in the adjacent recording channel so that the electro-encephalographer will see an apparent 180° phase difference between them. This "phase reversal focus" is accepted as the most reliable means of localization of discrete phenomena.

UNCOMMON EEG DISPLAY MODES

The voltage/time graph was used to originally display the EEG because oscillographs were available to the electrocardiographer. There is no certainty that these are the optimum ordinates to use in studying the EEG and a number of other techniques have been proposed.

Some of these give a form of map-like presentation and allow the potential gradient over the head to be studied either in a "snapshot" fashion as used by Remond or as a synoptic display over a short time interval. Such devices generally speaking, are good indicators of change in EEG activity. But we get very poor for quantization. especially in amplitude. The use of more sophisticated methods of display is increasing because of advancement in technology in signal processing. On-line, real time digital computers which have permitted data transformation in a number of increasing ways.

SPECTRUM ANALYSIS FOR EEGs

A spectrum analysis system has been occasionally used in research applications to present the EEG using amplitude and frequency co-ordinates. Most conventional sampling type instrumentation spectrum analyzers are not suited for direct EEG analysis. This is due to low frequency performance characteristics are inadequate for the data and which is changing continuously as in the case of EEG. Real time-spectrum analyzers are the most desirable one but is very expensive. Frequency analysis is rarely used for EEG in clinical use; it masks much useful information which a human operator, using our superb pattern recognition abilities, can see at a glance. Mathematically, the difficulty of spectrum analysis of an EEG is that is not time-invariant for a long period compared with the lowest frequencies present.

TAPE RECORDERS

Spectrum analysis of the EEG has been performed with conventional instrumentation and sampling type spectrum analyzers by utilizing an Instrumentation tape recorder as indicated in Fig. 4.9. With this system a standard tape recorder is operating in the speed of 47 cm per second records the EEG. A small section of this recorded EEG is formed into a tape loop. This tape is then played back at 150 cm per second. To effectively increase the frequency of the recorded information and to allow the use of a sampling-type spectrum analyzer, such as the Tektronix spectrum analyzer (3L5) in conjunction with a Tektronix storage oscilloscope. The simulated CRT display shown in Fig. 4.10, represents two separate tape loops, one recorded with a subject's eyes open and one recorded with a subject's eyes closed but with a subject awake. This display clearly shows the predominance of alpha activity with the eyes closed and the shift from alpha predominance with the eyes open.

INTRACRANIAL ELECTRODE PLACEMENT

In some diagnostic procedures, the EEG recording electrodes are placed directly on the exposed surface of the brain. Under these conditions, the output voltage will be considerably higher than the voltage obtained with a normal EEG electrode placement. Thus the gain of the recording instrument must be correspondingly reduced. Standard EEG electrodes cannot be used under these conditions as they are non-stable and physically unsuited, thus special electrodes are used.

During neurosurgery, needle electrodes are often used to place the electrode deep within the subject's brain. These "deep electrodes" may consist of a needle insulated over its entire length with the exception of a small area at the tip. Or they may consist of concentric needles of varying length to effectively provide many electrodes at regular intervals along the length of the needle. These are often called as "**insulated needle Electrodes**".

APPLICATIONS OF THE EEG

The EEG is primarily used in clinical neurology for assessing a subject's neurological state partially. The other uses are :

1. **Anesthetic level indicator.** When a brain cell is affected by anesthetic agents for example, and the EEG is a sensitive indicator of the depth of anesthesia. Some workers indeed have used the EEG signal in a closed loop controller to keep constant **anesthetic level.**
2. **Monitoring during surgery.** In many surgical procedures involving the heart, the ECG waveform cannot be monitored, thus the EEG signal is used as an indication of subject's well being. With these procedures the verification of death can no longer be related to the activity of the cardiac system, thus the presence of EEG activity is, in part, a useful indicator. EEG monitoring during surgery, does not require the use of multi channel EEG instrumentation. The EEG signal can be monitored using a single channel recorder or, more commonly, by using an oscilloscope. Many surgical monitors, including the Tektronix (type-410) physiological monitor, designed primarily for cardiac monitoring, include EEG monitoring facilities. This monitor simply requires two electrodes

placed on the head over the occipital regions and one ground electrode placed anywhere on the subject.

3. **Alertness Monitor.** The EEG is also a very subtle estimator of the differences between sleep and wakeness. Much of our present knowledge of sleep phenomena-and sleep is much more complex than it seems at first sight-EEG is observed for the sleeping subjects. A number of states can be distinguished. For those who must be alert as specified times during a task, piloting a spacecraft is a case in point, the EEG can be made the basics of reliable "state of alertness monitor".
4. **Stimuli responses.** Modern amplifier techniques and non-polarizable surface electrodes have established that the shifts in the DC potential are associated with voluntary responses to stimuli. It is very probable that such studies will extend the use of EEG techniques into the realm of psychophysiology; already a number of tentative relationships between mental state and variation of the slow expectancy waves have been established.

THE CHARACTERISTICS OF THE ABNORMAL EEG

For analyzing the EEG for various disease states, it is important that very few single clinical tests are themselves sufficient to make a diagnosis. Thus, the EEG is only one of many procedures used by the clinician in assessing the neurological state of a subject. The most common condition in which the EEG is valuable is **epilepsy.** Strictly speaking, one should refer to "the epilepsies" since many varieties are found. The EEG is of great help in forecasting the outcome of an epileptic illness and is valuable in establishing the optimum course of treatment.

Brain Injury. For example, injury in a specific region of the brain can leave a permanent scar on the cerebral cortex. Such scar tissue is electrically inert but has an irritative effect on nearby healthy cortex. The EEG will often show a localized spike discharge and will suggest, among other possibilities, surgical removal of the damaged tissue.

Inborn Epilepsy. When epilepsy is inborn, and in some forms of this is hereditary, the abnormal electrical activity generally contains signals at many frequencies in the range of 1–50 Hz. There is no consistent phase relationship between the various components so that the EEG presents, to the eye, a "noisy" appearance. The signals are generally a good deal larger than the α rhythm and usually cannot be localized to any specific region of the brain.

Petit Mal. In this "petit mal" epilepsy, the manifestation of the illness is often a transient loss of consciousness or some automatic motor behavior. The EEG signals are wideband but have remarkedly consistent phase relationship between each component. The signal is thus seen as a regular pattern in which a sharp spike appears superimposed on a smooth low frequency wave (1–3 Hz). Although many hypotheses have been advanced to account for the remarkable phase consistency seen in this "spike and wave" phenomenon, none are entirely convincing and all are outside the scope of this chapter.

Tumors. When the brain is invaded with some form of tumor, a considerable portion of the active nervous tissue may be displaced by the electrically inert new growth. If this is very large, its presence can be inferred from the absence of organized electrical activity from the region of the tumor. Usually, a tumor detection is done with a detectable area of 'electrical silence' where it is associated with it. But the other technique of tumor detection is done by analyzing the EEG signals. This gives a better detection of brain tumors at a much earlier stage itself. The expanding new growth can interfere with the blood supply to neighboring areas and the consequent malfunctioning of nerve cells around it manifests by a large, slow discharge i.e., the a rhythm. There may also be significant differences in the electrical activity in the affected hemisphere, perhaps as a result cf interference with the internal communicating pathways within the brain. This technique of detecting brain tumor through EEG depends on many factors; one of the more important factors is the rate at which the tumor is growing; secondly, its spatial relationship to the recording electrodes and the skill of the electroencephalographer.

With the above conditions noted, the EEG is a more frequently used technique for brain tumor detection. In some other circumstances, such as certain toxic conditions and some psychological states, the EEG can add to the overall amount of clinical information with significant benefits to the subject and physician.

INTENTIONAL MODIFICATION OF THE SUBJECT'S EEG

Up to this point, we have assumed that the electroencephalographer plays an entirely passive role and is content to study the brain in its normal physiological milleau. In practice, a number of techniques are used to increase the yield of meaningful information; some of these apply external stimuli to the subject and record their effect on the EEG. Because the excitability of various parts of the nervous system is critically dependant on the acid-base balance and thus on the oxygenation of the body blood, it is general practice to modify this balance by asking the subject hyperventilate, that is, to breath rapidly and deeply while at rest. For the normal subject, this method produces a nominal slowing of the α rhythm and some small increase in the overall signal level. When the subject is epileptic, then the record is dramatically changed to an extent that the seizure may be provoked. Some epileptics are markedly affected by lowering their blood sugar and for this reason many clinical records are obtained from fasting subjects.

Another important means of modifying the EEG is the rhythmic sensory stimulation. One or more of the senses is stimulated by short repetitive stimuli; light flashes are the most commonly used., because they are easy to generate and also because the visual cortex is large and the source of the α rhythm. Sensory stimulation of this kind can emphasize latent abnormalities in the resting EEG and help in the interpretation of the tracing.

CIRCUITS FOR E.E.G.

The E.E.G. signal, being in the microvolts range, needs a sensitive pre-amplifier, with the same requirements of input impedance over 2 meg-ohm and CMRR of 100 dB.

Earlier instruments used tube circuits which could provide the requirements of high gain and low noise in addition to high common mode rejection with good twin triode tubes employed at the front end.

Now-a-days, the dual FET is a commonly used front end pre-amplifier circuit. The use of a constant current source for the differential amplifier's tail, with a special constant current JFET is able to give the required common mode rejection.

The EEG signal itself should be free from much hum or noise and therefore, the patient and leads are often kept inside a shielded cage which is earthed.

After the initial pre-amplifier stage which fulfils the high gain, CMRR and input impedance requirements all in one, the further amplification and filter incorporation are done using suitable operational amplifier based circuits.

The EEG machine is generally having 8 or 16 channels of records, giving simultaneous signals from various electrode pairs. In the all–analog instrument, there will be 16 such pre-amplifiers and associated parts.

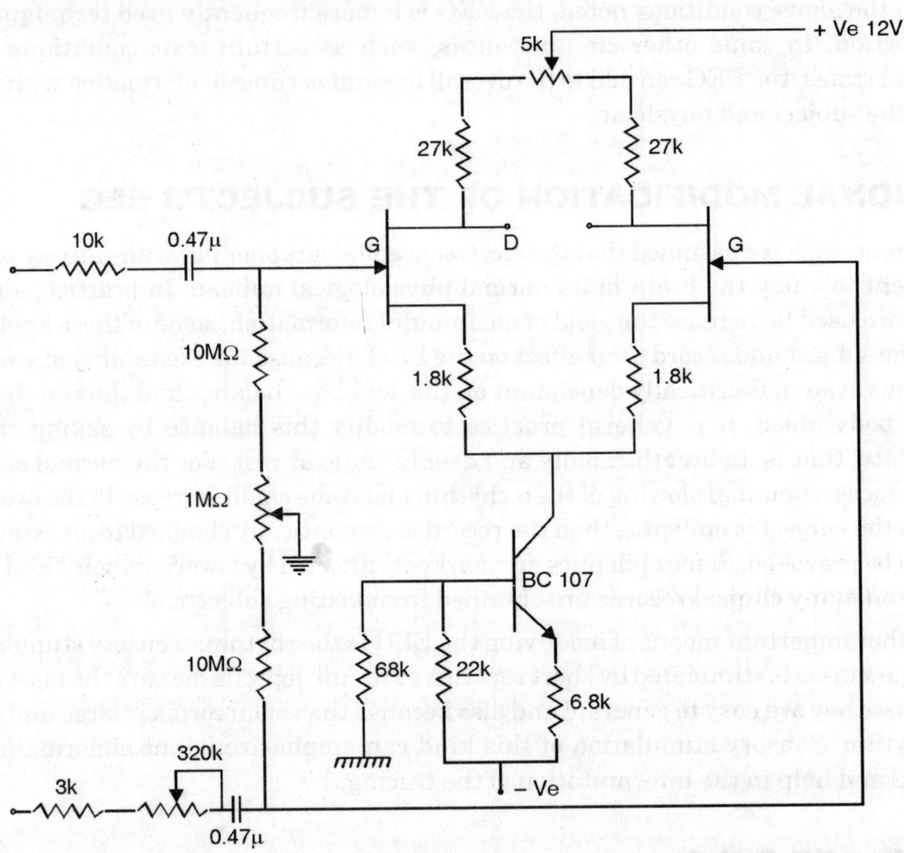

Fig. 4.10. Shows a typical analog instrument Pre- Amplifier circuit.

The C.C.S is a constant current source FET, available as a two-pin device. Instead of the bipolar BC107 constant current source, this can be used, because, Siliconix Inc. supplies two pin(the gate already wired internally to source) FETs as constant current sources. Using a C.C.S., the high CMRR is achieved.

Further to the Pre-amplifier, there are circuits which cut down the low frequencies and this is the time constant filter. It is arranged using capacitor resistor and an op-Amp in a Sallen-Key configuration.

Provision is given through a switch for selecting the time constant, which is useful in eliminating low frequency artifacts.

Then the low pass filter which cuts the low frequencies above 50 Hz is provided. This is also a sharp cut-off filter using at least-40 dB per decade slope with an op-AMP. The active twin-T notch filter for mains noise is also provided and is switch selectable for cut -off or no cut-off.

After these three filters stages, there is a master gain control switch which can uniformaly change all the channel gains. This is made possible by a multiple wafer switch having as many ways as we require the several choices of sensitivities; say 25, 50, 100 or 200 µV per division on the final recorder paper.

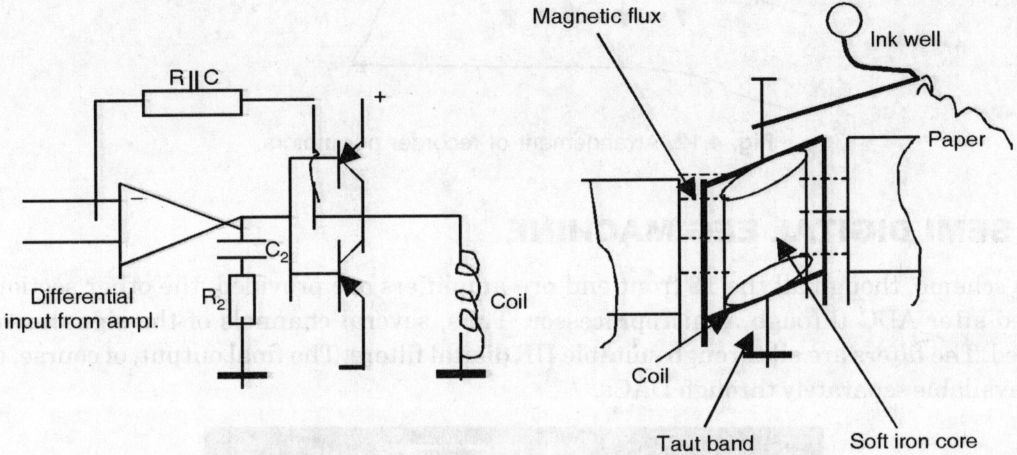

Fig. 4.11. Shows the Pen motor drive circuit.

The Pen motor drive amplifier is a complementary pair transistor driver.The feedback is from the coil. The damping circuit is R_2 and C_2. Nowadays, audio amplifier ICs such as LM380, TBA 810 etc., are usable. There must not be any DC in the output but a separate DC current may be passed through the coil of the pen motor to center adjust its pen.

The coil current feed back is required because of the inductance of the coil so as to adjust the transient response of the square wave signal to be free from overshoot.

THE PEN MOTORS

In a multi channel machine, there will be only one powerful hard magnet of alnico that provides the flux for all the coils (for 16 channels). The soft iron pole pieces as shown below enable the magnet to concentrate the flux in all the coil gaps.

The coil hangs in the air gap between the central fixed soft iron cylindrical case and the radial gap provided by the chamfered S.I pole pieces. The coil comprises of an Aluminium light former, over which enamelled copper wire of about 200 to 500 turns of the 34 to 38 SWG are wound. The former is attached to the sheet of phosphor bronze thin flat which carries the current and also provides the control torque. Fig. 4.12. shows the coil hanging in air-gap.

To the top end of the coil is fixed the pointer carrying a fine groove for ink to flow, from flexibly connected inkwell of the size of 0.5 cm through a thin PVC tube. The pen moves on the paper to be driven from a pulsed stepper motor drive through gears, to vary the paper speed.

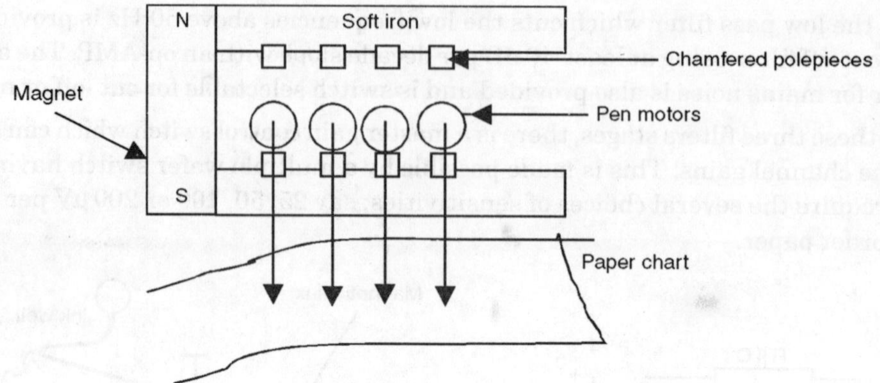

Fig. 4.12. Arrangement of recorder per motors.

THE SEMI DIGITAL EEG MACHINE

In this scheme, though all the 16 front end pre-amplifiers are provided, the other sections are handled after ADC through a microprocessor. Thus, several channels of the signals are also digitized. The filters are all through suitable IIR digital filters. The final output, of course, are all made available separately through DACs.

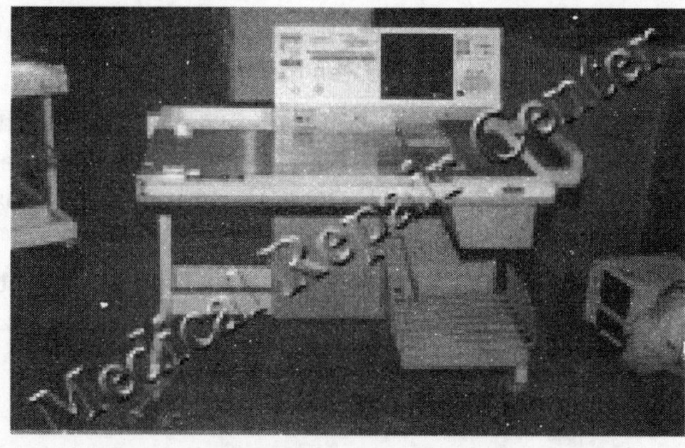

Fig 4.13. Shows a typical digital EEG machine.

Since the paper chart record is standard method of observation, it is provided right from the early day machines to even these modern instruments.

EEG FREQUENCY/WAVE ANALYSER

To analyze the frequency components in any chosen two channels of the EEG into Bands for a fixed pre-determined time, this is useful.

For this bandpass filters are used in the analog machines, while the semi-digital ones do it by bandpass IIR filter programs.

The wave analyzer unit is often equipped with a low frequency oscillator to calibrate and then check the bandpass filters.

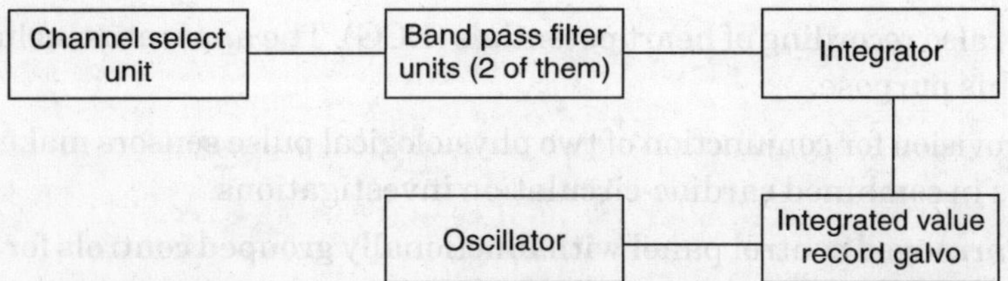

1. The unit is designed to select any desired channel out of a multi-channel EEG and supply the signals to the bandpass filters through a gain control.
2. **Band pass filter units.** Each of the two channels is selectable and has five filters between 2 to 30 Hz. Plug in type and easily replaceable.
3. Provided with ten channels of capacitor circuits and an electrical switching circuit.

The output voltage from each BP filter is simultaneously charged in the capacitor for 5 or 10 secs. (Integ. Period Selector) after amplification and rectified.

The integrated value is amplified and recorded by the pen motor in the next 5 to 10 secs. Meantime, another capacitor circuit does the integration. Hence, a couple of capacitors are used for each, switched by a switching circuit.

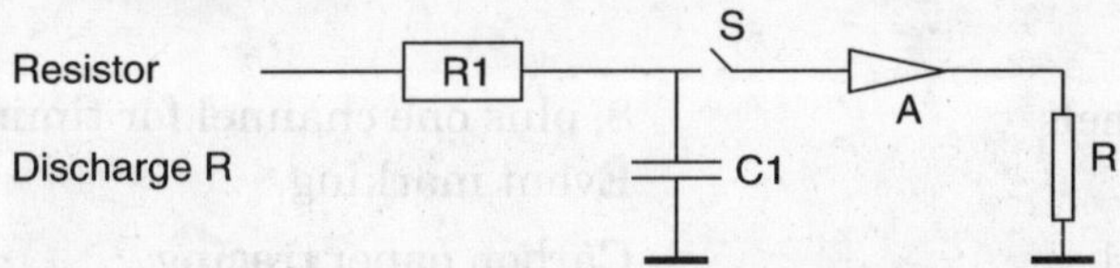

In the standard Mark II EEG machine of the early times, 8 channels are recorded and there is a low frequency wave analyzer built in. The relative amounts of various frequencies will be recorded on this channel.

There is one time marker pen showing one sec intervals.

The paper speed is 30 mm per second, with additional settings for 15 and 60.

One other time marker pen records stroboscope flash speed. A stroboscope which pulses light flashes is used to test epileptic prone patients.

The wave analyzer in this machine has 1.5 Hz to 30 Hz relative amounts of frequency on one strip of EEG. The channel no. being analyzed is also indicated on red ink pen used on the time marker trace.

A TYPICAL EEG MACHINE SPECIFICATIONS AND REQUIREMENTS

The Photograph shows actual recording of the EEG signal with a subject using EEG-8,III model machine from RFT.

This model-EEG 8, III is a highly sophisticated version featuring remarkable convenience of operation and modern styling is widely used available for clinical use.

Using the inherently robust, cost saving and reliable carbon-paper tracing method for long, the EEG 8, III enables recording of eight different bio- electric potentials simultaneously. Its specific application is seen in EEG for recording of electrical activity emanating from the brain, whereby the leads are taken from the intact scalp. The amplifier time-constant of 1.5 second permits in addition also recording of heart potentials (ECG). The apparatus includes patient cable input sockets for this purpose.

A further provision for conjunction of two physiological pulse sensors makes the unit equally well suited for uses in combined cardiac-circulation investigations.

The clearly arranged control panel with functionally grouped controls for ease of operation allows the attending staff to concentrate fully on the patient.

A number of up to 26 electrodes can be connected. Apart from programming on a manually operated single-lead keyboard, there is also choice of up to 21 routine programs.

Timing as well as stimulus and event marking with the alternatives of applying internally or externally preset signals is possible through an additional ninth channel, writing a separate trace on the record.

The EEG international standard paper speeds can be set by simple push - button pressing.

Each amplifier channel is provided with an output for display units.

SPECIFICATIONS

RECORDING UNIT

Number of Channels	8, plus one channel for timing, stimulus and Event marking.
Recording Method	Carbon paper tracing
Writing system	Differential armature pen drives
Frequency range	0.1–130 Hz.
Maximum write amplitude	± 14 mm
Paper speeds	7.5, 15, 30, 60 mm/sec. (0.3, 0.6, 1.2, 2.4 in./sec.)

AMPLIFIERS

Number of amplifiers	8
Maximum sensitivity	0.5mm/μV
Sensitivity setting	1. 8 steps at a ratio 1:2 2. continuously variable at a ratio of 1:2
Common sensitivity setting	3 steps (x1, x0.3, x0.1)
Parasitic voltage	1 μV average
Rejection factor	≥ 10,000
Time-constant	0.01, 0.1, 0.3, 1.5 sec; discrete setting for each channel.
Frequency Filters	15, 30, 70, 200, 2000 Hz; Selectable for each channel
Input impedance	≥ 600 kΩ
Internal reference voltages	10, 20, 50, 100, 200, 500, 1000 μV

OPERATIONAL FACILITIES

Programming	Up to 21 routine programs and Unrestricted programs selection from 26 Patient lead positions; additional programs For ECG and physiological pulse recording, Or combined program.
Measurement of electrode Contact resistance	Unpolarized, by AC voltage over range from 5 kΩ–200 kΩ
Time marking	Internal timer, 1second intervals, separate marker channel 9 .
Event and Stimulus marking	Marker pulses in channel 9 by 50 Hz voltage (push-button operated) or by externally fed signals.

GENERAL CHARACTERISTICS

Mains supply	110 VAC, 220 VAC, ± 20% 50 Hz or 60 Hz.
Mains frequency	50 Hz.
Power consumption	≤550VA
Dimensions	1100 mm × 710 mm × 820 mm approx.
Weight	230 kg (506 lb.)
Testing potential	4000 V (protective isolation)
Model N"	

THE ELECTROENCEPHALOGRAPH-GENERALIA

Our nervous system contains just over 10^{10} nerve cells most of which are in the brain, remainder through out the body. Our eyes, for instance, contain over 250 million receptors (the center of the spleen is practically nerveless). Each brain cell is estimated to have connections with 5,000 to 50,000 brain cells. No one knows how these brain waves are produced, though it is almost certain that they arise in the huge nerve populations of the fore and mid brain.

Electrodes: Rubber suction caps
Silver/silver chloride disc
Pad electrode

Even two channels enough - for example, during surgery, surgeon and anesthetist rely on the EEG and one EKG. 8 channels are in common use.

Electrodes have internationally recognized positions for EEG electrodes. All points except those on the mid line (P_Z,C_Z and F_Z) are symmetrical with similar points on the left side of the head (*e.g.*, FP_1 and FP_2).

The eyes have aqueous humor (in front of the lens) which is 100mV (cornea is) positive compared to the vitreous humor (behind lens) and causes artifacts when patient blinks.

If electrode is placed on a small artery over the scalp, we get a pulse artifact; so move electrode 2.5 mm away.

To illustrate, the following is the specification of a typical analog EEG machine.

ECEM Data : (RFT-German Make)

High sensitivity : 1 mm/μV

Display : The oscillographs (pen needles) operate without the paper unwinding. In this position, any interference can be observed before tracking begins (power line, drift etc.).

Stop : Simultaneous stop of record and paper drive.

Motor : Paper alone unwinding, oscillographs at rest.

Chart : Normal working position–The oscillographs operate and paper unwinds.

Paper Drive : 15–30–60 mm/sec.

Oscillograph : These narrow bore pens trace out a fine line. They are supplied with ink wells with individual plungers.

0.5–70 c/s.

Trace Linearity : For an input level increasing, the track amplitude increases linearly, with 10% up to 2cm P-P deflection.

The following is another EEG machine specification data.

TOSHIBA MODEL

They uses pattern selector-the pattern is chosen from among five representative types.

I	Channel	1–E_L	2–E_R	5–E_L	6–E_R	13–E_L	14–E_R	9–E_L	10–E_R
II	Channel	1–11	11–13	13–15	15–9	2–12	12–14	14–16	16–19
III	Channel	1–3	3–5	5–7	7–9	2–4	4–6	6–8	8–10
IV	Channel	11–19	19–12	13–5	5–20	20–6	6–14	15–21	21–16
V	Channel	20–3	3–4	4–20	20–7	7–8	8–20	13–20	20–14

Sensitivity of EEG : 10 mm pen deflections / 25 μV input

Step Gain : 8 steps, 6 dB and vernier

Overall frequency characteristic : – 4dB over 1-60 c/s

No-9 Channel : DC

Time constants : ECG 1.7 sec minimum

: EMG 0.03–0.05 sec

All channels : EEG 0.3 to 0.4 sec

Input impedance	:	5 MΩ min
Discriminator	:	60 dB min
Equ. Noise voltage	:	3 μV PP maximum.
Calibrate voltage	:	20, 50, 100, 200, 500 μV and 1 μV.
Time Marker	:	10.1 sec ± 2%
Pattern marker	:	Symbols representing the type of patterns can be placed on chart paper.
Extension input terminals	:	Terminals are provided for receiving the output signal of a frequency analyzer.
Output terminal	:	for driving a CRT
Electrode	:	24 selective electrodes 5 pattern
Contact resistance of electrode	:	Can be measured up to 100 kΩ
Recording Speed	:	10 mm/sec and 30 mm/ sec
Capacity for recording	:	500 meters max, 245 mm wide.
Power consumption	:	190 Watts

And a Compact high sensitivity galvo is provided.

ACCESSORIES

Electrode Junction box

Cranial electrode of pasting type with leads

Ear electrode

EEG- 8-III

The description and spare parts list of the typical EEG machine is given below.

Requirements and Specifications

- Clearly arranged **EEG lead selector panel** fitted with highly reliable Rotary switches, enables operation from seated position.
- Automatic control unit provides for rational EEG recordings.
- Protective insulation withstanding 400 volts ensures maximum safety for patient and attending staff.
- Direct writing method gives minimal operating costs and contrasting traces at all paper speeds.
- Insertion of stimuli and event markers in additional timing channel.

Ordering Information

Item	Description
1.	8-channel electroencephalograph EEG 8, III
	Accessories required :

Accessories set 19-20

Accessories set 17-18

1. One EEG Distributor
2. One Label with routine program
3. Five Labels, blank
4. One Lead schematic
5. One paper guide
6. One paper take-up arm
7. Two earth wires
8. One connecting cable for ninth channel
9. One mains lead
10. Drivers spare parts
11. Drivers special tools
12. Drivers fuses and lamps
13. Nine spare styli
14. Five tubes of electrode paste
15. 30 lead cords, short
16. 4 lead cords , long
17. one roll of recording paper
18. 10 stacks of fan folded recording paper
19. 4-Rolls carbon paper
20. ECG Plug-in program unit, non-wired
21. EEG scale
22. Instruction manual
23. Instrument cover

Optional Extras for Neuro-diagnostics

1. EEG distributor stand
2. Distributor holder
3. Rubber strap cap
4. Distributor for lead modes with central point
5. Electrode set
6. Screening mat
7. Fan-folded recording paper ;
8. 240mm wide, stack of 200 sheets, each 300 mm long
9. Recording paper rolls-240 mm wide, 50 m long, white, blank

10. Bio-monitor (single channel unit)
11. General purpose display unit
12. Photo-phono stimulator

Optional Extras for Circulation Diagnostics

Patient cable

Plate electrodes

Standard chest electrodes

Straps

Buttons

Suction electrodes

Arterial pulse transducer

Venous pulse transducer

Stand for pulse generator

Fine adjustment for stand ST-1

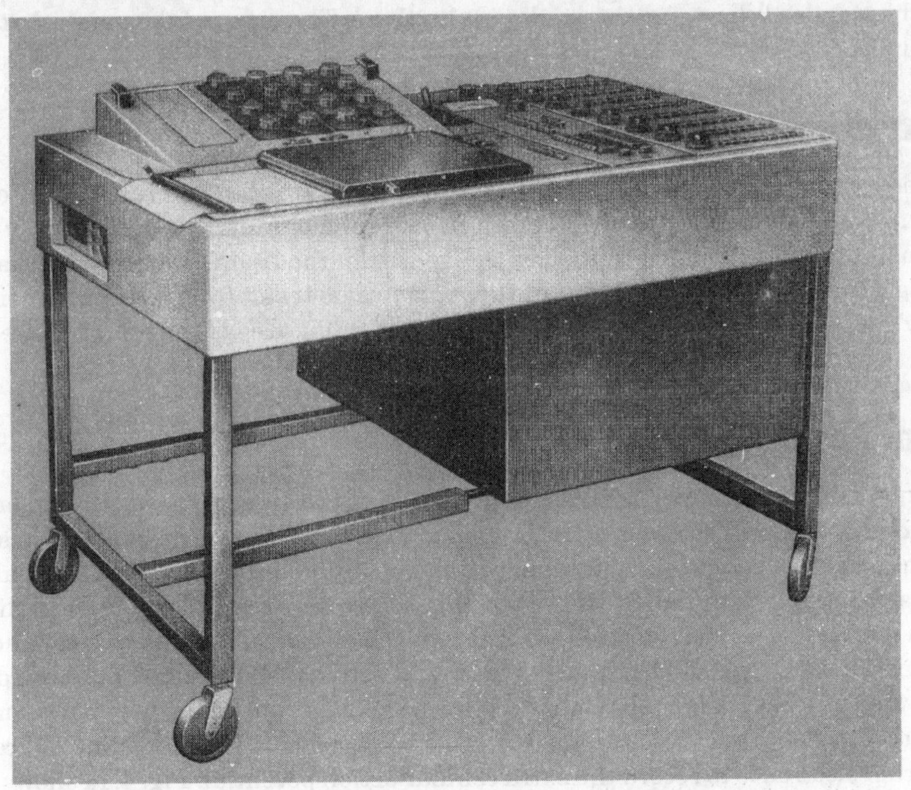

Photograph shows a typical EEG machine and the electrode positioning with the Patient/Subject

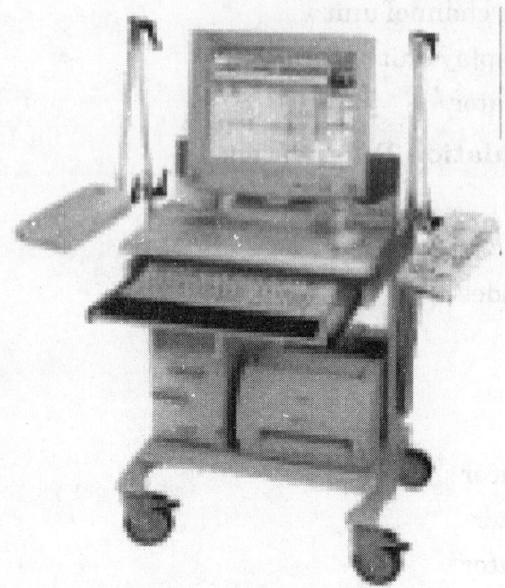

Figure above shows a modern EEG machine with monitor (Color LCD) display and in addition, the standard chart paper recorder is also there. The view is taken and whatever needs printing can be done on it.

EVOKED CORTICAL RESPONSE

The electroencephalogram (EEG) discussed so far is a measure of the overall activity of the brain with the subject when they are at rest. The electroencephalogram (EEG) is probably associated with the computation process continuously active within the brain. Evoked potentials are also potentials generated within the brain. But these potentials result from a stimulus being applied to the body's sensory system and are localized to a particular area of the brain. These potentials are known to be "evoked" by the stimulus.

EVOKED POTENTIAL

As mentioned in the previous paragraph, stimulation of the subject's sensory system produces electrical activity in a localized area of the brain. For analyzing this stimulus effect, it is necessary to record the electrical potentials generated within individual brain cells. This is usually done by intracellular recording techniques. These techniques are only used in research applications on nonhuman subjects. External electrode will record the electrical activity of a cell, however, as many adjacent cells may also be producing electrical activity, the results obtained could not be attributed to in any particular cell. Under certain conditions, particularly when recording from the spinal cord rather than from the brain, it may be possible to isolate individual cell activity using external electrodes to record the extra cellular action potential. Fig. 4.14 shows the action potential generated by a single cell with both internal and external electrodes and shows the time and voltage relationship between these two recording techniques.

Normally, when recording the intracellular potential with an internal electrode, about 110mV is generated during a cell depolarization/repolarization process and this signal is known as the **intracellular action potential.** It is possible to record still lower amplitude signals generated within the cell, such as results of excitation and inhibition stimuli. This intracellular action potential is shown in Fig. 4.15. It is evident, that, after a period where the cell is receiving excitatory stimuli which decreases the cell resting potential at a linear rate, this continues till the cell threshold is reached, at which time the rate of change of potential increases, indicating regenerative depolarization. The cell subsequently repolarizes.

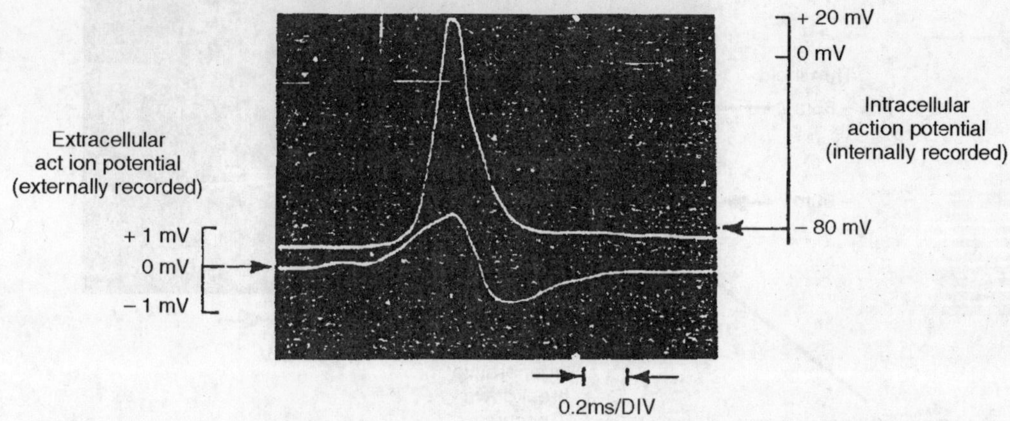

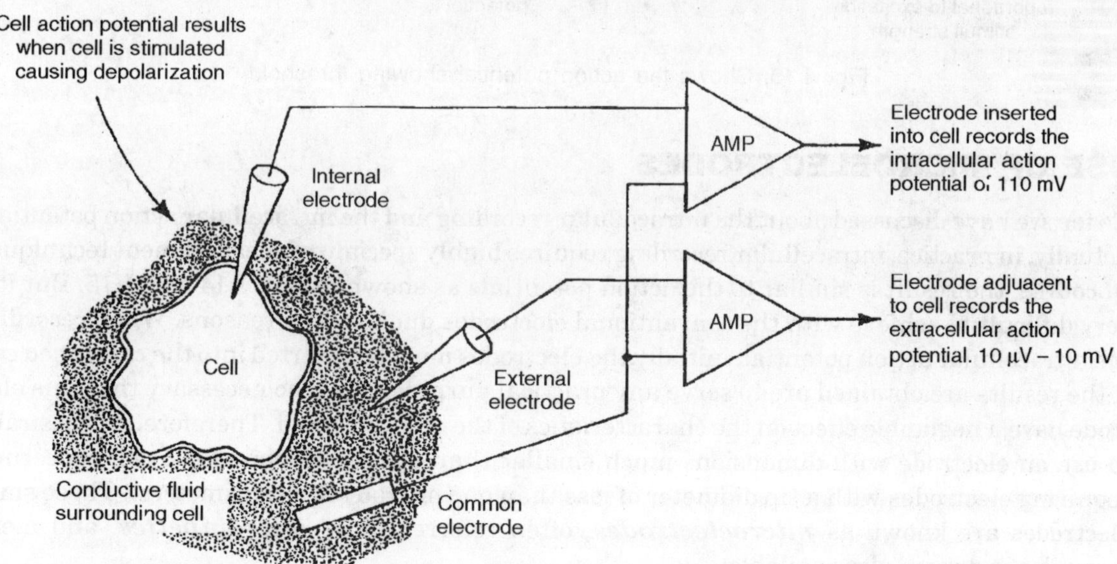

Fig. 4.14. Shows the cell action potential-internally and externally recorded.

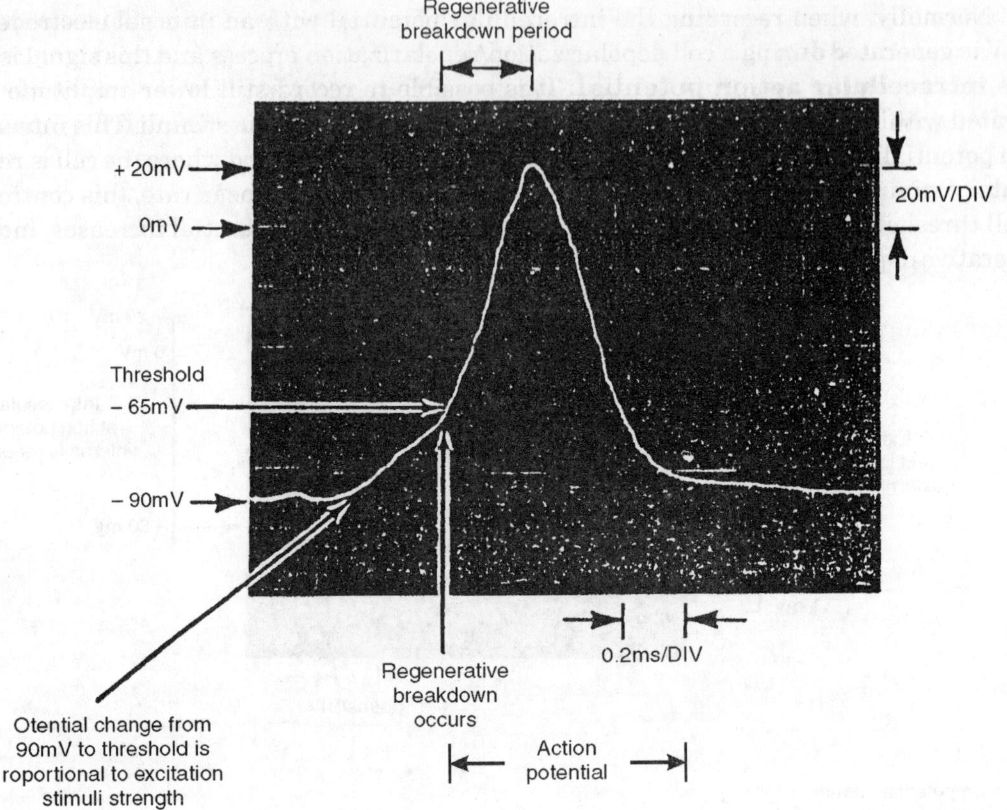

Fig. 4.15. Shows the action potential showing threshold.

USE OF MICROELECTRODES

So far, we have discussed about the intracellular recording and the intracellular action potentials. Actually, in practice, intracellular recording requires highly specialized measurement techniques. Of course, the result is similar to the action potentials as shown in Fig. 4.14 and 4.15. But it is very difficult to achieve with the conventional electrodes due to many reasons. When recording the intracellular action potential, initially the electrodes must be inserted into the concerned cell. If the results are obtained are to serve any practical purpose, it is also necessary that this electrode have a negligible effect on the characteristics of the cell concerned. Therefore, it is desirable to use an electrode with dimensions much smaller than the dimension of the cell concerned; requiring electrodes with a tip diameter of less than one micron (10^{-4} centimeters). These small electrodes are known as ***microelectrodes***, often referred to as ***micropipettes***, and metal microelectrodes are also available.

There are various type microelectrodes are available and it can be chosen according to the requirement. The main two types microelectrodes are:

1. Metal microelectrode and
2. Glass microelectrode

The basic difference between these two is , that in the metal microelectrodes the metal is in direct contact with the biological tissues whereas in the glass microelectrode, an electrolyte is interspersed between the tissue and the metal electrode. Thus, **metal microelectrodes** have a lower resistance, but they polarize even with smaller amplifier input currents and they may develop unstable electrode offset potentials. Unless extreme precautions are taken, they are, therefore, unreliable for steady state potential measurements.

GLASS MICROELECTRODE

This type interposes an electrolyte between the tissue and the metal electrode. This gives improved stability. The electrolyte can be chosen so that small, steady currents can pass through their junction without modifying the electrical properties of the electrodes. The surface contact area between the electrolyte and the metal is large so that the current-carrying capacity of the electrode is substantial. The glass microelectrode is, therefore, usually preferred .

Fig. 4.16 shows a typical tip dimension of a glass microelectrode, having a overall tip diameter of about 0.6 microns with an internal diameter of 0.2 microns. The glass microelectrode

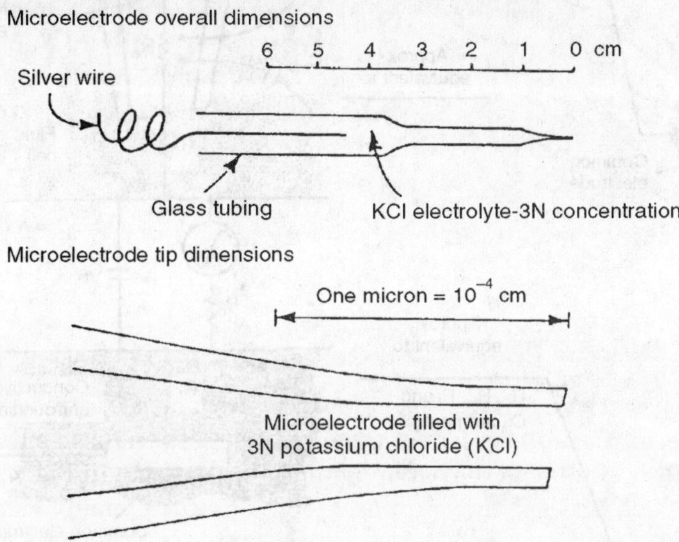

Fig. 4.16. Shows the glass microelectrode geometry.

is formed by heating special glass tubing and drawing it out over several stages of reduction. Although the tubing is reduced to less than one micron diameter, it still remains hollow. Potassium chloride solution is introduced into the microelectrode as the electrolyte. Since it is not possible to fill the microelectrode by pressure (surface tension) or by capillary action, boiling it with or without reduced pressure is often employed. Ideally, one would like to use an electrolyte within the microelectrode having the same concentration as the potassium chloride within a typical cell (0.1 Normal). It is, however, impossible to use an electrolyte of this concentration as it increases very much the resistance of the microelectrode. The resistance of the microelectrode will be more than 1000 MΩ in such a concentration. It is, thus, common practice to use 2 or 3 normal potassium chloride in the microelectrode. This electrolyte has a resistivity of 3.3 Ω centimeter which gives the microelectrode similar as shown in Fig. 4.16, a typical resistance value of 10 MΩ. Some microelectrodes are specially designed with much smaller tip diameters and using a less concentrated electrolyte having a resistance value of typically 100 MΩ. Special recording techniques are necessary to accommodate this extremely high series resistance of the electrodes.

The equivalent circuit of a typical microelectrode inserted into a cell is shown in Fig. 4.17. The equivalent electrical circuit is formed between this microelectrode and a common electrode placed elsewhere on the subject. Fig. 4.17 can be further simplified to the microelectrode resistance with distributed capacity and an RC load on the microelectrode formed by interconnection capacitance, amplifier input capacitance and amplifier input resistance. As we know, the dimensions of the microelectrode tip are extremely small. The most of the microelectrode resistance is located within one millimeter of the microelectrode tip. Therefore the distributed capacities associated with the electrode resistance are less than one picofarad.

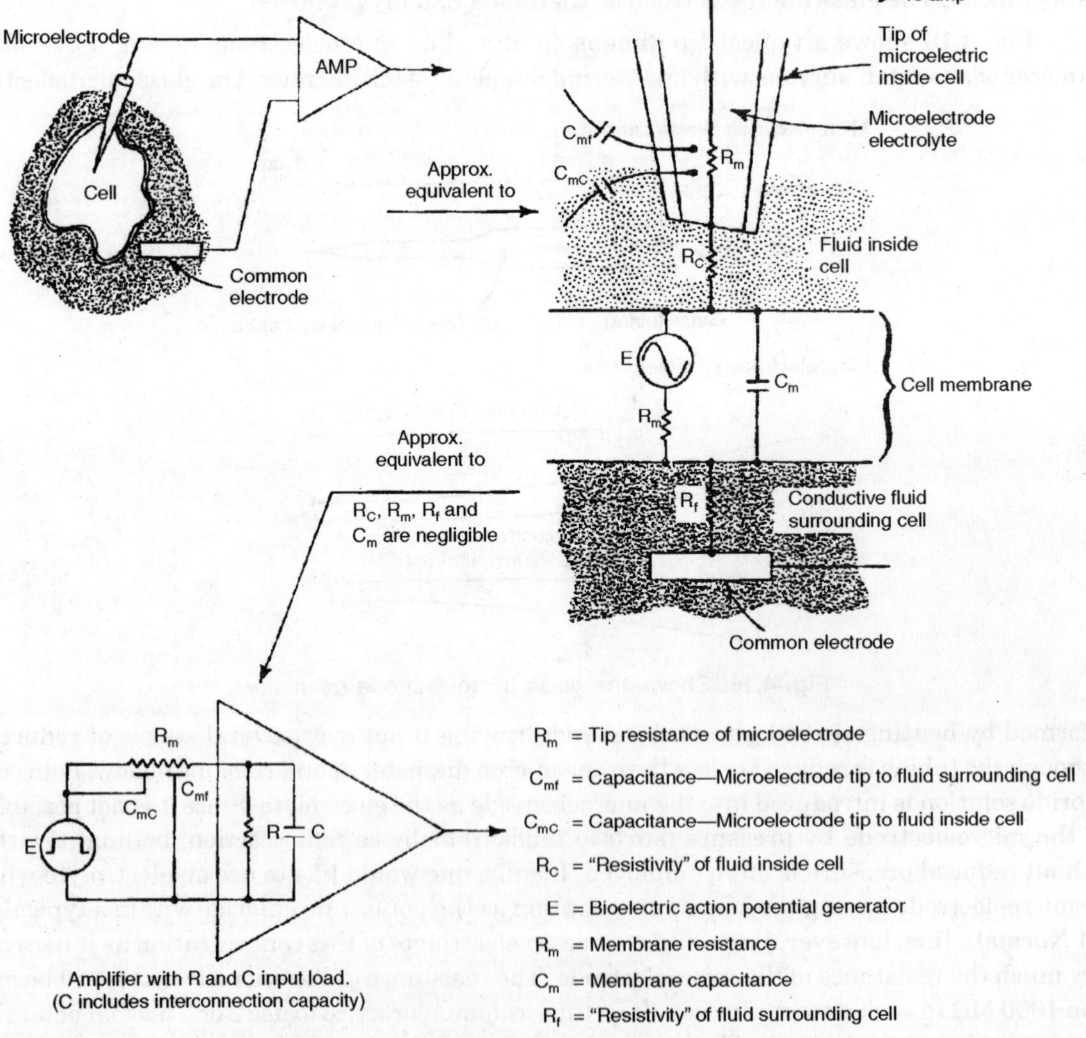

Fig. 4.17. Shows the cell microelectrode equivalent circuit.

Fig. 4.18 shows a typical microelectrode equivalent circuit together with a typical values for the impedances concerned. This equivalent circuit represents a low-pass filter and an attenuator. It is necessary to know the characteristics of this circuit so as to determine the fidelity expected for the systems when recording the action potential. This equivalent circuit can be modified using a pulse generator in place of the cell and using discrete impedance in place of the microelectrode resistance and capacitor. Fig. 4.18 shows the degradation that can be expected form an input action potential having a rise time of 0.1 millisecond and a fall time of 0.2 millisecond for various values of electrode internal resistance when using an amplifier having an equivalent input capacity of 1pF and an equivalent input resistance of 1000 megohms.

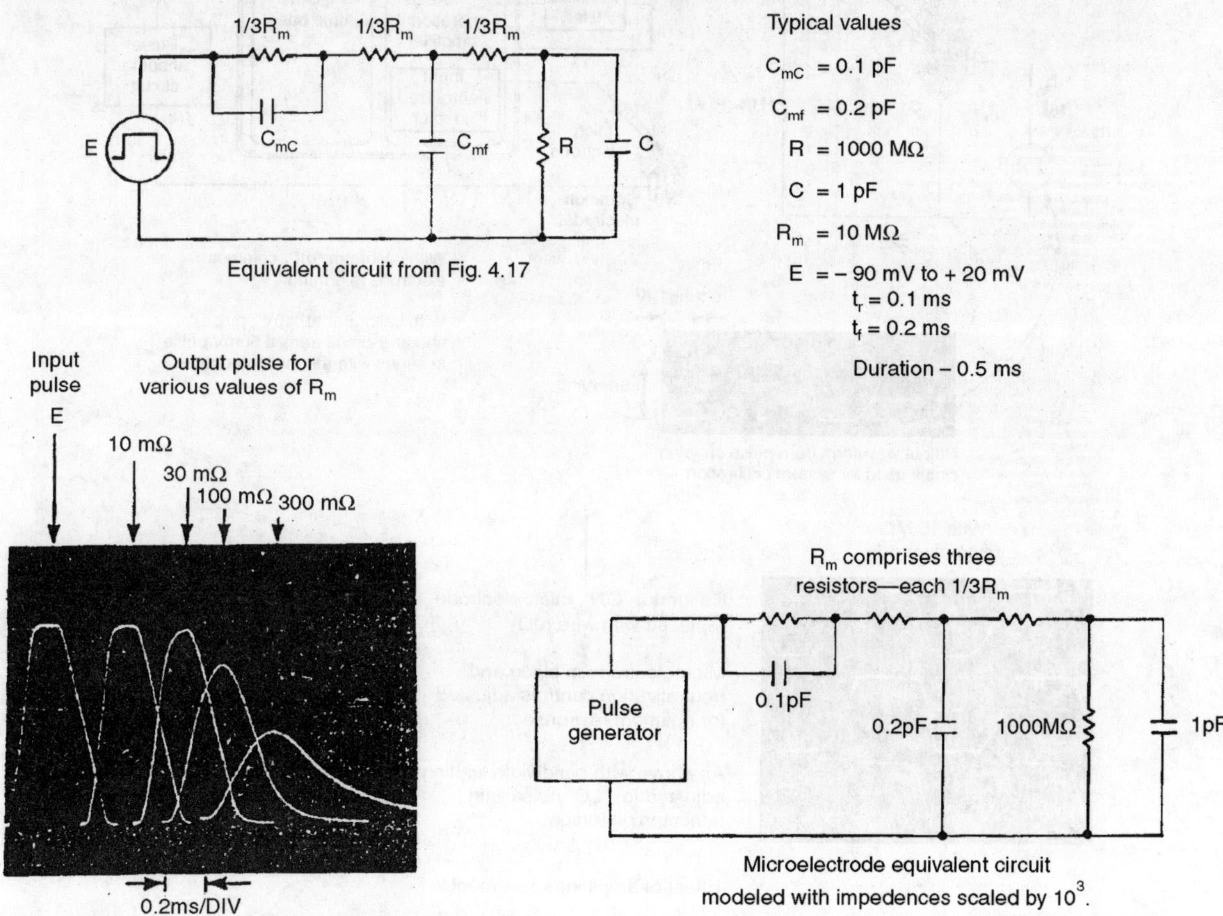

Fig. 4.18. Shows the microelectrode model and resultng pulse response.

It may be noted from the Fig. 4.18, a 100 megohm microelectrode used in the above system reduces the amplitude of the action potential by 20% and degrades it rise time and fall time. It is thus desirable to either reduce the resistance of the microelectrode to 30 MΩ or perhaps even 10 MΩ to increase fidelity or else increase the input impedance of the amplifier and interconnection network. Since decreasing the microelectrode resistance is not possible unless the size of the microelectrode is increased, it is preferable to increase Z_{in}.

INPUT NEUTRALIZED AMPLIFICATION

The impedance load on the microelectrode can be increased by using an active feedback amplification to provide input impedance neutralization raising the Z_{in} to 10000 MΩ. Fig. 4.19 shows a typical

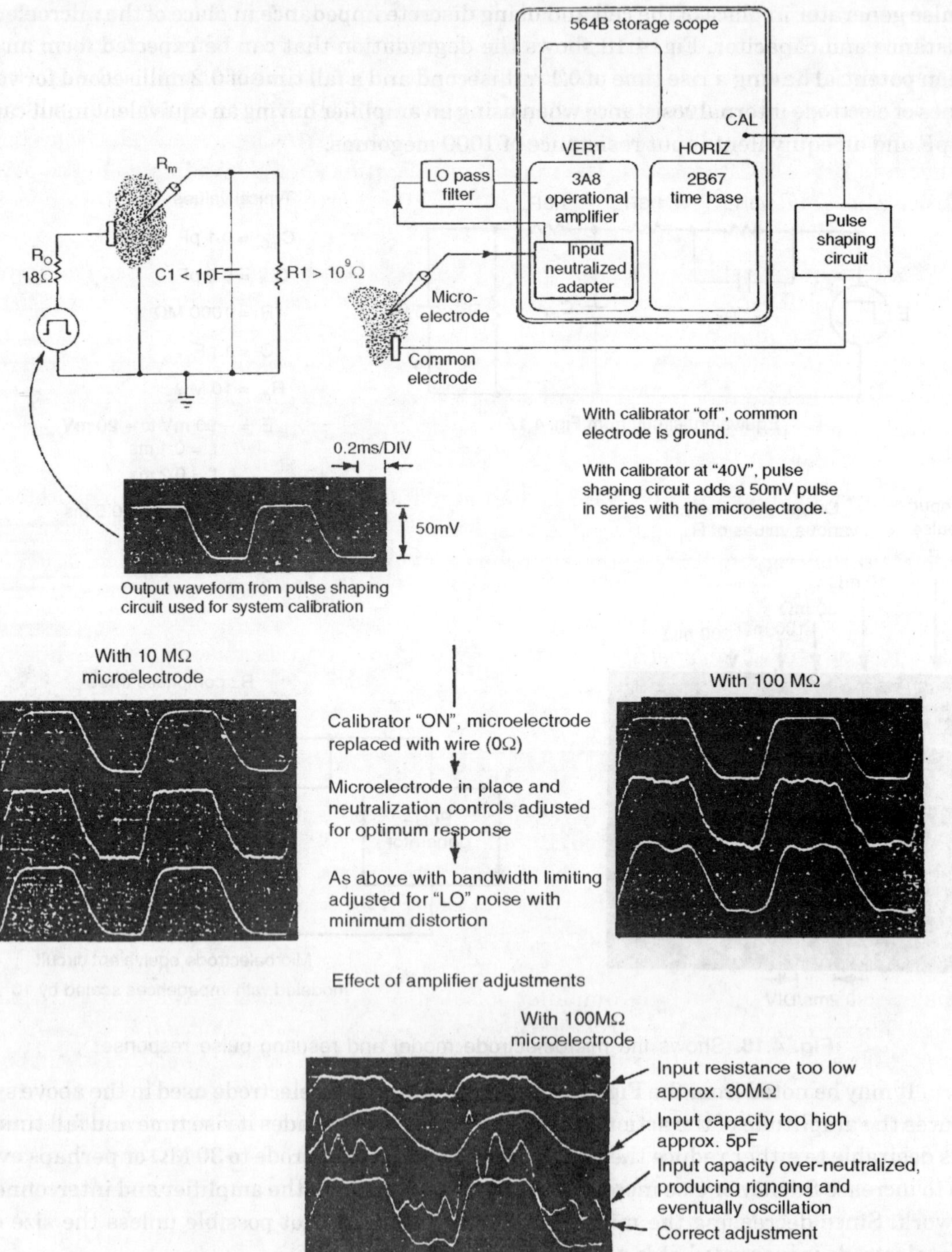

Fig. 4.19. Shows an input neutralized amplifier and scope system.

microelectrode system utilizing a Tektronix type 3A8 OP-AMP plug-in unit operating in an "input neutralized" mode. This requires the use of an input neutralizing adapter in conjunction with the 3A6. This microelectrode recording system also incorporates a series calibration waveform. By switching the 564B calibrate from OFF to 40V, a 50 mV, 1000 Hz, signal is added in series with the microelectrode. This signal has a controlled rise time of about 0.1 milliseconds and a controlled fall time of 0.2 millisecond and is used in conjunction with two input neutralization controls (–R and –C) to check the amplitude and time calibration of the system. When the calibrator is returned to its OFF position, this signal source is essentially replaced by a short circuit. This calibration waveform and the response of the system for various settings of the input neutralization controls are shown in Fig. 4.19. In practice, the input neutralization should be adjusted to the point at which overshoot and ringing are reduced to less than 10%. Further reduction of the overshoot and ringing will degrade the rise time of the system.

The dynamic resistance of the neutralized amplifier may be above 10^{10} ohms. The amplifier input current must be $< 10^{-12}$ A or else it will thus not operate. Since the dynamic input resistance of any device is determined by the change in the input current for an incremental change in input voltage; $R = \Delta V/\Delta I$; and as amplifier input current does not change with an incremental change in input voltage, this amplifier input current is not reflected by the input resistance specification of the amplifier and must be specified separately. Any neutralized amplifier should have an amplifier input current below 10^{-12} amperes.

The system shown in Fig. 4.19, has an amplifier input current of approximately 10^{-13} Amps. These extremely small currents are necessary when using the amplifier for intracellular recoding as the current will cause potassium ions to migrate from the microelectrode into the cell. This upsets the intracellular concentration, which may change the cell resting potential. Small changes in resting potential due to extremely small currents cannot be avoided, and it may not be significant. However, it is obviously desirable to maintain the current below the level required to cause cell depolarization.

NOISE REDUCTION IN NEUTRALIZED AMPLIFIERS TANGENTIAL NOISE

The noise in neutralized amplifier is proportional to the degree of neutralization required; a tangential noise of several millivolts is not uncommon. The system shown in Fig. 4.19, when neutralized correctly, produces a tangential noise of 1 mV when used with an electrode having a resistance of 10 MΩ and 2.5 mV when used with an electrode having a resistance of 100 MΩ. This noise can be eliminated when recording the intercellular potentials since these potentials will be in the order of 100 mV. For extracellular measurements, however, the extracellular action potential may be as low as 20 μV and the amplifier noise will completely swamp away any extracellular signals. This situation also occurs when using intracellular recording at high sensitivity in an attempt to observe the excitation and inhibition potentials. The signal-to noise ratio can be substantially improved by a low pass filter following the neutralized amplifier. Such a filter is included in the system shown in Fig. 4.19. Even using a filter for extracellular measurements, the noise level obtained may still completely swamp the signal and at best will be extremely objectionable. Thus, particularly when working at sensitivities below 100 μV per division, some more effective noise reduction technique should be adopted.

AVERAGING TECHNIQUE FOR NOISE REDUCTION

A single response evoked by one stimulus is usually too small to be seen above the on going EEG activity and the noise inherent in the system. However, when we assume that the response always follows the stimulus after a fixed delay, "signal averaging" technique can be employed using computers which can improve the signal to noise ratio. Normally, when this technique is used for noise reduction, this extracts a wanted signal from a background of unwanted noise. It can only be used effectively if the desired signal, with its accompanying noise, can be generated a number of times either periodically or aperiodically. That means, one has to do repeated measurements and averaging the signal, so as to get effective noise reduction accompanying with the signal of interest. In addition, a trigger pulse is required that has a fixed time relationship to the desired signal. The stimulus, or trigger pulse, initiates a scanning device which samples the signal at fixed intervals. These time-sequential samples are stored in discrete storage channels or memory locations, each channel collecting data over a small time segment. When the stimulus is repeated, the responses are added to the values stored at each location. During readout, each of the channels displays the sum of all the previous samples fed into it. If the background activity is random with respect to the stimulus, the time-locked response will add linearity with the number of samples (n) while the background will add only as the square root of ***n***. If the stimulus is repeated 64 times , then the response to noise ratio will have been improved by a factor of

$n/(\sqrt{n}) = (\sqrt{n}) = 8$ if $n = 64$ which is fairly a common number.

Filtering to the maximum permissible extent should always precede the averaging device.

SIGNAL-TO NOISE RATIO IMPROVEMENT

The signal-noise ratio improvement by averaging is shown in Fig. 4.20. The noise has a peak value about equal to that of the signal, equivalent to an RMS S/N ratio of about 4. Averaging is an

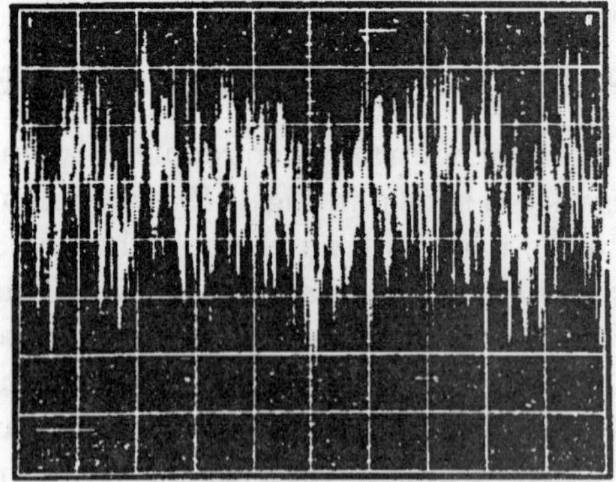

Raw signal output from neutralized amplifier
vertical 100μ V/DIV (referred to input)
horizontal 0.2ms/DIV

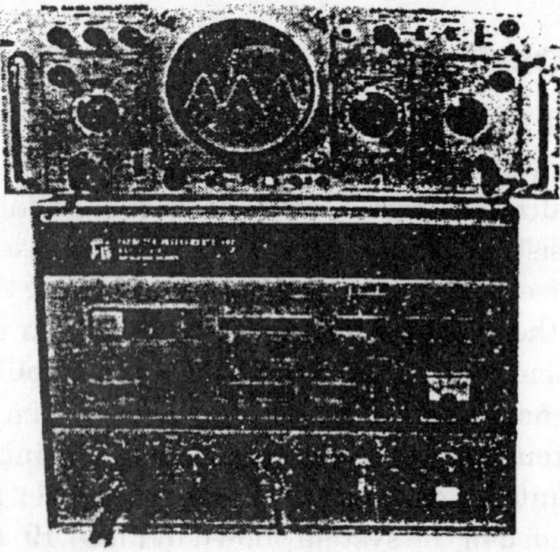

Signal averager and readout oscilloscope

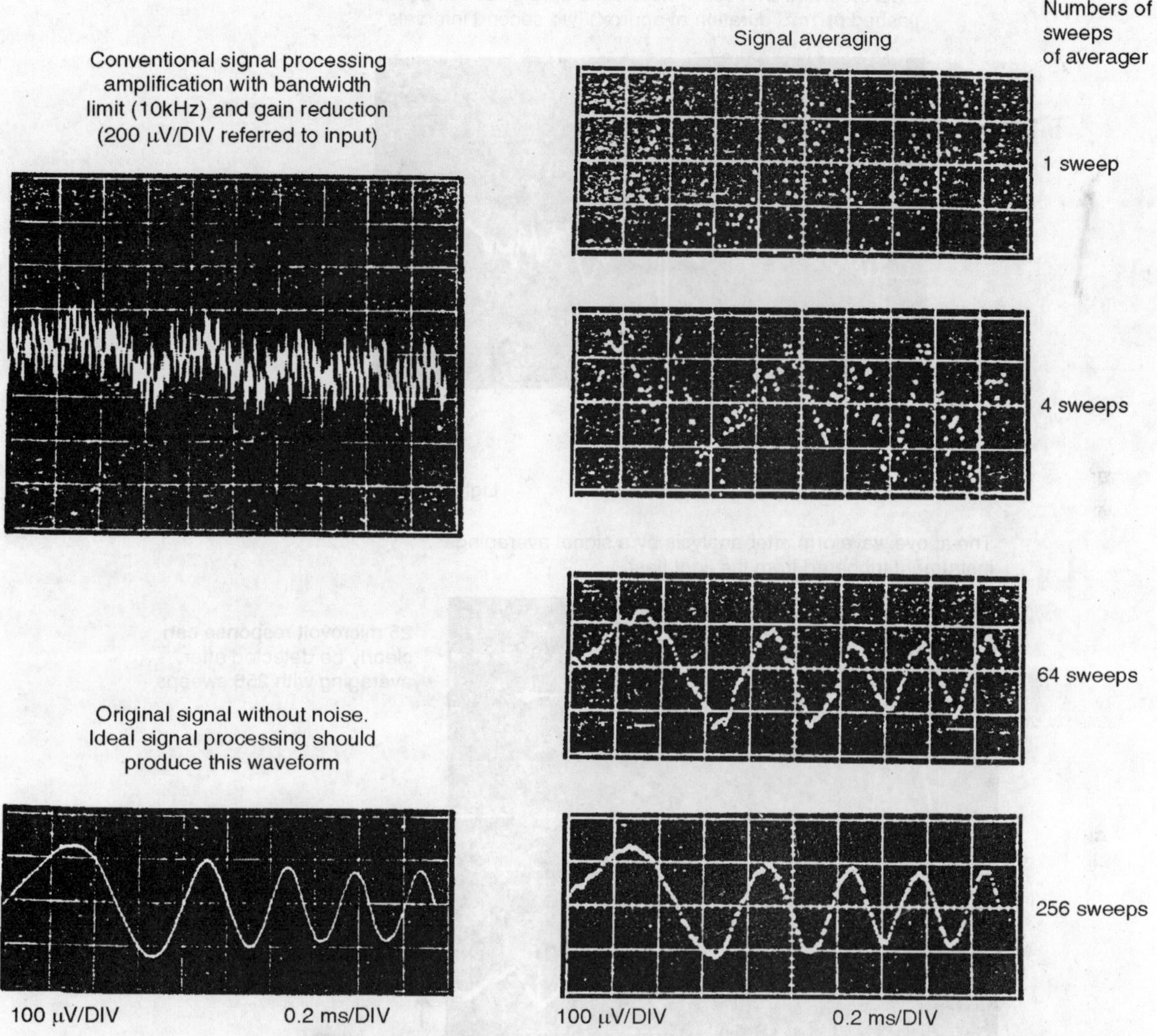

Fig. 4.20. Shows the techniques involved in the signal-to noise improvement (with averaging).

ideal technique under these conditions. For greater noise levels, the signal content is reduced, because the peak noise plus signal must still not overdrive the averager; difficulty then arises because signal component alone is not being digitized to a sufficient number of bits to give a useful output.

In many circumstances, averaging can be carried out in the absence of the trigger pulse if it is possible to use part of the response itself as the stable point. This is an aspect of averaging which is currently of great interest to physiologists. Fig. 4. 21 shows the use of averaging technique to detect a response in the EEG.

EEG recorded with scalp electrodes during repeated light flashed of 1mS duration at approx. Two second intervals.

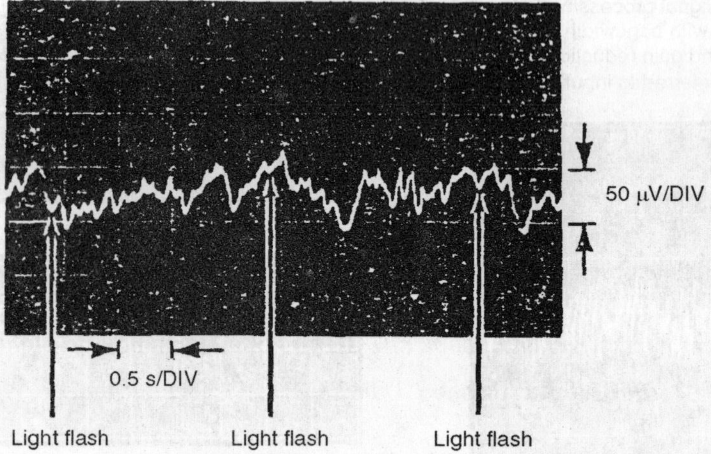

The above waveform after analysis by a signal averaging instrument triggered from the light flash.

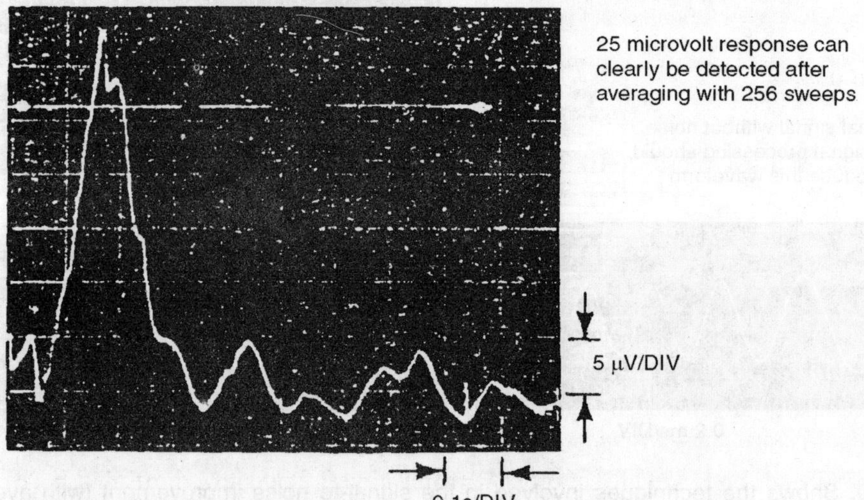

Fig. 4.21. Shows the use of averaging to detect response in the EEG.

The resolution of the signal averager is limited by the number of addressable channels; commercial units may contain from 64 to 1024 channels; the speed of the system is limited by the length of time required to store information into any one channel.

The signal averager relies on a trigger pulse being available with known relationship to the desired signal. When recording evoked potentials, it will be recalled that these potentials are generated in response to a stimulus being applied to the patient, this stimulus can be used as the trigger for the averager.

TYPICAL EVOKED RESPONSES

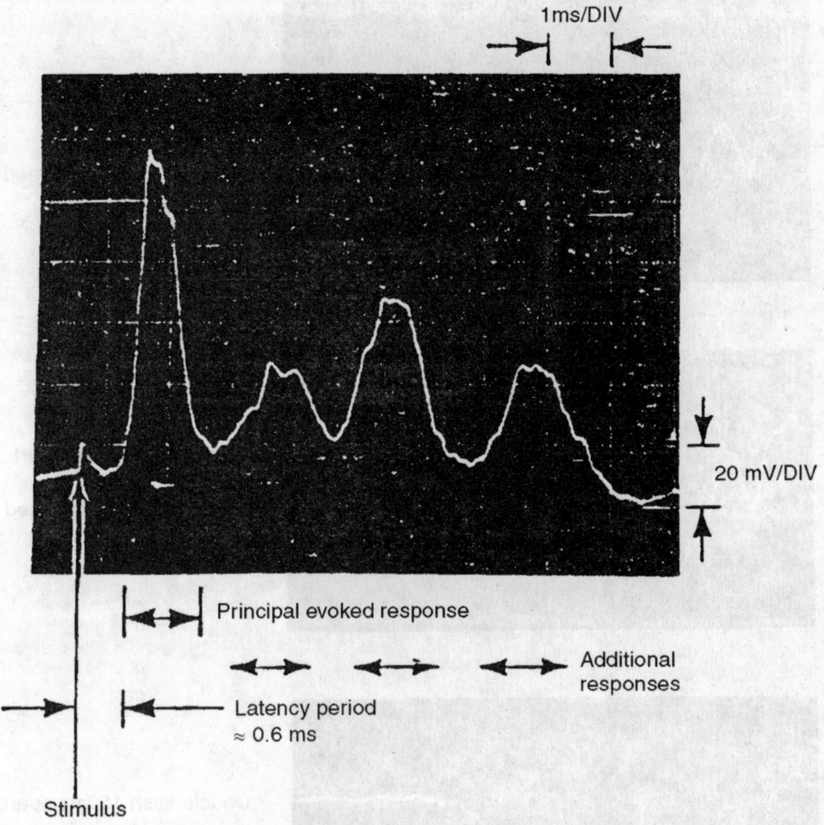

Fig. 4.22. Shows the Evoked response showing latency and additional parameter.

A typical evoked response obtained with a microelectrode on a laboratory animal is shown in Fig. 4.22. The response waveform is preceded by a small amount of stimulus artifact. Although it is desirable to reduce the level of stimulus artifact appearing on recordings, it is impossible to completely suppress it as it does provide some time relationship in the recorded evoked potential. The evoked potential begins sometime after the stimulus is received; this delay is known as latency and is approximately 0.6 milliseconds in the waveform shown in Fig. 4.22.

Typical evoked potential obtained with an extracellular microelectrode with stimulation of the visual cortex of a laboratory animal are shown in Fig. 4.23. Stimulus artifacts has deliberately been added to these recordings to provide time reference as discussed earlier. Fig. 4.23 shows the evoked response obtained for a single light flash and for multiple light flashes separated by various periods from one another. The 50ms pair of flashes is seen by the subject as one, whereas two flashes are perceived for the 150 and 250 millisecond intervals. Unlike the evoked response shown in Fig. 4.22, these responses were obtained with extracellular electrodes and show the effect of many cells within the visual cortex; thus the "time scale" of the responses is greatly increased as many cells involved.

Response to single and double flashes of light. Each flash is 10μs duration. (Arrows indicate light flash.)

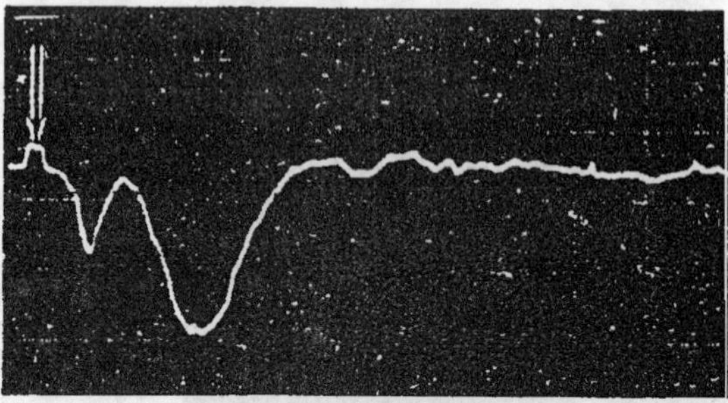

Single flash

Single response obtained

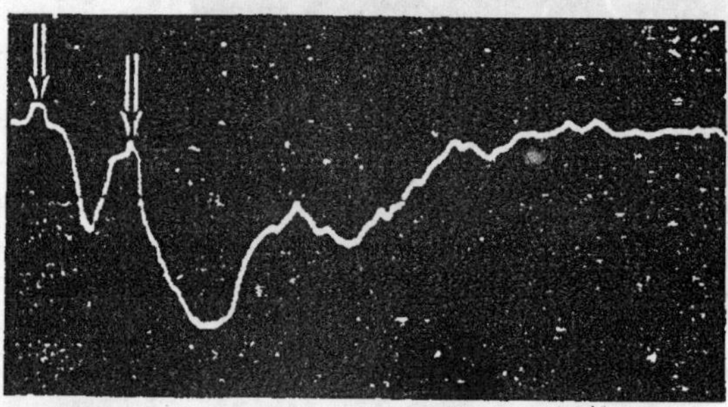

Double flash 50ms apart

Single response obtained

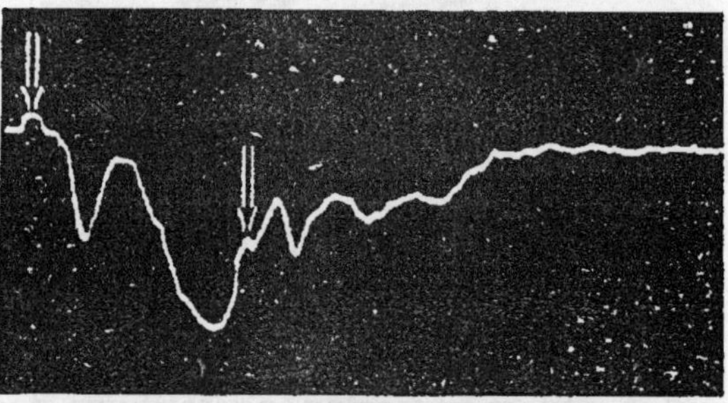

Double flash 150ms apart

Double response obtained

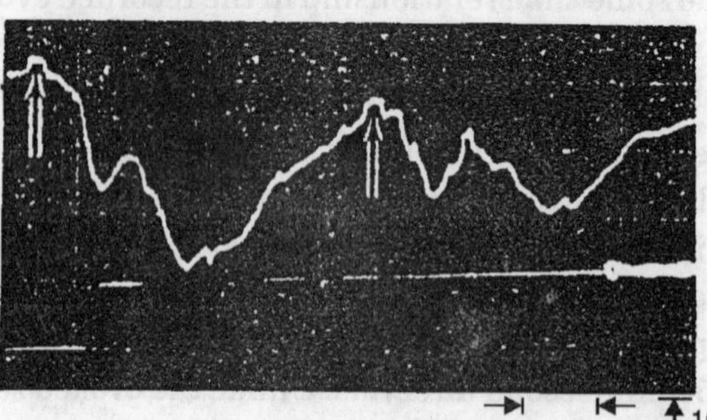

Double flash 250ms apart

Double response obtained

50ms/DIV 100μV/DIV

Fig. 4.23. Shows the evoked potentials from the visual cortex.

STIMULATION

As discussed earlier in this chapter, the potential are produced by a stimulation. But the techniques used to provide this stimulation have not been covered so far. The principles applied to stimulating the peripheral nerves and muscles also apply to the stimulating the cortex. It should be noted that the cortex stimulation may be carried out with the brain exposed with stimulation electrodes spaced by only a few millimeters so as to provide extremely localized stimulation. Under these conditions, a greater percentage of the stimulation current passes through the cells of interest and thus, overall stimulus current required to produce a response is far lower than in the case when stimulating through the skin and bone wit electrodes placed many centimeters apart. Generally, when stimulating with the cranium opened, stimulators capable of output up to ten volts are adequate. Stimulus electrodes are normally needles or concentric needless. The concentric needles provide stimulation between two electrodes less than one millimeter apart and also provides some degree of shielding to minimize the level of stimulus artifact appearing in the recorded response. Since electrical stimulation may create stimulus artifact potentials which camouflage the response, and since it appears to be desirable to stimulate via a sensory modality rather than to use direct stimulation, light stimulation or other sensory receptor stimulation is often used.

STEREOTAXIC SURGERY

The instrumentation system shown in Fig. 4.19 simply depicts a microelectrode inserted into a specimen. In practice, when recording the evoked potentials, the skull is held firmly in a jig and the microelectrode is positioned with a micromanipulator or stereotaxic instrument, usually with the aid of a microscope or X-ray techniques, as shown in Fig. 4.24. Although stereotaxic instruments are available commercially, many are constructed from precision microscope stages.

The stereotaxic surgery is a procedure to drill a hole in skull and after studying the evoked response, inject wax into those areas which are over excitable, thereby providing a cure for 'aggressive' patients with uncontrolled aggressive activity.

THE ELECTRORETINOGRAM (ERG)

As explained in earlier, it is almost not possible to detect the electrical activity produced by most of the sensory receptors on the body as they are too small and are dispersed. Some exceptional cases are the potentials resulting from stimulation of the middle ear by sound waves and of the retina by light. If a bright light is projected into the eye, the retina will be stimulated and will generate action potentials known as ERG, which can be detected by an electrode placed on the outside of the retina.

The human electroretinogram is recorded by using a silver / silver chloride imbedded in a contact lens , and a common silver/ silver chloride electrode placed on the subject's forehead, as shown in Fig. 4.25. Application of the contact lens electrode is painless and is thus suited to clinical use. The subject is placed in front of a light source which may simply be an incandescent light coupled to a photographic shutter or more commonly, a stroboscopic light as shown in Fig. 4.25. The Neon (red) or Organ (white) stroboscope is ideal for this application. Stimuli are presented in the form of flashes of light and the responses, which are obtained by means of the contact lens electrode, are displayed on a medical monitor such as any one of the physiological monitors. The 410 is operated in the EEG mode with the "EEG electrode" formed by the contrast lens and common electrode. Careful technique is required in affixing EEG electrodes and recording the ERG. It is of paramount importance that the input current of the amplifier used to record the ERG be extremely low as serious damage can occur to the eye if DC current is allowed to flow through the ERG electrode. Since stimulus artifact is not involved, AC-coupled amplifiers can be used and a capacitor may be used in series with the ERG electrode to eliminate DC currents.

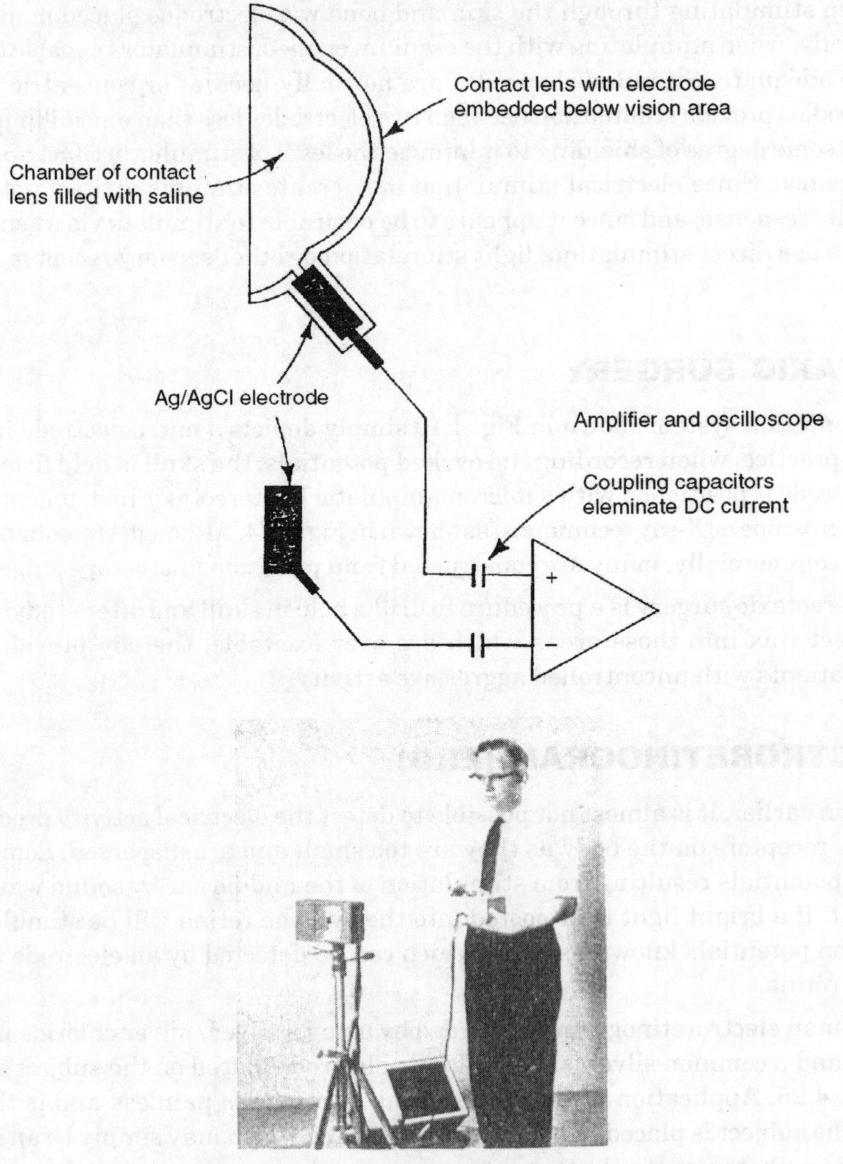

Fig. 4.25. Shows the contact lens ERG Electrode.

Fig. 4.26 shows a typical electroretinogram (ERG) together with a diagram showing general characteristics of the ERG. Variations in the characteristics of the stimulating light, as well as variations in the level of the state of light adoption of the retina, will affect the response characteristics. The electroretinogram (ERG) shown in Fig. 4.13 was recorded after the subject had become adapted to room lighting. The general characteristics of the electroretinogram consist of an initial ***A*** wave, followed by a positive ***B*** wave, a more slowly developing positive ***C*** wave (which is dependant upon duration of the stimulation) and a ***D*** wave or off-effect.

Chapter 5

Electromyography (EMG)

MUSCLE ACTION AND THE SENSORY SYSTEM

There is a fundamental relationship that exists between muscle function and the sense receptors, the brain the nervous system and the peripheral nerves. This chapter discusses about the nervous system and the peripheral nerves. The brain is at this stage, regarded as a processor and was discussed in the separate chapter on Electroencephalography (EEG).

The biological unit of muscle function is named as motor unit. A motor unit consists of a motor nerve arising from motor neurons in the brain-stem or spinal cord and branching into various motor end-plates. These motor end plates are each connected to an individual muscle fiber. Stimulation of these motor end-plates causes contraction of the single muscle fiber attached to it as shown in Fig. 5.1. The number of motor units varies between the different muscles of the

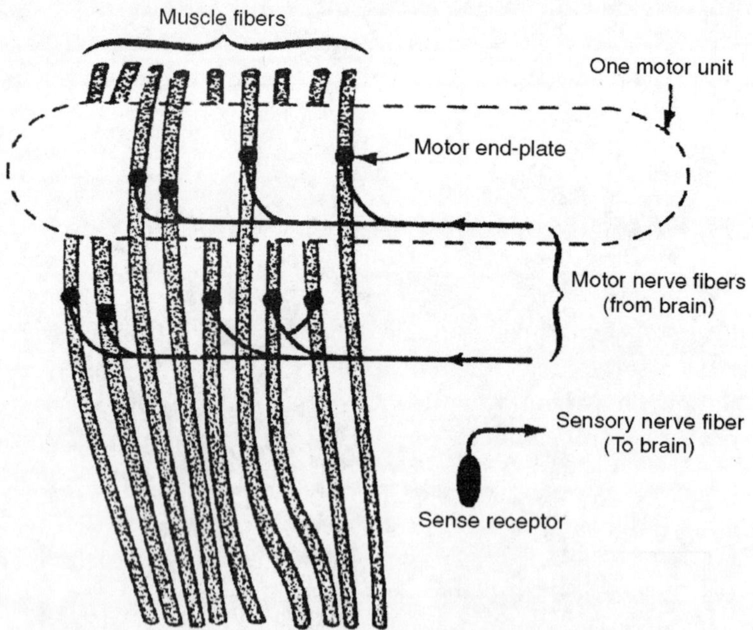

Fig. 5.1. Shows the relationship between nerve and muscle.

body. Almost in all cases, the larger the muscle, the more motor units will be found for that muscle. The size of the motor unit, that is, the number of muscle fibers activated by the name nerve fiber, can be quite different for different muscles. In man, one motor unit may contain from 25 to 2000 muscle fibers. The force developed by a motor unit may range from 0.2 to 250 grams weight. The muscle fibers of a motor unit are joined together in one part of the muscle, but rather the muscle fibers of different units are interlaced as shown in Fig. 5.1.

FORCE GENERATED BY MUSCLES

As discussed in chapter-1, a cell can only exist in its polarized or depolarized state; that is, it is a bi-stable device and intermediate potential levels are not stable. Motor nerves are also cellular in nature. So, any individual motor nerve can only exist in polarized or depolarized state. This will transmit only two potential levels to the motor end-plates causing a bistable "on-off" action of the muscle fiber. Thus, the individual muscle fibers of one motor unit exist in only two states, namely relaxed state and a tensed state. Normal muscular activity is characterized by smoothness of movement, steadiness and precision. These characteristics are due to the large number of motor units comprising of one muscle. If a small muscular effort is required, only one motor unit will be called into action; when more muscular effort is required, many more motor units are called into action until the muscle is providing maximum effort, at which time all the motor units connecting to this muscle are being used. In this way, some smoothness of movement is taking place.

Fine movement is achieved by modulating the number of muscle fiber contractions per unit time. Although an individual motor unit can result in only one level of muscular contraction, the number of times that this contraction occurs per unit time (the number of depolarizations and repolarizations executed by the motor end-plate cells) will effectively increase the power of these muscle fibers. Thus, the smoothness of movement of a muscle is controlled both by the number of motor units activated and by the rate at which these motor units are being activated.

THE SERVO-MECHANISM IN MUSCLE ACTION

Brain Control

The block diagram of the nervous system controlling muscle action is shown in Fig. 5.2. The system is similar to a servo-mechanism control system; A sensor or transducer produces position or velocity signal. This signal is sent to the brain via the sensory nerve. The brain in turn initiates an "error" or control signal by comparing the measured position with the desired level stored in the memory. This signal is sent via the motor nerve to the muscle to control its action.

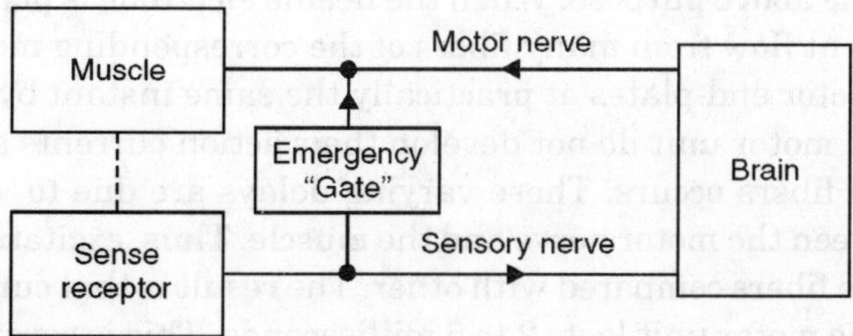

Fig. 5.2. Shows the block diagram of the nervous system.

This servo-system can be demonstrated by the following way. Let one place his finger onto a cool object. The sense receptor in the finger senses the temperature and relays this information to the brain. The brain interprets this signal as coming from a cool object and thus does not necessarily initiate any signal to the motor nerves. If the finger is then placed on a warm object, the brain will interpret the information received from the sensory nerves as relating to a warm object and will activate the motor nerves controlling muscles in the arm and the hand causing the finger to be lifted from the warm object. There is a time delay of several hundred milliseconds between the time that the sense receptor feels the warm object and the time that finger is lifted form the warm object. This delay is governed largely by the degree of attention that the subject is paying to the warm object. Now, if the finger is placed on a hot object, a reflex response is obtained and the finger is removed from hot object in about 150ms. This reflex is active at all times although it is most marked for the hot object.

Emergency gate and Reflex response

An emergency gate has been shown in Fig. 5.2. This gate is not very much involved in normal receptor / muscle operation. When a reflex response is called for, then this emergency gate bypasses the signal path to and from the brain and initiates a reflex response. This emergency gate is usually located within the spinal cord. Thus, a reflex response results form a "large signal". That means a high repetition rate signal being received from a sense receptor. This signal bypasses the brain in the initiation of muscle action. These reflex responses are to protect the body from serious damage.

Muscle Potential generated

Depolarization is initiated within a sense receptor which travels to the brain along the sensory nerve fiber as a series of travelling depolarization waves. The brain then initiates another series of travelling waves of depolarization along the motor nerves. This causes a series of depolarization of the motor end-plates. Depolarization of the motor end-plates depolarizes the cells within the muscle fiber causing contraction of these fibers.

The actual internal cell potentials are due to the normal cell polarized potential of – 90 mV and the normal cell depolarized potential of the value of + 20 mV.

Types of Electrodes

Needle electrode and surface electrodes are more commonly used ones for the measurement of potential generated during muscle action.

Needle electrodes are used to record the net result of a number of cells, such as one motor unit; surface electrodes are used to record the results of many motor units. Micro electrodes are not generally used for the above purpose. When the needle electrode is placed near these muscle cells, it will detect current flow from many fibers of the corresponding motor unit. These fibers are being fired in the motor end-plates at practically the same instant by the branching nerve. The different fibers of a motor unit do not develop their action currents simultaneously; small time variation between fibers occurs. These varying delays are due to varying lengths of the terminal branches between the motor nerve and the muscle. Thus, excitation, as it travels along, is slightly ahead in some fibers compared with other. The result is that current flow in any small area from the cells of one motor unit lasts 2 to 5 milliseconds. This is several times the duration of the current from any single muscle fiber. This asynchronous action helps to produce smoothness of muscle action.

The best method to the detect the potentials from a single motor unit is by a concentric-needle electrodes. This is often called as insulated needle electrode. This is shown in Fig. 5.3.

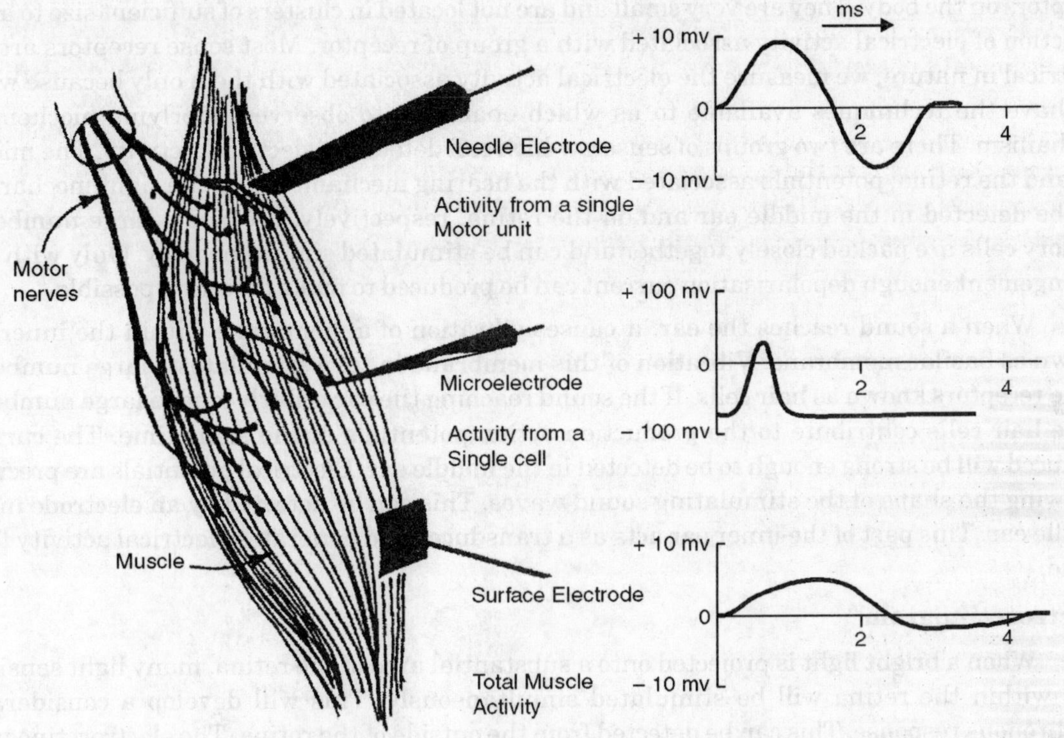

Fig. 5.3. Shows the EMG obtained with various electrode types.

Single motor unit activity may sometimes be detected by placing a small electrode on the skin over the muscle. The volume of muscle influencing such an electrode is, however, the total activity from many motor units having random relationships to one another. The potential produced by muscle action, whether recorded by needle electrode or surface electrodes, is known as the **electromyogram or the EMG.** Measurement techniques for electromyographic recording are explained later in this chapter.

The Sense Receptors

When a sense receptor or a transducer cell is activated by a physical distortion, a temperature change or some other effect, a series of nerve impulses are produced. The time between the individual nerve impulses becomes more and more when various factors come into play. After a while, even with continuation of the physical stimulus, no nerve impulses are generated. It is certain that the sense receptors generate discrete potential levels. These are more or less logarithmically related to the stimulus strength. These potentials in turn produce a series of nerve impulses in the nerve fiber. Impulse repetition frequencies will vary from a few impulses per second to 1000 per second; rates above 50 per second are most unusual in human subjects. Since the sense receptors generate an approximate logarithmic response to the stimulus, they can respond over an enormous range (1:10^7 or more) of stimulus energy levels.

The potential generated by sense receptor stimulation

It is almost impossible to detect the electrical activity associated with most of the sense receptors on the body. They are very small and are not located in clusters of sufficient size to allow detection of electrical activity associated with a group of receptor. Most sense receptors are not electrical in nature; we measure the electrical activity associated with them only because we do not have the techniques available to us which enable us to observe underlying biochemical mechanism. There are two groups of sensors which can detect the electrical activity. The middle ear and the retina; potentials associated with the hearing mechanism and the sight mechanism can be detected in the middle ear and on the retina, respectively, because a large number of sensory cells are packed closely together and can be stimulated simultaneously. Only with this arrangement enough depolarisation current can be produced to make detection possible.

When a sound reaches the ear, it causes vibration of a membrane within the inner ear known as basilar membrane. Vibration of this membrane in turn stimulates a large number of sense receptors known as hair cells. If the sound reaching the ear is fairly loud, a large number of these hair cells contribute to the production action potentials at the same time. The current produced will be strong enough to be detected in the middle ear. Electrical potentials are precisely following the shape of the stimulating sound waves. This can be detected by an electrode in the middle ear. This part of the inner ear acts as a transducer and generates electrical activity form sound.

Electroretinogram

When a bright light is projected onto a substantial area of the retina, many light sensitive cells within the retina will be stimulated simultaneously. This will develop a considerable synchronous response. This can be detected from the outside of the retina. The electroretinogram (the External Electrical Response to Light Stimulation) may be detected by an electrode consisting of a small, flat silver plate fitted to the inner surface of a small contact lens.

STIMULATION-ELECTROMYOGRAPHY-NERVE CONDUCTION

We know that the bioelectric signals are generated within the individual cells when these cells are stimulated. Stimulation refers to an external force being applied to the cell. This results in the cell depolarizing and then repolarisation takes place. Cells in the eye are sensitive to light stimulation; the cells in the ear are sensitive to sound stimulation. And of course nerve cells are sensitive in electro-chemical stimulation. All cells are sensitive to one degree or another to artificial electrical stimulation. The passage of electric current through the cell will cause it to depolarize.

Artificial Stimulation

When analyzing the bio- medical phenomena, it is often desirable to artificially stimulate a group of cells. A pulse generator is used for the above purpose. The pulse generator passes current through the cells concerned, for a small duration. Suppose, for example, one wishes to cause the ulnar nerve in the arm to propagate a depolarization pulse. Then the particular nerve can be stimulated by passing current through the arm with the aid of two surface electrodes placed so that part of the current flow between them passes through the ulnar nerve.

It is impossible to localize stimulating current to a particular cell or small group of cells. Current is passed through the bulk tissue surrounding these cells. A finite, but unpredictable, portion of this current will pass through the cells. Since it is impossible to localize current flow to a particular cell, it is impossible to know how much current will flow through it.

Type of stimulators

The following two types of the stimulators are extensively used.

1. Constant current stimulators
2. Constant voltage stimulators.

Stimulators provide an output from either a constant current source ($Z_0 > 10,000\ \Omega$) or from a constant voltage source ($Z_0 < 50$ ohms) (Fig. 5.4). Arguments for and against both stimulators have existed since very early days of physiology. Many modern pulse generators intended for tissue stimulation provide constant current and constant voltage output characteristics. A pair of stimulating electrodes immersed in tissue fluid typically has an impedance of about 500 ohms at the frequencies involved in the stimulus part.

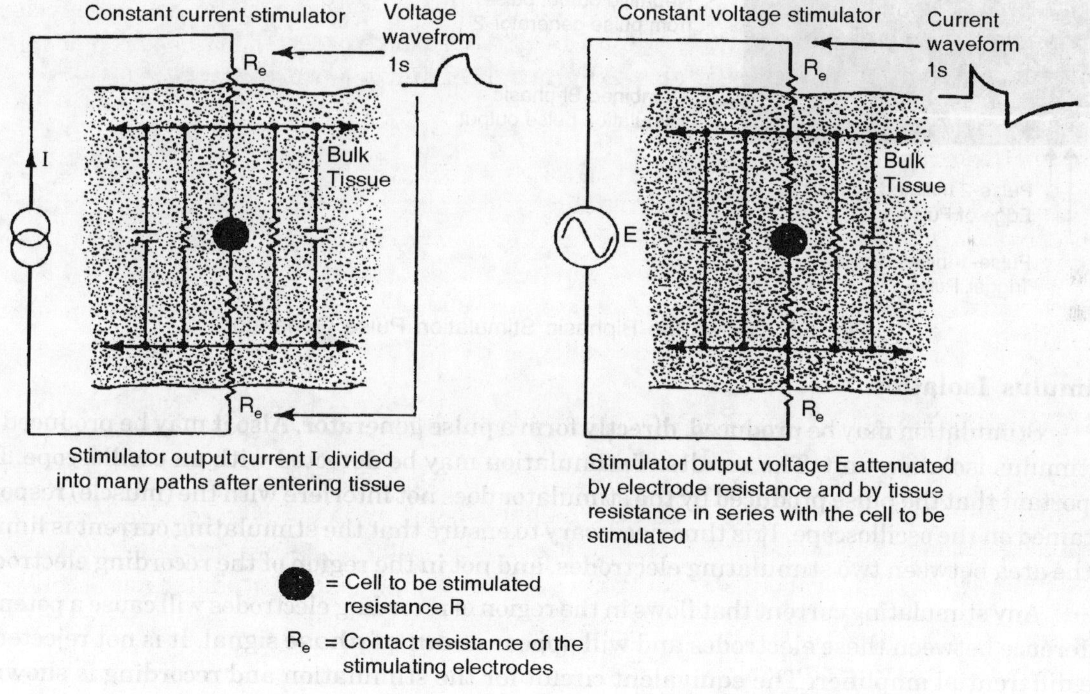

Fig. 5.4. Shows the constant current and constant voltage stimulation.

If a stimulus current of insufficient intensity to cause cell depolarization is applied to a cell, the cell membrane resting potential will be reduced from its normal value of - 90millivolts. If an additional pulse of the same intensity is then applied to the cell within the next few milliseconds or so, the cell may then depolarize, as the cell membrane potential has not yet returned to its normal resting potential as discussed in chapter 1. The cell would appear to be more sensitive to stimulation for the second pulse than from the first. It has been suggested that cell recovery from the effect of a stimulus current can be hastened by the passage of an opposing lower intensity current for an appreciably longer period so that the net quantity of electricity is zero. This feature is incorporated in the biphasic stimulation shown in Fig. 5.5. Biphasic stimulation also neutralizes recording electrode polarization. In the waveform shown in the figure, the stimulating pulse is followed by a pulse of opposite polarity, of one-tenth the amplitude and ten times the width.

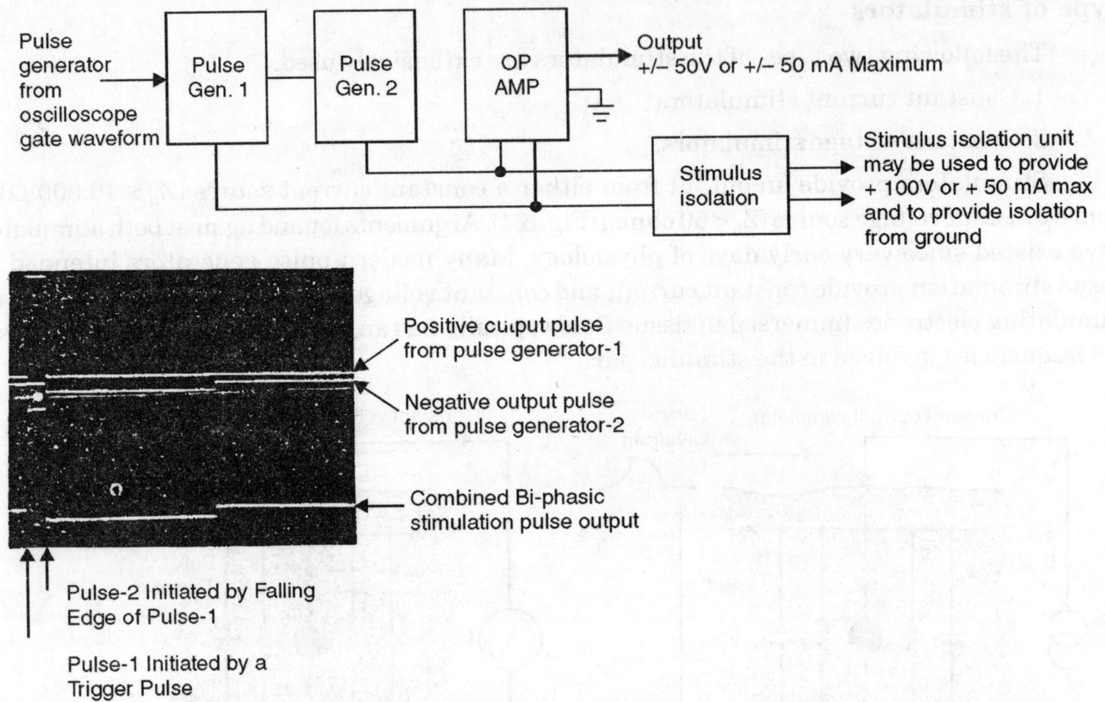

Fig. 5.5. Shows the Biphasic Stimulation Pulse Generator.

Stimulus Isolation

Stimulation may be produced directly form a pulse generator. Also it may be produced via a stimulus isolation unit. The results of stimulation may be detected with an oscilloscope. It is important that the pulse produced by the stimulator does not interfere with the (muscle) response obtained on the oscilloscope. It is thus necessary to ensure that the stimulating current is limited to the area between two stimulating electrodes, and not in the region of the recording electrodes.

Any stimulating current that flows in the region of recording electrodes will cause a potential difference between these electrodes and will appear as **out of phase** signal. It is not rejected by the differential amplifier. The equivalent circuit for the stimulation and recording is shown in Fig. 5.6.

Impedance Matching

In this circuit (Fig. 5.6), most of the stimulating current flows through the impedance formed by the tissue between the stimulating electrodes. It is apparent that two alternating current paths exist; via the tissue impedance Z_1 and Z_2 and the amplifier input impedance to ground. If it were possible to make $Z_1 = Z_2$, then no in-phase signal would be produced at the recording electrodes. These impedances are not controllable however, and it is impossible in practice to balance them even by careful placement of the recording electrodes.

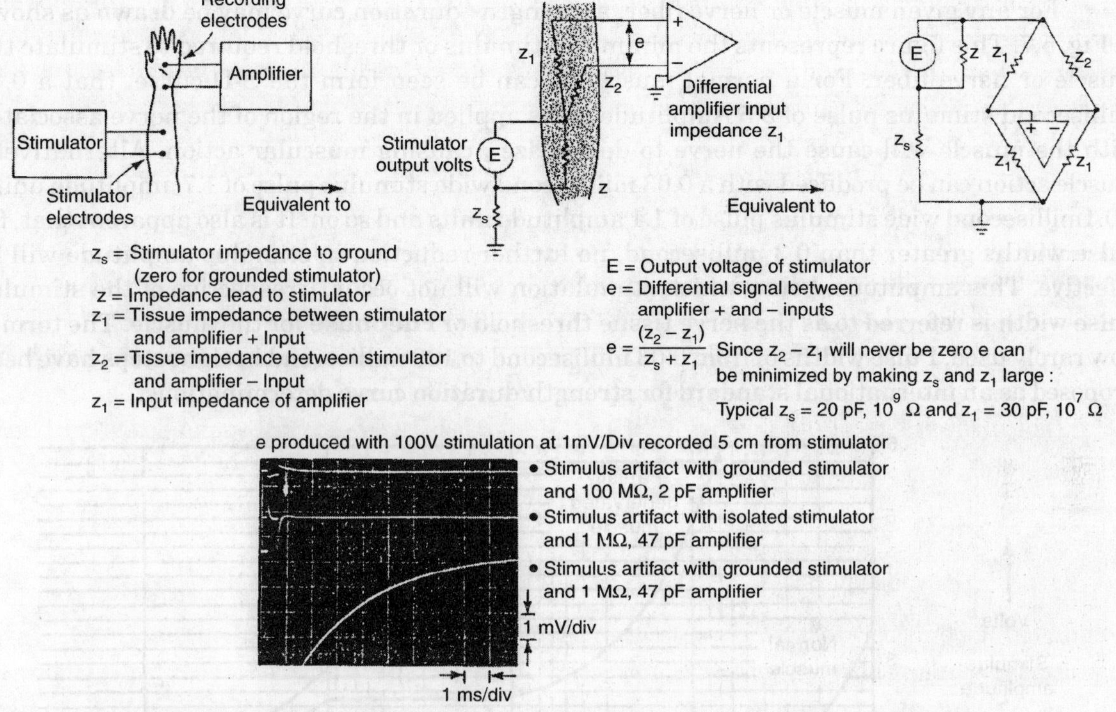

Fig. 5.6. Shows the equivalent circuit of stimulator, subject and amplifier.

Isolated Stimulator

Since it is not possible to balance the tissue impedances, then one must reduce the stimulating current passing through these impedances to as low as a value possible in an effort to reduce the differential signal processing at the recording electrodes. To reduce these currents, it is necessary to either increase the input impedance of the differential amplifier or to increase the impedance between stimulator and ground. It is easy to make both these impedances as large as possible practically in an effort to achieve the maximum reduction in the level of stimulus signal appearing at the recording electrodes.

High input impedance Amplifier

With a non-isolated stimulator, the impedance between stimulator and ground is zero. However, with an isolated stimulator this impedance can be made very high, typically in the order of 10^9 ohms.

If a grounded stimulator is used in tissue, the ground electrode should always be placed between the hot electrode and the recording electrode, to minimize stimulus artifacts.

Strength/Duration curves

Strength/Duration curve shows the excitability characteristics of muscle or nerve fibers. Stimulation of a cell is achieved by the passage of a certain quantity of electricity through the cell. Stimulation is dependant on charge rather than on current. Stimulation can be achieved by passing a large current for a short period or with a lesser current for a longer period. Since diffusion within the cell tends to oppose the stimulating current, a lower limit of current is reached below which stimulation will not occur, no matter how long the current is maintained.

For any given muscle or nerve fiber, a strength / duration curve may be drawn as shown in Fig. 5.7. This figure represents the minimum stimulus or threshold required to stimulate the muscle or nerve fiber. For a normal muscle, it can be seen form the S-D curve, that a 0.01 millisecond stimulus pulse of 3.5 Amplitude units applied in the region of the nerve associated with the muscle will cause the nerve to depolarize , causing muscular action. Alternatively, muscle action can be produced with a 0.03 millisecond wide stimulus pulse of 1.7 amplitude units, a 0.1millisecond wide stimulus pulse of 1.1 amplitude units and so on. It is also apparent that, for pulse widths greater than 0.3 millisecond, no further reduction in stimulus amplitude will be effective. This amplitude, below which stimulation will not occur, irrespective of the stimulus pulse width is referred to as the nerve tissue threshold or **rheobase** for the muscle. The term is now rarely used. Pulse widths of from 0.03 millisecond to 100 millisecond in eight steps have been proposed as an international standard for strength/duration curve determinations.

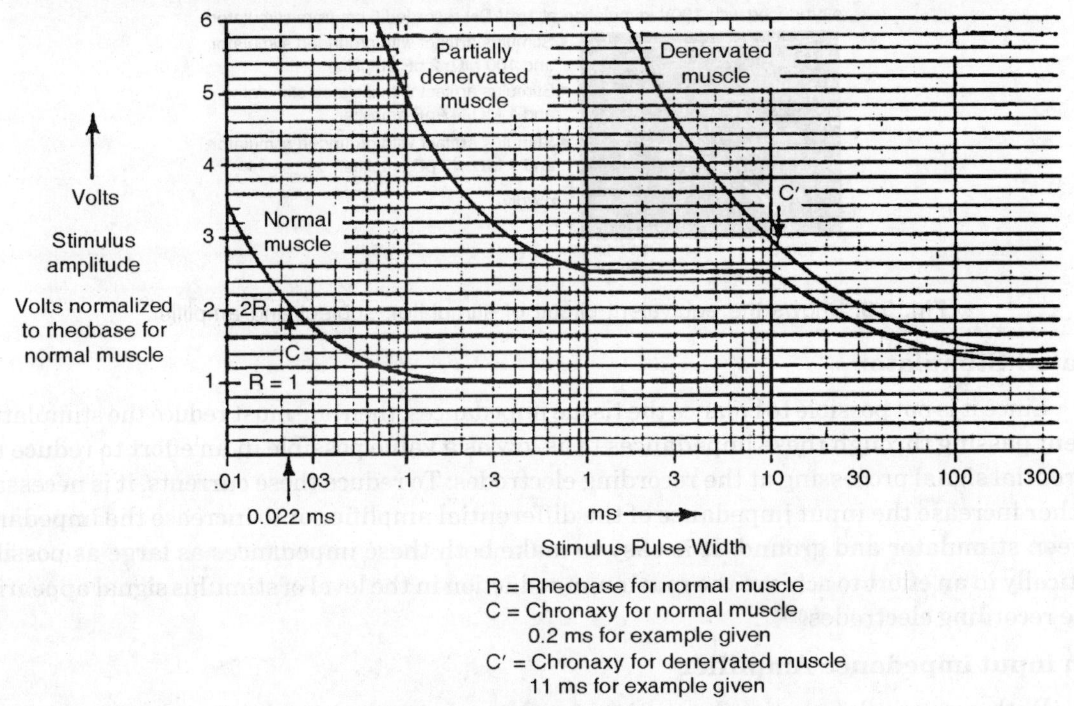

Fig. 5.7. Shows the strength/duration or S-D curve.

PULSE AMPLITUDE NORMALIZED TO RHEOBASE

In the particular example shown in Fig. 5.7, this rheobase occurred when using a constant voltage stimulator set at 30 V. As discussed earlier, this absolute voltage level has little meaning. For instance, a 30 Volts is equivalent to 1.0 unit of stimulus amplitude and 2.0 units of stimulus amplitude being equivalent to 60 volts etc.

Chronaxy

Once a strength / duration curve is determined, it is desirable to have a technique whereby curves for various muscles can be compared. S-D curves may be compared by comparing the chrnoaxy obtained form the curve. The chronaxy is the minimum pulse width required to excite the tissue for a stimulus of twice amplitude of the rheobase. The chronaxy, in the example shown in S-D curve (Fig. 5.7) is 0.022 millisecond for normal muscle.

Denervated Muscle Action

The S-D curve for a denervated muscle is shown in Fig. 5.7. A denervated muscle exists when the nerve connection to the muscle has effectively been interrupted. This may be achieved by impairing the motor end-plates action with drugs such as *curare*. It can be seen form S-D curve, that a denervated muscle is less sensitive to stimulus than a normal muscle. In a normal muscle, the stimulating potential excites the more sensitive nerve fibers which in turn excites the muscle whereas in a denervated muscle, the stimulating current must stimulate the muscle directly. Thus, the S-D curve for a muscle shows the excitability characteristic for a single motor neuron; however, the S-D curve for a denervated muscle shows the excitability characteristics of a single muscle fiber.

Fig. 5.7 also shows a S-D curve for a partially denervated muscle. It can be seen for pulse width up to 10 milliseconds, muscle action is due to stimulation of the nerve, whereas for pulse width greater than 10ms, muscle action is due to stimulation of the muscle directly. The S-D curve is, thus, displaying excitability characteristic of the component which has the lower threshold for a specific pulse width.

When preparing S-D curves, muscle action is determined by viewing the muscle concerned in a well lit environment. When stimulating with a hundred millisecond pulse, the muscular contraction produced is brisk and pronounced when the contraction is due to excitation of the nerve fibers, but sluggish when stimulating muscle fibers directly. When stimulating with a narrower pulse, the muscle action is characterized by a twitching of the muscle concerned only.

Muscle action can also be determined by using some form of force gauge attached to the muscle concerned showing muscular movement, or, more commonly, by recording the electrical activity produced within the muscle when the muscle is stimulated by the nerve.

In some instances, the plotting of the S-D curve is somewhat tedious and abbreviated S-D curves are obtained by determining the stimulus amplitude required for a 100 millisecond pulse and a 1 millisecond pulse and expressing these as ratio.

In a normal muscle, this ratio should be approximately unity, in a partly denervated muscle, it will be between 1.5 and 4. In a fully denervated muscle, it will be between 4 and infinity.

Denervated S-D curves may also be obtained by determining the rheobase and then determining the chronaxy directly by doubling the stimulus amplitude and reducing the pulse width to a point where the tissue can no longer be stimulated. This point will represent the chronaxy.

MYOGRAPHY

Myography is a study of muscular contraction and a myograph is an apparatus for recoding the mechanical effects of a muscular contraction.

A myograph may simply consist of a displacement transducer or a force transducer mechanically coupled to the muscle under investigation. As shown is Fig. 5.8, an elastic strip is paced around the muscle concerned and a strain gauge is bonded to this elastic strip. Muscular contraction causes a tension increase in the elastic strip with resulting resistance change in the strain gauge. The muscular contraction may be initiated voluntarily or produced by electrical stimulation. The output form a recording system, a series of muscular contractions over a 20sec. period is also shown in figure-8. Force myographs are particularly suited to exercising subjects or for the study of muscular fatigue over prolonged periods.

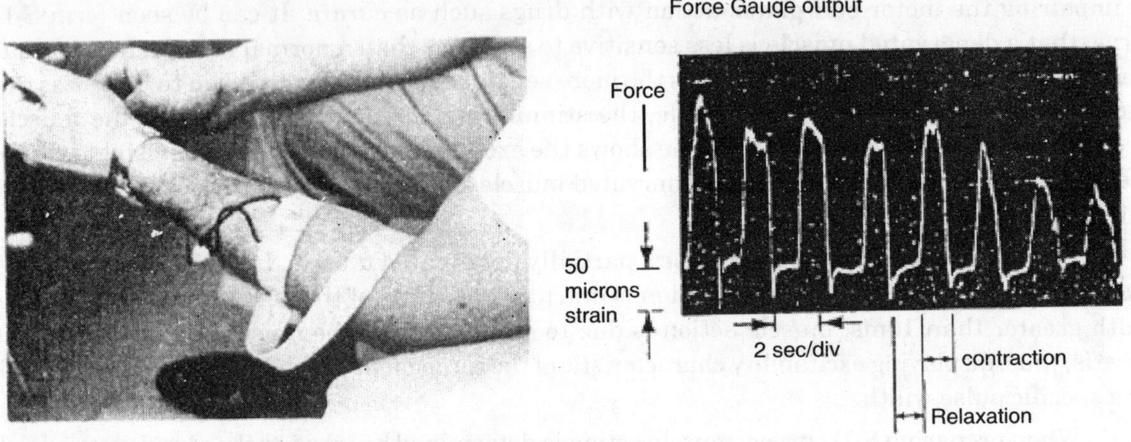

Fig. 5.8. Shows how a myograph with a strainage is used.

ELECTROMYOGRAPHY

The myography records are for the study of muscular contraction, the EMG records the electric effects of such a contraction. Muscular contraction is caused by depolarization of the muscle fibers. The depolarization produces action potentials as discussed in earlier chapters. This muscular action potential is known as the electro myogram or EMG. An electromyogram will be produced in a muscle where the muscle contraction is caused either by voluntarily muscle action or by electrical stimulation of the muscle.

Electromyography with Voluntary Muscular Action

A typical system of recording the electromyography produced by voluntary muscle action is shown in Fig. 5.9. The muscle action potential is picked up by a needle electrodes inserted into the muscle or by surface electrodes placed over the muscle concerned . Then the signal is amplified by a suitable differential amplifier. The EMG can then be detected audibly by using a speaker in conjunction with an audio amplifier. The EMG may also be displayed directly on an oscilloscope. Or this may be converted to an absolute integral and then displayed on an oscilloscopes. Both direct displays and integrated and displays are shown in Fig. 5.10.

Referring to the Fig. 10, the upper trace is on the top photograph shows the EMG produced by a mild voluntary contraction. The action potential produced by a single motor unit can clearly be differentiated from other action potentials. The absolute integral of this activity is displayed on the lower trace in the same photograph. The integral displays the quantity of electricity involved in the muscular contraction. The quantity of electricity associated with the single motor unit action potential can also be determined.

With a more forceful voluntary contraction, as shown in the Fig. 5.7*b*, many motor units are involved and the EMG obtained is the result of the action potential produced by all these motor units; the resulting integral being greater than the integral obtained for a single motor unit. By using a slower sweep speed in conjunction with the system shown in Fig. 5.9, the EMG and absolute integral for a series of contraction may be displayed as shown in the Fig. 5.10.

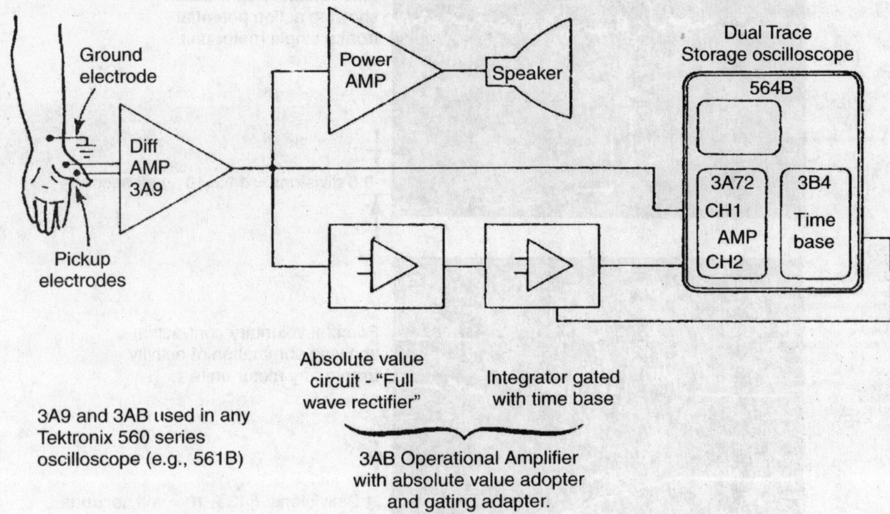

3A9 Differential amplifier set at 1 mV/div. Provides A gain of 1000X to the 3AB operational amplifier and 3A72 channer 1.

3A72 Channel 1 set at 1 V/div providing a sensitivity referred to the electrodes of 1 mV/div

3A8 Operational amplifier #1 used in conjunction with an absolute value circuit as shown in chapter 29

3A8 Operational amplifier #2 used in conjunction with a low speed gating adapter as shown inchapter 29. z_1 set at 1 MΩ, z_f at 0.1 μF for integration.

3A72 Channel 2 set at 0.1, 0.2 or 0.5 V/cm providing varying integration sensitivities.

Integrator calibration–Oscilloscope amplifier #2 at 0.2 V/div

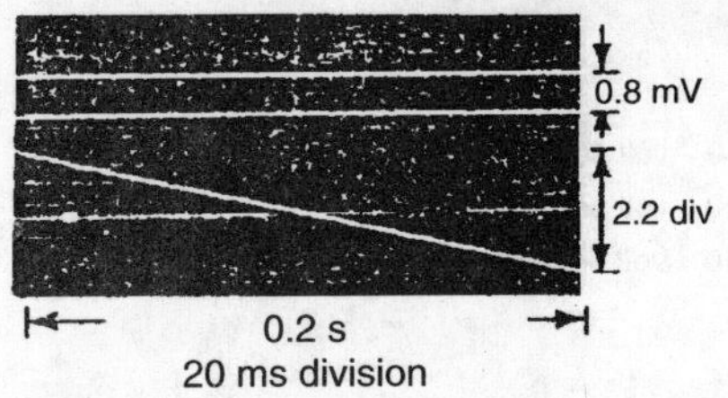

4mV calibrator signal from oscilloscope calibrator connected to differential amplifier.

Differential amplifier gain reduced by 5X (from 1 mV/div to 5mV/div) providing a calibration voltage relative to the EMG system of 0.8 mV.

Calibrator duty factor is 50%.

Calibrator input shown $= 0.8 \times 10^{-3} \times \frac{50}{100} \times 0.2$ volt seconds

$= 80 \times 10^{-6}$ volt seconds.

2.2 Div of integrator output $= 80 \times 10^{-6}$ volt seconds

$\therefore$ Integrator calibration is 36×10^{-6} volt seconds/div with oscilloscope amplifier 2 at 0.2 V/div.

Integrator output $= 180 \times 10^{-6}$ volt seconds input/volts output

Fig. 5.9. Shows an electromyograph system.

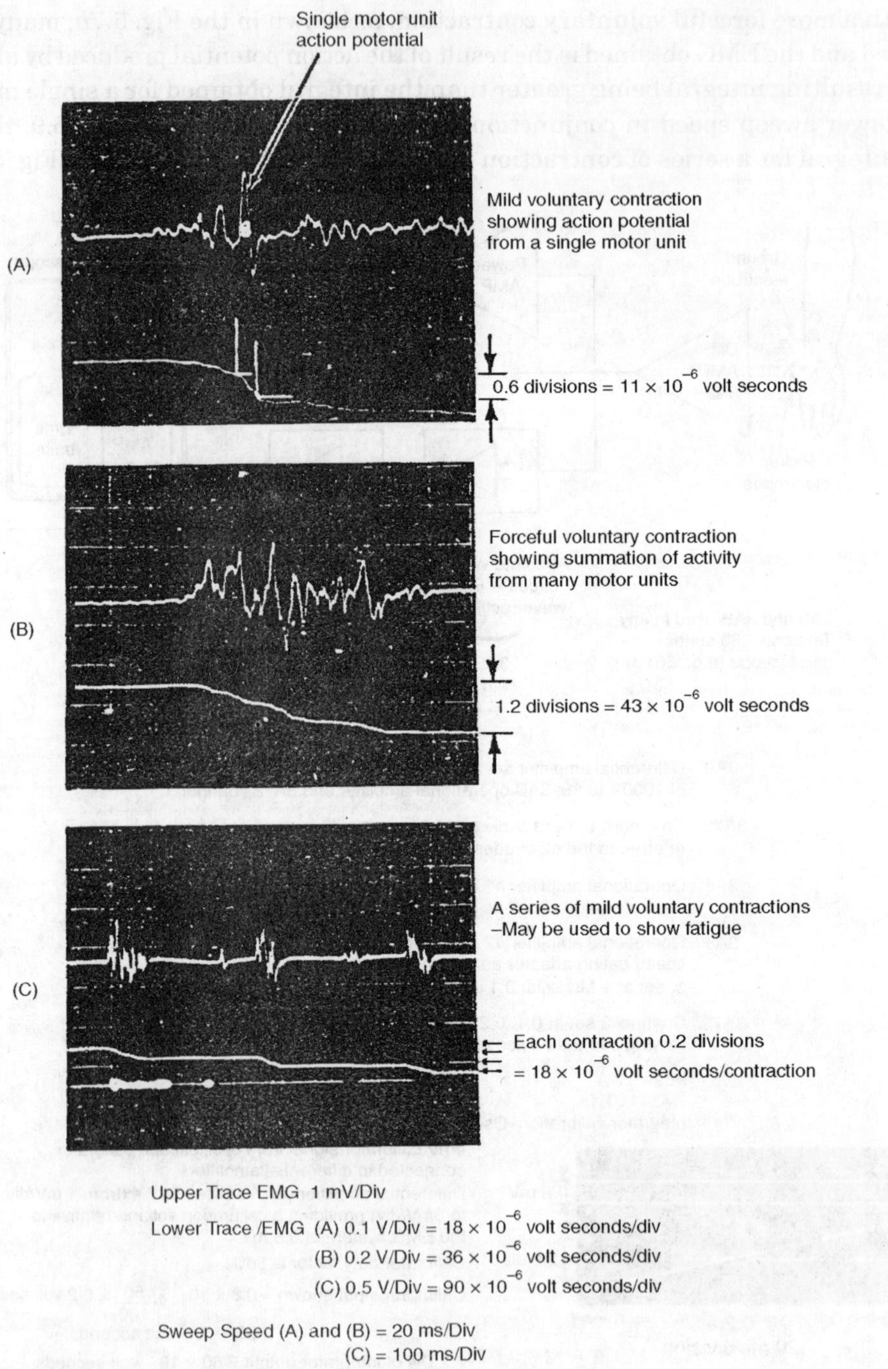

Fig. 5.10. Shows the results obtaned with the system shown in Fig. 5.9.

The quantity of electrical activity produced by a muscular contraction is a monatomic function of strength of the contraction. Since it is difficult to estimate this quantity from an observation of the EMG waveform, the absolute integral of the EMG is used as a measure of this quantity. The integrator output is calibrated in units of electrical quantity, i.e., volt seconds.

Since 1 volt second is a substantial quantity of electricity, it is preferable to refer to EMG's in smaller units, one "unit" being equal to 10 -6 volt seconds. It can be seen from Fig. 5.10, that for a particular subject and a particular muscle, 11 units are produced by a single motor unit, 18 units by a mild muscular contraction and 43 units by a forceful contraction.

Calibration

Referring to Fig. 5.9, the absolute integral is obtained by full -wave rectification of the electromyography. The integrating of this rectified signal is done by full wave rectification. Then integrating this rectified signal is with an integrator gated "on" for the duration of the oscilloscope sweep. The whole system consist of the differential amplifier, the full-wave rectifier, the integrator and oscilloscope for displaying the signal.

The EMG is often presented audibly in clinical applications. And the trained listener can judge the condition of the muscle by the volume and characteristic tones produced by the audio system during a muscular contraction.

ELECTROMYOGRAPHY DURING ELECTRICAL STIMULATION

The EMG produced during a voluntary twitch is spread out over a period of 100 millisecond or more as the nerve impulse to various motor units are not time coincident and as the propagation delay from the spinal cord to the muscle concerned is different for all nerve fibers. Also, since the contraction is voluntary, any one motor unit may produce several action potentials. The frequency of discharge is determined within the spinal cord. Such is not the case when recording EMG produced by electrical stimulation. All neurons with threshold above the stimulating intensity are simultaneously stimulated by the electrical impulse. Thus all muscle fibers discharge simultaneously, producing substantial activity for a brief period of time, typically less than 10 milliseconds. Although the response obtained when stimulating is referred to as an EMG, it is an unnatural occurrence and should perhaps be correctly referred to as a "myographic response" or a "muscle action potential". The stimulus pulse used to initiate this response usually has an amplitude of > 100 V and is either 0.1 millisecond, 0.3 ms or occasionally, 0.5 ms wide.

A typical EMG produced by electrical stimulation is shown in Fig. 5.11. A 0.3 millisecond stimulus pulse width was used to initiate the response. A delay occurred between the stimulating pulse and the response; this delay is referred to as latency. The action potential shown in Fig. 5.11*a* has a latency of 4 milliseconds and produces an action potential covering the following 7 milliseconds. This action potential is referred to as **diphasic** as it shows a single positive deflection followed by a single negative deflection.

Monophasic Response

The action potential shown in Fig. 5.11*b* is referred to as monophasic as the action potential appears to be comprised of only one positive deflection. This action potential is partially camouflaged by the amplifier recovery characteristics due to the use of non- isolated stimulator. If a grounded stimulator is used on tissue , the ground electrode should always be placed between the "hot" stimulating electrode and the recording electrodes, to minimize stimulus artifacts.

Triphasic Response

The EMG shown in Fig. 5.11*c* is referred to as triphasic as two positive deflections and one negative deflection are exhibited. This EMG was recorded using a concentric needle pickup electrode

which effectively locates two electrodes less than one millimeter apart in the muscle in an attempt to record the action potential produced by a single motor unit rather than by the complete muscle. All three EMG's shown in Fig. 5.11, are considered acceptable and basically serve to show that the nerve and muscle relationship is functioning correctly as the latency is not excessive and action potential is, in fact, generated.

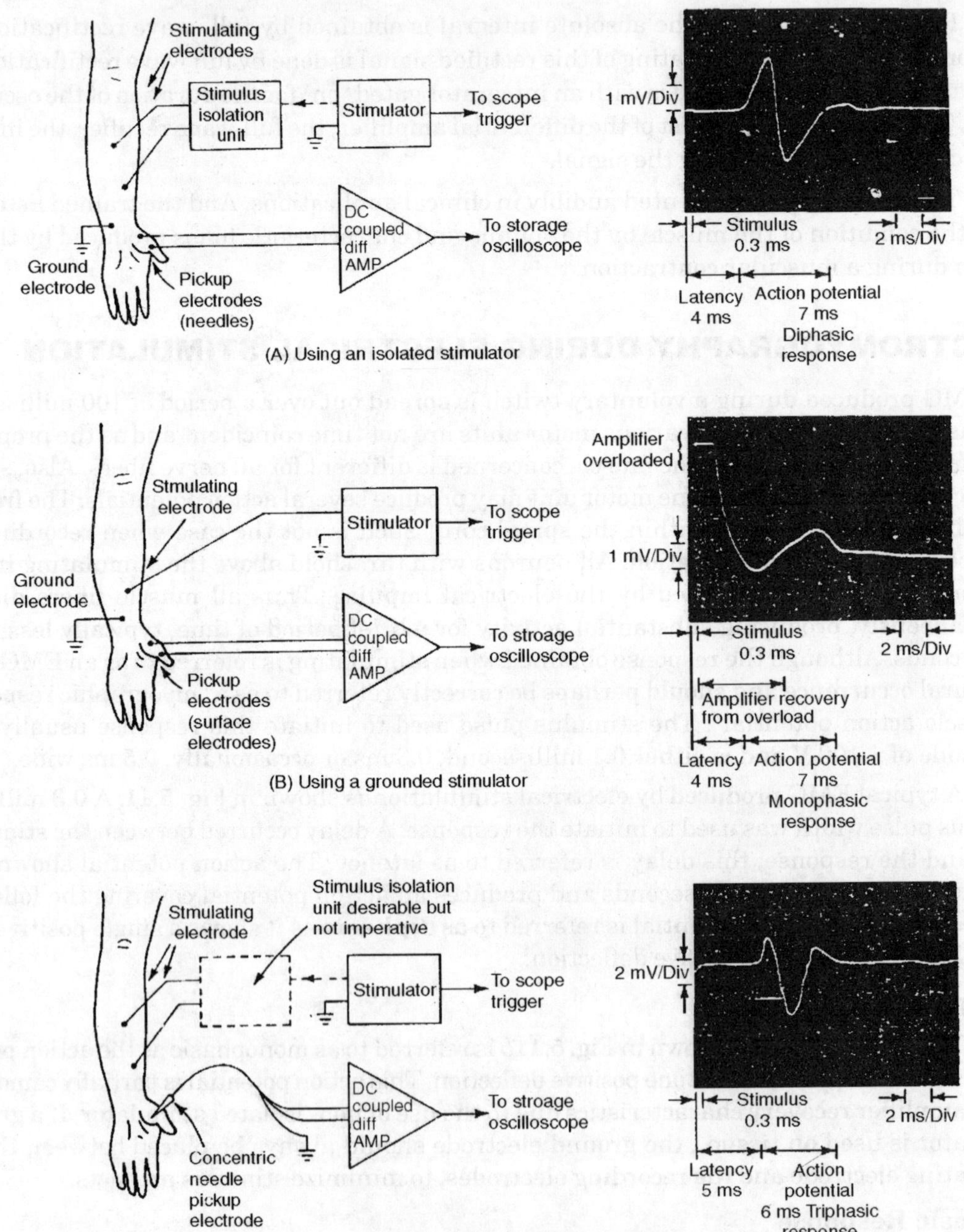

Fig. 5.11. Shows the EMG produced by electrical stimulation.

The H-reflex

The muscular reflex response generated within the spinal cord was covered in earlier in this chapter. When recording EMG's produced by electrical stimulation, the stimulating current excites the motor nerve which in turn initiates a response in the muscle concerned. This stimulation current also excites the sensory nerve. It is possible to decrease the stimulus level to a point, where

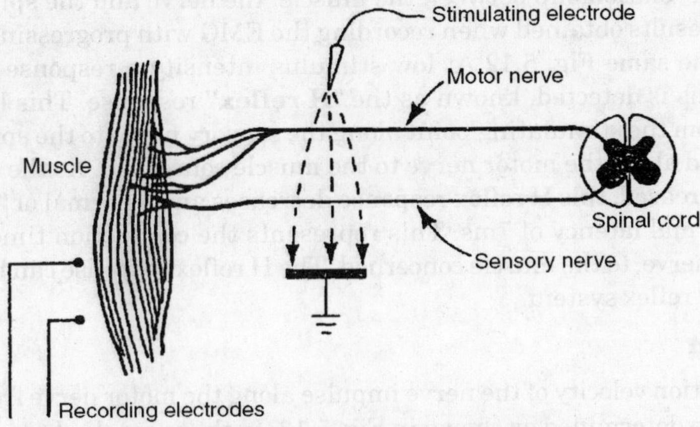

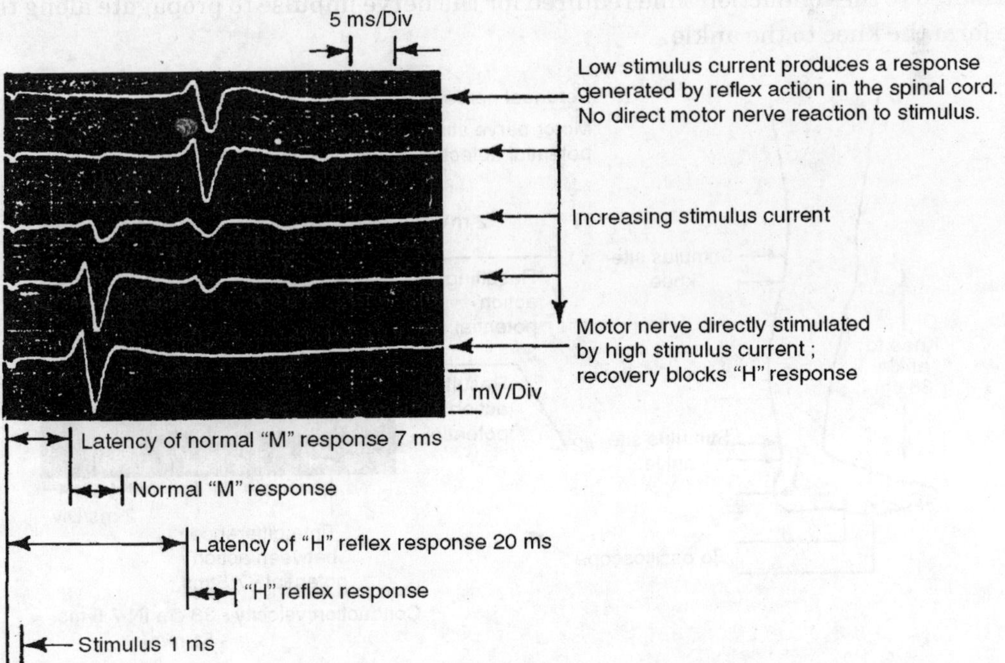

Fig. 5.12. Shows the H-Reflex response.

the stimulus intensity is insufficient to excite the motor nerve but is sufficient to excite the more sensitive sensory nerve. The depolarization pulse propagated in the sensory nerve as a result of this stimulation travels to the spinal cord. The spinal cord generates the reflex response which is propagated to the motor nerve. This reflex response is in turn propagated along the motor nerve to the muscle concerned, initiating a muscular response.

The physical relationship between the muscle, the nerve and the spinal cord is shown in the Fig. 5.12. The results obtained when recording the EMG with progressing stimulus intensity is also shown in the same Fig. 5.12 At low stimulus intensity a response having a latency of approximately 20ms is detected, known as the **"H reflex"** response. This latency is due to the conduction time from the stimulating point along the sensory nerve to the spinal cord and thence from the spinal cord along the motor nerve to the muscle concerned. As the stimulating current is progressively increased, this H reflex response decreases and a normal or **"M reflex"** response appears with a normal latency of 7ms. This represents the conduction time from the stimulus site, via the motor nerve, to the muscle concerned. The H reflex response can be used to determine the condition of the reflex system.

Nerve conduction

The propagation velocity of the nerve impulse along the motor nerve from the stimulus site to the muscle can be determined as shown in Fig. 5.13. In the example shown, the *peroneal* nerve of the left leg is stimulated behind the knee and a muscular response is detected on the foot, using either surface electrodes or the needle electrodes. The response shown in the figure has a latency of 11.5 ms. The stimulus electrodes are then moved to a point behind the ankle and a response obtained in the foot, having a latency of 4 milliseconds. The difference between these two latencies is attributed to the conduction time required for the nerve impulse to propagate along the motor nerve form the knee to the ankle.

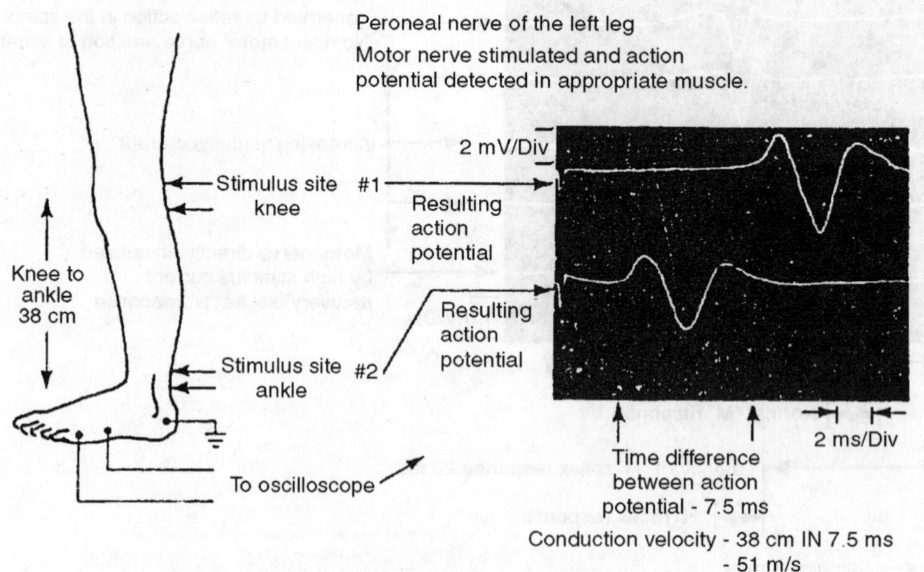

Fig. 5.13. Shows the motor nerve conduction velocity determination.

The propagation velocity can be determined by measuring the distance form the knee stimulation point to the ankle stimulation point and dividing it by the difference in latencies. A 100 volt stimulus pulse, 0.3 millisecond pulse width, is usually used. Occasionally, pulse widths of either 0.1 or 0.5 millisecond are used. The stimulus should be repeated several times to ensure that the response obtained is consistent.

A similar technique can be used to measure sensory nerve conduction velocity as shown in Fig. 5.14. In Fig. 5.14, we moved the stimulus site with respect to a fixed recording site. When attempting to record sensory nerve conduction velocity, it is necessary to stimulate at a fixed sense receptor site. To record the propagation of this stimulus pulse along the sensory nerve, it is done by detecting the nerve impulse or "traveling wave of depolarization" at various sites of nerve.

Fig. 5.14 shows the results obtained when stimulating the hand and recording the propagation of this pulse along the ulnar nerve at four points along the length of the nerve using a four-channel oscilloscope. The vertical position of the four channels on this oscilloscope are adjusted to represent distance in centimeters from the stimulus site. The various latencies obtained should be directly proportional to the distance , resulting in the straight line shown in Fig. 5.14. Any deviation in straightness in this line would then represent a change in conduction velocity. Injury to the nerve will normally result in decreased conduction velocity in the injured part of the nerve.

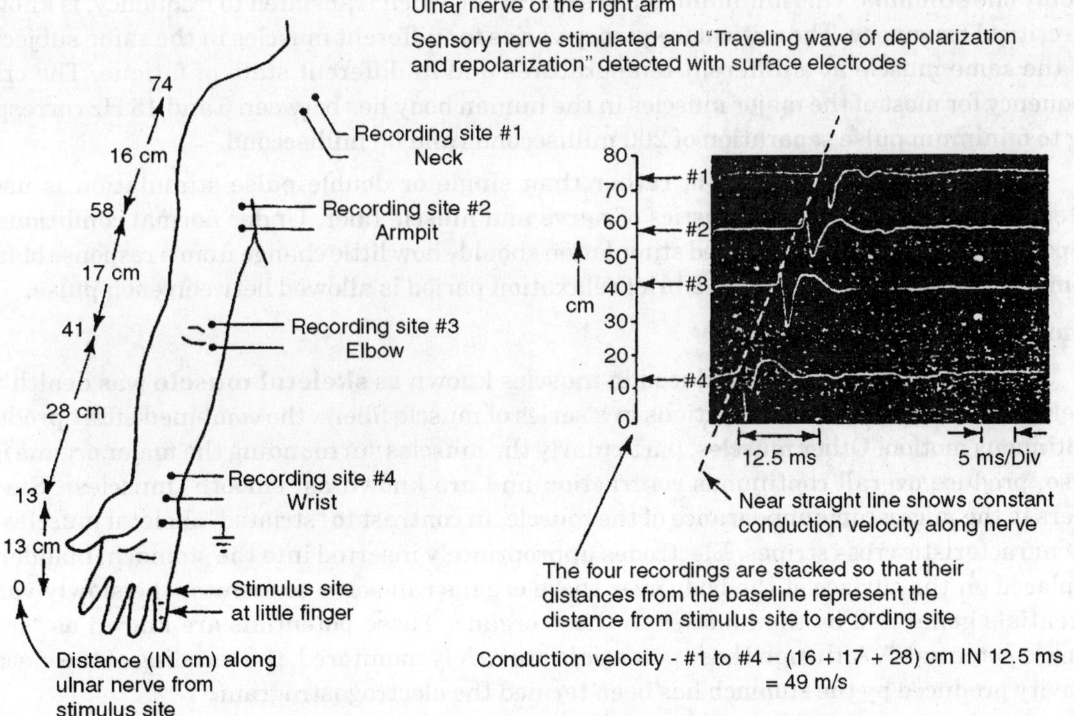

Fig. 5.14. Shows the sensory nerve conduction velocity determination.

Limb Nerves Investigations

When measuring conduction velocity, four nerves are principally investigated. The ulnar, and median nerves of the arm and the peroneal and tibial nerves of the legs. The ulnar, peroneal and tibial nerves perform both general sensory and motor functions. However, the median nerve primarily performs a sensory function. Response from the ulnar nerve are normally detected on the back of the hand or on the fingers, the median nerve on the thumb or on the thick fleshy part of the hand near the thumb, the peronel nerve on the four smaller toes or the top of the foot and the tibial nerve at the side of the foot near the larger toe or on the larger toe.

Normally, conduction velocity is measured, or EMG's are recorded to diagnose an abnormality in the subject. Since this abnormality usually manifests itself in only one side of the subject at a time, the limb on the other side of the subject may be regarded as normal and the conduction velocities or EMG's compared between the two limbs. As we know, the conduction velocity depends on the nerve under investigation. But the conduction velocities for a healthy nerve is given as in the range of 40 to 60 meters per second; injury or abnormality being indicated by the lower conduction velocities, typically, in the order of below 10 meters/second. The term electrodiagnosis as applied should include most of the techniques covered in this chapter.

Repetitive Stimulation

So far, in this chapter, we have dealt with the effects of a single stimulating pulse on muscle and nerve fiber. When we want to determine the recovery characteristic of a motor unit, it is necessary to stimulate with a double pulse. That is to determine the delay required between the two pulses for the stimulus pulse to be seen by the muscle as two separate stimuli rather than as only one stimulus. This minimum pulse separation, when translated to frequency, is known as the critical frequency. The critical frequency varies for different muscles in the same subject and for the same muscle at a different temperatures and in different state of fatigue. The critical frequency for most of the major muscles in the human body lies between 5 and 15 Hz corresponding to minimum pulse separation of 200 milliseconds and 66 millisecond.

Multiple pulse stimulation, rather than single or double pulse stimulation is used to determine the fatigue characteristics of nerve and muscle fiber. Under normal conditions, the response obtained during prolonged stimulation should show little change from a response obtained from a single stimulus as long as a brief relaxation period is allowed between each pulse.

Smooth Muscle Potentials

The electrical activity produced in muscles known as **skeletal muscle** was dealth with. Skeletal muscle produces contractions in a series of muscle fibers, the combined effect producing continuous motion. Other muscles, particularly the muscles surrounding the major organs in the torso, produce overall continuous contraction and are known as "smooth" muscles. "Smooth" refers to the microscopic appearance of the muscle, in contrast to "striated" skeletal muscles with its characteristic cross stripes. Electrodes appropriately inserted into the stomach, bladder etc., or placed on the surface of the body over these organs can serve to monitor the slowly varying potentials generated by the muscles in these organs. These potentials are known as "smooth muscle potentials". Although these potentials are rarely monitored, the recoding of the electrical activity produced by the stomach has been termed the electrogastrogram.

Electrogastrogram

The electrogastrogram is characterized by a slowly changing DC potential (below 1Hz) which would normally be recorded on a DC coupled instrument at a sensitivity of 10millivolt per division and at a sweep speed of perhaps 1second per division.

EMG INSTRUMENTATION

The EMG signal requires essentially a long persistence CRO or presently, a storage oscilloscope. The Y-input amplifier should have provision for differential input, with a common ground. The sensitivity requires to be up to 20 μV/division. The frequency response is required, unlike the ECG/EEG signals, to be much high into the audio-frequency range. In fact, under certain muscle pathologies, tremor frequencies will have such values and may need recording.

Clinical Electromyography is of value chiefly in the diagnosis of diseases which affect the lower motor neurons, neuromuscular junctions, or skeletal muscle fiber. The electric activity detected by a needle electrode is displayed on a CRO and played over a loud speaker for simultaneous visual and auditory analysis. Deviations from normal of activity are evidence of abnormality of the nerve or muscle and to some extent can interpreted in terms of the nature and location of disease process.

EMG SPECIFICATIONS

CRT	:	Long-persistence type or storage CRO
Sensitivity	:	5 μV/mm
Response	:	40Hz to 3000 Hz, 90% down
CMRR	:	2000 : 1,
Input Impedance for 1mm and less diameter needle tips	:	500 k to 2 MΩ with 25 pF.
Cable capacitance	:	<250 pF
For microelectrodes Z_{in}	:	10 MΩ
Audio output on speaker	:	3 Watts with fine control
Extremely low noise		
Pre amplifier	:	Solid state , dual channel pre-amplifier with extremely low noise, high input impedance, high common mode rejection ratio and selectable bandwidth.

Other features of the EMG Machine include the following

- Direct measurement of nerve condition velocity
- Excellent isolation of stimulator pulse reducing artifacts
- Visual display as well as hi-fi audio output.
- Accessories
- Bipolar needle and nerve stimulator electrodes.
- Sweep speed of 1 ms to 100 ms/ cm in steps,2,5,10,20,50,100 ms/cm
- Triggering modes : Free running EMG mode
- Triggered by stimulator in nerve conduction mode
- Triggered by + 5V pulse in external mode.
- Markers-stimulus markers and variable time interval marker

- Stimulator modes of operation are : single auto, single manual
  Double auto and double manual.
- Plug in module for heart sound amplifier
- Double isolation from Ground.
- Power requirement : 230 V, 50 Hz.

PULSE GENERATORS AND STIMULATORS

As covered in various chapters in this book, the passage of electric current through various type of cells may cause these cells to depolarize and to generate as action potentials. This passage of electric current is achieved by a biological nerve impulse propagated from within the central nervous system; however, it may be stimulated or artificially produced by the stimulator. The stimulator may be a self contained instrument of it may be a separate pulse generator. For the purpose of disconnection of stimulus system, the pulse generator portion will be defined as that part that generates the pulse wave shapes required for stimulator and stimulation will be defined as that part that amplifies the signal to a level sufficient for artificial biological stimulation. Typically, a pulse generation may generate 10 volts; this pulse is then amplified within the stimulator to 100V or more for stimulation.

STIMULUS SYSTEM

A typical physiological stimulus system is shown in Fig. 5.15. The pulse generator section of this stimulus system uses a ramp generator to control two pulse generators. These pulse generators

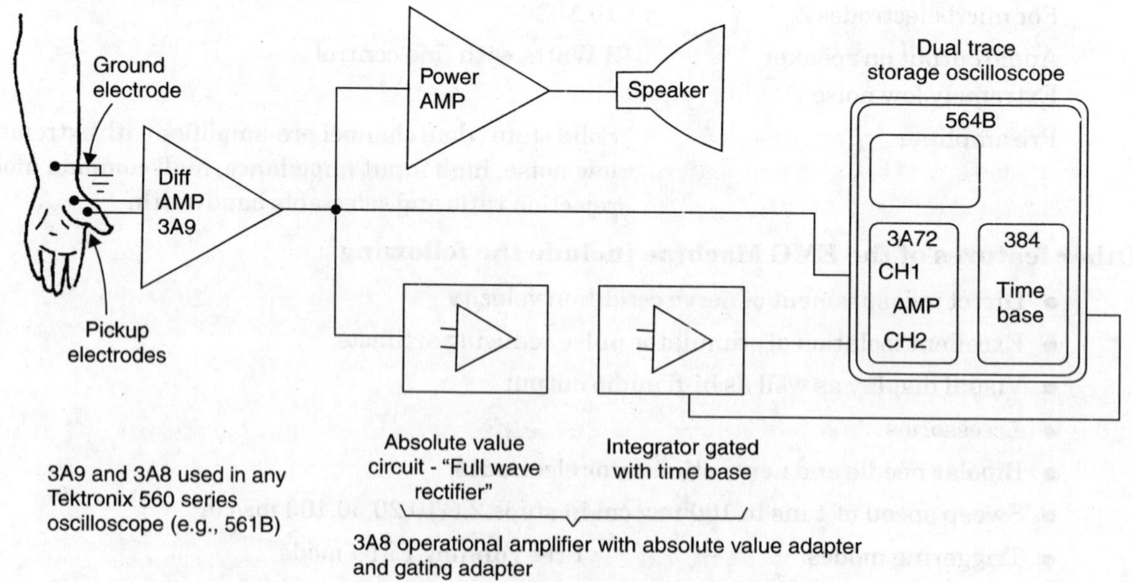

Fig. 5.15. Shows the 3A9 differential amplifier at 1 mv/Div. provides a gain of 1000X to the 3AB operational amplifier and 3A72 channel.

are triggered at discrete ramp levels, thus providing delay between the initiation of the Ramp and the initiation of the pulse. With this system shown in Fig. 5.15, the ramp can either be generated repetitively, generated via an external trigger source or can be initiated manually from a push button on the waveform generator. The output pulses from the pulse generator are combined to produce two positive pulses or a positive/ negative pulse pair.

A stimulus system suited to most bio physical measurement requirements may have the following characteristics.

Pulse generation

- Double pulse capability with each pulse independently controlled
- Pulse widths from 0.1 ms to 300 ms.
- Pulse rise time and fall times lesser than 1 μs.
- Pulse repetition rate, controlled by ramp rates, from 1,000 Hz to 0.1 Hz with single pulse capability.
- Delay between pulses in double pulse format from 0 to 300 ms.
- Output pulses from constant current sources to allow mixing. Current amplitude and voltage compliance must be compatible with power operational amplifiers and similar isolation unit. Usually, 10 mA current with compliance to 10 volts is adequate.

Stimulation Using Power Operational Amplifier

- Input configurations to allow summation of either voltage source or current source outputs.
- Slew rate of > 50 V/ms
- Up to ± 50 V/ ± 50 mA capability as either a voltage or as a current source.

Stimulation Via Stimulus Isolation Unit

- Tristable output capability for stimulation with pulses having positive and negative components.
- Isolation between output and source of < 5pF, > 10^{10} Ω and between output and ground of < 33pF, > 10^{10} Ω .
- Up to ± 100V/± 50mA as either a voltage or as a current source.

For stimulation of the exposed brain (for open cortical stimulation) it requires sufficiently less stimulus energy than peripheral stimulation (stimulation of arms and legs). Cortical stimulation requires from 0.1 to 10 V / 0.1 – 10 mA but peripheral stimulation requires from 10V to 200V/1-50mA. Cortical stimulus energy should be maintained below 1Watt peak and 0.3 μ coulombs to avoid thermal and or electrolytic injury to brain cells. Peripheral stimulation energy should be maintained below pain thresholds.

A typical Pulse generator system (Tektronix 160 model)

A typical pulse generator (Tektronix type 160) is shown in Fig. 5.16. This can be operated in three modes as given below;

1. Recurrent mode
2. Gated mode and
3. Triggered mode.

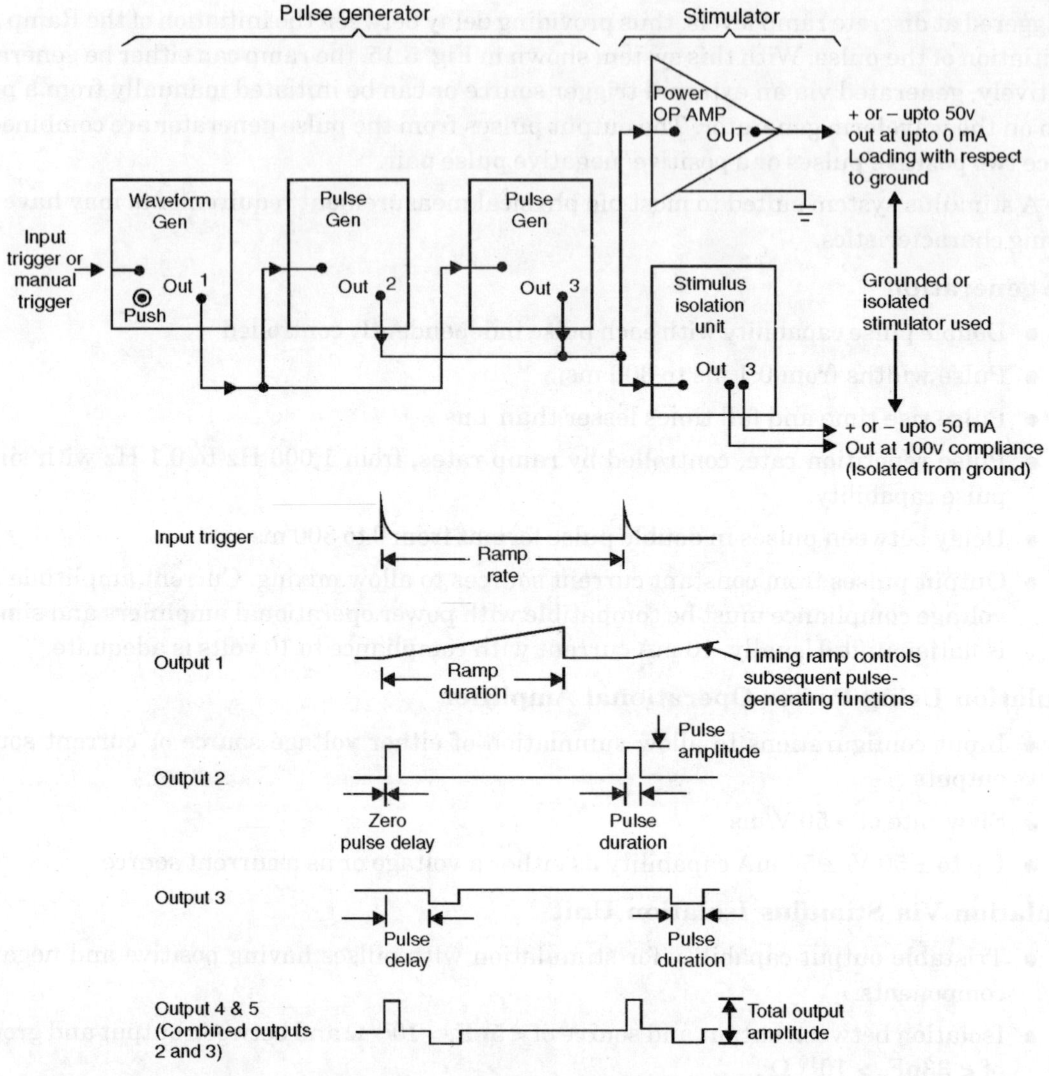

Fig. 5.16. Shows a typical physiological stimulus system.

1. Recurrent Mode

In this mode, the ramp will immediately reset itself to zero after completing a ramp cycle and begin a second ramp. This process is done continuously and repeatedly. (Fig. 5.17*a*).

2. Gated mode

In this gated mode, the ramp generator will free run for the duration of the input gate pulse. The ramp begins when the input gate pulse goes positive and after the last ramp being completed after the gate pulse again returns to zero.(Fig. 5.17*b*).

3. Triggered Mode

In this mode, the ramp generator operating may be triggered from external positive trigger pulses or by internal trigger pulses generated or by manually operated push button. (Fig. 5.17*c*).

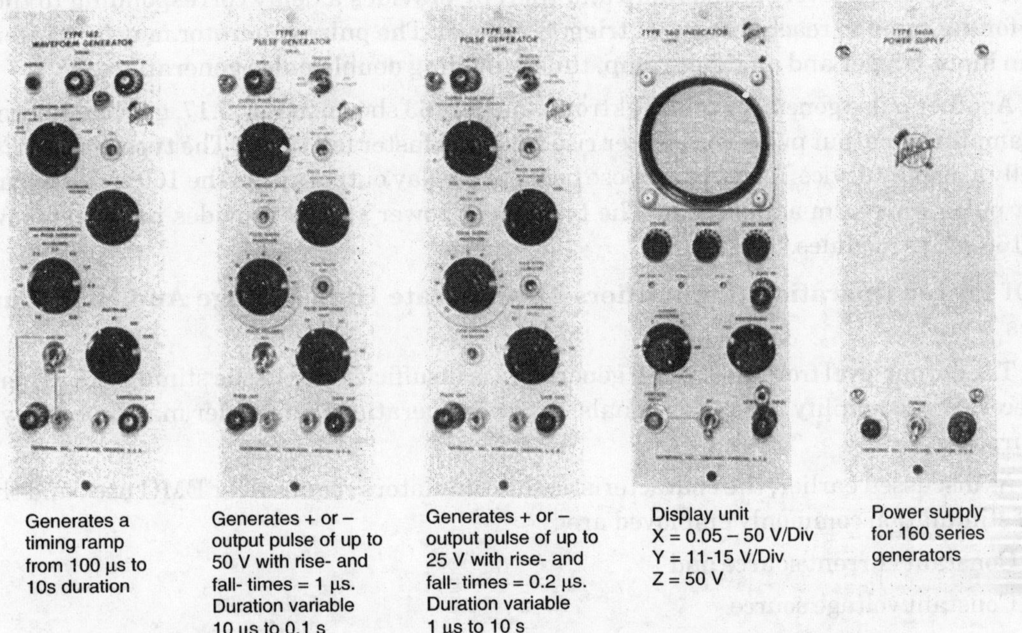

Fig. 5.17. Shows the Tekronix "160" series pulse generator system.

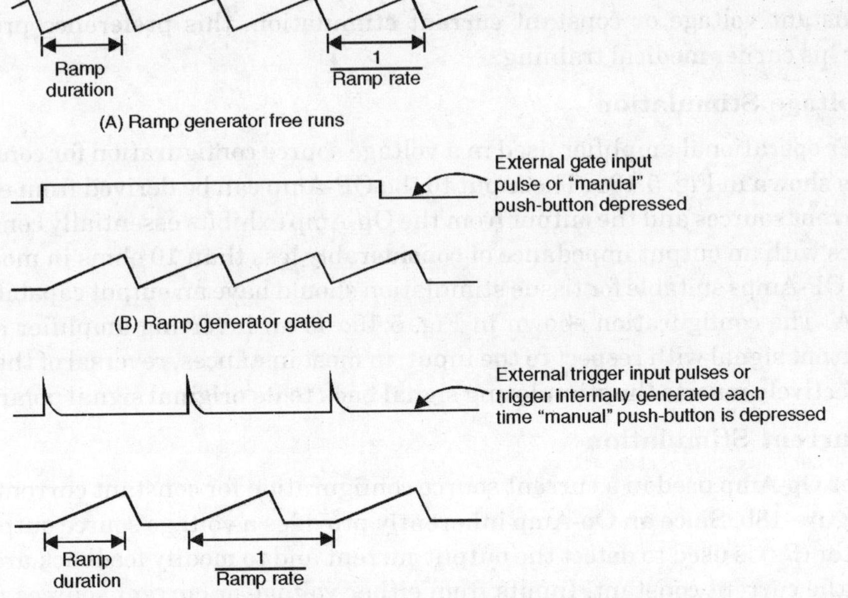

Fig. 5.18. Shows the timing ramp control.

The various operating modes of the pulse generator system (Tektronix) is shown in Fig. 5.18. The pulse generator may be triggered from external positive trigger pulse source, in which case, the pulse output will begin when the trigger pulse goes positive. The pulse generation circuit may be initiated by an input ramp. Level sensitive trigger circuitry within the pulse generator triggers at a precise level on this ramp and thereby provides a delay corresponding to the time taken for the ramp to reach the preset triggering level. The pulse generator may be triggered by both an input trigger and an input ramp, thus providing double pulse generation..

Another pulse generator from Tektronix-model 163 shown in Fig. 5.17, gives comparatively lower amplitude output pulse with faster rise time and faster fall times. The type 360 indicator is basically a display device; its main purpose being to display outputs from the 160 series to simplify output pulse waveform adjustment. The type 160A power supply provides regulated power to other 160 series modules.

Use Of Power Operational Amplifiers To Generate High Voltage And High Current Pulses

The output level from most pulse generators is insufficient for tissue stimulation. Therefore, it is necessary to amplify the pulse signals. A power operational amplifier may be employed for this purpose.

As discussed earlier, the characteristics of stimulators required for EMG use , and the two type of stimulation commonly employed are :

Constant current source and

Constant voltage source.

A tissue may be stimulated by using either of the above two sources. But it is difficult to correlate results obtained when using these different stimulating sources. Thus, while both systems are entirely adequate, the clinical electromyographer or physiologist will normally have preference for either constant voltage or constant current stimulation, this preference probably being influenced by his earlier medical training.

Constant voltage Stimulation

A power operational amplifier used in a voltage source configuration for constant voltage stimulation is shown in Fig. 5.19*a*. The input to the OP-Amp can be derived from either voltage sources or current sources and the output from the Op-Amp exhibits essentially constant voltage characteristics with an output impedance of considerably less than 10 ohms in most power OP-Amps. Power OP-Amps suitable for tissue stimulation should have an output capability of at least 50V at 50 mA. The configuration shown in Fig. 5.19*a* is an inverting amplifier and hence, it inverts the output signal with respect to the input; in most instances, reversal of the stimulating electrodes effectively inverts the stimulating signal back to its original signal polarity.

Constant Current Stimulation

A power Op-Amp used in a current source configuration for constant current stimulation is shown in figure-18b. Since an Op-Amp inherently provides a voltage source output, a current sensing resistor (Rs) is used to detect the output current and to modify feedback around the Op-Amp to keep the current constant. Inputs from either voltage or current sources may be used. The output which has a constant current characteristic should have an output impedance typically in excess of 0.1 MΩ. An Operational amplifier suitable for constant current stimulation should have an output capability of up to 50mA with a voltage range of to at least 50 V.

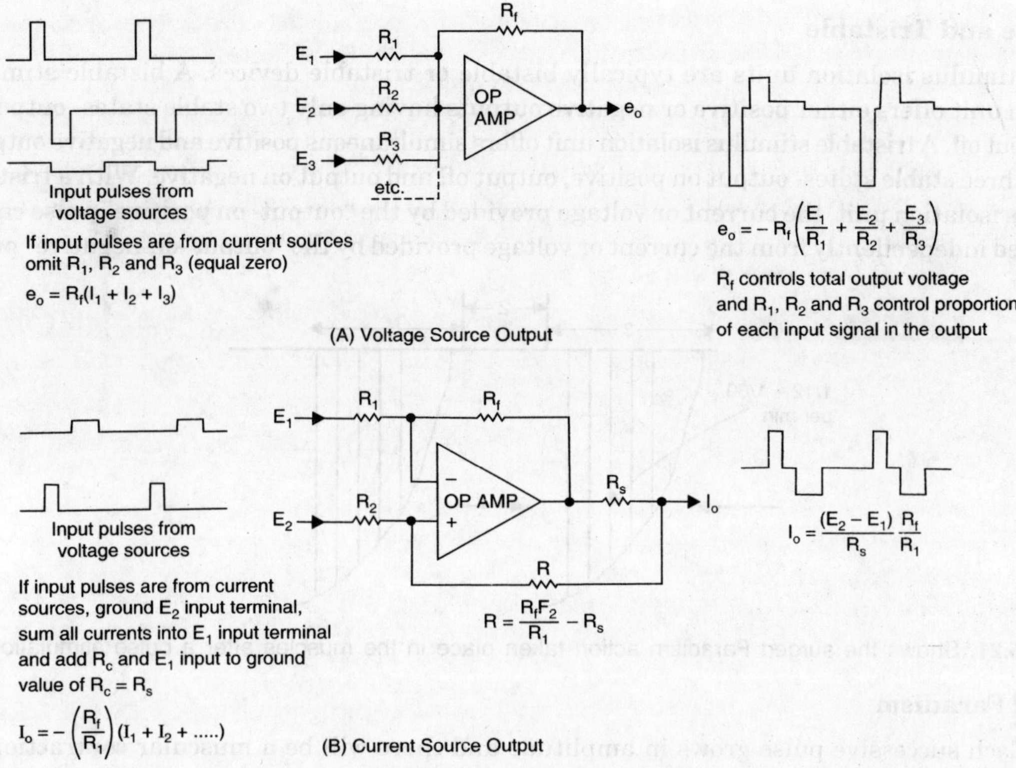

Fig. 5.19. Shows the pulse combination and amplification with a power operational amplifier.

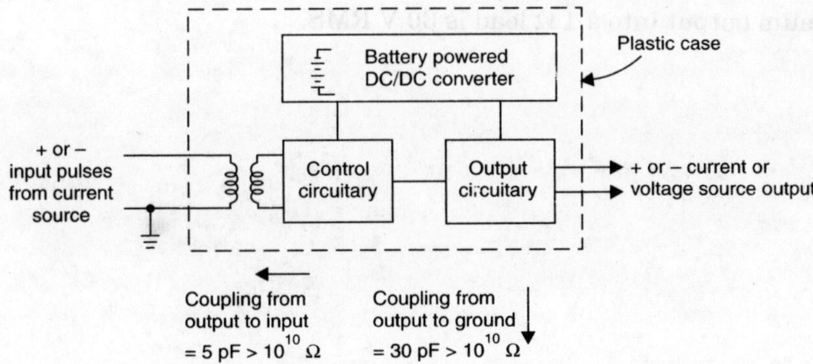

Fig. 5.20. Shows the equivalent circuit of a stimulus isolation unit.

Stimulation Isolation Unit

A stimulus isolation unit provides amplification of an input pulse or pulses and isolates the output from both ground and the input pulse source. The reasons for output pulse isolation are already discussed. An equivalent circuit for a typical stimulus system is shown in Fig. 5.20. A typical stimulus isolation unit operating in a constant voltage stimulation mode may provide voltage output of up to 100 V with a current capability of 50 mA. Similarly, when operating in a constant current stimulation mode, it may provide a current of up to 50mA with compliance up to 100 V.

Bistable and Tristable

Stimulus isolation units are typically bistable or tristable devices. A bistable stimulus isolation unit offers either positive or negative outputs having only two stable states- output on and output off. A tristable stimulus isolation unit offers simultaneous positive and negative outputs, having three stable states- output on positive, output off and output on negative. With a tristable stimulus isolation unit, the current or voltage provided by the "output- on positive" pulse can be controlled independently from the current or voltage provided by the "output -on-negative" pulse.

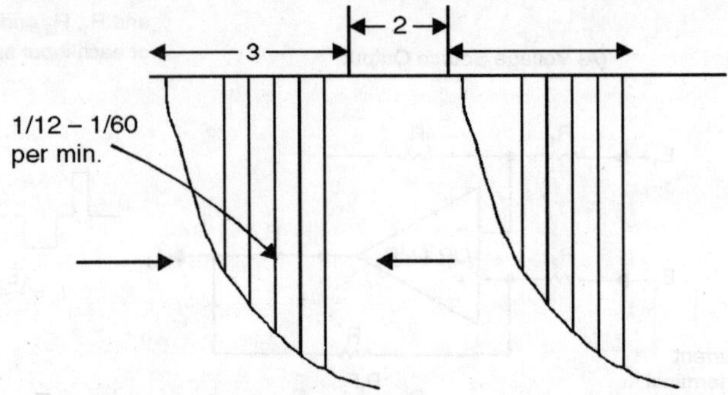

Fig. 5.21. Shows the surged Faradism action taken place in the muscles after a pulse stimulation.

Surged Faradism

Each successive pulse grows in amplitude and there will be a muscular contraction for each surge. Each surge wave has 1/12 to 1/60 per minute., after relaxation of the muscle has taken place. The on-off ratio is 3:2.This is shown in Fig. 5.21.

The maximum output into a 1 Ω load is 30 V RMS.

Chapter 6

Respiratory Testing Instruments

So far, we have not covered the physiological aspects of the respiratory system. In this chapter, the physiology of the respiratory system is going to be discussed.

RESPIRATORY SYSTEM

The primary functions of the respiratory system are to oxygenate the blood; that is to dissolve oxygen into the blood; also to remove carbon dioxide from the blood. If the blood is not oxygenated sufficiently due to failure of the circulatory system, then the oxygen content of the blood decrease rapidly. After 60 to 90 minutes, the subject will become unconscious, death occurring in 4 to 5 minutes.

THE LUNG

The lungs are the major component of the respiratory system. Oxygenation of the blood occurs at the lungs. When the lungs are forced to expand by muscular contraction of the diaphragm and

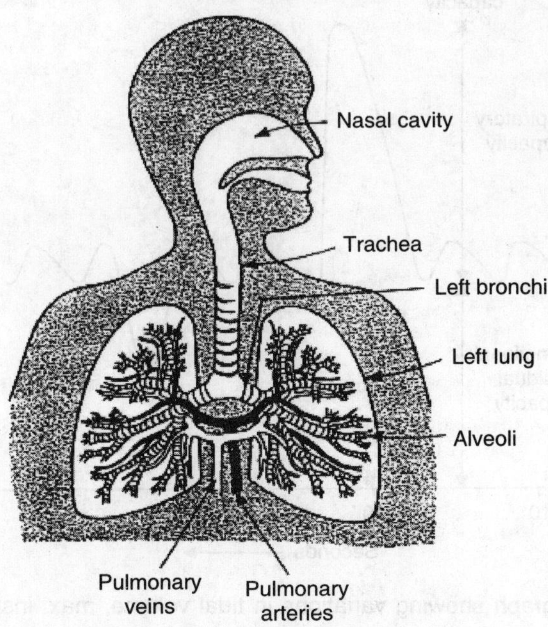

Fig. 6.1. The respiratory system.

expansion of the thoracic cage by contraction of the rib muscles, air enters the lungs via the bronchi and is diverted to millions of small air sacs known as alveoli. The membrane comprising of alveoli is moist and the oxygen contained in the air is dissolved by this moisture. Interspersed with the alveoli are fine capillaries, branching from the circulatory system. Through the circulatory system, blood is continuously flowing. The oxygen dissolved in the moist surface of the alveoli diffuses into the blood stream via these capillaries. The carbon dioxide contained in the blood stream is also diffused through the alveoli membrane to be expelled with expired air. Fig. 6.1 shows some of the principal components of the respiratory system.

Lung Capacity

A normal grown up man at rest inhales about 500 cubic centimeters of air with each breath (during inhale) and takes between 12 to 15 breaths per minute. During periods of moderate exercise, he may inhale one liter or more with each breath and take up to 25 breaths per minute. At maximum exercise, the vital capacity of 4 to 5 liters is reached.

Lung Volume

The breathing action is controlled by muscular action causing the volume of the lung to increase and decrease. During normal breathing, the lung does not contract to its minimum possible volume, nor does it expand to its maximum possible volume. Maximum lung volume is obtained when inhaling with maximum effort. Fig. 6.2 shows diagrammatically the changing lung volume that can be expected for a resting man and the lung volume that may be achieved during maximum inspiratory and expiratory effort.

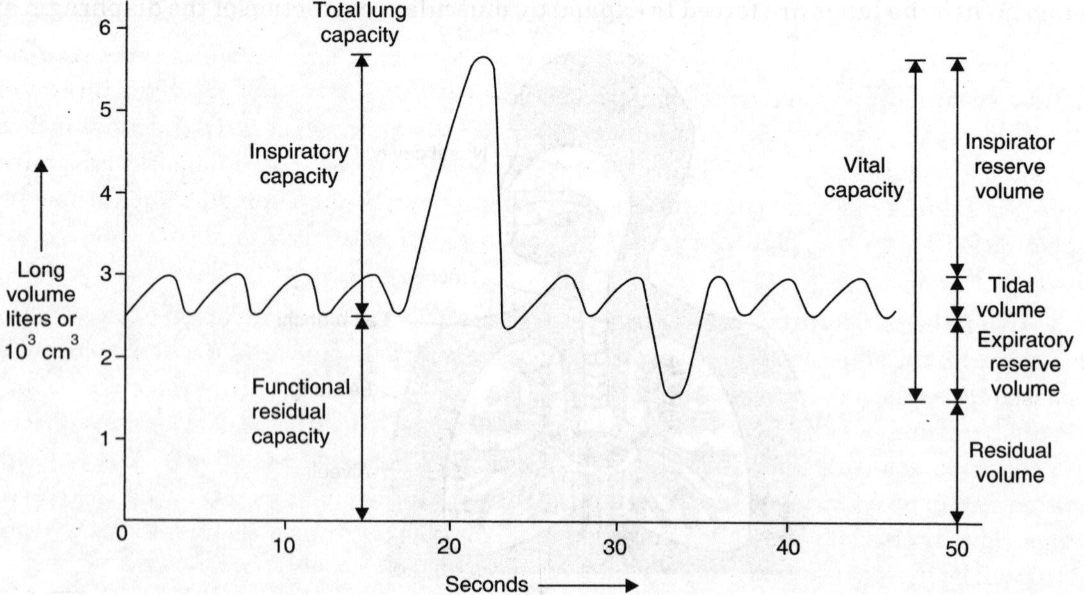

Fig. 6.2. The graph showing variations in tidal volume, max. inspiratory lung volume and expiratory lung volume, residual lung volume.

LUNG VOLUME MEASUREMENT

Lung volume is measured by a spirometer. Recording of lung volume changes with time is knows as a Spirogram. Instruments that simply detect respiratory activity are referred to as pneumographs and the resulting recording of respiratory activity changes with time is known as Pneumogram. A Spirogram is normally required only when attempting to analyze the respiratory system or to detect a malfunction of this respiratory system . This is very rarely used for routine monitoring. A Pneumogram may be used for routine monitoring and is basically used to indicate the fact that the subject is breathing. Breathing rate could be obtained from either Spirogram or Pneumogram.

Respiratory Activity

Relative Respiratory activity may be detected in following ways;

1. by detecting the physical changes in the torso associated with breathing or
2. by detecting the flow of air through the nostrils.

Since no absolute measurements are required, the measurement techniques involved have been simplified to allow easy application of the devices concerned to the subject.

Thermistor Pneumograph

The simplest form of pneumograpgh employs a thermister placed in the nasal package to detect the temperature different between inspired cool air and expired warm air. This technique satisfies the majority of clinical needs including those of operative and post operative subjects. If the subject breaths through his mouth, or if he wishes to converse, the thermistor may be placed in the mouth or in such a position as to detect the flow from either the nose or the mouth. The thermister concerned should be supplied form a constant current source at a low current to maintain thermistor self heating below one degree centigrade or so. Sensitivity is adequate with 5mW of thermistor dissipation. Excessive thermistor heating can cause subject discomfort. Therefore, the thermistor dissipation should be limited to 40mW for small bead-type thermistors. A thermistor pneumograph suitable for use with a Tektronix-410 monitor, together with a typical pneumogram obtained from this system, is shown in Fig. 6.3.

When the temperature of the outside air is same as the temperature of expired air (body temperature), the above system is said to be unsatisfactory. In this case, enough current should be passed through the concerned thermistor so as to raise the temperature somewhat above the body temperature, but still below a temperature which may cause discomfort for the subject. This can usually be achieved with thermistor dissipations of between 5 to 25 mW. The flow of both inspired and expired air over this thermistor will tend to cool it, thus producing the resistance change. Since both inspiration and expiration decreases the thermistor temperature, the resulting output will be twice the respiratory frequency.

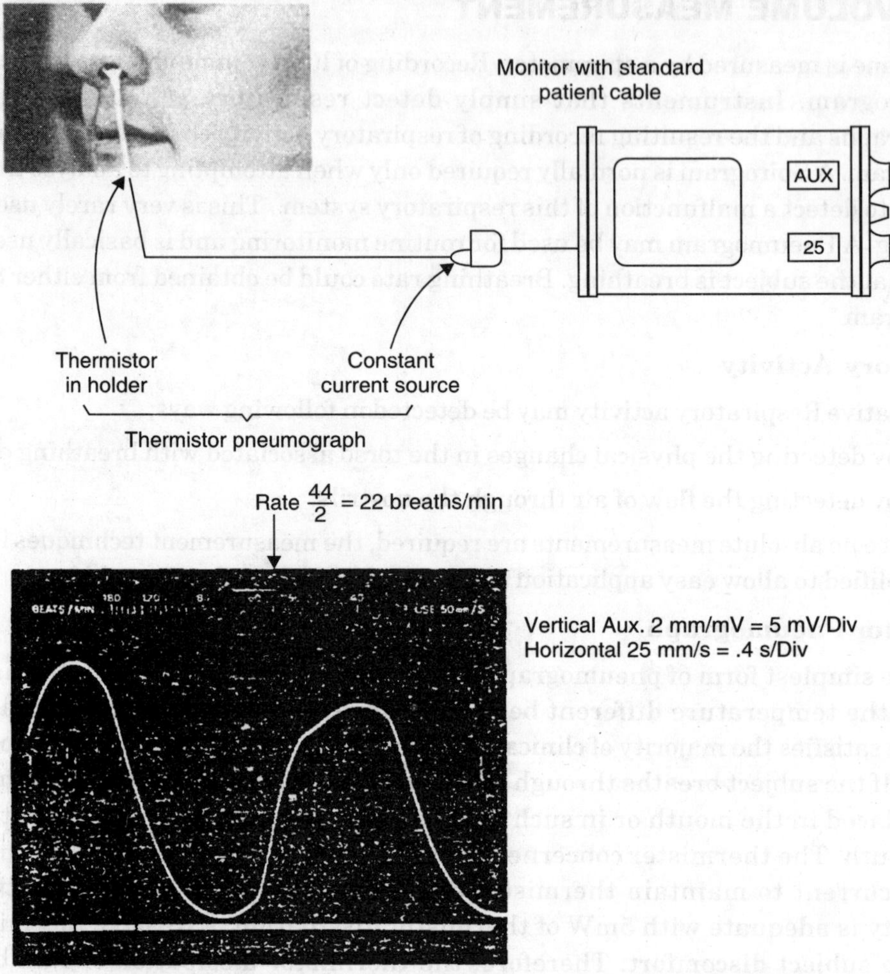

Fig. 6.3. Showing Thermistor Pneumogram with the Monitor.

Detection of Chest Size Changes

Changes in the physical size of the torso with respiration may also be detected to indicate respiratory activity. A strain gauge attached to a piece of elastic is used to form a band around the chest. Since the circumference of the chest varies with the respiration, the elastic band will stretch causing a change in resistance in the strain gauge. This resistance change is detected by a DC-excited Wheatstone bridge method or by use of an carrier amplifier. Such a system and the resulting pneumogram obtained is shown in Fig. 6.4.

Changes in chest circumference may also be detected by a rubber tube filled with mercury, fastened firmly around the chest. When the chest expands, the rubber tube increases in length and thus the resistance of the mercury from one end of this tube to the other changes. This resistance change may be detected using a constant current source in the same way as the thermistor resistance change was detected in Fig. 6.3. The main disadvantage of this mercury filled rubber tube pneumograph is its extremely low resistance requiring large currents and sensitive detecting instruments. These disadvantages can be largely overcome by replacing the

mercury with a conductive solution such as copper sulphate solution (with copper plugs in the ends of the rubber tube) or with some of the less viscous type of electrode paste commonly used to apply electrodes to the skin. Commercial electrode paste vary greatly in resistivity; however, a 45 inch long and 1/8 inch diameter rubber tube filled with electrode paste should have a resistance of between 1000, and 100,000 ohms.

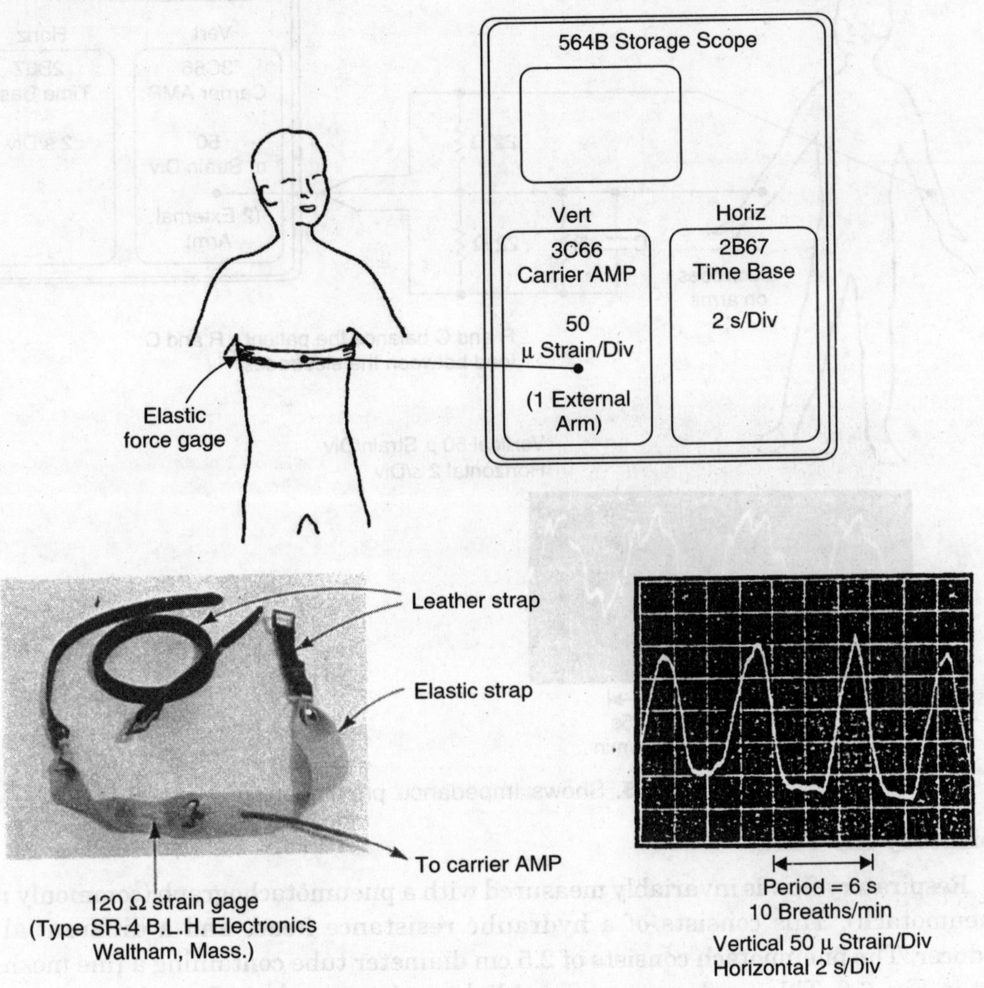

Fig. 6.4. Strain Gage respiratory transducer.

Resistivity of the Torso : Impedance Pneumogram

Respiration activity may be detected by measuring the change in resistivity across the torso. This technique is similar to the technique used to measure cardiac activity. The resistance changes or the impedance changes are used to detect the cardiac activity whereas the capacitive component of the impedance change is used to detect the indication of the respiratory activity. A typical impedance pueumogram system together with a typical impedance pneumogram obtained from this system is shown in Fig. 6.5. There appears to be little practical use for this system as the variations produced by the heart in record prevent a good recording from being obtained.

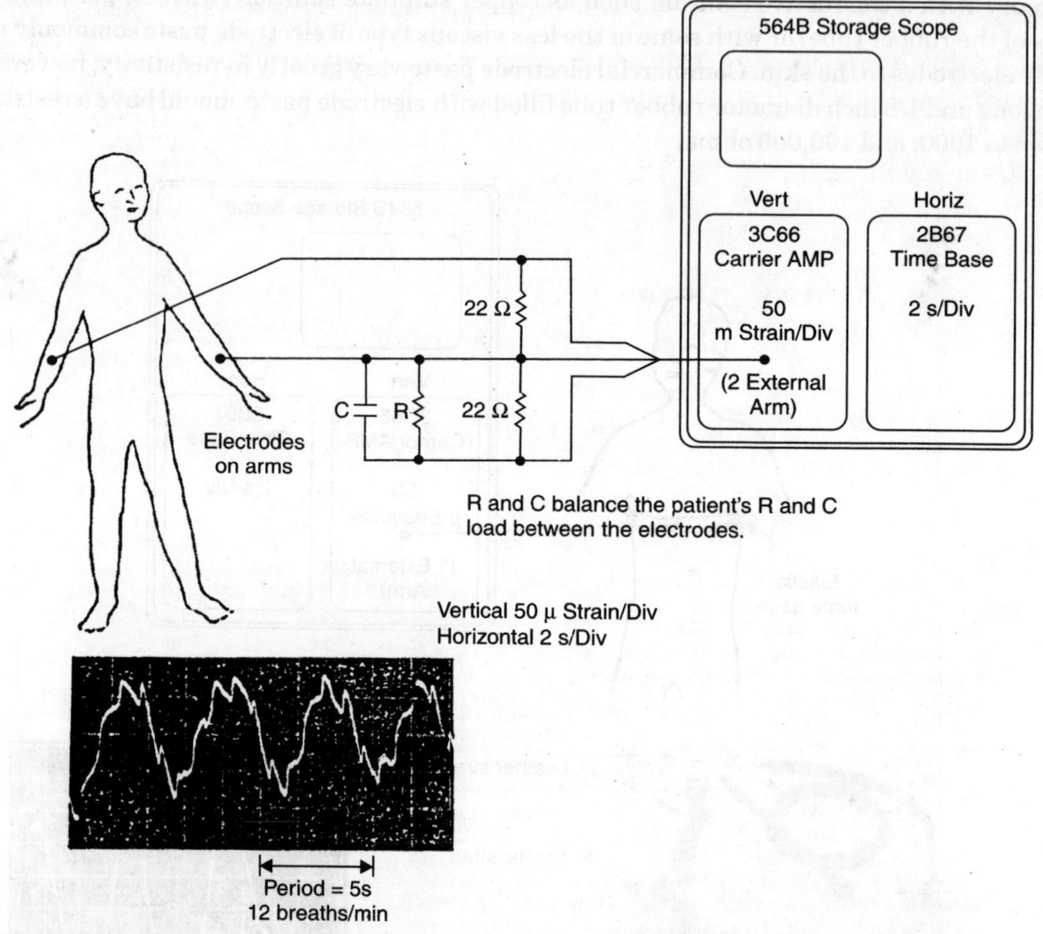

Fig.6.5. Shows Impedance pneumogram.

Respiratory Air Flow

Respiratory flow is invariably measured with a pneumotachograph (commonly referred to as pneumotach). This consists of a hydraulic resistance head, and a differential pressure transducer. The pneumotach consists of 2.5 cm diameter tube containing a fine mesh screen as shown in Fig. 6.6. This mesh screen offers slight resistance to air flow; this resistance to flow produces a pressure differential across the mesh screen which is proportional to the mean flow velocity. A Sensym make (Semi-conductor strain gauge used) pressure transducer can be used. This pressure differential is detected by the differential pressure transducer. The sensitivity of the device can be varied by varying the size of the mesh screen or by using several mesh screens. However, the total airway resistance offered to a subject should never exceed about 1 cm H_2O if normal respiration is not to be affected by the measuring device. A typical pressure differential across the screen would be 0.09 cm H_2O per 10 liters per minute flow using 5 cm diameter, 160 per cm, stainless steel gauze in the head.

Differential Pressure Transducer and Calibration of Measurement System

The differential pressure transducer can be used in conjunction with a carrier amplifier (Tektronix-3C66) along with a storage oscilloscope. The complete flow measuring system consists of the following:

1. Pneumatic unit
2. Pressure transducer unit (Differential pressure transducer)
3. Amplifier
4. Oscilloscope (Tektronix- 564B)

The above unit may be calibrated with a known flow.

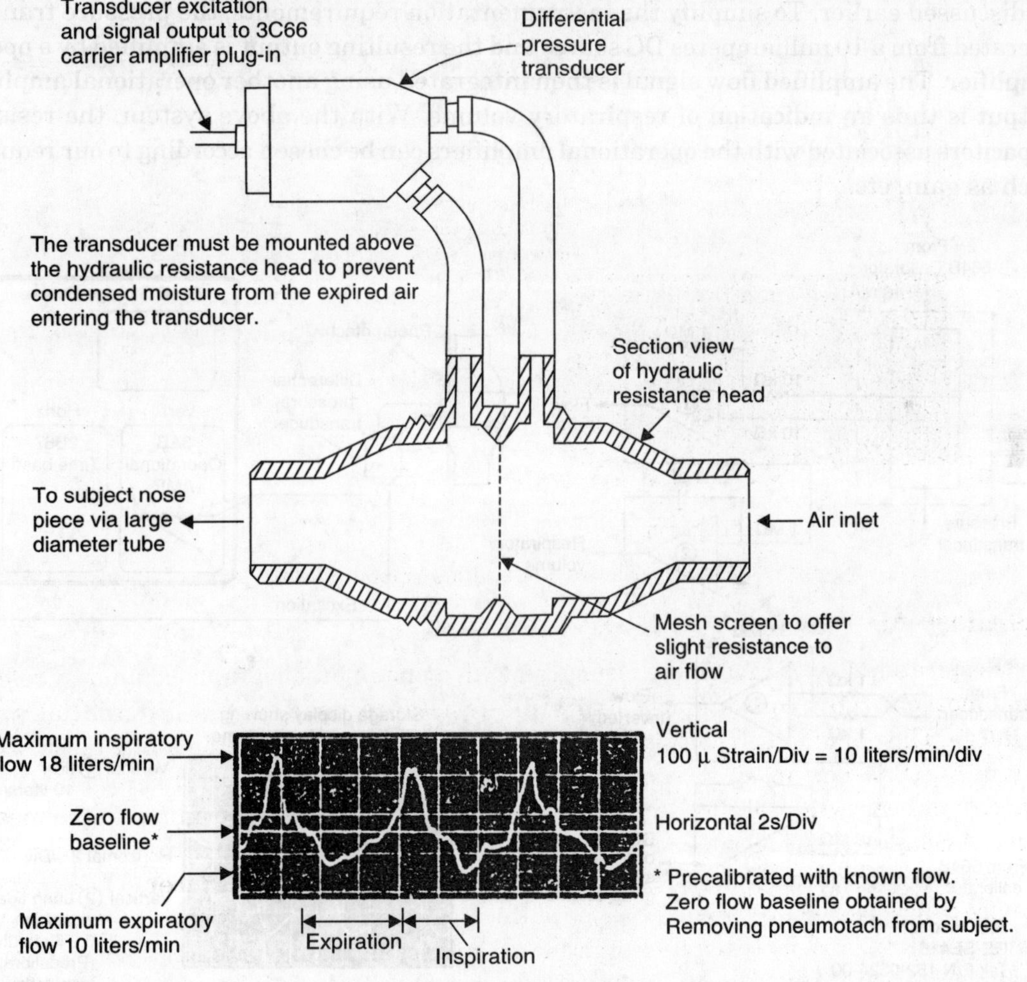

Fig.6.6. Shows the Pneumotach air flow transducer.

Commercial pneumotachs usually provide a calibration of the differential pressure produced per 10 liters per minute flow. This information, when related to the sensitivity of the pressure transducer, can be used to provide a calibration factor and this will be discussed later.

A typical flow Pneumogram is shown in Fig. 6.6. A zero base line was added to the display to provide zero flow reference by simply removing the subject from the Pneumotach system and adding an additional sweep to the previously stored Pneumogram.

Respiratory air flow measurement is frequently used to estimate a subject's respiratory function. Flow measurement also allows respiratory volume to be easily obtained

RESPIRATORY VOLUME

Since air flow is simply a measurement of volume per unit time, respiratory air flow information may be integrated to provide respiratory volume. Such a system is shown in Fig. 6.7. The pneumatic and the differential pressure transducer produces an output proportional to the respiratory flow as discussed earlier. To simplify the instrumentation requirements, the pressure transducer is operated from a 10 milliamperes DC source and the resulting output is amplified by a operational amplifier. The amplified flow signal is then integrated using another operational amplifier. The output is thus an indication of respiratory volume. With the above system, the resistors and capacitors associated with the operational amplifiers can be chosen according to our requirements such as gain, etc.

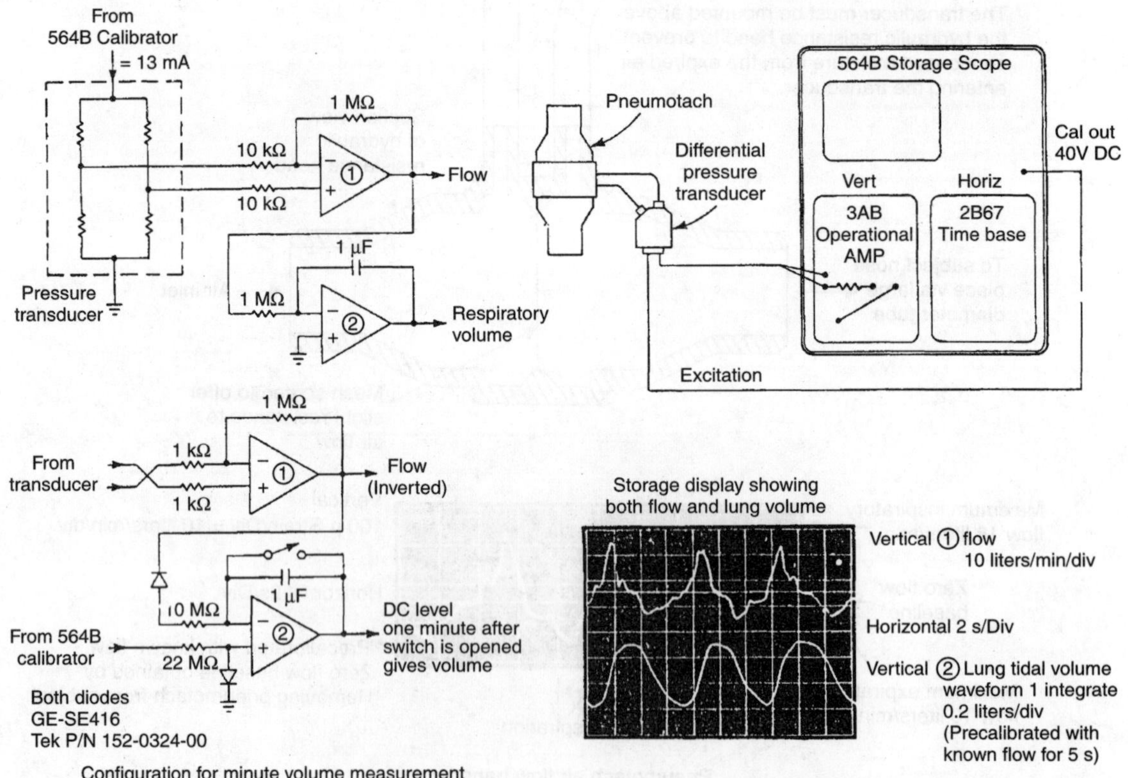

Fig. 6.7. Showing a spirogram obtained with an integrating pneumotach.

One minute respiratory volume may be measured by modifying the above procedure. Minute respiratory volume is the amount of air that a subject inhales in a minute period. It may be measured by integrating inspiratory flow only, over a one-minute period. Referring to Fig. 6.7, the output of the second operational amplifier in the same operational amplifier, will register minute volume if the flow signal is coupled to the integrating circuit via a diode and the integrator is gated ON for a one-minute period.

Conventional Spirometer

A more conventional spirometer is shown in Fig. 6.8. In this unit, inspiration and expiration raises and lowers a counterbalanced bell located in a container with full of water. Movement of

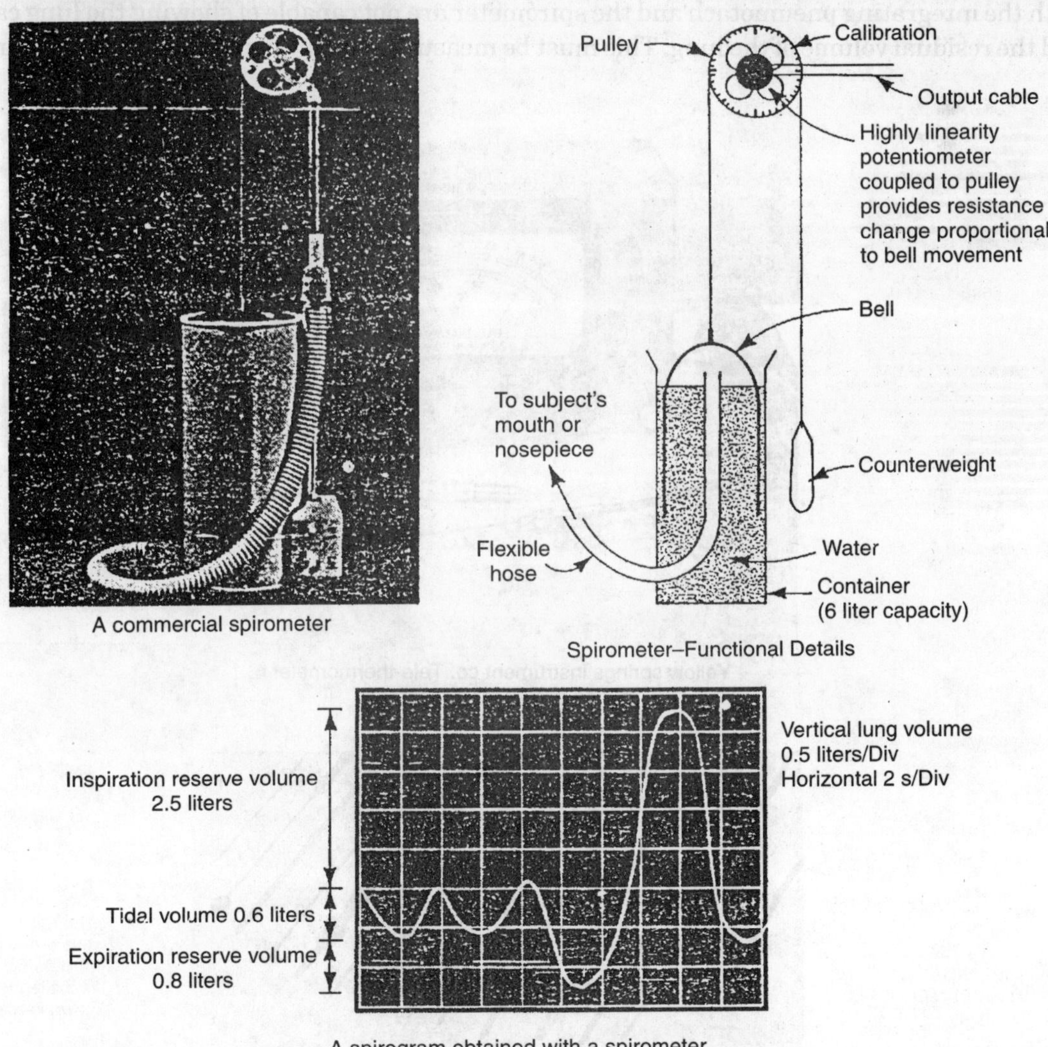

Fig.6.8. Shows a spirogram obtained with a Spirometer.

this bell is transferred to a pulley whose periphery contains a calibration of bell displacement which is, of course, related to bell air volume. Respiratory volume may be read directly form this calibrated pulley. This pulley may also be coupled to a high-linearity potentiometer and the resistance change in this potentiometer used to indicate respiratory volume. A DC output from a current calibrator is used to provide a constant- current source for this potentiometer; the output voltage will then be proportional to the changing resistance. A spirogram recorded with this system is also shown in Fig. 6.8. A spirometer is inherently a heavily damped device, containing appreciable hysterisis, so small subtle changes in inspiration and expiration volume are not recorded with this device.

Fig. 6.9 shows the theoretical changes in total lung volume with inspiration and expiration. Both the integrating pneumotach and the spirometer are not capable of showing the lung capacity and the residual volume of the lung. This must be measured only by using gas-dilution techniques.

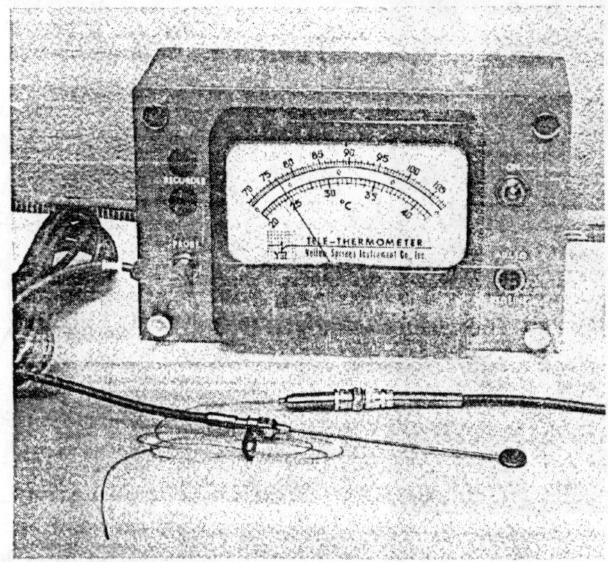

Yellow springs instrument co. Tele-thermometer with an output for a recorder.

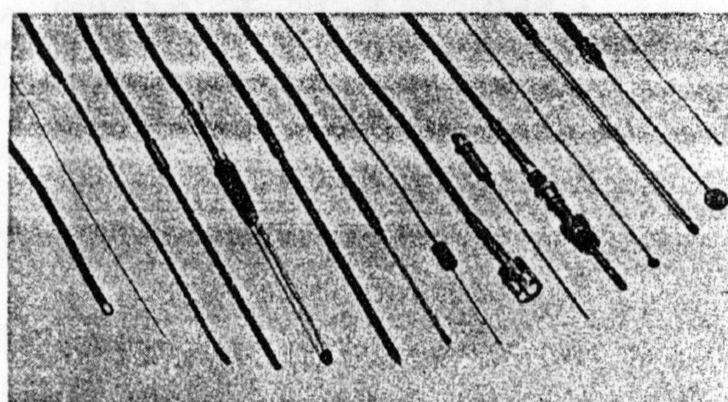

Various thermistor probes available from yellow springs instrument co.

Fig. 6.9. Thermistor telethermometer and sample probes.

TEMPERATURE MEASUREMENT

In most cases, temperature does not vary at very appreciable rate and, thus, may be displayed using a moving coil meter. Such a thermometer, using thermistors in conjunction with a moving coil meter, is shown in Fig. 6.9. For some applications, however, the meter display is inadequate and thus an oscilloscope or chart recorder is required. The meter shown in Fig. 6.9 provides and output for use with an oscilloscope. Clinical thermometers based on semiconductor diode sensor with LCD display are now available.

THE RADIOACTIVE LUNG TESTING METHOD

In this method a radioactive gas is inhaled by the patient and its distribution is followed by placing scintillation counters on the chest wall in suitable positions. Such a method has the great advantage that it need not interfere in the slightest with the normal course of breathing and any of form anesthesia is avoided.

The radioactive gas is used as tracer. Of the various gases available 133 Xenon has proved to the most suitable for most purposes. It has a half life of approximately five days in vitro, and emits gamma rays having an energy equivalent to 0.081 mV. The radioactive isotopes of argon and oxygen have also been used for special purposes.

I.D.L. (**Isotope Developments Ltd.**) first supplied their instrument to the Brompton Hospital, London. The equipment has the instrumentation shown below in Fig. 6.10.

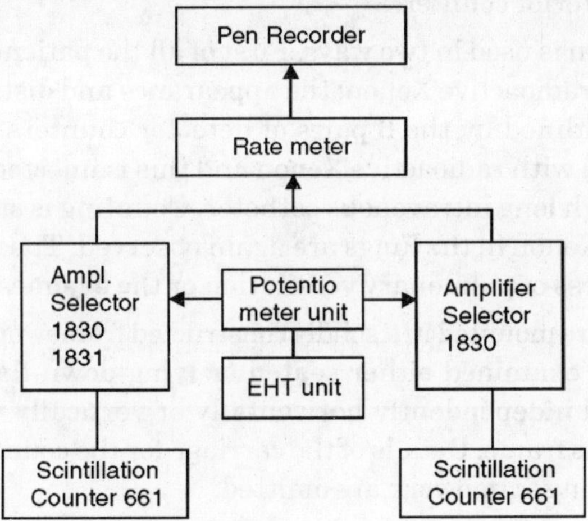

Fig. 6.10. The Radio Isotope lung testing-I.D.L. modules.

The system has basic standard units of known reliability combined to make the complete equipment suitable for a specialized application.

13 nos. of Scintillation counters type 661 with Sodium iodide crystal type 2004.

12 nos. of Amplifier selector type 1830.

6 nos. of rate meter type1810.

2 nos of EHT P. Meter type 532D.

1 no. scaler unit type 1700 D.

1 no. bench scintillation counter type 6006.

1 no well sodium diode crystal type 2003 B.

2 nos of 4 channel Recorder.

A mechanical console stand mounting frame for the 12 calibrated detectors is part of the system.

These component circuits have been mounted in a movable console to simplify operation of the complete assembly and make it maintenance simple.

The unit is designed to allow simultaneous recording of the output of 12 Scintillation counters. These are arranged in pairs which are applied at pre-determined points to the chest wall in such a way that the two counters in each pair are in line facing one another. The output of each counter is fed with one amplifier-Selector 1830 and the resulting signals are combined and fed into a single rate meter. The output of the latter, is in turn, supplied to one channel of the 8-channel direct writing recorder. In this way, changes in counting rate of the pair of scintillation counters are recorded, breath by breath, during the whole course of the test. The distribution of radioactive gas in six regions of the lungs can thus be recorded simultaneously.

At the same time, it is possible to record tidal air on the seventh channel and the radioactivity of the mixed expired air on the eighth. For the above purpose, a Scintillation counter is used together with a 1700 scaler. A bench Scinti is provided for other radioactive measurements. Switching arrangements have been fixed whereby the counters used on the chest wall may be isolated from one another thus allowing comparison of anterior counting rate with counting rate from the corresponding posterior counter.

The radioactive Xenon is used in two ways. First of all the patient breathes the air from the Spirometer which contains radioactive Xenon; the appearance and distribution of this is detected and followed as already outlined by the 6 pairs of detector counters. Secondly, about 5 ml. of normal saline are saturated with radioactive Xenon and this is injected into the **Superior Vena cava** or right atrium through long intravenous catheter. Counting is started and the appearance and the distribution of the Xenon in the lungs are again observed. The two sets of tracings can be used to estimate the evenness of pulmonary ventilation or the evenness of blood flow into lungs.

The paired counters are mounted in a solidly constructed framework which has been designed to allow the patients to be examined either seated or lying down flat or on either side. Each counter may also be moved independently horizontally or vertically within the frame. Special collimators are built into this frame. Details of the carriage for the counters, the electronic console and various type of supporting framework are omitted.

HEART-LUNG MACHINE

INTRODUCTION

Heart-Lung Machine. One of the truly revolutionary pieces of medical equipment has been the invention and development of the heart-lung machine. Before its introduction to medicine in the 1950s, heart surgery was unheard of; there was no way to keep a patient alive while working on the heart. Today, about 750,000 open-heart procedures are performed each year. During an open-heart surgery, such as bypass surgery, the heart-lung machine takes over the functions of the heart and lungs and allows a surgeon to carefully stop the heart while the rest of the patient's body continues to receive oxygen-rich blood. The surgeon can then perform delicate work on the heart without interference from bleeding or the heart's pumping motion. Once the procedure is over, the surgeon restarts the heart and disconnects the heart-lung machine. The first heart-lung machine was built in 1937 by physician John H. Gibbon, who also performed the first human open-heart operation in 1953. Motivated by the death of a young patient in 1931, Gibbon pursued total artificial circulation for almost three decades in his laboratory at the Jefferson Medical College in Philadelphia. His first experimental machine used two roller pumps and was designed to replace the heart and lung action of a cat. But Gibbon's initial machine was massive, complicated, and difficult to manage. Its action often damaged or destroyed blood cells, causing bleeding problems and loss of viable blood. Improvements came in 1945, when scientist Clarence Dennis built a modified Gibbon pump, but Dennis' machine was hard to clean, caused infections, and never reached human testing. A Swedish physician, Viking Olov Bjork invented a blood-oxygenating device with multiple screen discs that rotated slowly in a shaft, over which a film of blood was injected. Oxygen passed over the rotating discs and provided sufficient oxygenation for an adult human. Bjork, along with the help of a few chemical engineers, one of whom was his wife, developed a blood filter and an artificial material that they applied to all parts of the perfusion machine to delay clotting and save platelets. Bjork took the technology to the human testing phase. About the same time, Dr. Forest Dodrill, a surgeon at Wayne State University's Harper Hospital in Detroit, was developing a machine to detour blood while he repaired patients' hearts. In a move that combined engineering and medicine, Dodrill teamed with engineers at General Motors to help him design the device, which resembled a 12-cylinder engine. The six cylinders on each side of the "engine" were separate chambers for pumping blood. Doctors later used Dodrill's machine to perform an open heart surgery in human clinical trials. After an interruption in research by his service in World War II, Gibbon joined forces with Thomas Watson in 1946. This merger also demonstrated the benefits of using engineering to solve a medical problem. Watson, an engineer and the chairman of International Business Machines (IBM), provided the financial and technical support for Gibbon to further develop his heart-lung machine. Gibbon, Watson and IBM engineers improved the original machine to reduce damage to the red blood cells and prevent air bubbles from entering the blood. Their new device used a refined method of cascading the blood down a thin sheet of film for oxygenation, rather than the original whirling technique that could potentially damage blood cells. This new device kept twelve dogs alive for more than an hour during heart operations. Then, in 1953, Dr. Gibbon performed open-heart surgery with artificial circulation by closing a hole between the upper heart chambers in an 18-year-old girl. Since those early years, the safety and ease-of-use of heart-lung equipment has gradually improved. Advances in materials and computing have led to safer, more effective machines. It is now commonplace for surgeons to stop the heart for several hours while modern heart-lung machines maintain circulation. Basically, heart-lung machines work by withdrawing bluish, unoxygenated blood from the upper heart chambers through a tube into a reservoir. From there, the blood is pumped through an artificial lung designed to expose the blood to oxygen and permit the blood cells to absorb oxygen molecules directly. Then the blood, now red and rich with oxygen, is pumped back into the patient through a tube connected to the arterial circulation. The heart-lung circuit is a continuous loop; as the red blood goes into the body, blue blood returns from the body and drains into the pump to complete the circuit. Modern heart-lung machines can do a number of other tasks needed for a safe open-heart operation. Any blood that escapes the circulation and spills around the heart can be suctioned and returned to the pump. This greatly preserves the patients own blood stores throughout the operation. Also, the patient's body temperature can be controlled by selectively cooling or heating the blood as it moves through the heart-lung machine. Thus the surgeon can use low body temperatures as a tool to preserve the function of the heart and other vital organs during artificial circulation. Medications and anesthetic drugs can be given via separate connections. In this way, medications arrive to the patient almost instantly by simply adding them to the blood within the heart-lung reservoir. But despite all its advantages, heart-lung machines still carry some substantial risks. These include the formation of small blood clots in the blood, which, in extreme cases, can cause stroke, heart attack or kidney failure upon return to the body's bloodstream. The machine can also trigger an inflammatory process that can damage many of the body's systems and organs. Post-operative bleeding may be a serious complication, occasionally requiring a return to the operating room. Problems with temporary confusion or memory loss have also been reported in some cases. Those risks push today's biomedical engineers not merely to improve the heart-lung machine, but to develop advances that would eliminate the need for the machine altogether. One such advance is minimally invasive surgery. Minimally invasive heart surgery is any of several approaches for bypassing critically blocked arteries that are less difficult and risky than conventional open-heart surgery. These procedures have the potential benefit of avoiding complications associated with the heart-lung machine, such as increased risk of stroke, lung complications, kidney complications and problems with mental clarity and memory. Other benefits are faster recovery and reduced hospital costs. Biomedical engineers are developing the surgical tools, imaging and robotic technology necessary for minimally invasive surgery. Another approach is "beating heart" surgery, where the surgeons operate on the heart while it still beats and moves blood throughout the patient's body. Recent clinical studies suggest that there may be benefits to beating heart surgery, such as less trauma to the blood; decreased risk of adverse events, such as stroke; and a quicker return to normal activities. One of the greatest challenges in beating heart surgery is the difficulty of suturing or sewing on a beating heart. A stabilization system makes it possible for the surgeon to carefully work on the patient's beating heart, and in the great majority of cases, eliminates the need for the heart-lung machine.

DESCRIPTION

It maintains arterial pressure high enough to nourish the brain and deeply relaxed tissues as well to keep the kidneys active. Also maintains the blood PO_2 and PCO_2 at appropriate levels. This can be used on any one patient for only a few hours.

Lot more blood cells in the stream are destroyed (>1000 per second). Blood protein gets denatured due to direct contact with oxygen owing to strong shear forces when disks spin or bubbles rise through blood.

A heart-lung machine is meant for temporary extra corporeal support to circulation. In one type, it consists of roller- type peristaltic pumps, rotating-disc oxygenator and a heat exchanger. The oxygen feed through the hollow axial shaft permits use of disc diameters close to that of the oxygenator cylinder resulting in maximum film area for a given blood priming volume. An electronic photoelectric sensor is used to detect level changes in the oxygenator and thus control the pump flow rates compensating for fluctuations in venous return.

A variety of pumps and artificial lungs have been developed during last 20 years, with a view to extend the safe period of total body perfusion. A roller-type peristaltic pumps and rotating-disc oxygenator are simple to design. Other important parts of the heart-lung machine are a heat exchanger and a level sensor for the blood in the oxygenator.

DESIGN ASPECTS OF HEART LUNG MACHINE

To serve the functions of natural heart and lungs, the heart-lung machine should be able to arterialise upto 5 liters per minute of venous blood from 65% oxygen saturation to above 95% oxygen saturation, the carbon dioxide elimination being adequate. It should cause least trauma and the damage to blood particles should be within biologically compensatable limits. Its priming volume should be minimum and yet sufficient to maintain a constant volume of blood in the perfused patient, compensating for minor transfusion or hemorrhage that might occur.

PUMPS

The pumps must be designed to have flow rates upto 5 litres per minute with a pressure head upto 200 mm Hg. The roller occludes the tube and displaces the fluid. This roller pump shown in Fig. 6.14 is a 180° double roller, with different tubing within the pump head and the tube is guided ahead of the rollers. The pump has wide flow range. The flow is varied by varying the rotating speed of the pump head between 0-180 rpm. The flow rate varies linearly with speed the occlusion of both rollers can be adjusted in a single setting by means of the knob provided at the top of the pump head. The lever mechanism changes occlusion settings of both rollers simultaneously even when the pump is running. Each pump head is driven individually by a 1/8 H.P. single phase A.C. motor. The speed variation is accomplished by varying the voltage setting on the variac. The direction of rotation of the pump head can be reversed using the three position reversing switch provided. The modular pump unit system permits use of varying number of pumps as per perfusion requirements.

DESIGN OF THE OXYGENATOR

The oxygenator must be able to oxygenate about 5 litres per minute of venous blood from 65% oxygen saturation to above 95% oxygen saturation before the blood enters the physiological system. The natural lungs have a wide surface area of about 50–100 m^2 so that blood as a film of thickness 0.005–0.010 mm gets oxygenated in a contact time of 40–50 ms. The inability to provide such extended surface area and thin blood film offers the greatest resistance to the oxygen transfer. To offset these draw-backs, the disc oxygenator has a continuously renewable film 0.1–0.3 mm thick having contact time of 0.2–0.3 second under oxygen partial pressures of about 650 mm Hg.

The disc oxygenator shown in Fig. 6.15 consists of a cylindrical glass vessel of 15 cm internal diameter, 38 cm long in which 80–100 stainless steel discs of 0.6 mm thickness and 14 cm diameter are mounted axially with 3 mm spacers between discs. The shaft on which the discs are mounted is hollow and is supported by three ball bearings at the ends. The oxygen is fed through the axis of the shaft and it enters the oxygenator through the distributing apertures on the circumference of the shaft. The oxygen feed system permits use of disc diameters close to the diameter of the oxygenator cylinder so that for a given blood priming volume maximum utilization of the available surface area is made. The optimum blood level in the oxygenator that provides the maximum film area for a given priming volume is 0.7 R where R is the radius of the disc (see below for the derivation). For this blood level in the oxygenator the values of the various design parameters viz. number of discs, diameter of discs, length of the oxygenator, are determined for given requirements of oxygenation.

For this disc oxygenator, with a blood level of 0.7 R ,the available film area is 1.47 m^2 and the priming volume is 2.19 litres. To oxygenate 5 litres per minute of blood would require a rotating speed of about 150 rpm. The oxygenation capacity can be varied by varying the rotating speed of the oxygenator during perfusion of the patient or by changing the number of discs otherwise.

The blood level in the oxygenator is monitored by a photo-electric level sensor. The sensing element is a photo conducting cell which conducts depending upon the light radiation it receives. A light source is fixed on top of the oxygenator as shown in Fig. 6.16 and the light reaching the photodiode depends on the blood level in the oxygenator. Knowing the signal corresponding to a blood level of 0.7R, one can suitably adjust the pump flow rates to compensate for any fluctuation in this signal. Manual control is replaced by a feedback control of the power supply of the motor using the signal from the photo sensor.

HEAT EXCHANGER

The heat exchanger is a single pass, shell and tube heat exchanger with blood flowing on the shell side and water flowing on the tube side. The priming volume of the heat exchanger is about 250 ml and blood flows as a thin film in the annulus between the shell and the tube. The temperature of the blood stream and the water stream are monitored at both inlet and outlet with thermocouple sensors.

THE CARDIOPULMONARY BYPASSCIRCUIT

The circuit for heart-lung bypass is shown in Fig. 6.17. One of the pumps is connected on the suction line and the other on the arterial line. Oxygen flow is regulated in the range 0–15 litres per minute with a rotameter and needle valve flow controller. The arterial and venous pressure gauges are provided. The blood from the heat exchanger is passed through a bubble trap before it is returned to the patient.

The role of physical factors such as oxygen saturation of incoming blood, the blood distributing system in the oxygenator, oxygen carrying capacity of blood under given conditions, the blood flow rates, oxygen flow rates, temperature of oxygenation, partial pressures of oxygen etc., all tell upon the performance of the oxygenator.

CALCULATION OF OXYGENERATOR FILM AREA-APPENDIX

Maximisation of film area for a given priming volume

Let us disc of radius R dip into the blood pool of height H. As the disc rotates it carries a blood film of width r = R = H on it.

Area of the segment upto the liquid level is

$$A_{segment} = R^2 \cos^{-1} r/R - r \quad \sqrt{R^2 - r^2}$$

Area of the annular film is

$$A_{film} = \pi(R^2 - r^2) - R^2 \cos^{-1} r/R + r\sqrt{R^2 - r^2}$$

Maximizing A_{film} with respect to r, we get, for $dA_{film}/dr = 0$,

$$r = R/\sqrt{\pi^2 + 1} = 0.3\ R$$

hence the liquid level that maximizes the film area for given priming volume is H = 0.7 R

for this liquid level,

$$A_{film} = 1.886\ R^2 \text{ for one side of a disc}$$

$$A_{segment} = 0.97\ R^2$$

Total film area $= A_{film} \times 2N$, **where N is the number of discs**

$$= 3.772\ R^2\ N$$

Priming volume $= A_{segment} \times L$, **where L is the length of the oxygenator**

$= 0.97\ R^2L$ **+ any annular volume between the oxygenator body and the outer edge of the discs.**

PRACTICAL CONSIDERATIONS

The efficiency of the gas exchange per unit volume must be increased. Modern machines have around 1litre volume small enough to prime them with sterile plasma-like fluids without diluting the patients blood too much. Others with greater than 1.5 litre volumes, will be primed with bottled blood (danger of infection of jaundice and sensitization to serum proteins).

Measurements in Heart Lung Machine

Control parameters are fairly easy to measure; Arterial and venous pressures, blood flow rate, blood gas tensions. They are displayed on the machine. PCO_2 is frequently measured by a pH meter, PO_2 is fairly clear form the colour of the blood.

The machine can not be auto regulated because of it biological unsuitability.

If we can get a small machine which may be built with a breathing membrane that allows O_2 and CO_2 to dissolve in it and then to pass through, we would have a 'closed circuit' machine. Present day 'master' machine are only "open"-the level of blood in the oxygenator part of the circuit can rise and fall independently of the patients' blood volume. The closing of the circuit will remove the danger that can arise, when, for instance, the surgeon inadvertently leans on or moves venous lines, which drains blood from the patient, this makes the machine input fall below its output and the level of blood in the oxygenator falls. This would lead to inefficient oxygenation. And at very low levels it could create a danger of pumping a fatal mixture of air and blood into the return line. Much of the technician's time is spent in maintaining adequate level in the oxygenation.

Finally, if membranes are designed and stacked properly, oxygen can be pulsed through and blood is massaged through between twin membranes as long as a bubble of oxygen passes synchronously above and below from inlet to outlet.

In the actual lungs, the tension of CO_2 and O_2 in alveoli and in the capillaries causes a gradient for transfer. The resting PCO_2 in the venous blood is around 46 mm of Hg, that in the alveoli is around 40 mm of Hg. The gradient across the alveolar/capillary membranes in 6 mm of

Hg; comparable figure for PO_2 are 40 mm Hg, venous and 100 mmHg alveolar. The gradient is 60mm Hg-10 times greater. Yet, identical quantities of each gas pass in opposite direction per minute (240 ml). In short, the alveolar capillary membrane is at least 10 times more efficient at transporting CO_2 than transporting oxygen.

Actually, from measurement, during exertion we know it to be 15 times more efficient but the above is from resting measurement.

Relative permeability of various polymer membranes to O_2, the silicones top in the list. Rubber and cellulose are biologically unsuitable.

A membrane's permeability to a gas is a product of the solubility and the diffusion rate and is closely related to molecular diameter (some gases with diameter between those of O_2 and CO_2 are listed at the base of the first graph).

The combinations of silicone's fairly flat diffusion rate graph for gases and increased solubility for CO_2 than O_2 allows it to breath 6-times effectively than oxygen.

The polydimethylsiloxane molecules are considered to be arranged in the membrane with hydrogen bonds between chains, which are weak. There are also the $-Si(CH_3)_2O-$groups. This basic unit of–Si–O–Si–O imparts flexibility to the membrane. The Si–O angle can vary from 140° to 160°.

The membrane can be strengthened by incorporating phenyl or vinyl groups in the polymer. These unite molecules of neighboring chains with stronger covalent bonds,

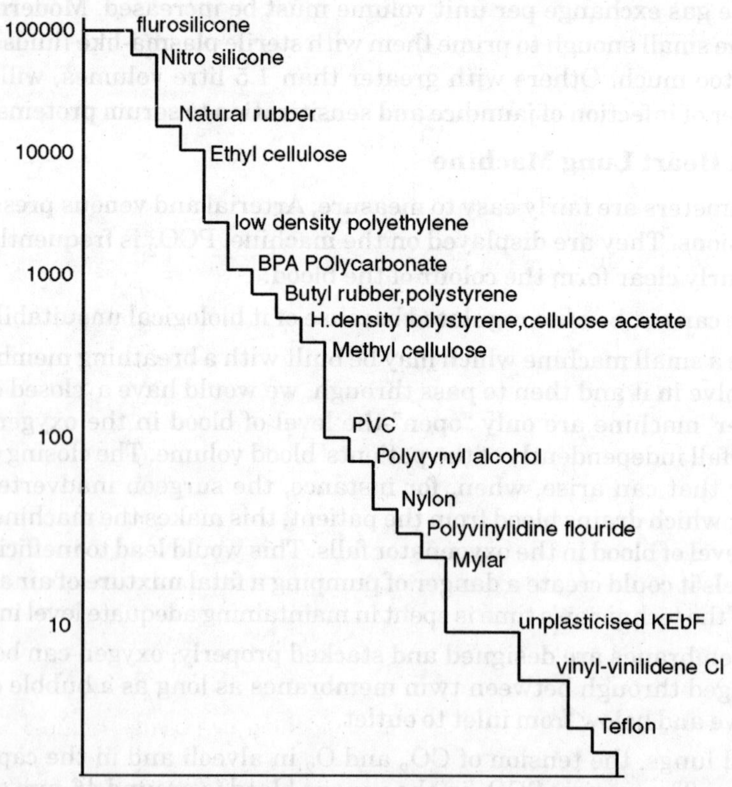

Fig. 6.11. Shows the relative permeability of various polymer membranes.

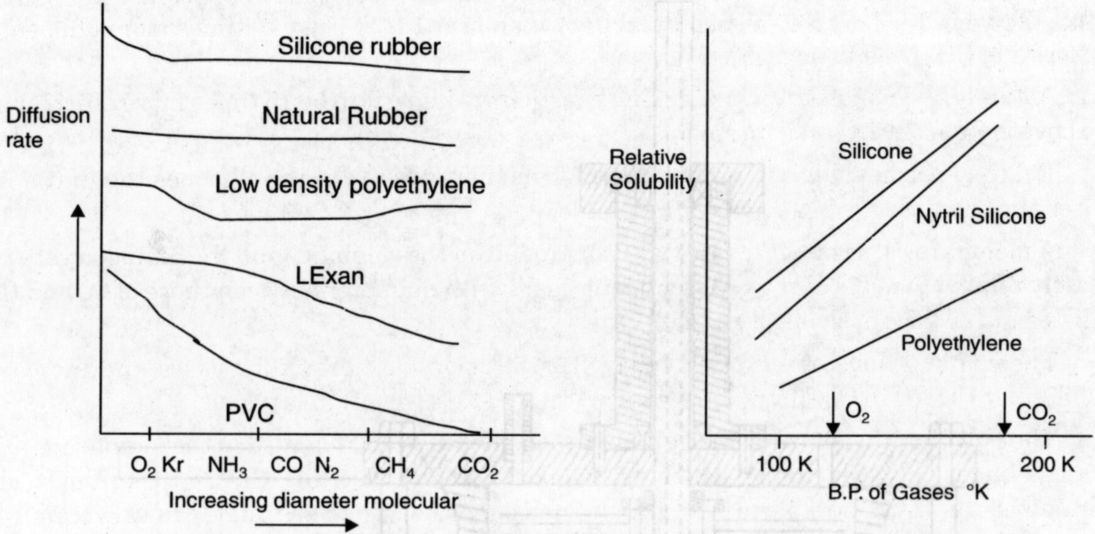

Fig. 6.12. Shows the graph for diffusion and solubility of various membranes.

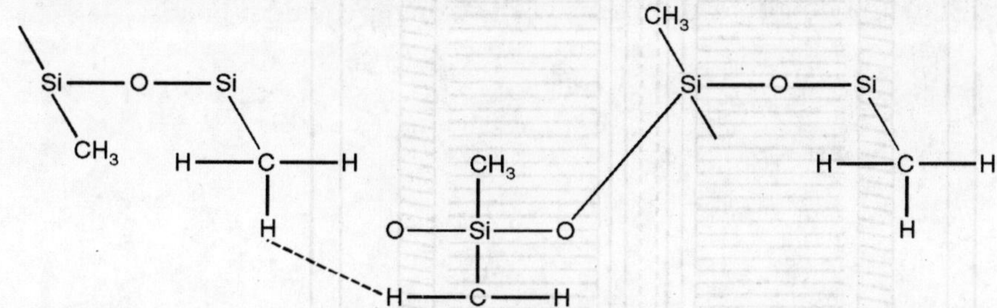

Fig. 6.13. Shows the arrangement of molecules for polydimethylsiloxane membrane.

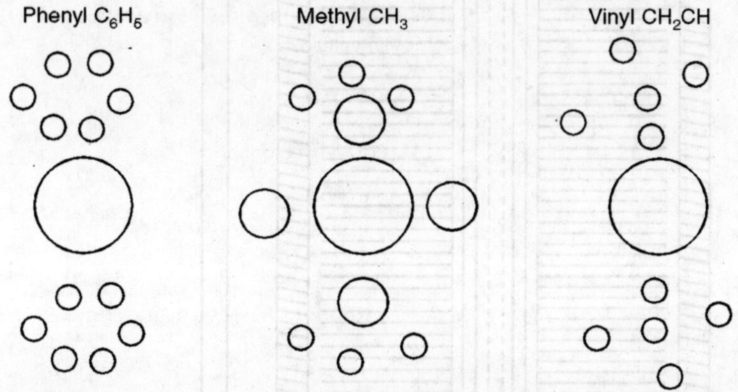

Fig. 6.14. Shows the membrane strengthening by polymer groups.

These unite molecules of neighboring chains with stronger covalent bonds, but cause a drastic reduction in breathability. Incidentally, 3% of methyl groups are added even in "pure" silicone rubber.

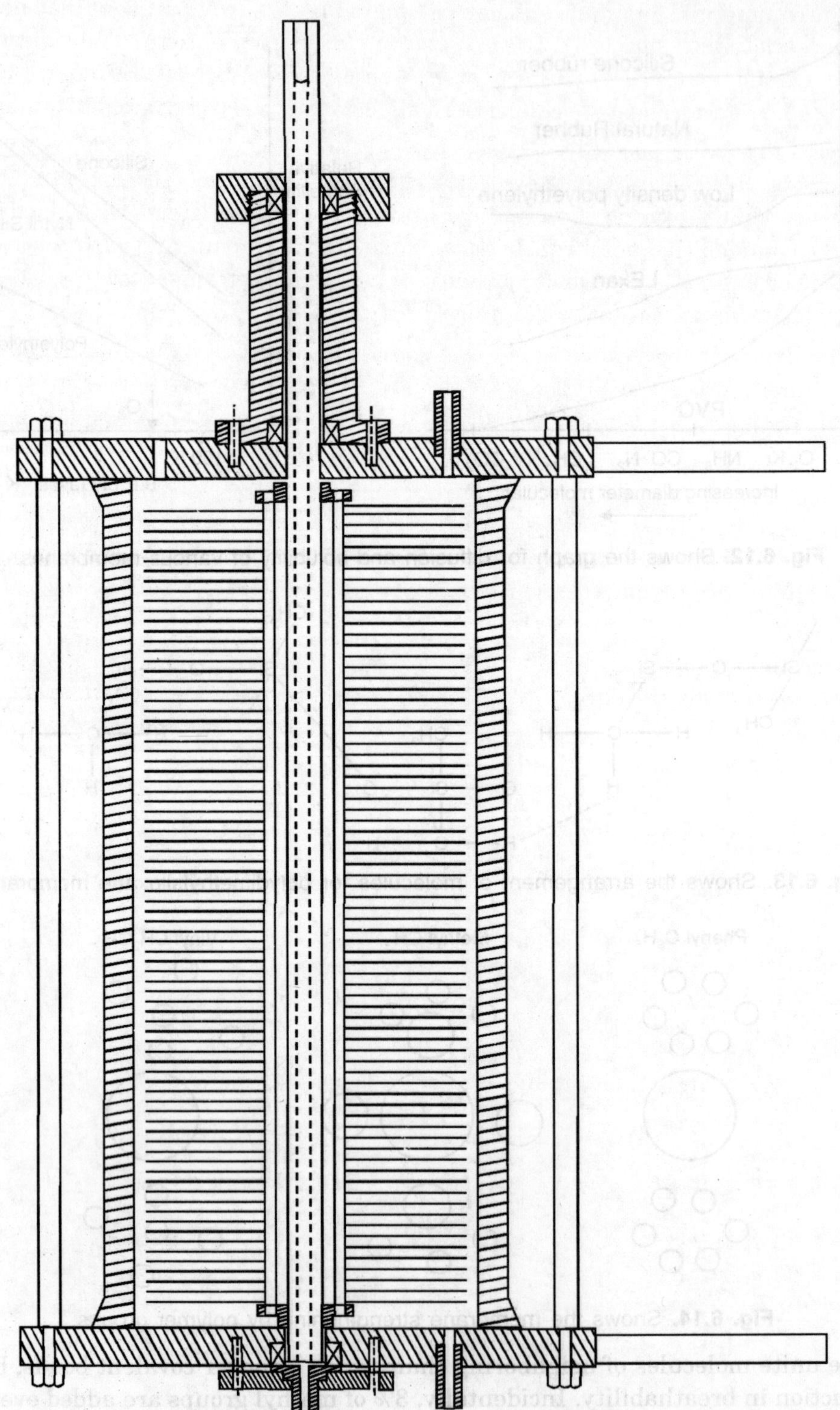

Fig. 6.15. Showing the Disc Oxygenerator.

The commercial available silicone polymers breathe so slowly that they need areas as big as 7 square meters to supply O_2 to and remove CO_2 from a patient. The volume of the circuit would be around 1 liter. The Royal post graduate Medical School, Hammeyharh, London are producing 12.5 micron sheets of rubber with almost unimpaired breathability and easy handling qualities.

Various 'flat-bed' oxygenerator qualities are being used in various centers. The simplest of these consist of pairs of rectangular silicone rubber membrane sheets with blood in at either end and air (O_2) outside the membranes. Others use disks of membrane with central to peripheral blood flow. The flat-bed oxygenerator, in one type has rocking arrangement to release the supporting boundary layer fluid adjacent to the wall.

The Bramson oxygenerator led by the team of Frank Gerbode in Los Angels has a radial flow type. Another uses the bubble oxygenerator, led by Walter Lillehei of the Minneapolis group.

Life support machines to aid a failing heart or lung will be used using membrane devices. One works by sucking blood form the main arteries in the groins during the ejection phase of the heart and replacing it under pressure during the filling phase. If this technique is to succeed, it presupposes that reliable EKG triggering is available to prevent the device from discharging while the heart is ejecting. Life support machine for heart or lung failure will eventually be in the form of small membrane pump oxygenerators to partly by pass and do the work of both ventricles and the lungs.

Another use for small membranes heart lung machine is for organ storage. Here, we have to be even more careful to avoid denaturing proteins. The reason is that there are no other organs in the system (such as lever, kidney) to mop up and process the products of blood destruction as in a complete organism. Organ banks would use such machines.

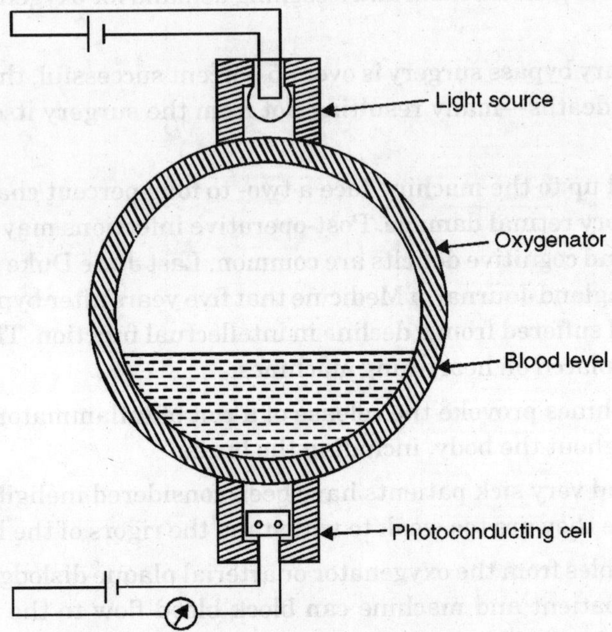

Fig. 6.16. Showing the blood level photosensor.

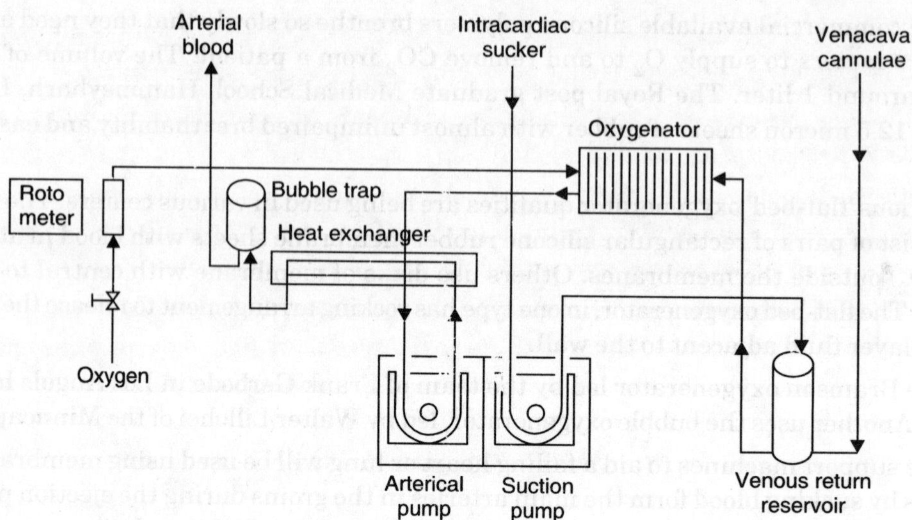

Fig. 6.17. Showing the bypass circuit system of heart lung machine.

NEW SURGERY ON THE BEATING HEART-NO HEART LUNG MACHINE

In conventional bypass surgery, the heart is flooded with cold fluids rich in potassium, an ion that arrests muscle contractions. The patient's blood is then rerouted into a heart-lung machine. There, it is forced over cheesecloth-like membranes of porous plastic, through which oxygen percolates. The blood is also cooled to about 82 degrees F, then pumped back into the body. Body temperature drops, slowing metabolism and lessening demand for oxygen. After surgery the body must be rewarmed.

Although coronary bypass surgery is over 95 percent successful, there remain serious side effects and occasional deaths—many resulting not from the surgery itself, but from the heart-lung machine.

Patients hooked up to the machine face a two- to four-percent chance of stroke and a 25-percent risk of transitory retinal damage. Post-operative infections may be more of a risk when the machine is used. And cognitive deficits are common. Last June Duke University researchers reported in the New England Journal of Medicine that five years after bypass surgery, 42 percent of patients studied still suffered from a decline in intellectual function. The risk was greatest for the patients who were placed on heart-lung machines.

Heart-lung machines provoke the release of a riot of inflammatory molecules capable of harming organs throughout the body, including the brain.

Many elderly and very sick patients have been considered ineligible for coronary bypass surgery simply because they are too weak to withstand the rigors of the heart-lung machine.

Microscopic bubbles from the oxygenator or arterial plaque dislodged during placement of the tubes connecting patient and machine can block blood flow to the brain or other organs. Mechanical damage to fragile blood cells can result in clots.

The beating-heart bypass—likened by some to cutting a gemstone while on horseback—was pioneered in 1965 by a Russian cardiac surgeon, Vassily Ivanovich Kolessov.

Although Kolessov achieved good results, the technique was considered too radical and was never adopted by surgeons of the day.

But with the development of new instrumentation in the mid-1990s, the approach was revived. The new instruments stabilize a small area of the heart, allowing a cardiac surgeon to safely place a bypass graft, while the rest of the heart thrashes away normally.

One device looks like a sewing machine foot. Another uses tentacles fitted with a series of suckers that grip the heart muscle with a vacuum seal. More than 45,000 bypass surgeries have been performed worldwide using the latter system alone. Today about 20 percent of cardiac surgeons in the United States have been trained in beating-heart surgery, up from 1 percent just five years ago.

At the annual meeting of the International Society for Minimally Invasive Cardiac Surgery in Atlanta last June, Duke researchers reported on the first 32 patients to receive off-pump surgery at their institution. The off-pump patients spent much less time on a ventilator and in the ICU. The average cost for respiratory care services was $936 versus $1,634. Overall ICU costs were $2,716 versus $5,009.

Other studies have shown similar cost savings among off-pump patients, along with reduced need for blood transfusion, less respiratory dysfunction, and lower rates of stroke, kidney failure, retinal bleeding, cognitive problems and wound infection.

BLOOD ACIDITY VERSUS RESPIRATION

Since blood is oxygenated by respiration, its pH changes with it and hence lungs and kidneys share their role in maintaining the alkalinity (slight) of blood

Acidity and alkalinity of blood and urine is of great diagnostic value.

They depend upon hydrogen ion concentration (H^+).

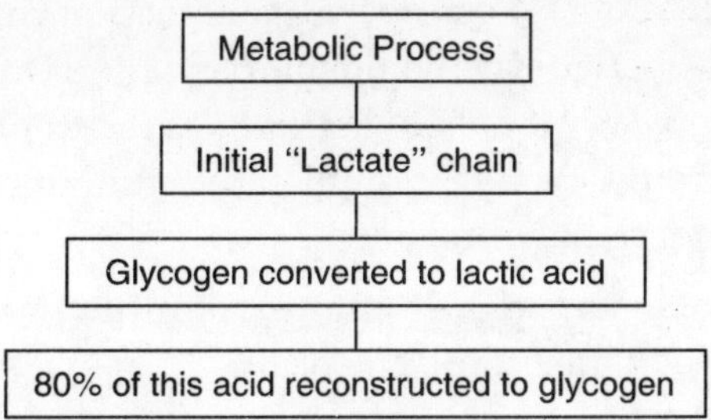

A strong alkali has only 10^{-14} of gm H^+ per liter.

A strong acid has 10^0 (*i.e.*, 1 gm) of H+ per liter.

Take a log scale, we get 0 to – 14.

By conversion, $pH = -\log(H^+)$

The mid point is 7, the pH of pure water

Acids – 0 to 7 , alkaline 7 to – 14.

The meter uses a 'Glass Electrode'—tubular membrane of special glass (5.0mm dia, 0.4 mm thick).

Blood volume needed is 1 cc in a typical blood of pH meter.

In healthy blood, pH never strays for long outside 7.37–7.45. (i.e. alkaline even though the end products of membrane are acidic).

Remaining parts together with proteins and fats goes through a complex cycle, called 'Kerb's cycle', whose end product are CO_2 and water

$$CO_2 + H_2O \rightleftharpoons H_2CO_3$$

Further details of lung gas chemistry is given in the Chapter on Chemical measurements.

Chapter 7

E.N.T. and Opthalmic Instruments

Speech and hearing are the most important means by which we communicate with each other. Through hearing we receive speech sounds from others and also listen to ourselves. In some ways it is more of a handicap to be born 'stone deaf' than to be born blind. Any child who cannot hear the sounds from his own vocal cords cannot learn to talk without special training. In earlier times a child deaf from birth was also mute, or dumb and since so much of our learning takes place through hearing , he often was not educated.

The sense of hearing is in some ways more remarkable than the sense of vision. We hear a range of sound intensities of over a million million (10^{12}), or 100 times greater than the range of light intensities the eye can handle (Fig. 7.1). The ear can hear frequencies that vary by a factor of 1000, while the frequencies of light that eye can detect vary by only a factor of 2.

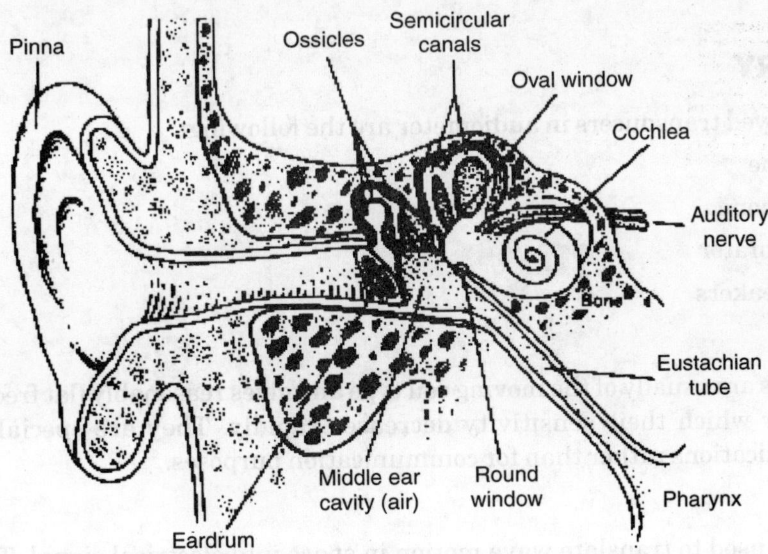

Fig. 7.1. The cross sectional view of the human ear showing parts.

The sense of hearing involves

1. the mechanical system that stimulates the hair cells in the cochlea;
2. the sensors that produce the action potentials in the auditory nerves;
3. the auditory cortex, the part of the brain that decodes and interprets the signals from the auditory nerves.

Deafness or hearing loss results if any of these parts malfunctions.

The ear is a cleverly designed converter of very weak mechanical waves in air into electrical pulses in the auditory nerve. Fig. 7.1 shows most of the structures of the ear involved with hearing. The ear is usually thought of as divided into three areas;

The outer ear consists of the ear canal, which terminates at the eardrum (tympanic membrane).

The middle ear includes the three small bones (ossicles) and an opening to the mouth (Eustachian tube).

The inner ear consists of the fluid filled spiral shaped cochlea containing the organ of Corti. Hair cells in the organ of Corti convert vibrations of sound waves hitting the ear - drum into coded nerve pulses that inform the brain of these sounds.

Fig 7.1. Shows the cross section of the Ear. (note that the connection to the middle ear to the pharynx)

STETHOSCOPE

Perhaps no symbol is more associated with the physician than the stethoscope hanging his neck or protruding from the pocket. This simple "hearing aid" permits a physician or nurse to listen to sounds made inside the body.

AUDIOMETRY

Generally employed transducers in audiometer are the following:

1. earphone
2. microphone
3. bone-vibrator
4. loud speakers

Earphones

Earphones are usually of the moving coil type and gives reasonably flat frequency response upto 6KHz after which their sensitivity decreases rapidly. They are specially designed for audiometric applications rather than for communication purposes.

Microphones

These are used to translate wave motion in space into electrical signal. Two types which are carbon button changes resistance with the pressure.

The second one is the electrodynamic type in which the voltage is induced in a coil by its motion relative to a magnet.

The third one is the condensor in which the capacitance of a condensor is varied by vibration of one of the condensor plates. High quality microphones of diameter 12.5, 6.25 and 3.15 mm are currently used depending on the frequency to be measured. For special purposes, microphones can be fitted to the earpiece used in reciprocal arrangment to transmit sound to the ear.

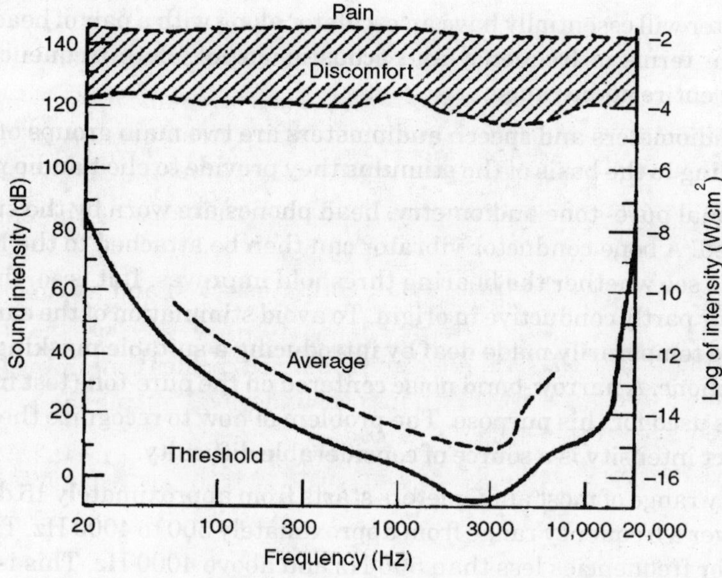

Fig. 7.2. Showing the sensitivity of the Ear.

BASIC AUDIOMETER

An Audiometer is a machine, which is used to determine the hearing loss in an individual. The audiometer must be capable of making all measurements quickly, precisely, with no discomfort to the patient. Pure Tone Audiometer works on the principle of presenting specific pure tone signals to the subject and determining the intensity at which they can barely hear these signals. Coming from India, where more than seventy percent of the population is rural, and the doctors attending to these masses have to often travel large distances on their two wheelers, it warrants that the Audiometer be extremely portable and rugged.

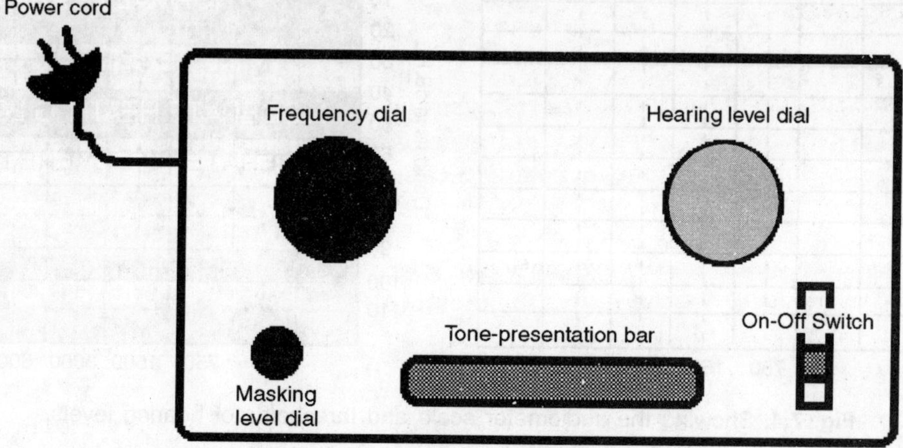

Fig. 7.3. A simple audiometer.

An audiometer will essentially have an oscillator along with a pair of head phones. Usually, this is calibrated in terms of frequency and acoustic output. Both frequency and output are adjustable over the entire audio range.

Pure tone audiometers and speech audiometers are two main groups of audiometers and are grouped according to the basis of the stimulus they provide to elicit audio response.

In conventional pure- tone audiometry, head phones are worn by the subject and a set of response is obtained. A bone conductor vibrator can then be attached to the head at the center forehead position to see whether the hearing threshold improves. If it is so, then the disorder is most likely wholly or partly conductive in origin. To avoid stimulation of the ear with the vibrator not tested, it can be temporarily made deaf by introducing a suitable masking noise in the non-test ear via an earphone. A narrow-band noise centered on the pure-tone test frequency or a wide band white noise is used for this purpose. The problem of how to recognize the need for masking and then the correct intensity is a source of considerable difficulty.

The intensity range of most audiometers starts from approximately 15 dB above normal to 95 below normal over a frequency range from approximately 500 to 4000 Hz. The intensity range is somewhat less for frequencies less than 500 Hz and above 4000 Hz. This is partly because of certain instrumental limitations imposed by the earphone or vibrator and partly due to the desirability of avoiding the threshold of feeling from stimulation at the lower frequency levels. The threshold of feeling is the sensation of pain or tickle in the ear which results form the sound pressures and limits the maximal sound intensity level at which the threshold of feeling is stimulated and varies with the frequencies. For example, the threshold of feeling is stimulated at the intensity level approximately 120 dB above the normal threshold of audibility from about 500 to 4000 Hz, but at 64 Hz the threshold of feeling is stimulated at sound pressures approximately 65 dB above the normal threshold value.

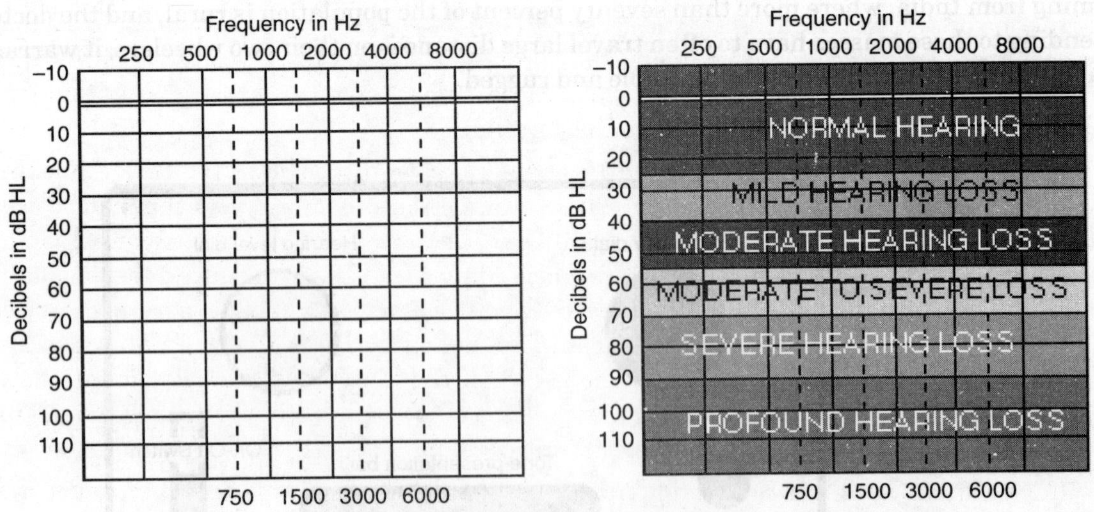

Fig. 7.4. Showing the audiometer scale and thresholds of hearing levels.

The stimulation dials on the audiometer provide variable intensity or volume controls. They are calibrated in decibels usually in discrete steps which differ by 5 dB in frequencies from step to step. Auditory acuity for each frequency is thus measured in dB above or below the normal-hearing-zero dB reference level for that frequency. This level is the minimal intensity at which each given frequency can be perceived by the normal ear in a noise free environment and is experimentally determined by averaging the results of measurement on a larger number of normal individuals between 18 and 25 years of age.

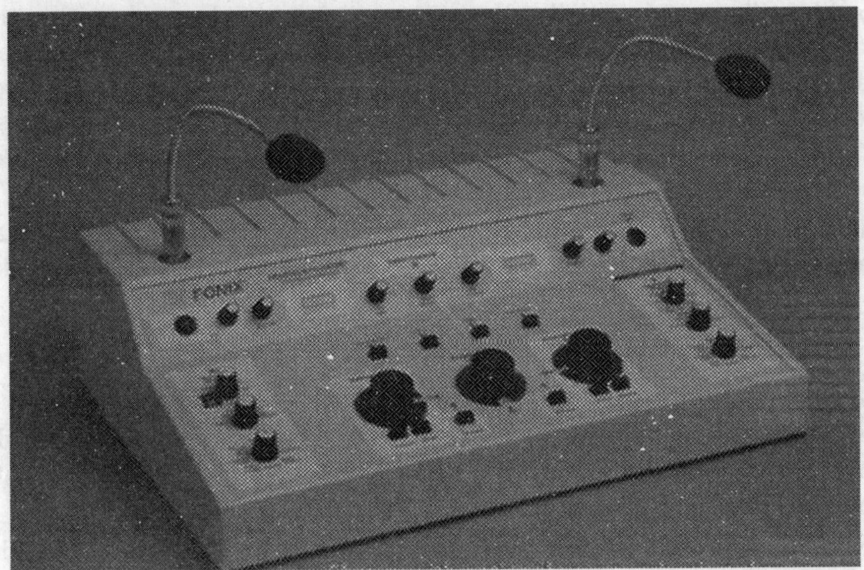

Fig. 7.5. A typical audiometer.

Audiometers usually have two channels, with a single pure tone generator. First channel has pure tone or speech output while the second channel has nominal masking. The pure tone and speech can be switched to both channels for special tests. Channel two can have either wide or narrow band masking. Each channel has an accurate independent attenuator output and the transducers are switched to each attenuator as required.

The specifications for audiometers allow a tolerance of threshold in the other. Masking efficiency depends upon the nature of masking sound as well as intensity. A pure tone can be used to mask other pure tones (Egan and Hake, 1950), but over a range of test frequencies masking efficiency of a pure tone is low compared to a noise composed of many frequencies, as usually provided in commercial audiometers. A restricted frequency bandwidth of white noise is also often used. An excellent complex masking noise can be obtained by using the thermal or random electronic emission from a semiconductor diode. When the tone is just audible against noise background, the total acoustic power of the narrow band is the same as that of the pure tone. This restricted range of frequencies is defined as the critical band.

If the difference in air conduction acuity between the two ears is 50 dB or more, it is advisable to place a masking noise over the better hearing ear while determining the threshold in the other.

PURE TONE AUDIOMETERS

Pure tone audiometers usually generate test tones in octave steps from 125 to 8000Hz, the signal intensity ranging from – 10 dB to + 100 dB.

A pure tone is the simplest type of auditory stimulus. It can be specified accurately in terms of frequency and intensity. These parameters can be controlled with a high degree of precision. Speech audiometry normally allows measurements to be made within the frequency range of 300–3000Hz. Some patients may have impaired high frequency response due to high intensity level occupational noise at 4000 or 6000 Hz. Pure tone measurements at these frequencies prove a more sensitive indicator of the effect of such noise on the ear than the speech tests. Changes in threshold sensitivity associated with various middle ear surgical procedures can be monitored more accurately with pure tone than speech tests.

The attenuators used in these instruments are ladder type, of nominal 10 Ω impedance. The signals are presented acoustically to the ear by an earphone or small loudspeaker.

SPEECH AUDIOMETER

It is sometimes necessary to carry out tests with spoken voices. These tests are particularly important before prescribing hearing-aids. A double band tape recorder is preferred to interface the two channel audiometer units. Masking noise is supplied by the noise generator. The two channels supply the two head-phones or the two loud speakers of 25 W each.

Calibration is effected in terms of the sensitivity relative to a stated threshold. Speech thresholds are not easy to define due to phonetic variations to different languages. Spondee threshold is defined as the level at which 50% of a spondee word list can be recognized and repeated by otologically normal subjects within the age group of 18 to 25 years.

The frequency response characteristics of a live voice channel should be such that with the microphone in a free sound field having a constant sound pressure level, the sound pressure level developed by the earphone of the audiometer in the artificial ear at frequencies in the range 250–4000 Hz does not differ from that at 1000 Hz by more than ± 10 dB.

BEKESY AUDIOMETER SYSTEM

An audiogram traced by the Beksy method represents the absolute threshold values at all frequencies in the range tested. In addition, it shows the intensity and those at which he just ceases to hear the signal when its intensity is decreasing.

The instrument generates a pure-tone signal which is presented to him through an air-conduction earphone. The subject is asked to press a switch when the tone is heard and to release the switch when it is not heard. A pen connected to the attenuator traces a continuous record of the patient's intensity adjustments on an audiogram chart, producing a graphic representation.

A block diagram of the audiometer consists of an electrical section and a mechanical section. The electrical section includes oscillator and modulator circuits for generation of the desired test signal, an automatic attenuator linked to the writing system, control circuits for the drive motors of the mechanical section and a master clock generator for control of all timing functions via a logic control circuit. The carriage drive and the writing system with their separate drive motors constitute the mechanical section.

Electrical section and Mechanical section

The electrical section includes oscillator and modulator circuits for generation of the desired test signal, an automatic attenuator linked to the writing system, control circuits for the drive motors of the mechanical section and a master clock generator for control of all timing functions via a logic control circuit. The carriage drive and the writing system with their drive motors constitute the mechanical section.

Electrical Section

This oscillator generates test signals with frequencies of 125, 250, 500, 1000, 1500, 2000, 3000, 4000, 6000 and 8000Hz. This sequence is first presented to the left ear automatically, each tone for 30s, and then to the right ear, the shift between the frequencies being noiseless. After both ears have been tested, a 1 kHz tone is presented to the right ear to provide a useful indication of the test reliability.

Modulator

Two models of modulators are available "Pulse" or "Cont" . In the 'Pulse' mode the test signal is modulated giving a signal which is easily recognized by the patient. In the 'Cont'mode no modulation is applied, giving a signal suitable for use, while calibrating the audiometer.

Attenuator

The attenuation range is 100dB, thereby covering the range of hearing levels from – 10 to + 90 dB. When the test is initiated, the attenuator starts at its top position of – dB and then increases the level with a rate of 5 dB/s.

The pen drive is controlled by means of the handswitch operated by the patient. Pressing the switch decreases the output from the potentiometer and thereby the level in the ear phones.

Earphones

The earphones are a matched pair with distortion which is typically less than 1%.

Mechanical carriage

Mechanical carriage with the writing system is driven by a stepping motor via a toothed belt. The speed and direction of rotation of the motor are automatically controlled via the logic control system. When the test is initiated and the patient indicates that he hears the signal by pressing hand switch, the carriage moves along the X-axis (Frequency axis) of the audiogram in tune with the frequency of the test signal. When the complete test is finished the carriage and writing system return to the start position.

Writing System

Writing System is operated by the pen drive, which is driven by a stepping motor. The pen drive moves the pen, and with it the wiper of the automatic attenuator, along the Y-axis (hearing level axis) with a constant speed corresponding to the change in attenuation of 5dB/s. The direction of movement of the pen is determined by the position of the hands witch operated by the patient. Limit switches are also included with the pen drive.

Audiogram Chart

The audiogram is printed in standard A5 format (148*210mm) .The recording space is large, 0.8dB /mm, to enable easy reading . For carrying out Fowler loudness balance test second channel is provided for the purpose. This channel also has a continuously variable intensity over the range 0 to 110dB and is calibrated in 1 dB increments.

Understanding Audiometric Symbols and the Concept of Threshold

- On this type of audiogram you will see several symbols. Most likely you will see a series of x's and o's. The **o's represent the right ear** and the **x's represent the left**. More specifically the symbols represent a person's hearing threshold. The hearing threshold is defined as the **lowest intensity that a person can detect about 50% of the time.**
- Make sure you know what the o's and x's represent.
- Be able to define hearing threshold.

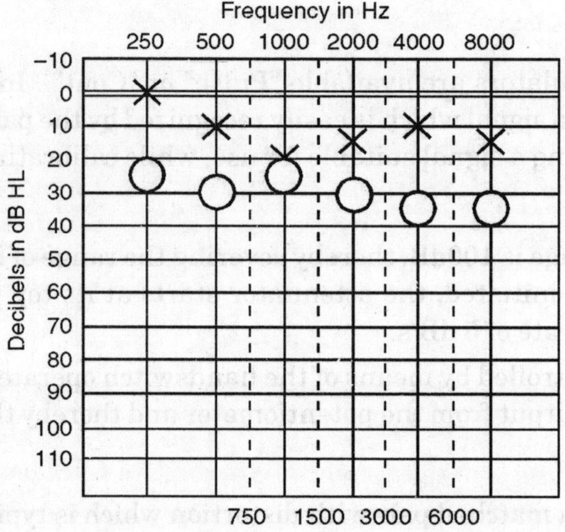

Fig. 7.7. Chart for Audiometery.

The Cyprus PSoC micro controller with its integrated analog and digital blocks is the right candidate for this kind of design. Using this micro controller it is possible to cut down on some of the support chips, thus automatically reducing the space and cost.

Key Features of Audiometer Extreme

1. Digitally generated Sine Wave with frequency up to 8Khz.
2. Noise generated using on chip PRBS modules.
3. Both Narrow band and Wide band noise available for masking.
4. The Narrow band noise is generated from Wide band noise using on chip Band pass filter modules.
5. A 16*2 line LCD displays all the necessary information in a clear and logical manner. LCD indication when input is tone. LCD indication when input is speech.

6. On chip ADC module is used to generate a Bar Graph display on the LCD module, when the selected input is Speech.
7. LCD contrast can be adjusted digitally.
8. An on chip DAC module is used to generate the control voltage for the voltage controlled amplifier. The DAC voltage is made to ramp up or ramp down with programmable slopes, so that the interruption of tone or speech is smooth.

Key Features of Hardware

1. The use of 48-pin microcontroller provided us with enough I/O pins such that no I/O expander needed to be used.
2. The LCD is interfaced in 4-bit mode using a total of only 7 I/O pins.
3. The clock for the Sine Wave generator module, which is 16 times the required frequency, and is as high as 128 KHz for 8 KHz Sine Wave, is generated using on chip 16-bit PWM module. This module is clocked by the internal 48 MHz signal, thus producing a very accurate Sine Wave frequency. Once the PWM registers are loaded, this clock is produced automatically without consuming precious CPU time.
4. Wide band noise is generated using 24-bit on chip PRBS modules, thus giving the PRBS generator a sufficiently long time period.
5. Narrow band noise is basically a band limited noise, about the tone frequency. Passing this wide band noise through an on chip band pass filter, whose center frequency corresponds to the tone frequency, generates this noise. Narrow band noise has a 3 dB bandwidth, which is about 1/10th, the value of the presented tone.
6. While generating Narrow band noise the clock to the PRBS module is changed to minimize aliasing in the following band pass filter module.
7. An on chip ADC module is used to display the peak levels of speech on a bar graph display created on the LCD module.
8. An on chip DAC module is used to generate the control voltage for TDA 7052A, which is 1-Watt mono BTL amplifier.
9. The speech tone attenuator is formed by using one Dallas DS 1267 digital potentiometer, which provides 80dB of attenuation and the TDA 7052A, which provides 60 dB of attenuation.
10. The masking attenuator is formed by using TDA 8551 IC, which is a 1-Watt audio amplifier with digital volume control. Using relay logic provides additional 20 dB of attenuation.
11. Second DAC module is used to control LCD contrast.
12. The ability of the flash memory to emulate an EEPROM is used for storing calibration data.

MICRO-CONTROLLER PROGRAM SET UP

Setup the modules required by the noise generator (i.e. PGA_1, BPF2_1, PSR24_1, Timer8_1.) but do not start the PRBS generator. Setup the DAC8_1 module. This module is used to generate the control voltage for the DC Volume control of TDA7052A IC Initialize the SAR6_1 but do not start it. Initialize DAC8_2 and start it.

Initialize Timer8_3 which is used as a system timer to interrupt 1200 times every second.

Setup the modules required by the tone generator (*i.e.* PWM16_1) but do not start the PWM module.

Initialize all system variables.

Initialize LCD in 4-bit mode.

Setup the LCD module to show horizontal bar graphs.

Get calibration values form flash memory to array in ram using EEPROM module routines.

Load the 1st Digital Pot with a calibration value for the current tone.

Reset TDA8551 used by the masking attenuator such that its attenuation is maximum (–80 dB)

Display the following information on the LCD.

Input (Tone, Speech) If tone is input display its frequency.

If speech is input show it as a Bar

Graph Display Format.

Input signal intensity.

Output (ACL, ACR, BONE)

Masking Type (NB, WB)

Masking Intensity.

Is Audiometer in calibration mode?

NO

YES

Display Calibration information on LCD module.

Is Audiometer in Speech mode?

NO

YES

Turn on SAR6_1 module and get sample form it. Use this sample to generate value for BAR GRAPH DISPLAY.

Interrupt Service Routine

Timer8_3INT

Is system timer variable = 0?

Decrement system timer variable. (So the main code of this ISR is executed only 30 times/ second from 1200 times/second)

YES

NO

System timer variable = 40

Scan Keyboard

1 > Make scan lines input, makes rows output.

2 > Read scan lines.

3 > Make rows input, make scan lines output.

4 > Read row lines.

Are HTL keys pressed?

YES

Incremet or Decrement HTL variable.

Are frequency keys pressed? YES

Increment or Decrement Frequency variable.

A

Are masking keys pressed?

YES

Increment or Decrement

Masking variable

YES

Increment or Decrement Masking variable.

Are noise select keys pressed?

Toggle between wide band & narrow band noise. By gating the PRBS signal either directly or via Band Pass Filter to noise output pin

Is input select key pressed?

YES

If input is speech set the speech flag. Is output select key pressed?

YES

Set the output variable.

Is interrupt key pressed?

YES

If input is tone set the interrupt flag.

If input is speech clear the interrupt flag.

Is PLUS 20dB key pressed?

YES

Set the plus20dB flag.

Set the port pins of the micro controller that controls the state ofthe output relays, depending on the output variable

Set the port pins of the micro

controller that controls the state of input select multiplexer depending on the state of the speech flag.

Depending upon the value of the frequency variable, load the PWM16_1 module to generate the displayed frequency.

Has frequency variable changed? (i.e. has frequency changed?) YES

Get new calibration value from calibration array in Ram for the new tone to be generated and send it to the digital pot used for calibration. Has HTL variable changed?

(i.e. has HTL changed?)

YES

Get new HTL attenuator value from flash look up table and update digital pot used for speech / tone attenuator.

Generate value to be loaded into the DAC8_1 module from the HTL attenuator look up table in flash. If 20dB key was pressed and 20dB head room available add a value 2db to the value to be loaded into the DAC. Depending upon the value of frequency variable update Timer8_2 period register. This timer determines the center frequency of the band pass filter used to generate narrow band noise.

Is interrupt flag set?

YES

Increment DAC8_1 value by up to16.

(Here we control the slope of the up going ramp.)

Is DAC8_1 value = its final value? (00h if interrupt off, above calculated value if interrupt on)

NO

Decrement DAC8_1 value by up to8.

(Here we control the slope of the down going ramp.)

A

Exit routine

Both models offer the standard features that you need: air, bone, speech, three kinds of masking noise, Stenger test, and hearing aid slopes. Both include a built-in amplifier for sound field speakers, and a built-in talk forward (talk over) function. The FA-10 has an Output Reverse feature, letting you control the frequency presentation to both ears from one side of the instrument. The FA-12 has a + 10 dB feature, extending the amplitude range of the instrument. Great care has gone into the design of these instruments so that they are easy to use and attractive to look at. They have the look of quality you want for your office.

The word "Digital" before Hearing Evaluator means that the FA-10 and FA-12 are microprocessor-based audiometers for the offices of the 21st century. They can be purchased as either 110V or 220V, making them compatible with nearly the entire global marketplace. With calibration that is stable over time, you can expect stable, dependable service with minimum maintenance and unusually tight technical specifications for an audiometer in this price category.

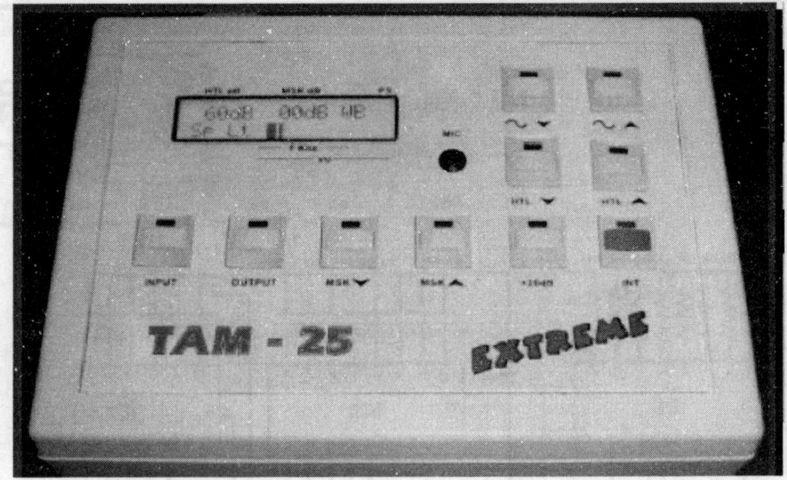

Fig. 7.8. Microcontroller based audiometer with 2 row LCD display.

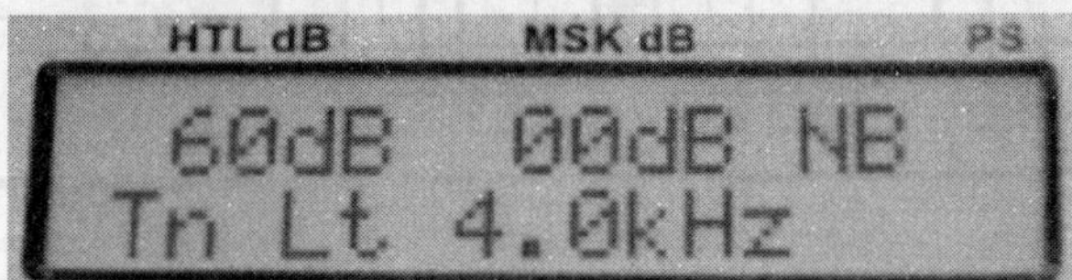

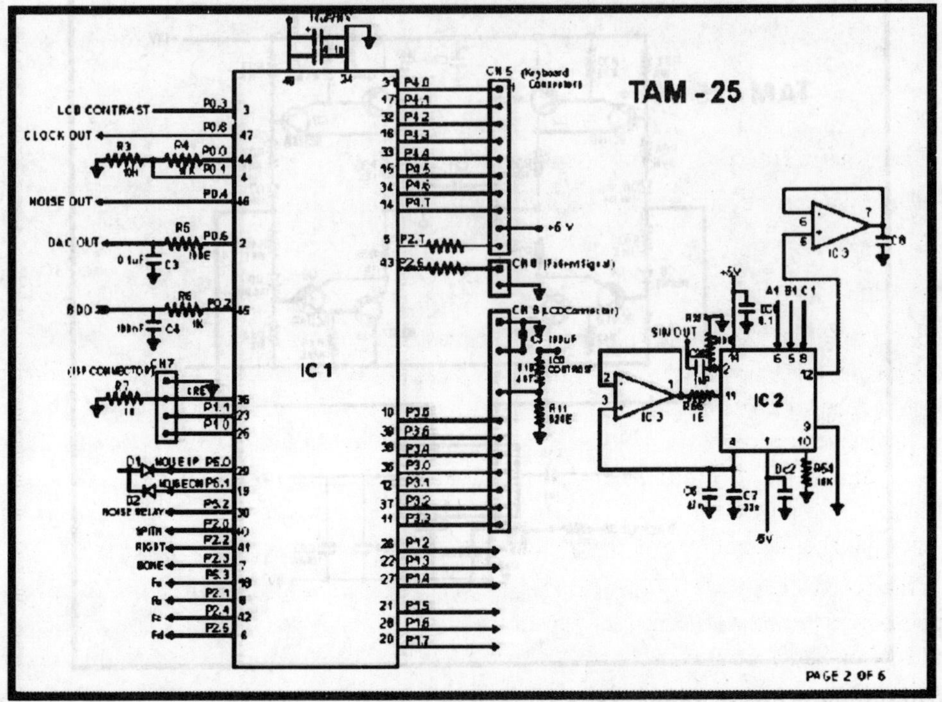

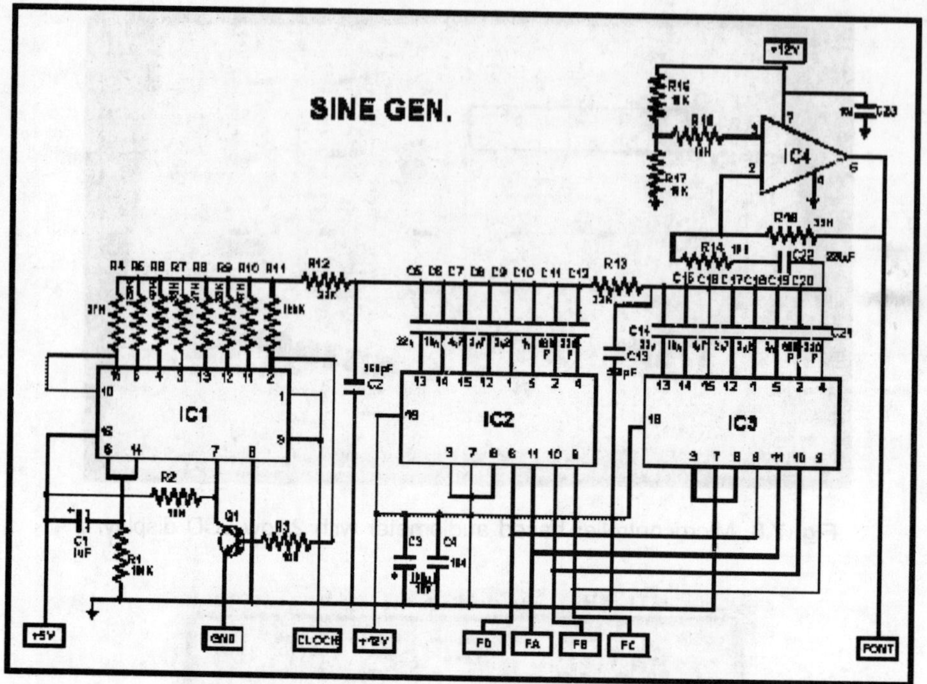

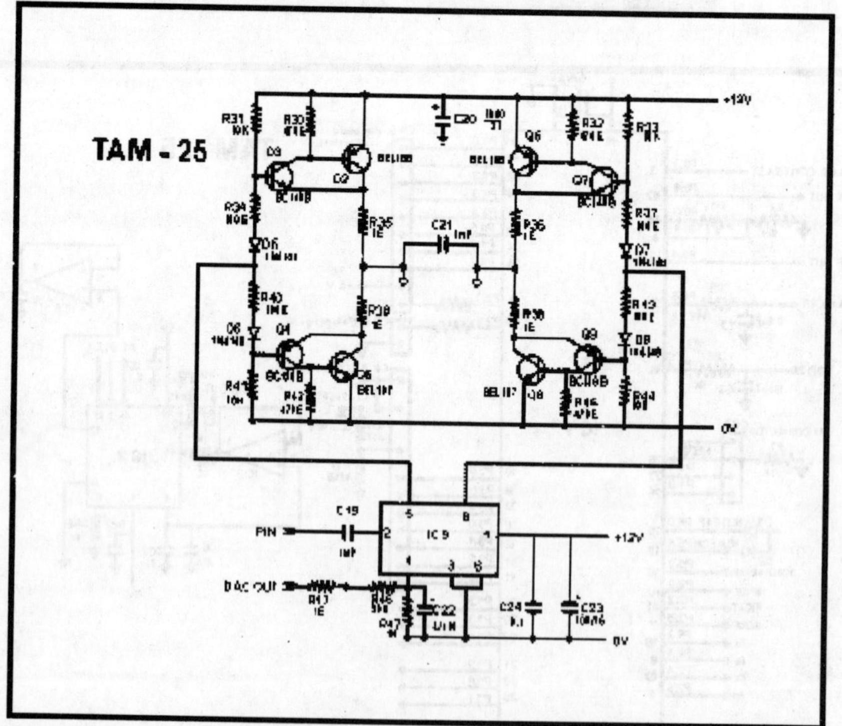

"An audiometer has to address the computerized office. The Hearing Evaluator does. The RS232 option lets you connect the Hearing Evaluator to a computer. Our WinCHAP program (also optional) will store your data and even let you run your tests from the computer."

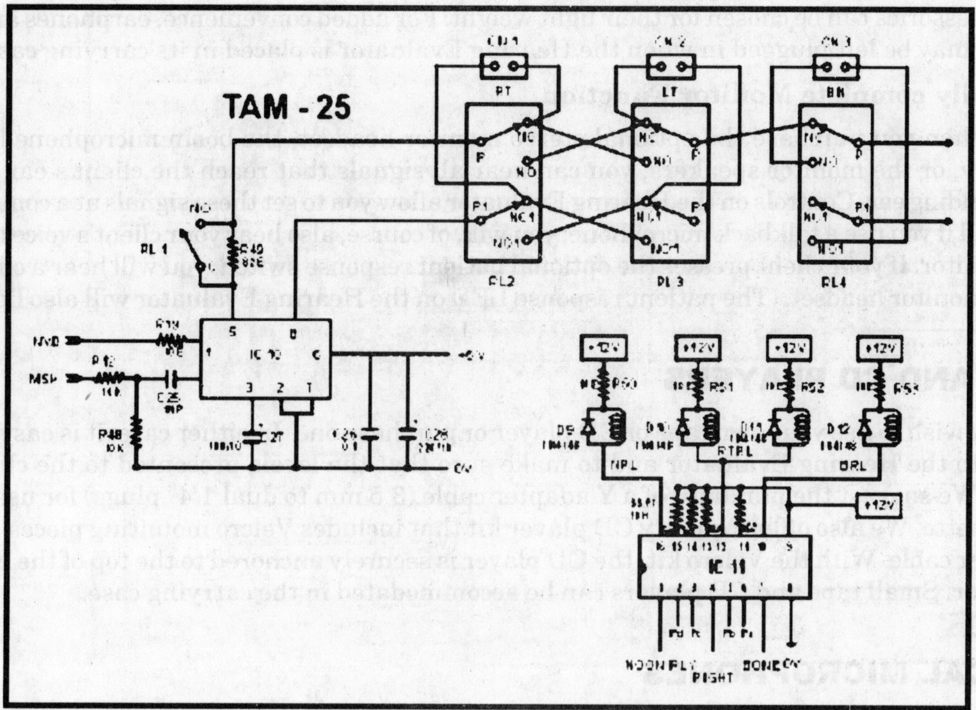

Fig. 7.9. Showing the typical circuitry of the audiometer using microcontroller.

DUAL CALIBRATION

With the Dual Calibration Option your Hearing Evaluator comes with calibrations for TDH 39 headphones and insert earphones. You can change the calibration with the turn of a dial. We also offer an earphone switch box, so that you don't need to plug and unplug the headphones or earphones each time you switch between them.

SPECIAL TESTS AT NO EXTRA COST

You may administer four special tests when using the FA-10 or FA-12: Stenger, ABLB, SISI, and MLB. These tests are included at no extra cost, so they are there when you need them.

CUSTOM LIGHTWEIGHT SOUND FIELD SPEAKERS

The optional high efficiency sound field speakers also fit into the carrying case and add very little weight. It is not necessary to purchase an additional amplifier for these speakers. The amplifier in the Hearing Evaluator will drive them to 85 dB HL at 1000 Hz when the client is located three feet from the speaker. Each sound-field frequency can be independently calibrated in HL (Hearing Loss)

SUITABLE FOR PORTABLE USE WITH SOFT CARRYING CASE

The Hearing Evaluator is quite light weight. Few dispensers will have trouble carrying its eleven pounds (5 kg). The optional custom-made soft case adds less than three pounds (< 1.4 kg) and other accessories can be chosen for their light weight. For added convenience, earphones and bone vibrator may be left plugged in when the Hearing Evaluator is placed in its carrying case.

Unusually complete Monitor Function

When you purchase the optional stereo monitor headset, the boom microphone/headset accessory, or the monitor speakers, you can hear all signals that reach the client's ear in your corresponding ear. Controls on the Hearing Evaluator allow you to set these signals at a comfortable level. And if you use a talkback microphone, you will, of course, also hear your client's voice through your monitor. If your client presses the optional patient response switch, you will hear a click/tone in your monitor headset. (The patient response LED on the Hearing Evaluator will also light up.)

TAPE AND CD PLAYERS

You may wish to use your own tape or CD player or purchase one. In either case, it is easy to plug them into the Hearing Evaluator and to make sure that the levels presented to the client are correct. We suggest the purchase of a Y adapter cable (3.5 mm to dual 1/4" plugs) for use with a CD/Cassette. We also offer a quality CD player kit that includes Velcro mounting pieces and the Y adapter cable. With the Velcro kit, the CD player is securely anchored to the top of the Hearing Evaluator. Small tape and CD players can be accommodated in the carrying case.

OPTICAL MICROPHONES

Should you wish the convenience of external microphones, you have two choices: the 12" gooseneck microphones and the convenient boom microphone/headset that combines the monitor and microphone functions. Whether you use the internal microphones or choose an optional microphone, you will be able to monitor your voice with the V.U. meters and the microphone control.

The talkback microphone is another optional accessory. The Hearing Evaluator has a control for this microphone too, so you can make adjustments for loud and soft voices.

Other Optional Accessories

Dust cover Speaker cables (6 ft./10 ft.) Patient response switch Talkback microphone Desk model mic stand, Lightweight mic stand, Speaker wall mounts, Monitor headset, Insert earphones External table top speakers CD/cassette player mount kit Otoscope.

The above details are from the leaflet TAM-25.

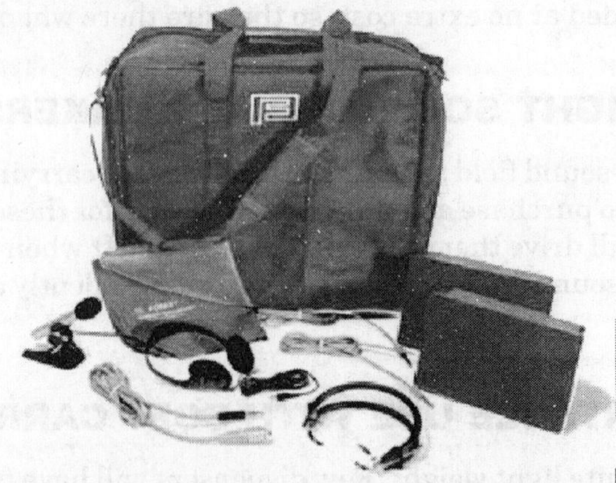

Fig. 7.13. Accesssories of an audiometer.

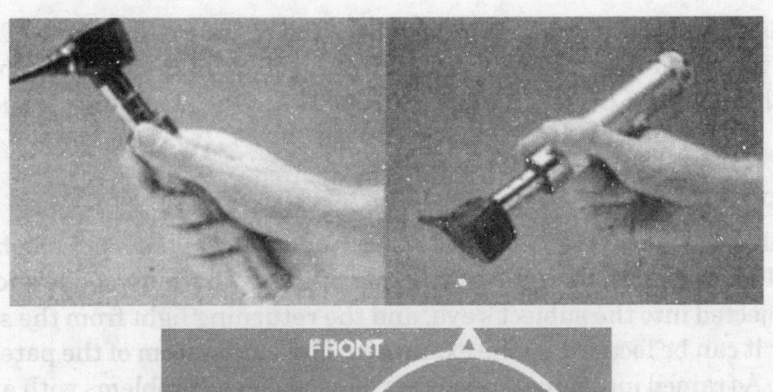

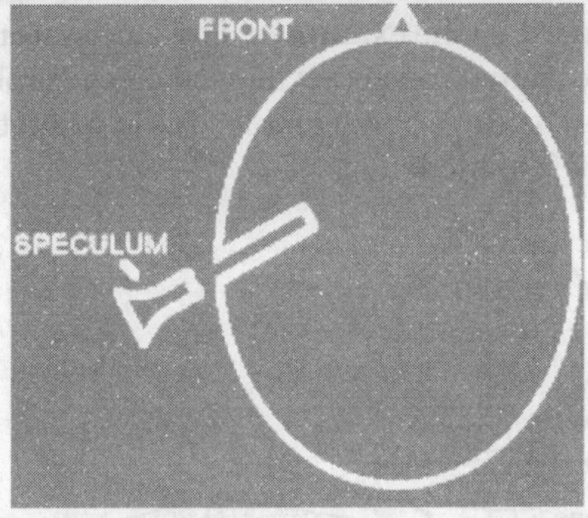

Fig. 7.14. Showing the Otoscope in Audio investigations by surgeon.

Calibration of Audiometers

Accurate Calibration of Audiometers is essential to ensure that the instrument produces a pure tone at the specified level and frequency, and that the signal is present only in the transducer to which it is directed. For pure tone and speech audiometers, the parameters, which are commonly checked, are frequency and intensity.

The specifications for audiometers allow a tolerance of ± 3 % for frequency output from a fixed frequency pure tone audiometer.

A typical example of an artificial ear is that of type 4153 artificial Ear from Bruel and Kjaer. It is designed in accordance with IEC 318. I* has a three cavity coupler and provides acoustic impedance which closely resembles that of the human ear. Different types of couplers are available fro use with artificial ears for measurements on headphones.

Audiometers test should be conducted in rooms which are reasonably quiet. As subject under test should not be disturbed either by sounds created within the room or by those intruding from outside. Such rooms are known as sound treated rooms.

INSTRUMENTS USED IN OPTHALMOLOGY

There are three major instruments used to examine the eye

1. **Opthalmoscope** which permits the physician to examine the interior of the eye.
2. The **Retinoscope** which measures the focusing power of the eye and
3. The **Keratometer** which measures the curvature of the cornea.

Another instrument, the tonometer measures the pressure in the eye. The lensometer is not used to study the eye; it determines the prescription of an unknown lens. These instruments are discussed in this chapter. Ultrasound measurements of the structures of the eye will also be discussed.

1. Opthalmoscope

The Opthalmoscope is by far the most used, and several versions have been designed. It was invented in 1851 by Helmholtz. The principle of the opthalmoscope is shown in Fig. 7.15. Bright light is projected into the subject's eye, and the returning light from the subject's retina is positioned so that it can be focused by the examiner. The lens system of the patent's eye acts as a built in magnifier. A trained individual can detect more than eye problems with an opthalmoscope since increased pressure inside the skull (for example, due to brain tumor) can cause a noticeable change in the interior of the eye (papilledemia).

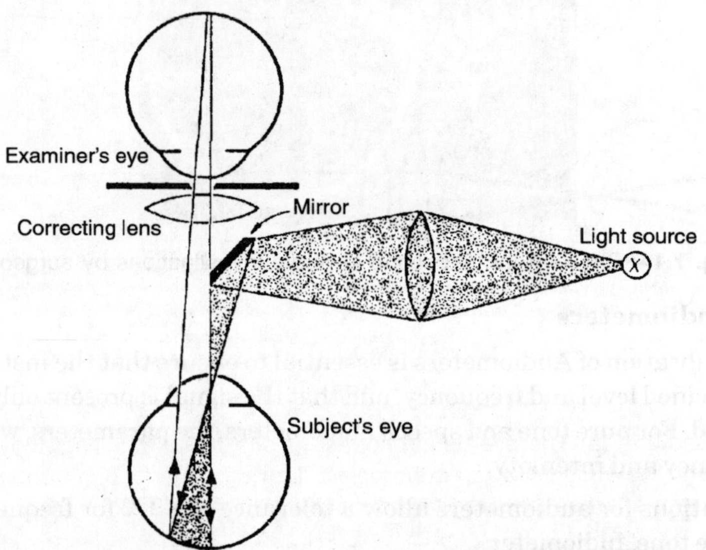

The ophthalmoscope permits the examination of the retina. Light is directed into the patient's eye to permit the examiner to view the retina through a correcting lens. (From T.N. Cornsweet, Visual Perception, Academic Press, New York, 1970, p. 62.)

Fig. 7.15. Shows the Ophthalmoscope principle.

2. Retinoscopy

The retinoscopy used to determine the prescription of a corrective lens without the patient's active participation, although the eye has to be open and in a position suitable for examination. The techniques can be used to determine for example, on an anesthetized infant. The retinoscope is also sometimes used to check the prescription determined by the usual "which is better the first or the second ?"

A streak of light from retinoscope is projected into the patient's unaccommodated diluted eye. This light beam is reflected from the retina and acts as a light source for the operator. The retina's function in retinoscopy is the reverse of its normal function (Fig. 7.16*a*). Since an object at the eye's far point would be focused at the retina of a relaxed eye, a light from the retina of a relaxed eye will produce a focused image at the far point. The operator views the patient's eye through the retinoscope and adds lens in front of the patient's eye (positive or negative, as needed) to cause the image from the patient's retina to be focused at the operator's own eye. (Fig. 7.2*b*). To determine the prescription needed to correct the patient's eye, the operator must change the lens power of these added lens by the dioptic power needed to focus the same eye at infinity. If the "operator distance" is 67 cm, – 1.5 D must be added.

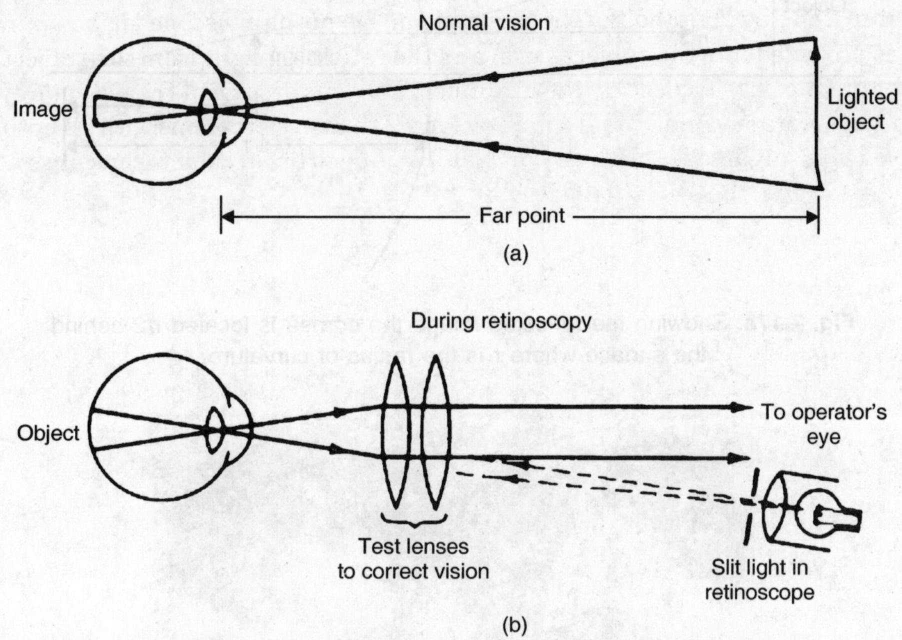

Fig. 7.16. Showing (a) The eye during normal vision (b) During retinoscopy, reflected light form the patient's acts as the object. Lenses are added in front of the eye to focus the image from the retina at the operator's eye.

3. Keratometer

The keratometer is an instrument that measures the curvature of the cornea. This measurement is needed to fit contact lenses. The keratometer produces a lighted object that is reflected from the cornea while the patient's head is held in a fixed position.

If we illuminate an object of known size placed a known distance from a convex mirror and measure the size of the reflected image, we can determine the curvature of the mirror. In keratometry, the cornea acts as a convex mirror. The reflected image is located at the focal plane, a distance $r/2$ behind the surface of the cornea (Fig. 7.17). The keratometer produces a lighted object that is reflected from the cornea while the patient's head is held in a fixed position. The operator adjusts a focus control to place the instrument a known distance from the cornea (Fig. 7.17*b*). Part of the reflected image passes through the prism that causes a second image to be seen by the operator. The operator determines the size of the reflected image by adjusting the angle of prism to produce a coincidence of marker lines in the two images. The position of the prism after this adjustment is indicated in diopters of focusing power of the cornea. The average value is 44D, which corresponds to a cornea with a radius of curvature of 7.7 mm. Because astigmatism is common the measurement of the image size is made in both horizontal and vertical directions.

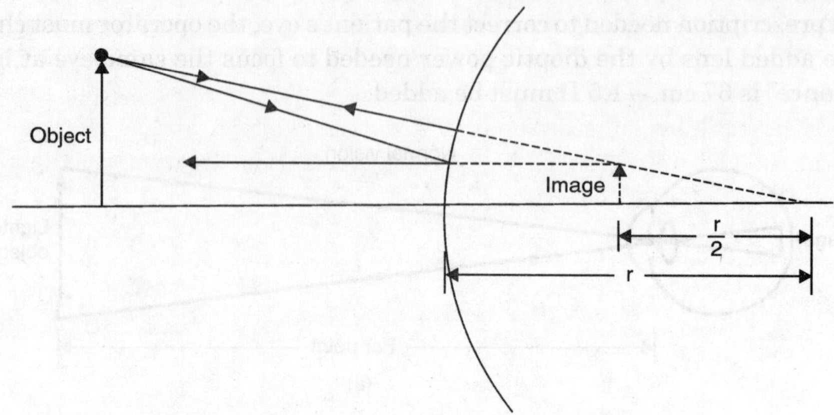

Fig. 7.17a. Showing the reflected image the cornea is located r/2 behind the surface where r is the radius of curvature.

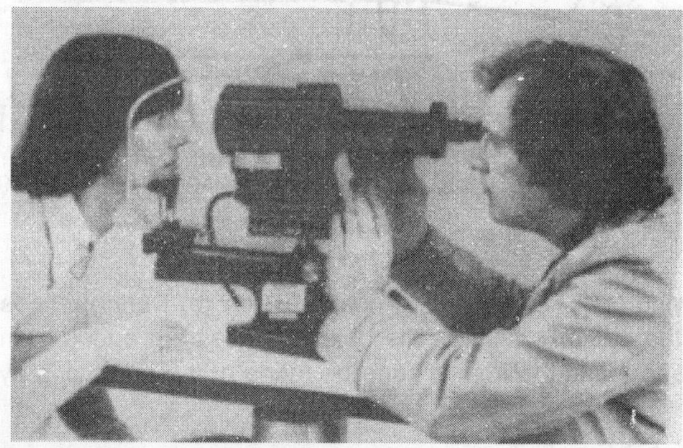

Fig. 7.17b. The Keratometer for prescribing lens (a) principle.

A simple experiment involves determining the focal length of a lens. If we have a positive lens (a magnifying glass), we can produce a focused image of a distant object (e.g., the sun). The image will be at the focal point of the lens. We can measure the distance from the lens to the image to determine the focal length. This technique will not work for a negative lens since no real image will be formed, but a simple modification will permit you to use the same idea. We can combine a negative lens with a strong positive lens of known strength and then produce an image of a distant object to get the focal length of the combination and from this its dioptric strength. Then, we can determine the diopters of the negative lens from

$$D_x + D_{known} = D_{measured}.$$

The above techniques for measuring the power of a lens are suitable for a physics laboratory, but eye can clumsy and inconvenient for an opthalmologist, opthometrist, or optician. For routine use, a commercial lensometer is more convenient (Fig. 7.18). It moves an illuminated object until it is at the focal point of a lens combination consisting of a fixed field lens and the unknown lens. The parallel trays emerging from the lenses are viewed by the telescope focused at infinity. The fixed field lens is placed a distance equal to its focal length from the unknown lens. This placement conveniently makes the position of the movable lighted object a linear function of the strength of the unknown lens. That is, the scale of diopters (Fig. 7.5) is uniformly divided. When the lighted object is at the focal focal point of the field lens, the lensometer reads 0D. As it moves further away from the field lens the lensometer reads in negative diopters, and as it moves closer the lensometer reads in positive diopeters. For a cylindrical lens (used to correct astigmatism) the strength of each lens axis is measured separately.

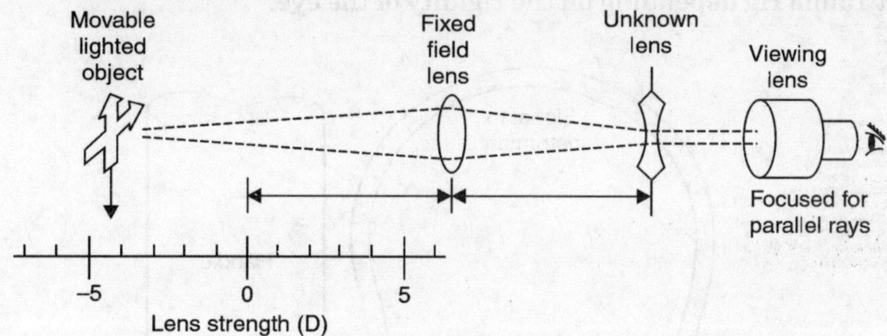

Fig. 7.18. A lensometer to measure power of unknown lens.

Intra Ocular Pressure

It has been known since before 1900 that high pressure is related to the condition of glaucoma. This disease narrows the field of view and leads to blindness if not treated. The production

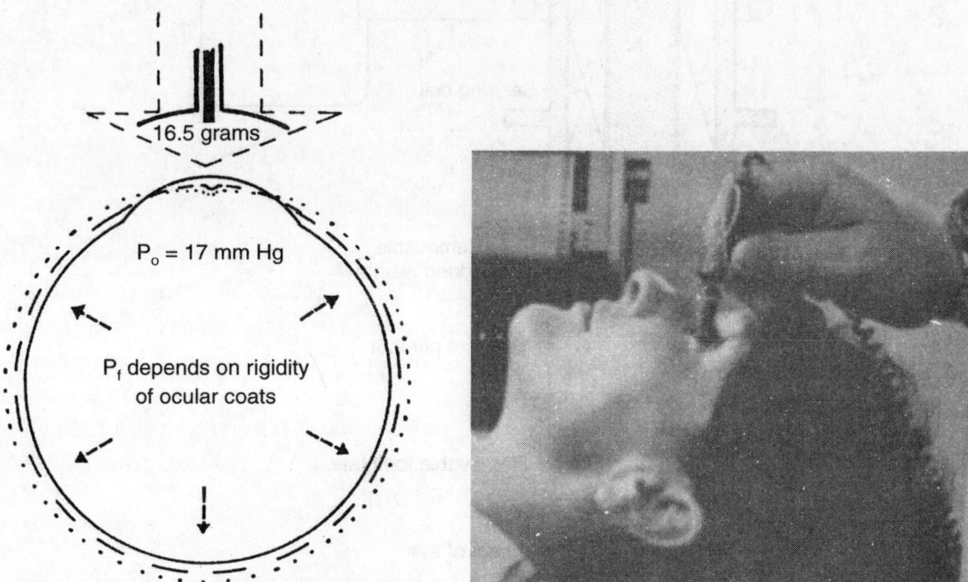

Fig. 7.19. Intra ocular pressure-significance.

and outflow rates of the aqueous humor (typically 5ml/day) determine the pressure in the eye. The fluids in the eyeball are normally under a pressure of 20 to 25mm Hg; in glaucoma, the pressure may go up to 85 mm Hg (the average arterial blood pressure).

In 1900, Schiotz (Germany) invented an instrument for measuring the intraocular pressure– the Schiotz tonometer. The basic technique is to rest the tonometer on the anesthetized cornea with a patient supine (lying face up). The center plunger causes a slight depression in the cornea (Fig. 7.19*a*). The position of the plunger indicates on a scale the internal pressure on the eye. The force on a plunger can be varied by adding various weights. The standard weights have masses of 5.5, 7.5, 10.0 and 15.0 g. The plunger alone has mass of 11.0 g. With the standard 5.5.g mass, there is a 16.5 g resting on a small area of the cornea (Fig. 7.19*b*). This increases the internal pressure about 15mm Hg depending on the rigidity of the eye.

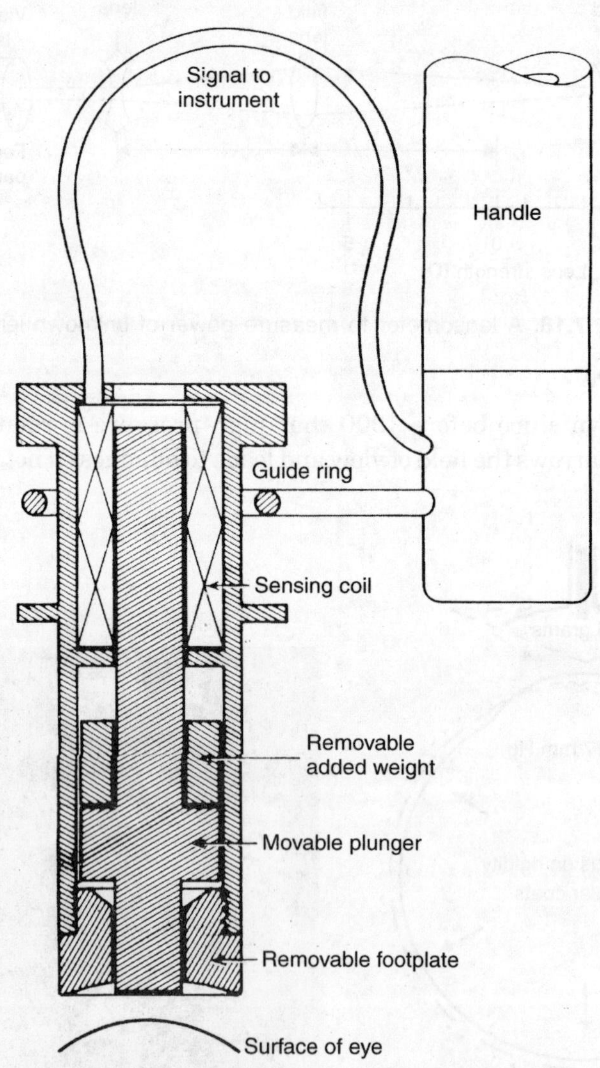

Fig. 7.20. The modified Tonometer after Schiotz.

The pressure measured by the tonometer is the original pressure , plus the increase due to the instrument. To remove the effect of the rigidity of the eye, another measurement is taken with a heavier weight or with a Goldmann tonometer. The two readings permit the operator to determine, with the help of tables, the original pressure and the rigidity of the eye. The rigidity has no diagnostic value.

The Schiotz tonometer was modified in about 1950 to give readings electronically. A coil magnetically senses the position of the plunger (Fig. 7.20). One advantage of this model is that it records the change of pressure with time. Fig. 7.21 shows such a record, called a tonograph. The fluctuations are noticeable due to the pulse in the arteries. The decrease in pressure indicates that the aqueous fluid is leaving the eye faster than normal under pressure produced by the tonographer. The outflow can be estimated from the slope of the tonograph. The outflow is normally 2 to 6 ml/min with the 15.0 g mass on the plunger. Patients with glaucoma often have an outflow of less than 1 ml/min.

The Goldmann applanation tonometer, developed in about 1955, gives a more accurate measure of the ocular pressure. The measurements usually taken with the patient in a sitting position (Fig. 7.22). The principle is simple; the force needed to flatten an area is 3.06 mm in diameter on the front of the cornea is measured. The operator looks through the optical system and adjusts the small force needed to cause the desired flattening. The force needed for a normal eye is equivalent to the weight of 1.7 g mass. The small force raises the internal pressure only 0.5 mm Hg, while the Schiotz tonometer increases 15mm Hg. The Goldmann tonometer is calibrated directly in millimeters of mercury of internal pressure. The rigidity of the eyeball has little effect.

A modified applanation tonometer is used somewhat like the Schiotz with the patient supine. The diameter of the area flattened with a standard weight is measured.

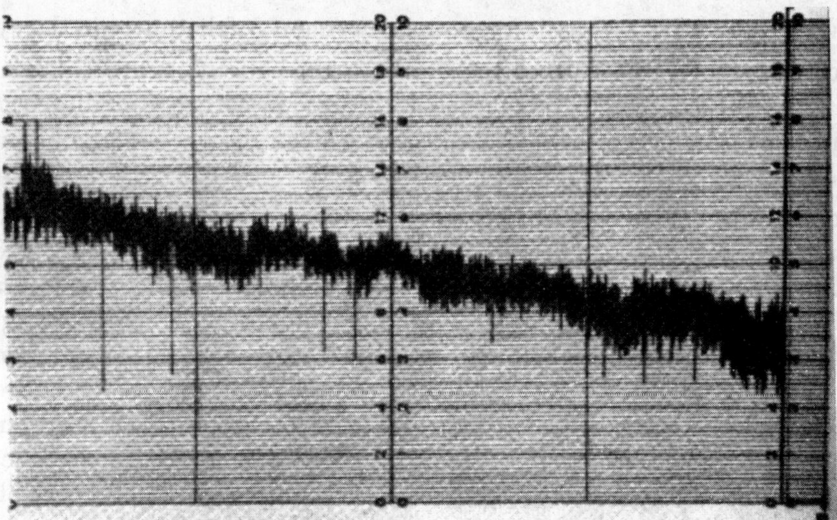

Fig. 7.21. Shows the tonometer record—decrease of pressure with time. Slope can be used to find flow rate.

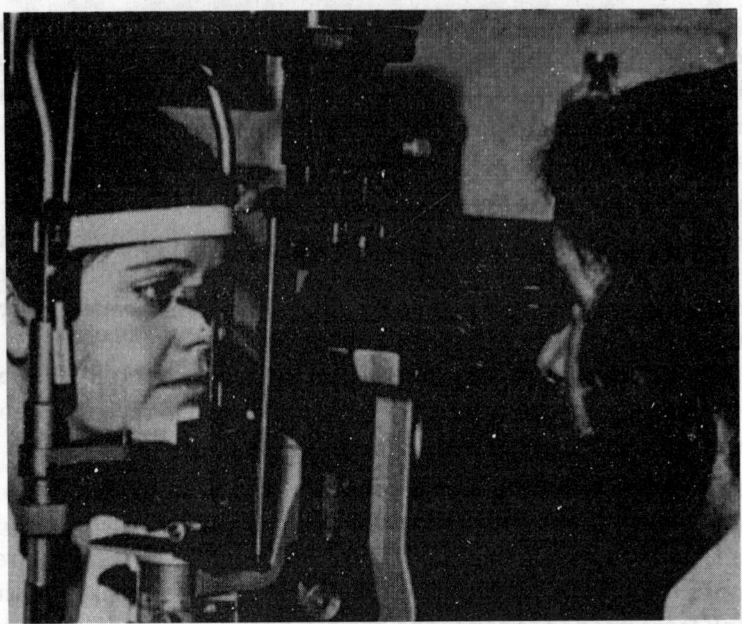

Fig. 7.22. Goldmann tonometer. Pressing and flattening a 3.06 mm dia of cornea, it finds the pressure needed.

Ultrasound in Opthalmology

Applications of A scans in Ophthalmology can be divided into two areas:

1. Is concerned with obtaining information for use in the diagnosis of eye diseaces;
2. The second one involves biometry, or measurements of distances in the eye.

At the low power levels used, there is no danger to the patient's eye. Ultrasound frequencies of up to 20 MHz are used. These high frequencies can be used in the eye to produce better resolution since there is no bone to absorb most of the energy and absorption is not significant because the eye is small.

Ultrasound diagnostic techniques are supplementary to the generally practiced ophthalmologic examinations; they can provide information about the deeper regions of the eye and are especially useful when the cornea or lens is opaque. Use of the A scan plus optical and even x-ray information may be necessary for a complete diagnosis. Tumors , foreign bodies, and detachment of the retina (the light sensitive part of the eye) are some of the problems that can be diagnosed with ultrasound. Fig. 7.23 is a schematic view of a normal A scan of the eye. Fig. 7.23*b* shows an A scan of a severe retinal detachment. Without ultrasound, the Ophthalmologists can look into the living eye up to the optic nerve (as discussed earlier). But measurements of the eye have been largely confined to the exterior segment. With ultrasound, it is possible to measure distances in the eye such as lens thickness, depth from cornea to lens, the distance of the retina, and the thickness of the vitreous humor. This information can be combined with other quantities such as the curvature of the cornea and the prescription of corrective glasses to determine the indexes of refraction of components of the eye.

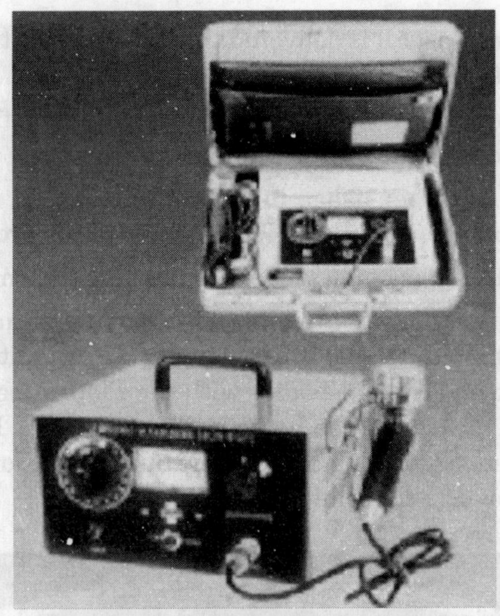

Fig. 7.23. Ultrasound equipment for therapy.

COMPONENTS OF A TYPICAL LASER SYSTEM IN OPTHALMOLOGY

The following are the four major Components of a typical Laser system in Ophthalmology. They are:

1. The laser system
2. The delivery system
3. The operator room
4. The patient

The laser system is the one which is in use depends upon the particular type of laser for particular application. The type of lasers and their uses are given below:

Sl No.	Type of Laser	Application
1.	Argon, Krypton Dye lasers	Photocoagulation
2.	The Carbon dioxide laser	Cutting
3.	Nd-Yag Laser	Photo disruption
4.	Excimer Laser	Photo ablation

Most Opthalmic lasers (except carbon dioxide laser) are delivered through an optical magnification device. The Argon, Krypton, Dye and Nd-Yag are delivered through a lamp microscope which requires no anesthesia by themselves. However for photocoagulation , a contact lens may need to be placed on the front of the eye and for this anesthetizing eye drops may have to be used.

In the case of the Excimer laser it is delivered through an operating microscope and requires the use of anesthetizing drops.

In addition, the Argon Laser, Diode etc., can be delivered by fiber optic cables within the eye during surgery in a procedure called Endo-photocoagulation.

In all the above cases of larger usage in Ophthalmology , it is important to protect the operator from the reflection of laser coming off lenses used in this procedure

Photo-phako-fragmentation is being studied as possible treatment of Cataracts.

Flourescein Antibody laser asepsis is a procedure in which a known organism infecting the Cornea is allowed to conjugate with topical drops that contain an antibody to the organism, that has been tagged with Florescien. The antibodies with the Flourescien tag attach themselves to the organism and with a non focused Argon beam is directed on the lesion for two minutes. The flourescein absorbs the laser energy raising the temperature of the Flourescien antibody organism complex to a temperature above its thermal death point.

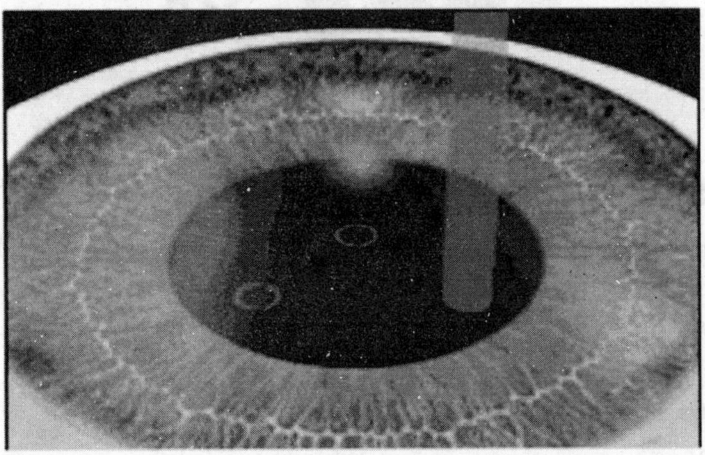

LADARVision®'s unique small-spot laser beam (less than one millimeter in diameter) offers micron size reshaping of the cornea resulting in an extremely smooth surface. LADARVision's ability to use a larger optical zone for treatments minimizes potential nighttime side effects of glare, halos, and starbursts. The feature is most important for patients with large pupils.

Chapter 8

Ultrasound Medical Diagnostic Instrumentation

PART-I

ULTRASONAGRAPHY

Ultrasonography is a technique by which ultrasonic energy is used to detect internal body organs. Bursts of ultrasound energy is transmitted from a transducer through the skin and into the internal anatomy. When the ultrasound energy strikes an interface between two tissues of different acoustical impedance, reflections are returned to the transducer. The transducer converts these reflections to an electrical signal. This electrical signal is amplified and displayed on an oscilloscope, each tissue interface appearing as a vertical deflection along the base line of the oscilloscope at a distance proportional to the depth of the interface. This ultrasonic technique is similar to the time domain reflectometry technique used to measure electrical cable length and the sonar technique used to detect objects under water.

While the use of pulse-echo ultrasonic energy is somewhat similar to the use of X-ray, the results obtained differ from an X-ray picture, being a cross sectional projection or simply a linear projection rather than a profile of the area examined.

ADVANTAGES OF ULTRASONOGRAPHY

Also, in contrast to the X-ray, ultrasonography uses mechanical energy at a level which is not harmful to human tissue. Thus, it may be used with safety on pregnant subjects and for frequent examination. It can detect materials that are not radio-opaque, thus angiographic dyes are unnecessary. As commercial ultrasonic diagnostic instruments are easy to operate, ultrasonography is rapidly becoming a valuable technique.

Among the applications of Ultrasound, medical diagnostics has been a very useful target area, which has been providing enormous scope for development during the past fifteen years. Today B-scan ultrasound machines are available with good imaging and Doppler flow measurement capabilities. Much of the work on the transducer part of the instrument is based on advanced sophisticated techniques of fabrication of the thin discs of transducer elements. Improved transducer arrays, linear and sector-scan multi element construction, possibility of varying the aperture, focusing and beam forming over two or three ranges of depths and signal detection on multiple elements with electronic delay elements are some of the contributions done recently. Further, high level signal processing and scan conversion have been incorporated into the machine using fast digital processing methods with the present day high speed DSP hardware. With all these improvements, today's B-scan machine is somewhat clear in giving the images of internal organs better than before.

Additionally, today's ultrasound technique also resorts to using the Doppler technique for combined information in the case of blood flow measurements particularly in echo-cardiography.

While the basic function of ultrasonic diagnostic equipment is to measure distances between interfaces that separate body structures by timing the echoes produced by these interfaces, this timed echo information may be processed in various ways to produce different forms of display. The technique is often referred as pulse echo method. In this, the three commonly used display modes are employed:

A-scan mode

B-scan mode

T-M-mode

The simplest of all the above three types is the "A" scan, which does not actually produce an image in the usual sense of the word. By transmitting a short pulse of sound into an object and then recording the echoes as a function of time, one can determine both its range and size information about the scattering centers in the object. In this mode (Fig. 8.1.), one transmits pulses on a periodic basis into an object, and synchronizes an oscilloscope to the transmitted burst. The echoes will appear on the screen. The horizontal axis will yield range while the vertical axis yield echo amplitude. Because **"A" scan** trace gives only an **one-dimensional spatial information**, it is not traditionally thought of as an image. However, by combining the "A" scan concept with careful raster movement, one can generate two dimensional spatial information and obtain a terrace that is suitably termed as "image".

The block diagram of 'A' scan Instrument is shown in Fig. 8.1. 'A' scan Ultrasonography displays the amplified echo signal on the vertical channel of an oscilloscope with the horizontal channel being deflected by a conventional sweep generator. This sweep generator is triggered form the impulse signal and the time delay between the beginning of the sweep and the echo appearing on the CRT screen is proportional to tissue depth. A conventional sweep generator may be used for this purpose; otherwise, a sweep generator which is specifically calibrated in tissue depth (centimeters) rather than in time per division. A sweep speed of 100 μs per division would correspond to approximately 6.25 cm of tissue per division. Faster sweep speeds would give correspondingly greater resolution. The fastest usable sweep speed would probably be 2 μs per division which would correspond to 1.25 millimeters of tissue per division. This faster sweep speed would only be usable with 10MHz transducers.

The most common usage of **'A'** scan ultrasonography is echo Echoencephalography. It detects brain midline position and possible displacement of this midline due to an abnormal space occupying mass within one side of the skull, such as a tumor. When performing an **'A'** scan with the transducer held against the side of the subjects's head, echos are received form the two halves of the brain as shown in figure-8.1b. The echo produced by the midline is termed the **'M'** echo and should be symmetrically placed between the echoes received from each side of the subject's skull.

Two decades ago, A-scan of the skull was performed in diagnosing brain injuries in accidents in Neurology Clinics by noting the mid line shift. Today, it is done by CT and MRI scans very much better.

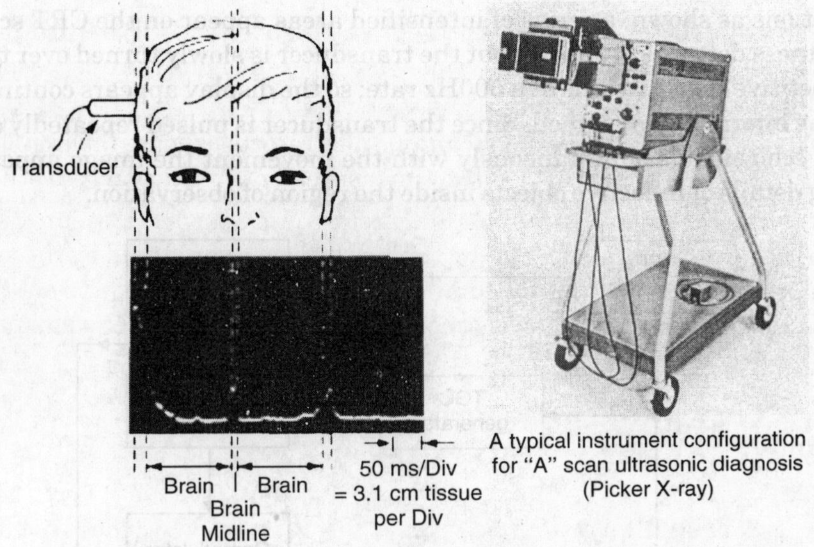

Fig. 8.1. (a) A-scan mode for finding the echo and showing a time plot.
(b) A scan of brain tumor in echo encephalography.

B-SCAN

The B-Scan ultrasound technique is one that has become a versatile diagnostic tool and has been developed over the past two decades considerably. B-scanning (brightness mode scanning) provide two dimensional cross section image of the object that is scanned. In this mode, the echo signal is connected to the Z-axis (brightness modulating cathode) of a monitor to provide intensification, while the X and Y directional signals are derived from a mechanical scanning systems. (presently electronic scanning systems are employed). This scanning system provides signals proportional to the position and direction of the probe. The resulting picture gives a two - dimensional cross sectional presentation of part of the subject. As seen in Fig. 8.2*a*, with a transducer placed in each

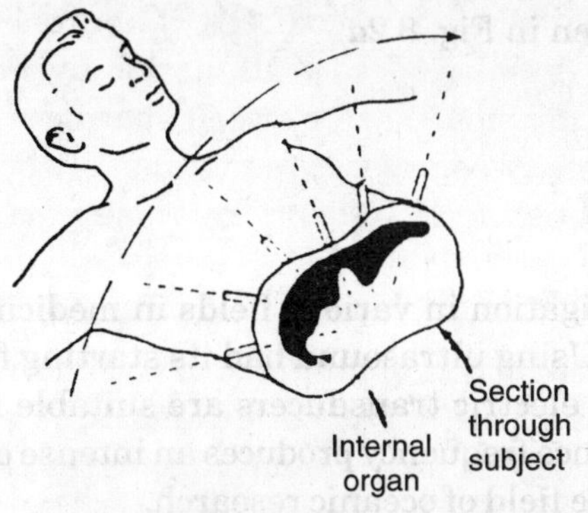

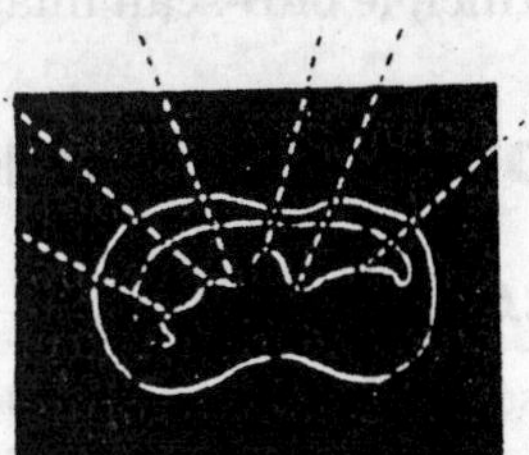

Fig. 8.2. (a) Shows the Principle of B-scan image formation. (b) Shows the block diagram of B-scanner with scan converter unit.

of the six positions as shown, a series of intensified areas appear on the CRT scan view, where only six brightness dots would appear, but the transducer is slowly turned over the object and is producing repetitive echo patterns at a 500Hz rate; so the display appears continuous instead of several dots, as informally presumed. Since the transducer is pulsed repeatedly at 500 Hz while collecting the echo signals simultaneously with the movement the image appears as a steady pattern giving details of reflective objects inside the region of observation.

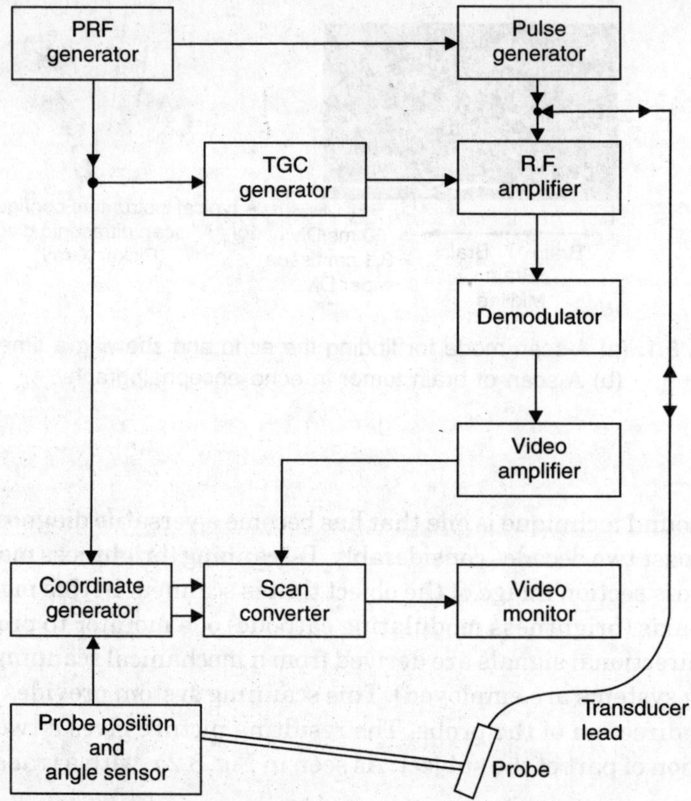

The principle of B-scan image formation is given in Fig. 8.2*a*.

ULTRASOUND SCANNING

MECHANICAL X-Y SCAN

Ultrasound has been an useful tool for investigation in various fields in medicine, non-destructive testing and also in defence applications. Using ultrasound had its starting from the year 1930 and has grown over these 70 years. Piezo electric transducers are suitable for such applications. The operation of transducer at its resonance frequency produces an intense outgoing acoustical beam. Initially this work was applied in the field of oceanic research.

Ultrasonography using the "B" mode technique is referred to as ultrasonic scanning. In this mode, the echo signal is connected to the Z -axis of a monitor to provide intensification as in the "Time-Motion" mode. However, the X and Y monitor input signals were derived from a mechanical scanning system (in early machines - today, by electronic scanning) and provide signals proportional to the position and direction of the probe to form part of a physical picture of the organs being examined. The result obtained is a two dimensional, cross- sectional presentation of part of the subject.

Generally, the same transducer is used both to send and receive the acoustic signals. An electronic pulse excites a transducer, so that a short burst of ultrasound is generated. Acoustic signals reflected from objects in the acoustic path impinge on the transducer, are converted to electronic signals and processed for display (Fig. 8.2*a*). A fundamental feature of a B-scan is that one of the dimensions is inferred from the arrival time of echoes of a short acoustic pulse as they reflect from structures along a straight line path. Signals received form structures close to the transducer arrive earlier than signals received from structures far from it. The other (transverse) dimension is obtained by moving the transducer (either physically or by mechanical means or apparently by physical means) so that, a different straight line path is continued until the entire object in the region of interest is scanned. Some means of tracking the propagation through the object is required in order to define the image. It is common practice to increase the amplifier gain for further echoes in order to partially compensate for the attenuation. This is known as time gain compensation (TGC). The position and angular direction of the ultrasound beam are determined by position monitoring. This keeps a position reference for the image signals to be displayed.

As the echoes are received by the transducer, they are amplified, rectified and filtered . The resulting signal is used to modulate the brightness of display. The early B-scan CT monitor used in conjunction with ultrasonic receiving systems was a bistable display type with a spot that was either on or off. A threshold control allowed the user to vary the value of a critical signal level above which all received echoes were shown as spots. With such a display, the resulting images were highly dependant on the threshold control and repeatability of images was difficult to achieve. In addition , since little more than contours were displayed , any interpretation of the images was subjective.

In 1976, a digital B-scan converter based on microcomputer was first developed. This System was capable of completing a single echogram in less than 15 seconds. The display had a raster density of either 80×100 or 160×200 pixels. This may be compared with the present day scanner resolution whose pixel sizes far exceed this. Today, it is common to find CRT with a grid size of 512×512 pixels and 16×32 shades of gray levels. Today's scanners, offer flicker free operation, increased reliability and also offer capabilities for image processing by gray level adjustment. Even portable types of B-scanners offer somewhat similar capabilities.

Time gain compensation is provided for the usual signals at large distances. This is a method of increasing the gain of the preamplifier with time and is set by a knob control or keypad control by the instrument user.

Additionally a threshold control enables elimination of weak signals or reflections to improve contrast or detail of the imaging. Today's machines do not employ any manual articulation of the transducer over the region in order to do the scanning. Earlier instruments ten years ago employed position encoders. Today, scanning is accomplished by two methods:

1. Linear array transducer scanning
2. Sector scanning

These two types of transducer are generally as shown in Fig. 8.3.

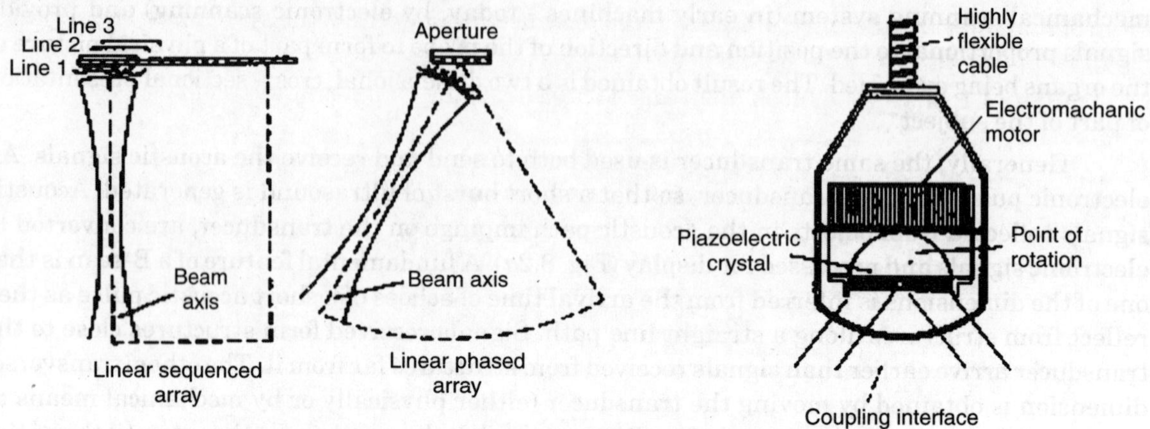

Fig. 8.3. Shows the Linear array and sector scan transducers.

The former employs an electronic method of scanning by exciting the various elements of the linear array in a phased manner so as to sweep the beam profile over the area under view. The latter has rotation (60–90°) mechanically performed inside an oil filled probe enclosure so as to vary the field of insonation and thus provide a scanning effect. Presently, the mechanical types have been almost replaced by the sonar beam-formed linear phased array transducers. Sonar beam forming is a method of adjusting the delays between adjacent lines in pulsing, so that the beam divergence is reduced.

A scan converter is the early machines was built of memory elements inside the C.R.T. The first digital scan converter was introduced by J. Ophir. Today digital signal storage and software enables fast scan conversion so as to view the image in the standard video format of 50 Hz frame sync, through actual scanning could take place at a much slower rate.

ULTRASONIC SYSTEMS

Ultrasonic energy for use in Ultrasonography is produced by exciting a piezoelectric crystal referred to as the ultrasonic transducer. These piezoelectric crystals normally have a self-resonant frequency of between 1 MHz and 10MHz; the most common types used for ultrasonography are having a self resonant frequency and produce a train of damped oscillations. Fig. 8.4*a* shows the input pulse used to excite a 2.5 MHz transducer and a reflected pulse detected by the same transducer. The amplitude of the input pulse of 200 volts with duration of 1 μ second. The transducer oscillates at 2.5 MHz, the damping factor being dependent on the transducer design and on the type of tissue in the transducer's path. As this transmitted damped oscillation reaches an interface between materials having different acoustical impedances, a reflection or echo is produced. By the time this echo has returned to the transducer, the transducer is passive and is then again excited by vibrations produced by this returning echo. This echo signal is then amplified and processed in a logarithmic amplifier and an envelope detector. This process is repeated at an approximate rate of 500 Hz. The time between the generation of the transducer exciting pulse and the detection of the received echo represents the time taken for the ultrasonic energy to travel form the transducer, to the interface, and thence from the interface back to the transducer. The velocity of sound waves, and thus of ultrasonic energy, in body tissue is about 0.125 centimeters per microsecond. It is rarely necessary to know this velocity accurately as relative interface distances are more important than actual interface distance. If these actual distances are required, the system can be calibrated against a known tissue interface distance.

Plate I.1. shows the block diagram of the Ultrasonic Diagnostic system.

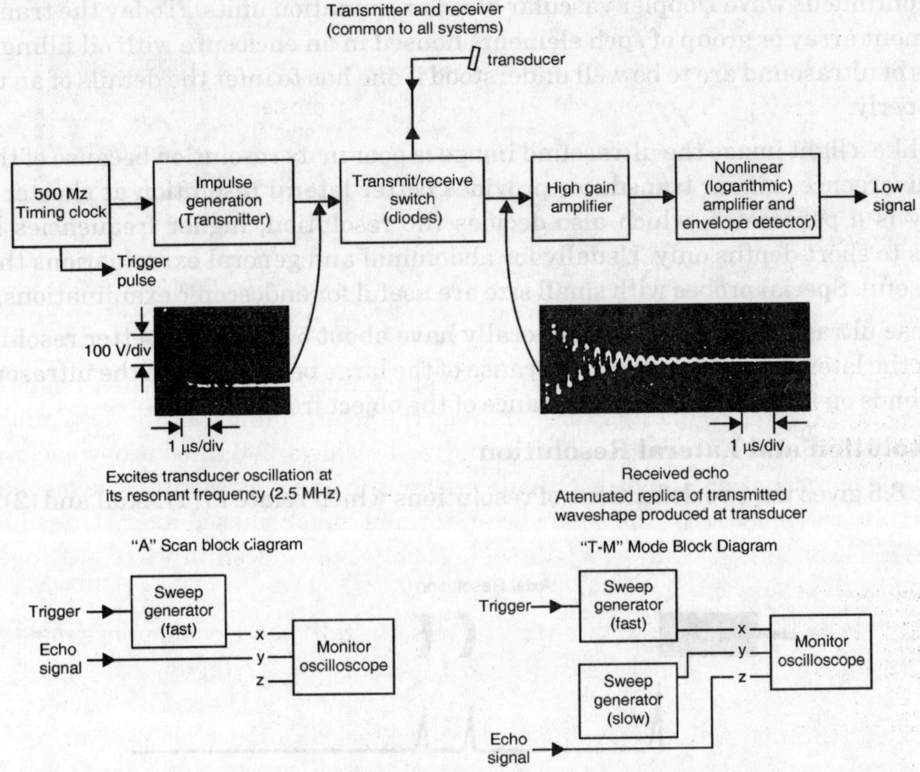

Fig. 8.4. Echo signal generation and block diagrams (T-M Mode and A-S Can)

Plate I.2. shows the usual spectrogram display for a material valve insonation. The curves are drawn by operator to evaluate pressure halftime and thence valve area.

DEPTH VERSUS RESOLUTION

Depth and resolution of the system depend on the crystal's resonant frequency. A 1 MHz crystal provides low resolution; however, reflections can be detected for tissue 50 centimeters from the transducer. The commonly used 2.5 MHz crystal can be used to at least 20 cm; whereas a 10 MHz crystal provides excellent resolution, however, it can not be used above about 5 cm. Relating distance to velocity, a tissue interface 5cm from the transducer will produce a reflection 80 μs after the impulse.

TRANSDUCER TISSUE-COUPLING

It is important that the transducer be firmly held against the tissue (skin) as any air in the transducer's path will severely attenuate the ultrasonic energy. A sufficient transducer/tissue coupling is more important and this can be assured by using a liquid coupler such as water. In certain ultrasonic scanning systems it is impossible to locate the transducer against the tissue and a substantial depth of water is used as a coupling medium.

PROBES FOR ULTRASOUND

A simple probe which has transmitter and receiver as separate parts as two semicircular discs was common in the early day ultrasound Doppler investigations. (This is even today in use in portable continuous wave Doppler vascular blood examination units). Today the transducer is a multi element array or group of such elements housed in an enclosure with oil filling. The basic properties of ultrasound are to be well understood if one has to infer the details of an ultrasound image properly.

Unlike a light image the ultrasound image is poor in its resolution because of the problem of beam divergence. Linear transducer provides better lateral resolution at shorter distances. Frequency is a parameter, which also decides the resolution, higher frequencies limit their usefulness to short depths only. Usually for abdominal and general examinations the 3.5 MHz probe is useful. Special probes with small size are useful for endoscopic examinations.

These ultrasound transducers generally have about 5 to 6 times better resolution in the axial than the lateral direction, mainly because of the large beam width in the ultrasound. Beam width depends on focusing as well as distance of the object from it.

Axial Resolution and Lateral Resolution

Fig. 8.5 gives the two definitions of resolutions which relate to (1) Axial and (2) Lateral as shown.

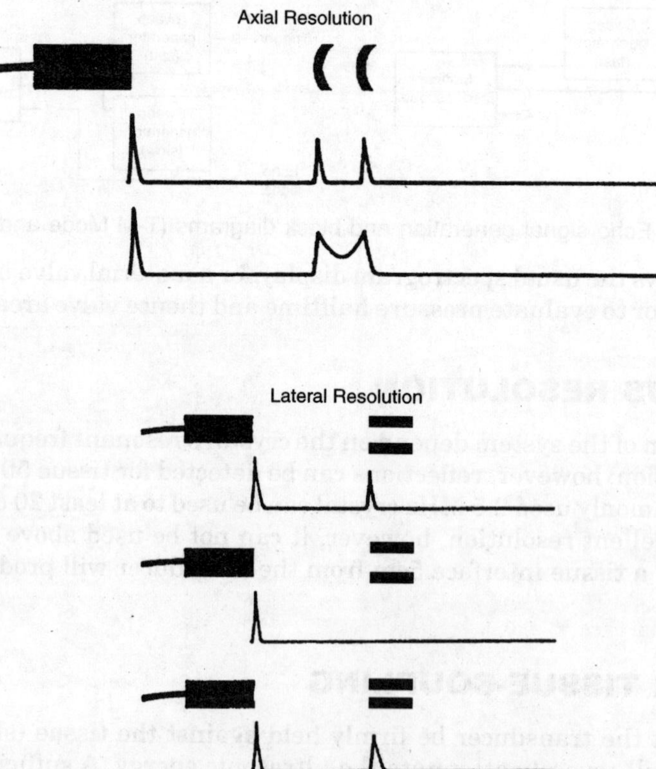

Fig. 8.5. Shows the two definitions of resolution which relate to (1) Axial and (2) Lateral as shown.

Fine transducer elements of small width can provide a good lateral resolution but still this resolution *ratio* is not altered anyway. So all images in Ultrasound have very poor lateral resolution and even today the instruments costing several tens of lakhs do not have any improvement in this part incorporated into them because this is a basic problem of ultrasound imaging.

As the AED (active aperture diameter) increases, beam width increases but width of the beam and also the region or zone of maximum sensitivity, allowing the transducer to the optimized for an application. Fig. 8.6 shows the Schematic illustration of an ultrasonic field, divided into three zones.

By a curved surface the focusing improves, so a facing material has to be applied to make it flat for contacting (Fig. 8.7*a*). Different foci can be had by changing the diameter (Fig. 8.7*b*). Further to this, multiple matching layers can also be considered.

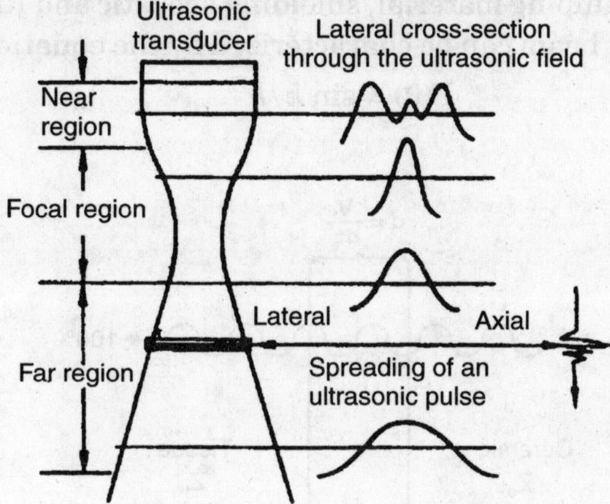

Fig. 8.6. Shows the Schematic illustration of an ultrasonic field, divided into three zones.

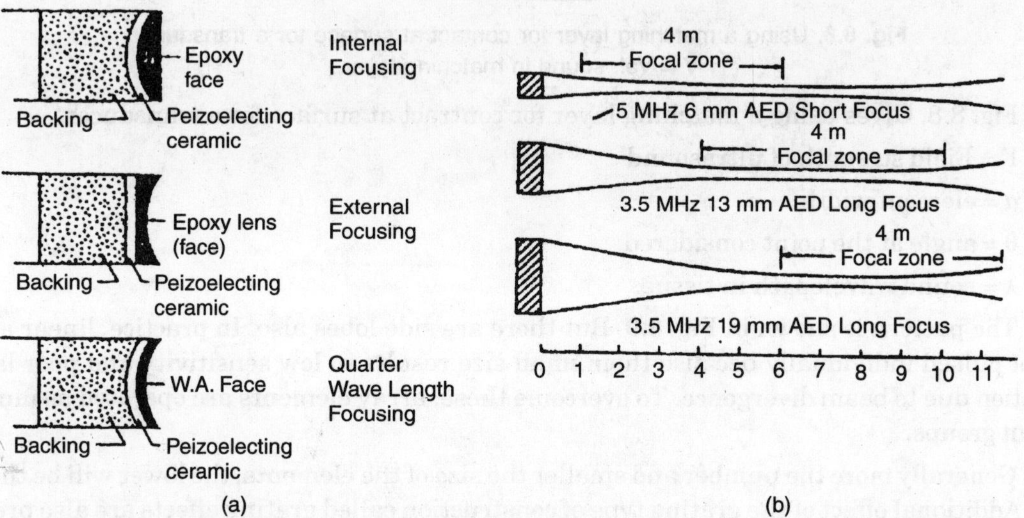

Fig. 8.7. (a) showing a curvature of transducer surface, (b) Different foci obtainable.

When a ceramic element with an acoustic impedance of 30 is kept in contact with body tissue having a similar impedance of 1.6, there is so much mismatch that result in considerable loss of energy and hence a weak signal results; this is improved by attaching a matching impedance layer of quarter wavelength (λ/4) for increased transmission at the interface. Such a material, usually a plastic, is chosen at the interface in the construction (Fig. 8.8).

Controlled focal characteristics can be obtained by using multiple matching layers also in a graded layer.

LINEAR ARRAY TRANSDUCER

Today most of the advanced ultrasound machines use a linear array or convex array transducer. Such an array comprises of several closely spaced rectangular elements arranged side by side along with inter-element damping material, shielding acoustic and RF focusing lens and plastic housing. If a single element beam can be characterized by the equation.

$$F(\theta) = \sin k / k$$

where $k = \pi a \sin \theta/\lambda$

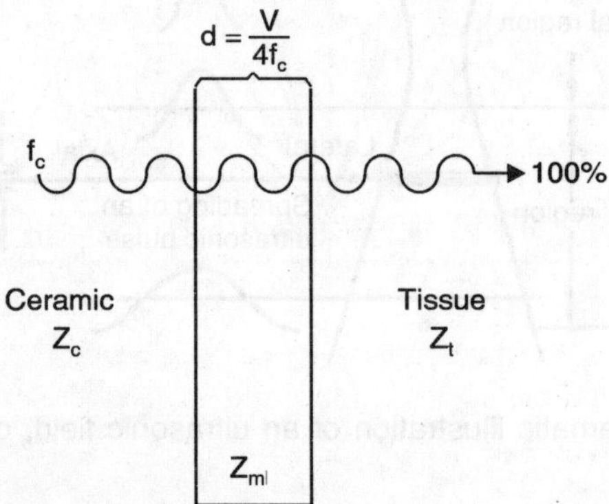

Fig. 8.8. Using a matching layer for contact at surface for a transducer. V = Vel. sound in matching layer.

Fig. 8.8. Gives using a matching layer for contract at surface for a transducer.

F = Field strength of ultrasound

a = element width

θ = angle at the point considered

λ = sound wavelength in tissue.

The pattern is shown in Fig. 8.9. But there are side lobes also. In practice, linear arrays are not pulsed individually because their small size results in low sensitivity and poor lateral resolution due to beam divergence. To overcome these, array elements are operated as multiple element groups.

Generally more the number and smaller the size of the elements, the lower will be the side lobes. Additional effect of the grating type of construction called grating effects are also present, (Fig. 8.9a) which is reduced by subdicing (Fig. 8.9b).

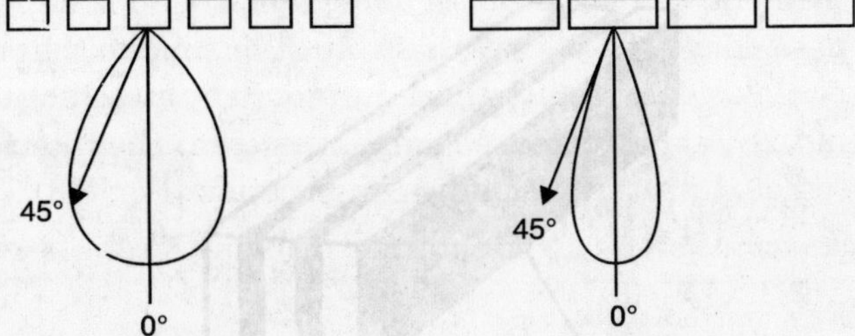

Fig. 8.9a. Shows the effect of width-size over the main lobe of radiation.

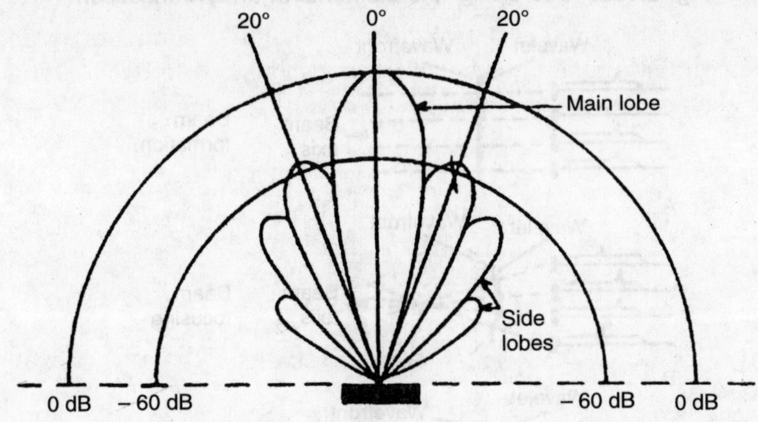

Fig. 8.9b. Shows the two-dimensional shape of the ultrasound signal showing main lobe and side lobes.

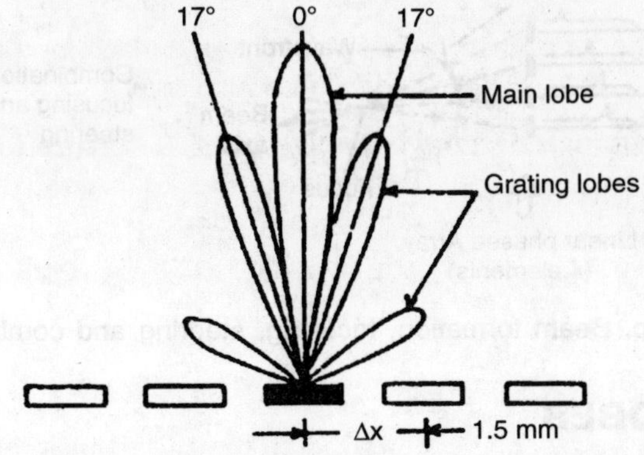

Fig. 8.10a. Locating grating lobes of greater angles reduces artefacts (ΔX is chosen).

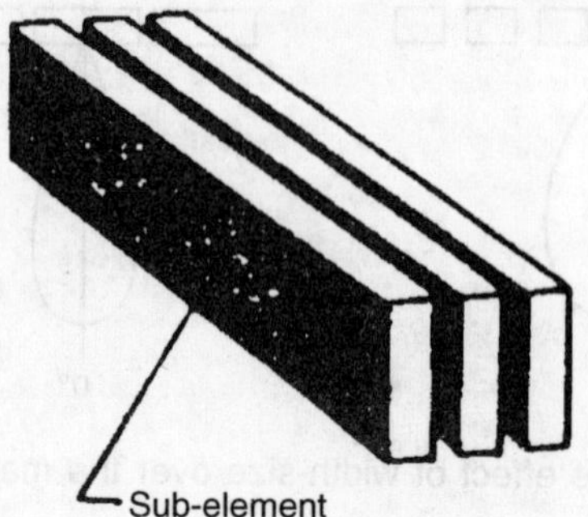

Fig. 8.10b. "Sub-dicing" the elements of array transducer.

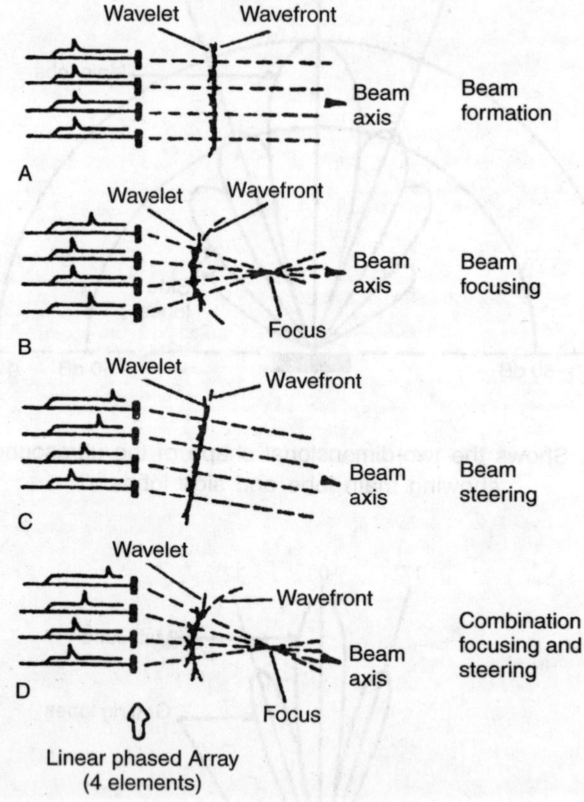

Fig. 8.10c. Beam formation, focusing, steering and combination.

SECTOR SCAN PROBES

In a linear array the drawback lies in its size. It needs a very big acoustic window. It is not always possible to provide such window for all organs. In order to scan for a larger field of view with a small window the sector scan transducer is preferable.

Three types are there:

1. Mechanical type
2. Electronic phased array
3. Radial Array

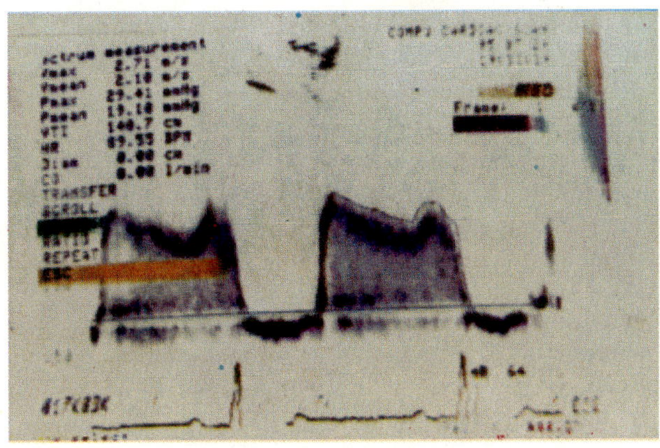

Plate I.1. Showing the Doppler Spectrogram of a region near mitral valve, showing the blood velocities with time. The profile of this is used to find the drop in pressure half-time and thereby evaluate the valve area.

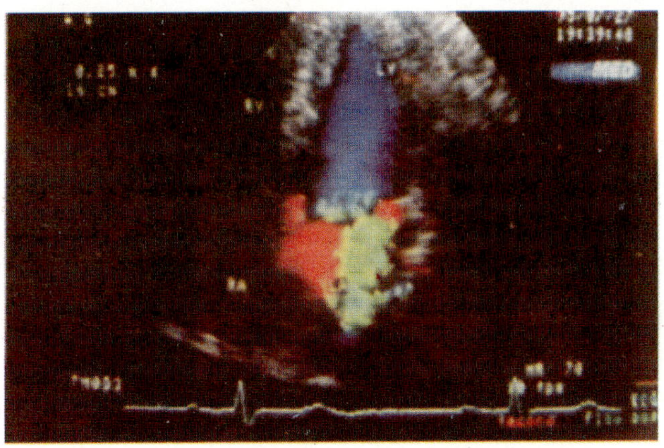

Plate I.2. Shows the scan near mitral valve, but the Doppler scan region is a smaller angle in the middle of the sector. The velocities are modulated as colours in the picture. Red shows one dircetion, blue another and those blood jets which have mixed velocities are shown in green.

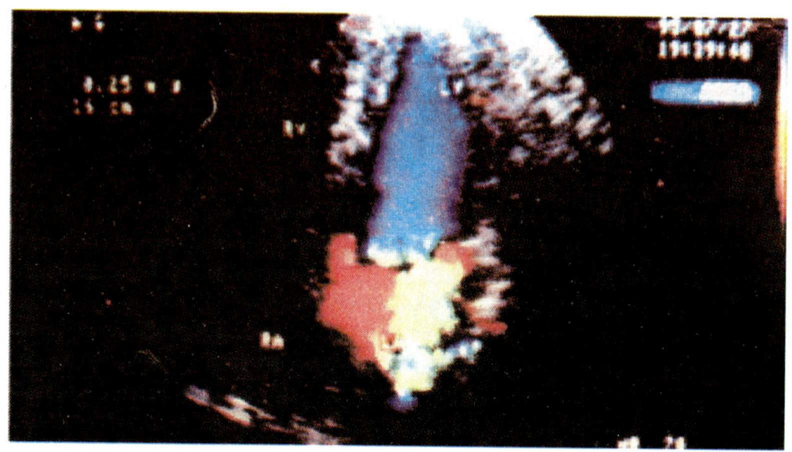

(a) Image B scan superposed with Doppler based colour view showing velocities of blood.

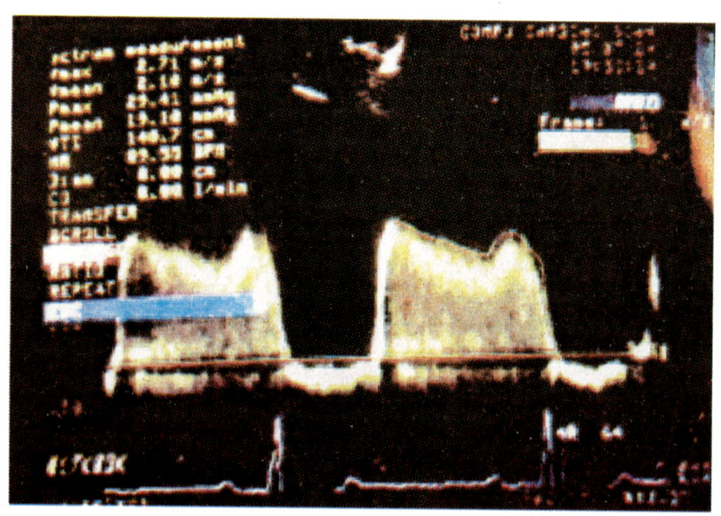

(b) Spectrogram plot on top. X-axis = time, Y-axis = frequency, + Y-axis is forward flow, – Y-axis is reverse flow. ECG waveform is shown below. Note the image view as a small region on top middle of screen.

Plate I.3

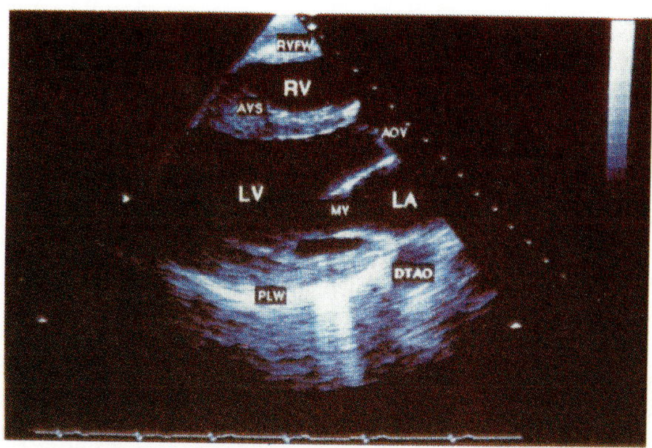

Plate I.4. Left parasternal long axis plane. AOV = aortic valve. AVS = anterior ventricular septrum. DTAO descending thoracic aorta ; LA = left atrium ; LV = left ventricle ; MV = mitral valve ; PLW = posterolateral wall ; RV = right ventricle ; RVFW = right ventricular free wall.

LONG AXIS M/Q 4 CHAMBER

Plate I.5. This study is from a patient with severe obstructive hypertrophic cardiomyopathy and severe mitral regurgitation (MR), some of which was independent of obstruction. *A*, Parasternal long-axis view showing turbulent left ventricular (LV) outflow tract jet and severe mitral regurgitation directed toward the posterior left atrial (LA) wall. *B*, Color M-mode study taken from apical four-chamber view with color M-mode line highlighted by white arrow in *C*. Flow toward transducer is shown in red and flow away in blue. Depth at which flow velocity is shown on M-mode corresponds to its position on simultaneous four-chamber view in *C*. Systolic flow at the midventricular level is homogeneously blue and thus laminar. As flow approaches the area of obstruction at the site of systolic anterior motion septal contact aliasing to red occurs over depth of about 1 cm. The obstructed area of the outflow tract then has a mosaic pattern indicative of turbulent flow within it. Systolic timing of events can be made with comparison to the electrocardiogram. In very early systole there is a narrow band of blue flow with brief aliasing to red followed by turbulent flow, indicating early development of turbulent flow, which was timed with onset of systolic anterior motion. AO = aortic root. IVS = Interventricular septum; LA = left atrium; LV = left ventricle; MV = mitral valve; PW = posterior wall. (From Rakowski H, Sasson Z, Wigle ED: Echocardiographic and Doppler assessment of hypertrophic cardiomyopathy. *J Am Soc Echocardiogr* 1:32–47, 1988.)

In the mechanical type, an array consists of three or four transducers. All of them are fitted on the edge of a wheel. The array is mechanically rotated by a motor. This motor is activated electrically or magnetically in an isolated condition. The whole array set up is immersed in an oil bath container for achieving high speed with low friction. The oil-bath container has a thin plastic material, which is placed on its surface where the cross-sectional image is need. Each one of the transducers is activated while it comes near the window. The transducer of different focal length can be placed in the sector- scan assembly for acquiring a clear image at different depths. But in these mechanical types dynamic focusing is not feasible.

Further there is a degradation in quality during the routine clinical use. Since the transducer is in motion while sending and receiving the signals there is a certain amount of uncertainty in the direction of the ultrasound signals.

In the phased array type of sector-scan transducer, the moving part of transducer system is eliminated. It is very light in weight and easy to handle. The strip of elements of this transducer are wired up like the linear array transducer and they are activated electronically to achieve the direction of the propagation of the ultrasound signals. The time of delay determines the direction of the signal and it can be achieved accurately. The dynamics of focusing for transmission and reception is performed without any problems (Fig. 8.10*c*). This is done by DSP and is called sonar beam forming.

Phased arrays are capable of electronic beam formation beam focusing, beam steering and any combination of these allowing dynamic focusing and steering (Fig. 8.10)

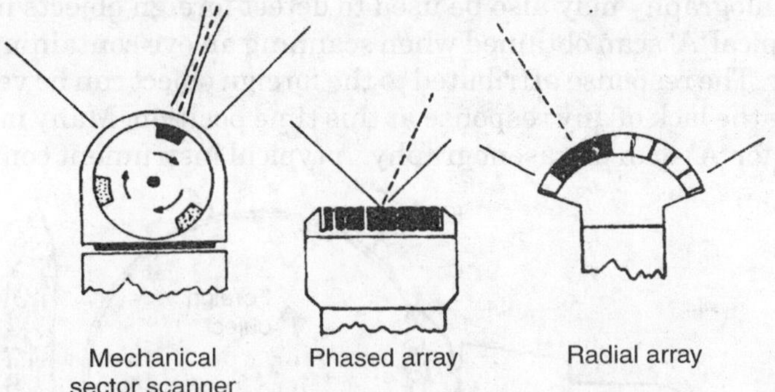

Fig. 8.11. Shows the different type of sector-scan transducers.

The problem with electronic phased array is the long delay times involved to trigger the transducer elements, while directing away the signal from the center of the field of view. This causes the image degradation like refraction errors due to the tissue inhomogeneity. In these types of arrays, grating lobe produces the degradation. The direction of such grating lobes is designed to be at a large angle. The transducer elements are all triggered at first time. If the direction of propagation has a small angle with the face of the transducer, then the grating lobe would be steered towards the face of the transducer itself.

The radial array is an array of elements serially arranged along predefined arc with a specific radius of curvature. It has been incorporated with the important features of linear array without sacrificing access or beam steering and dynamic focusing. It has no moving parts or liquid medium. Due to the curved nature, only one group of transducer elements are triggered for a particular angle. So there is no long delay time and the grating lobe remains to be at the fixed angle with respect to the main lobe.

The effective aperture of a phased array transducer decrease is 70% at 45° scanning. This decrease does not occur with this radial array, since the face of the array slowly changes direction and also faces the direction of ultrasound beam.

The most obvious advantage of the radial array is to achieve dynamic focusing which is not possible with the mechanical scanner in addition to its reliability for want of moving parts (Fig. 8.12)

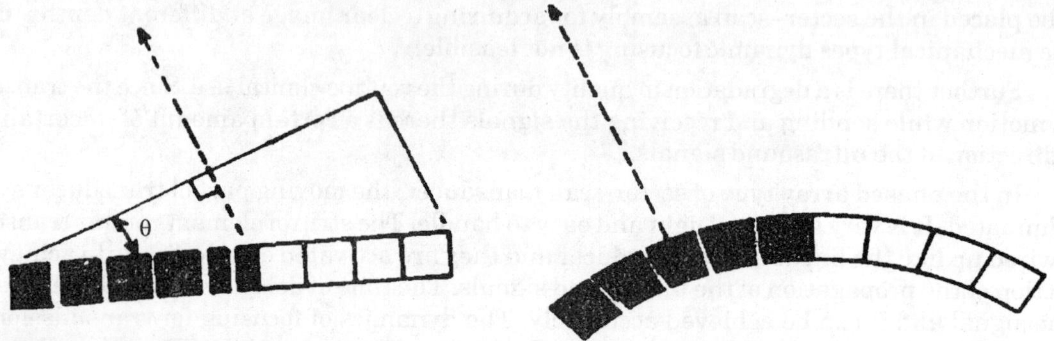

Fig. 8.12. Shows the effective aperture of the phased and radial array with increasing scan angle.

FOREIGN OBJECT DETECTION USING ULTRASOUND

'A' scan echoencephalography may also be used to detect foreign objects imbedded in a subject. Fig. 8.13 shows a typical **'A'** scan obtained when scanning an eye containing a foreign object with a 10MHz transducer. The response attributed to the foreign object can be verified by scanning the other eye and noting the lack of any response at this time position. Many manufacturers produce equipment suitable for **'A'** scan ultrasonography. A typical instrument configuration is shown in

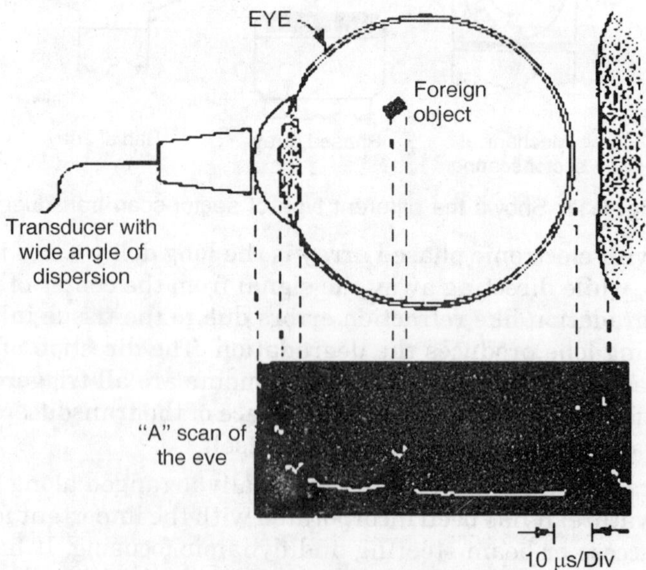

Fig. 8.13a. Shows "A" scan detection of a foreign object.

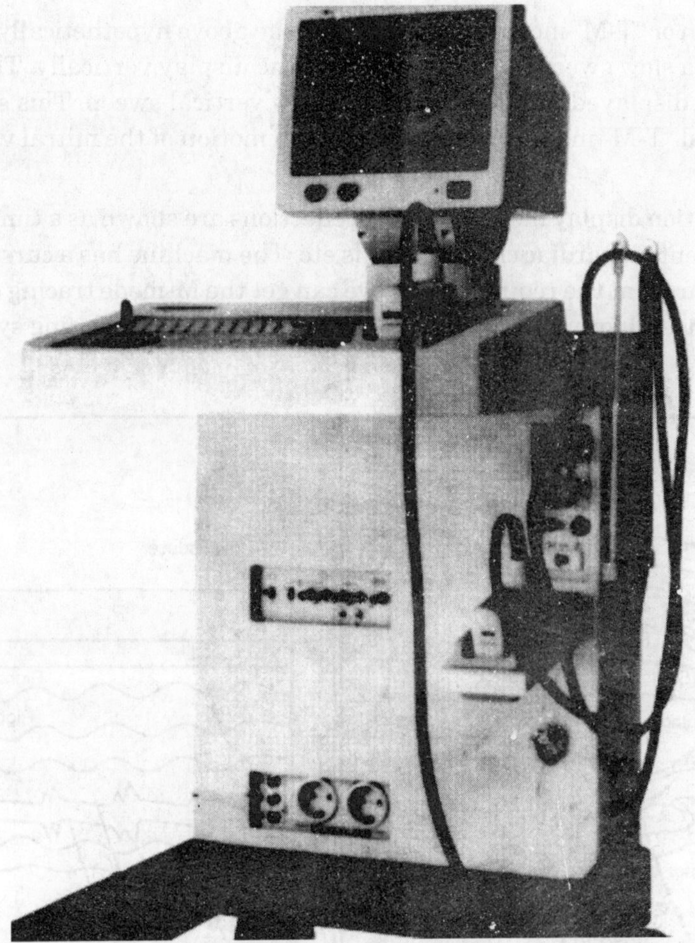

Fig. 8.13b. Showing a typical ultrasound scanner machine.

Fig. 8.13*a*; a Tektronix type 561B or 564B oscilloscope is used with a Tektronix type 2B67 time-base unit and a special vertical plug in unit, designed for echoencephalography, produced by the Picker- X-Ray corporation. Suitable probes are also produced by the Picker X-ray corporation. The complete instrument may be used in conjunction with w Tektronix scope-mobile® cart and Tektronix trace-recording camera.

TIME-MOTION (T-M) MODE ULTRASONAGRAPHY

Considering "A" ulrasonography as discussed earlier, if an interface producing an echo was moving in relation to the transducers, the response obtained in the CRT would also move horizontally relative to the beginning of the sweep. If this "A" scan system was to be modified slightly by removing the echo signal from the vertical channel (Y) and connecting it to the identifying channel(Z), am echo response would then appear as an intensified spot on the screen. Any motion in this echo response would appear as a horizontal motion of this spot between successive sweeps of the horizontal sweep generator. No vertical signal would be involved.

In time-motion or "T-M" mode ultrsonography, the above hypothetically modified " A" scan system is used with a slow sweep generator, moving the display vertically. Thus, any motion in the echo response is displayed in real time by the slow vertical sweep. This system is shown in Fig. 8.3, and a typical "T-M" mode ultrasonogram from motion of the mitral valve of the heart is shown below.

This is the motion display mode. Here the reflections are shown as a time course indicating for instance, movements of cardiac chamber walls etc. The machine has a cursor called M-cursor. By positioning the cursor at the required point we can get the M-mode tracing of the heart at that point. This mode is useful for measurement of chamber dimensions during systole and diastole. (Fig. 8.14)

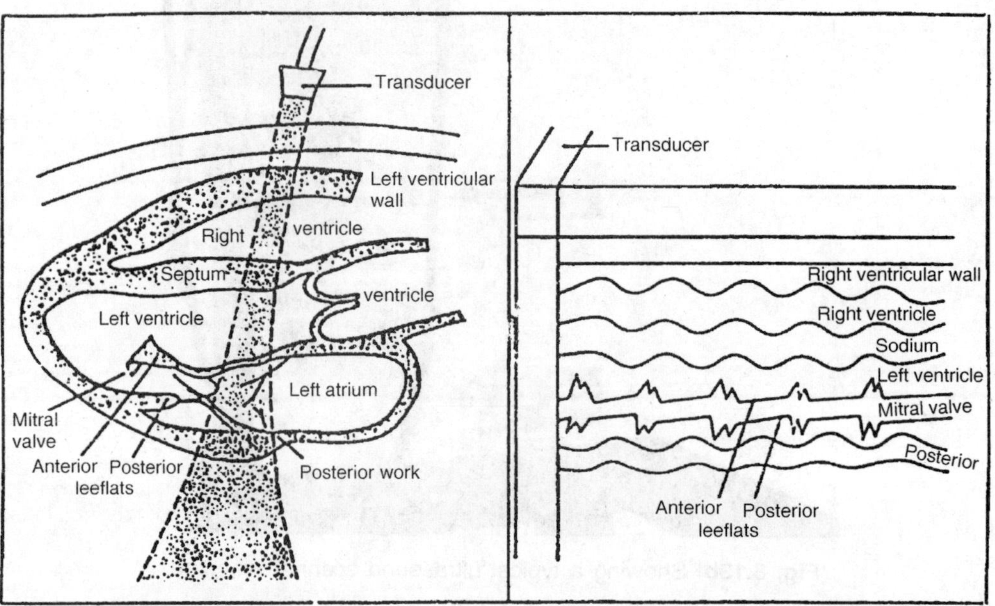

Fig. 8.14. M-mode echo cardiograph (a) shows heart chamber and insonation direction (b) shows the Motion mode display.

ULTRASOUND IN CARDIOGRAPHY

Referring to Fig. 8.15, the motion of the mitral valve is clearly shown on the vertically-swept trace on the screen of the CRT. Fig. 8.15, also shows that the motion of the walls of the heart, however echos from other interfaces in the transducer's path have been gated out in this instance. This particular application, known as "T-M" mode cardiography is particularly valuable in the detection of mitral stenosis. Since the actual movement of the mitral valve is shown in centimeters in real time (vertical sweep), the velocity of movement of this valve can be determined from the slope of the trace obtained. In the example shown in Fig. 8.15, the maximum velocity of the mitral valve is 16 centimeters per second, the overall movement of the valve is 2.2 centimeters and the heart rate is 86 beats per minute.

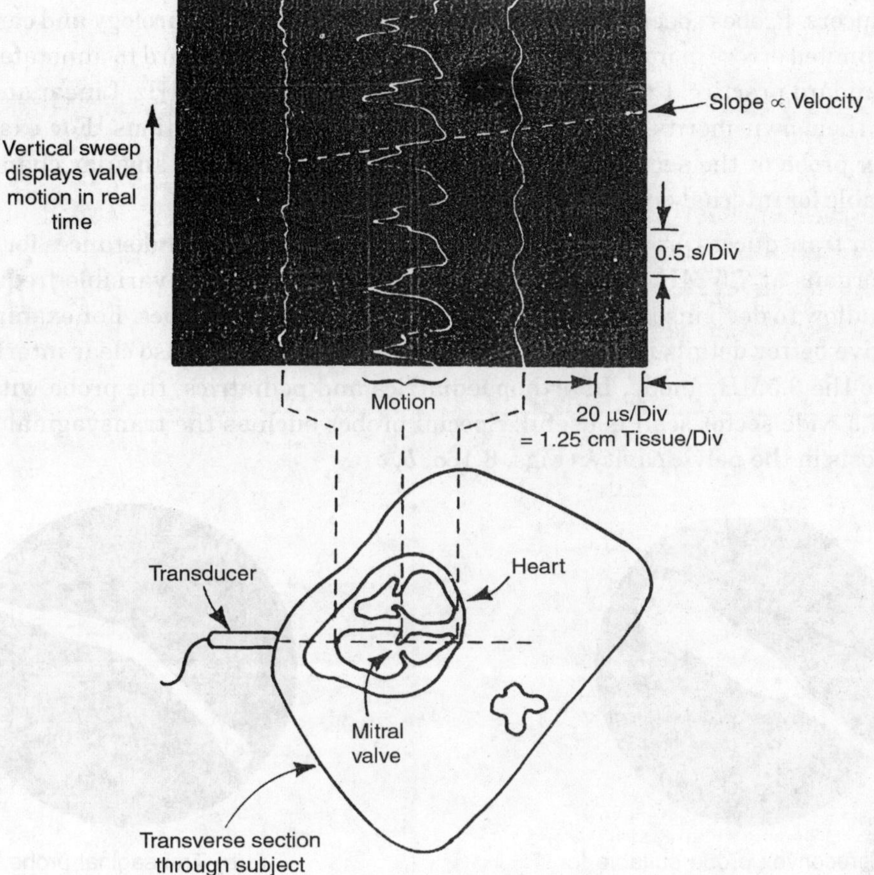

Fig. 8.15. Shows a typical "T-M" mode ultrasonogram from motion of the mitral valve of the heart.

SIGNAL PROCESSING

The generation of pulse signals and the gating of preamplifier to detect the echoes after the pulse are done with a microprocessor in the ultrasound machines.

In a plain ultrasound machine the signal processing comprises of the various filters, time gain compensation of signals for deep weak echoes and the storage of data in memory. The scan converter converts the data into the standard CCIR video signal which is given to the instrument monitor is also output for recording in VCR.

RECENT DEVELOPMENTS IN ULTRASOUND MACHNIES

The recent B-scan machines available from USA, Germany and U.K., give a blend of technology employing the latest microprocessors in signal processing hardware as well as transducers. Most of these latest machines provide a number of features that facilitate every day work and present view very clearly and visibly. Physicians are looking for machines having both linear and sector scan transducers. Probes specially made of Gynaecology / obstetrics, urology and cardiology have further eliminated errors in images considerably. Facility with keyboard to annotate an image for record is standard practice. Frequencies employed vary from 2 to 7 MHz. Linear and sector scan units have their own merits and demerits for their own examinations. For example, a fine microconvex probe of the sector type (Fig. 8.16*a*) with an internal angular change of 110° is ideally suitable for internal organs viewed between small costae.

Linear transducers provide better lateral resolution for shorter distances for examination of shallow organs at 7.5 MHz . Most of the present machines have variable frequency probes enabling shallow to deep insonation, even without changing the probes. For example, the same probe can give better details in the near distances at 7.5 MHz and also clear interior details by switching to the 3.5MHz mode. In orthopaediatrics and pediatrics, the probe with a high frequency and a wide sector scan is useful. Special probes such as the transvaginal probe allows clear diagnosis in the pelvic cavity. (Figs. 8.16*a, b, c*)

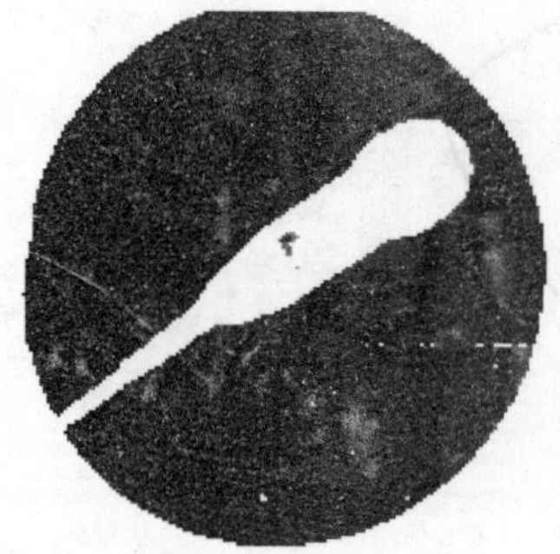

(a) Microconvex probe suitable for observation through narrow electronic scanning is most suited for organs located.

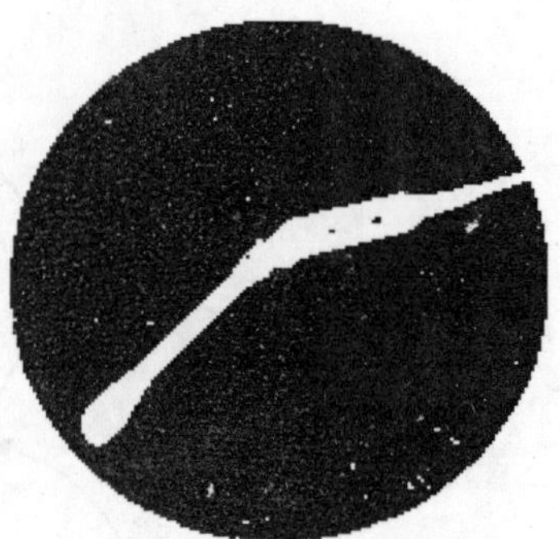

(b) Transaginal probe.

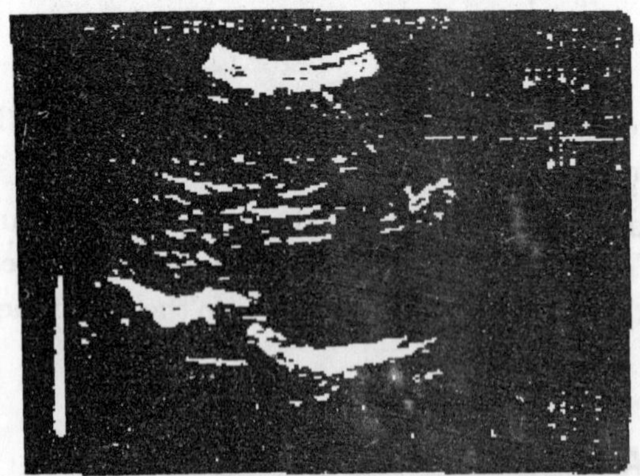

(c) Gestational week measurement.

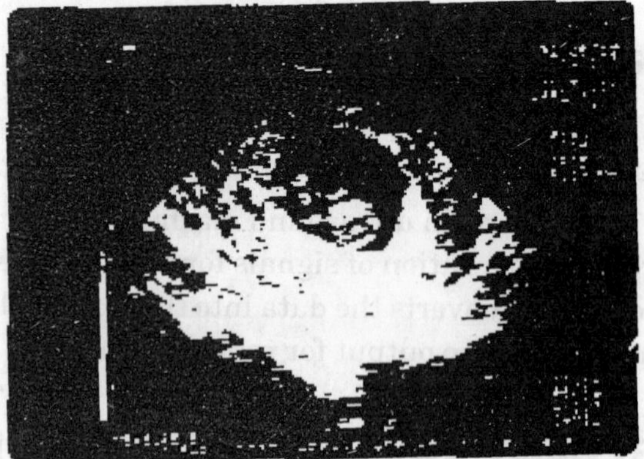

(d) Image of large ovarian cystoma.

Fig. 8.16

Display technology on CRT using high persistence phosphors have made possible high resolution pictures on small tubes. The microprocessor is used for transducer control, grey level adjustment, scan conversion, display of legends and storage of images in digital memory. Provision for multiple views (Fig. 8.17) in the two dimensional planes (transverse and sagittal) in one screen enables easy assessment of volume information. Additionally, some instruments provide for the measurement of length , area and volume (as in Fig. 8.15) by suitable built-in programs. The accuracy of such measurements depends on markings made by the doctor on the screen in-situ with the cursor facility provided. As the poor lateral resolution of plain B-scan images do not ordinarily permit directly visible clear outline of organs, inferences of pathology depend on the clinical acumen of doctor or sonologist. These measurements would vary with actual sizes, to an extant of 50%.

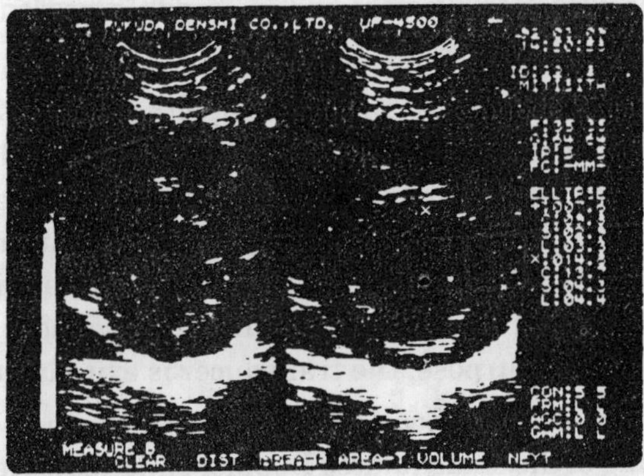

Fig. 8.17. Shows the dual image in B-mode to obtain areas of mitral valve in systole and diastole.

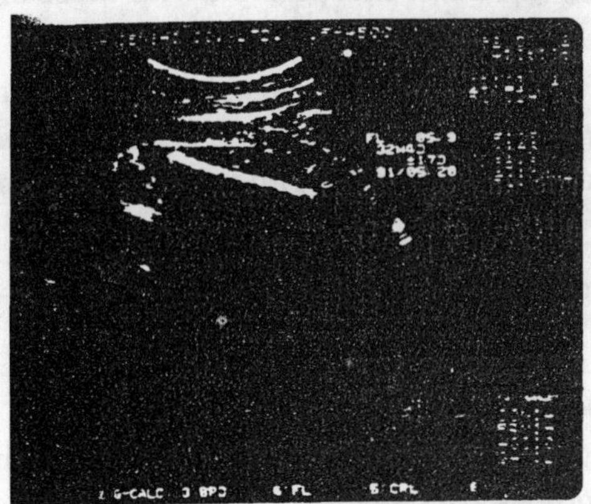

(a) Measurement of femur length

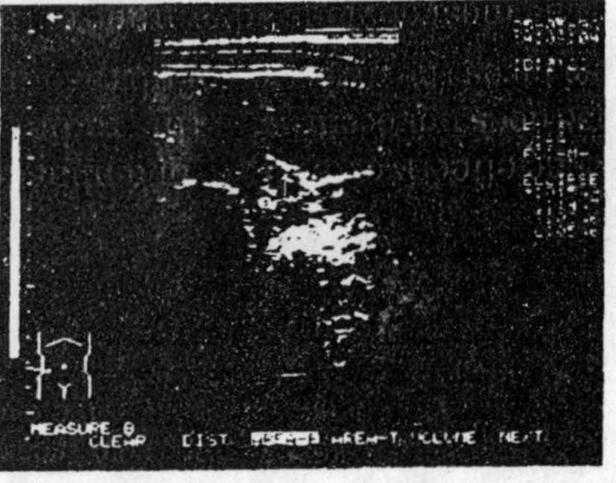

(b) Area/Circumference measurement

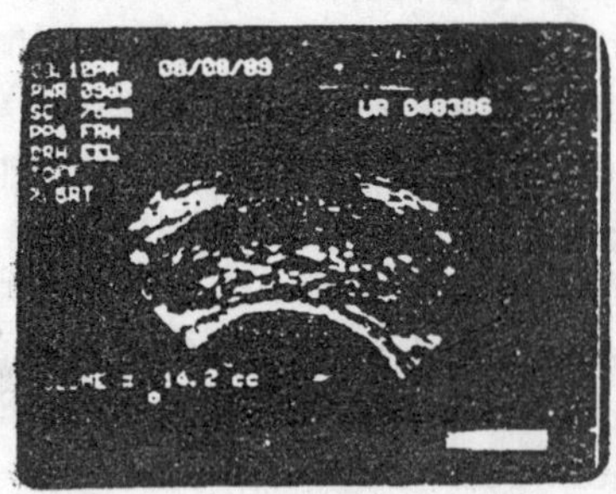

(c) Prostate gland showing volume measurement

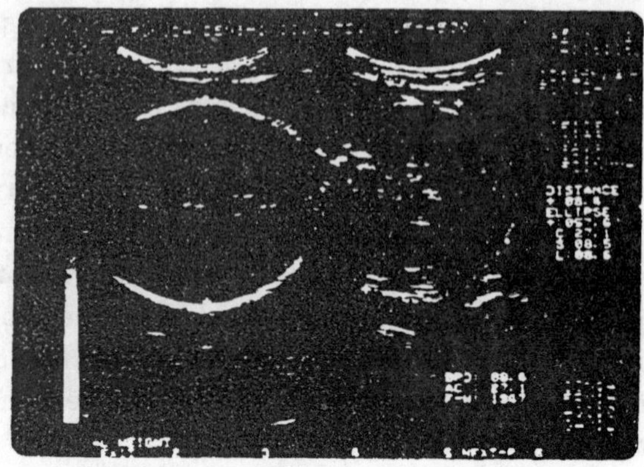

(d) Estimation of weight of fetus

Most instruments have provision for recording the screen video in a video cassette recorder (VCR). Optionally an electrocardiography(ECG) amplifier with provision of ECG display is available. The machines used for echo-cardiography provide Doppler spectra display also on the screen. Such Doppler probes are dual frequency type which enable a Doppler-shift of the signals at a particular point in the image to be recorded. As the sector- transducer scans its path, say 90° or 110°, the Doppler transducer is activated on a chosen line and the data is picked at a specific time-of flight, so that a limited region in the scanned transverse section. The flow of blood via the cardiac valve is covered. For this purpose, the transducer is exited with a pulse burst.

Every scan repeats this process. Scan occurs every fifteenth of a second repetitively. The Fourier Transform processing of the demodulated Doppler shift audio frequency signal is displayed as a real time spectrogram on the same screen which shows the B-scan also in real time. The use of high speed digital signal processing hardware only has made this possible with these high end class ultrasonic scanner machines.

The Zooming function in the region of interest have been provided by latest ultrasound machines, gives an effective diagnosis of early pregnancy and examination of the fetal heart as discussed earlier. Present day instruments have better magnification and clarity as given by:

1. Optimized line and pixel densities
2. Increased resolution by electronic focusing with linear arrays.
3. Increased frame rates with fast scanning
4. Increased image size with better cathode ray tubes.

In surgery, the positional accuracy and clarity of B-scan images render a proper application of puncture and biopsy needles possible. Moreover, probes are specifically designed for endoscopic applications as well. The forceps position can be monitored during surgery by real time B-scan views and the same can be steered to move it in the right direction.

ULTRASONOGRAPHIC APPLICATIONS

Fig. 8.18 shows a typical "B" mode displays obtained with a compound scanning system. These displays are self-explanatory and indicate some of the potential advantages of ultrsonography.

Neither of the three displays shown could have been obtained by conventional X-ray techniques as; for the fetus in vitro, fetal development is impaired by X-ray energy; for the breast cyst, such cyst tissue is not X-ray specific for the scan of the eye, resolution with X-ray techniques cannot be obtained if the X-ray plate cannot be located directly behind the region concerned.

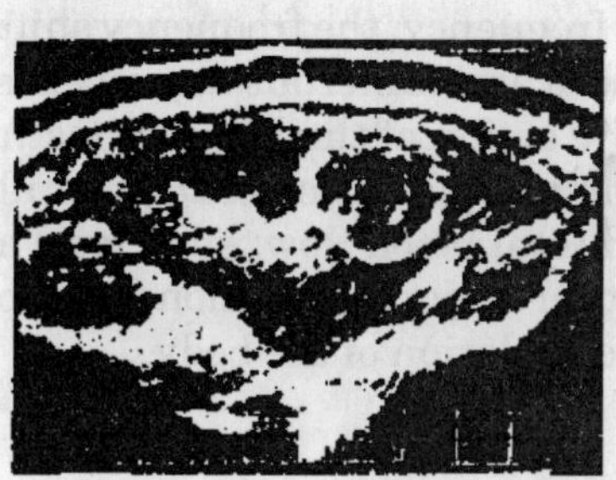

Position of Fetus in Utero

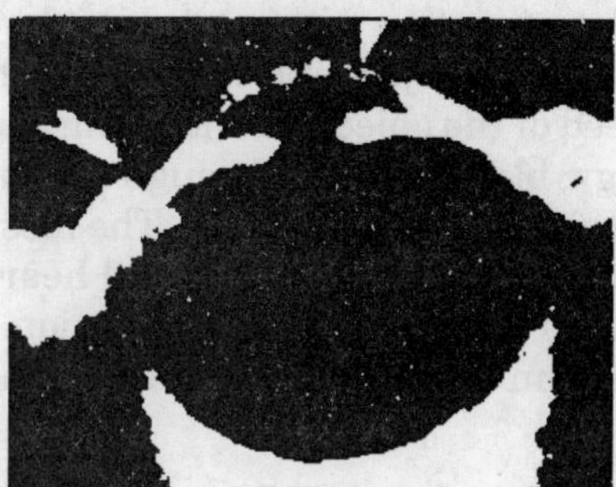

Corneal Thickness Determination

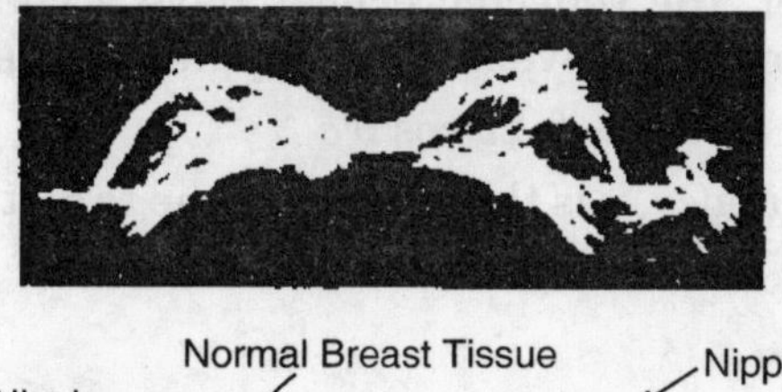

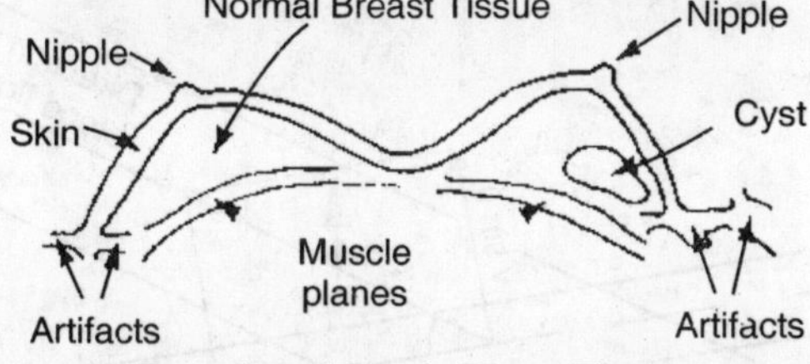

Detection of Cyst in Breast Tissue

Fig. 8.18. Shows typical "B" mode display from a compound scanning system.

PART-II

DOPPLER ULTRASOUND

Continuous ultrasonic energy, rather than bursts of ultrasonic energy is used in ultrasonography. This is used to detect motion within a subject by the Doppler principle. When ultrasonic energy is reflected from a moving object, it is shifted slightly in frequency, the frequency shift being proportional to the speed of the object. In the living body there are numerous movements which reflect ultrasonic energy; blood flowing through arteries, the action of the heart, intestinal movement and passage of urine and gastric juices. The most common application of Doppler ultrasonics is in obstetrics to detect movement of the fetal heart and fetal blood flow; such fetal activity can be detected as early as the tenth week of gestation. Another major application for Doppler ultrasonics is in the detection of blood flow in the peripheral circulation of the body.

DOPPLER SIGNALS FROM PROBE

Today's machines have built-up Doppler processing of the echo signals. When an ultrasound signal strikes a moving target, the reflected echoes have a change of frequency (or Phase) corresponding the motion of the target given by the Doppler frequency shift.

$$f_D = f_0 \, 2v \cos \theta / c \qquad \ldots(1)$$

where f_0 is the ultrasound frequency, v is the velocity of the target and q the inclination and c is the tissue sound velocity (usw. 1540 m/s) (Fig. 8.19)

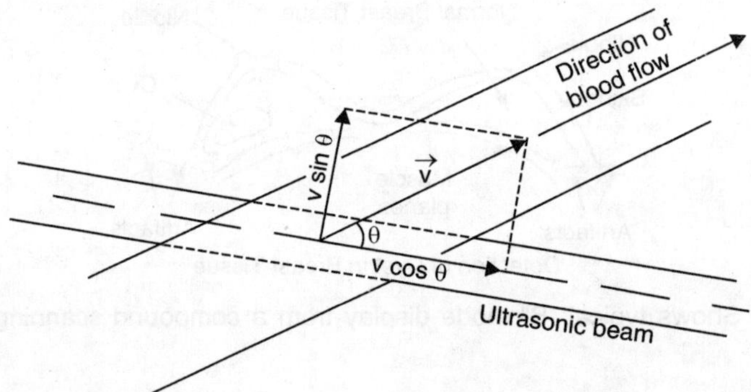

Fig. 8.19. Shows doppler relation for ultrasound signal in a blood vessel.

While scanning takes place over a region by the linear or sector transducer, typical paths of the beam could be chosen to process the Doppler sampled volume inside the region. The velocity information in that region can be processed by using the shift of frequency and plotting the spectrogram. The received signal generally comprises of reflections from blood vessels, walls and signal from the blood flow in arteries. The former two are low frequency shifts, while the latter, attributed to Raleigh scattering of the beam by the moving particles of blood, is of a higher frequency varying from 2 to 16 KHz depending on the nature of blood flow, laminar or turbulent or jet.

Echo cardiography analyses the pathology of valves and their narrowness in diseased or abnormal conditions by noting the velocity patterns during the systole and diastole in the heart beat cycle, which is usually accompanied with ECG waveform display also. Plate I.3*b* shows the usual spectrogram display given by a machine of a region of insonation under the mitral valve flow, giving forward high velocity flow patterns due to a narrowed (stenosed) valve. In some other pathologies there may be regurgitation also observable (negative frequencies), which would show high velocities in the spectrogram during the period when the valve closes. Plate 1.3*b* shows a colour Doppler view of the ventricular jet of blood flow.

Doppler attachment in many machines provides additional circuits. The choice of sample volume for which the Doppler signals are collected is related to the scan time course. Hence, it is possible to pick up the pulse echoes during that scan angle and do the processing. Note that in Plate I.3*a*, the Doppler angle is less than the sector scan angle.

Doppler processing is done usually with DSP hardware. Chirp-Z transform is performed using dedicated integrated circuits on the signals after demodulation. The RF demodulators separate the two components of the signals using phase sensitive demodulators using typical high frequency integrated circuits meant for the purpose. These two I and Q signals are in the audio frequency range and they can then be processed for the evaluation of the Complex Fourier Transform (Fig. 8.20). (Phase quadrature outputs)

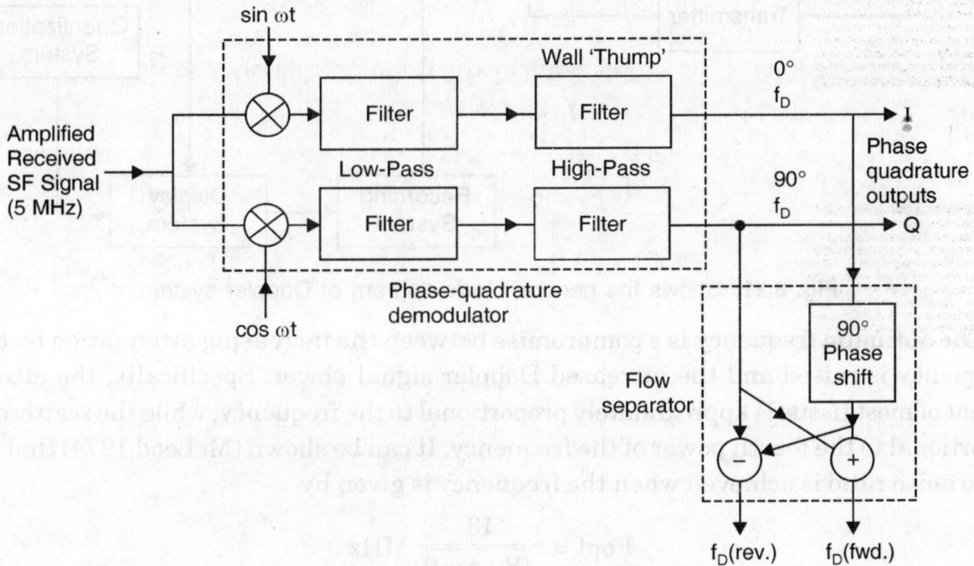

Fig. 8.20. Shows the phase quadrature scheme of doppler signal extraction.

DOPPLER ULTRASOUND

BASIC ASPECTS OF DOPPLER SYSTEMS

The basis of most Doppler ultrasound systems is shown in the block diagram (Fig. 8.21). Also we know that the transmitter portion is responsible for excitation of the Doppler probe crystal. For a continuous wave (CW) system, the excitation signal is sinusoidal at a frequency range of 3 MHz to 8 MHz typically, as per probe choice. For a pulsed system, the transducer is excited by a high amplitude sinusoidal burst whose duration is typically several cycles on, and this is repeated at the pulse repetition rate, which is often around 10 kHz. The received signal consists of reflected and scattered signals from fixed interfaces along with the Doppler signal from vessel wall movement, and the much weaker Doppler signal arising from scattering by red blood cells. This composite signal from the receiving transducer is first amplified and then demodulated in order to extract the forward and reverse Doppler signals. The Doppler signal arising from blood generally contains the frequencies considerably higher than those arising form vessel wall movement.

The function of the signal processor is to anlayse the Doppler signal by a method called real time Fourier analysis. Information from this analysis may be displayed along with the B-scan image so as to ensure probe position and insonation of the vessel. (See image on top middle of screen as a small picture in Plate I.3*b*)

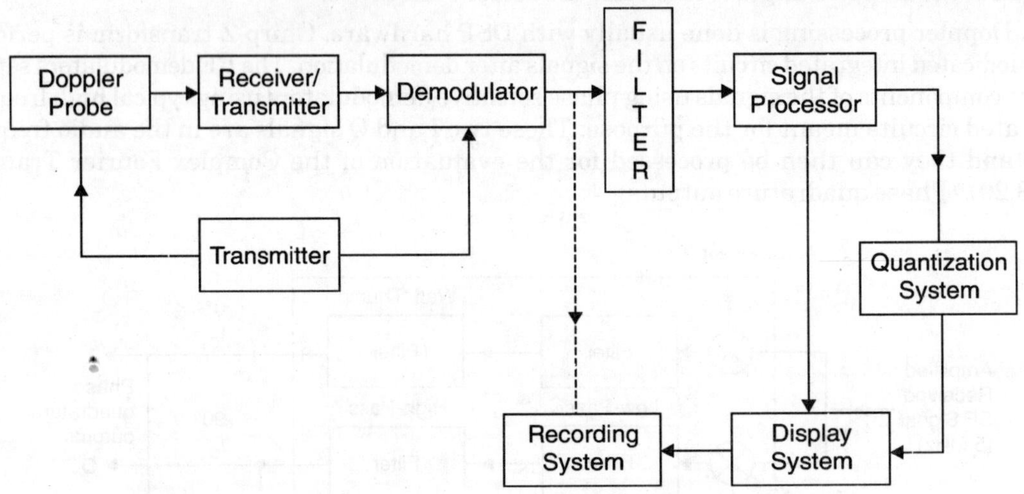

Fig. 8.21. Shows the general block diagram of Doppler system.

The optimum frequency is a compromise between the increasing attenuation by tissue as the frequency is raised and the increased Doppler signal power. Specifically, the attenuation coefficient of most tissue is approximately proportional to the frequency, while the scattered power is proportional to the fourth power of the frequency. It can be shown (McLeod 1974) that the best signal to noise ratio is achieved when the frequency is given by

$$\text{Fopt} = \frac{13}{\sqrt{R / \cos\theta}} \text{ MHz} \qquad \text{...(2)}$$

where R is the total tissue path length from the transducer to the vessel expressed in centimeters. For example, if the vessel is 1.5cm from the skin surface and the probe to vessel angle is 60° then *Fopt* = *7.5* MHz. In practice, other factors are also important, e.g., the dependence of the ultrasound beam pattern on frequency, and the reduction in the Doppler frequency shift as the transmission frequency is decreased. For pulsed Doppler, the spatial resolution increases at higher frequencies but, on the other hand, in situations where frequency aliasing is significant (deep structures with high associated velocities) a higher transmit frequency will increase this problem. In spite of these limitations, eqn. (2) serves as a useful design guide for the best choice of transmission frequency. In systems that combine B-mode imaging with Doppler, the imaging frequency and the Doppler transmission frequency may vary. For example, 7.5 or 10 MHz may be used for imaging in order to achieve improved spatial resolution, while the Doppler transmission frequency could be 4MHz. This choice of frequencies allows the examination of vessels for which the ultrasound beam tissue path length is less than 5cm.

TRANSDUCER DESIGN

The transducer for a simple, CW system generally consist of two piezo-electric crystals; one for transmission and one for reception (Wells 1974). Some examples of the crystal arrangement are shown in Fig. 8.22.

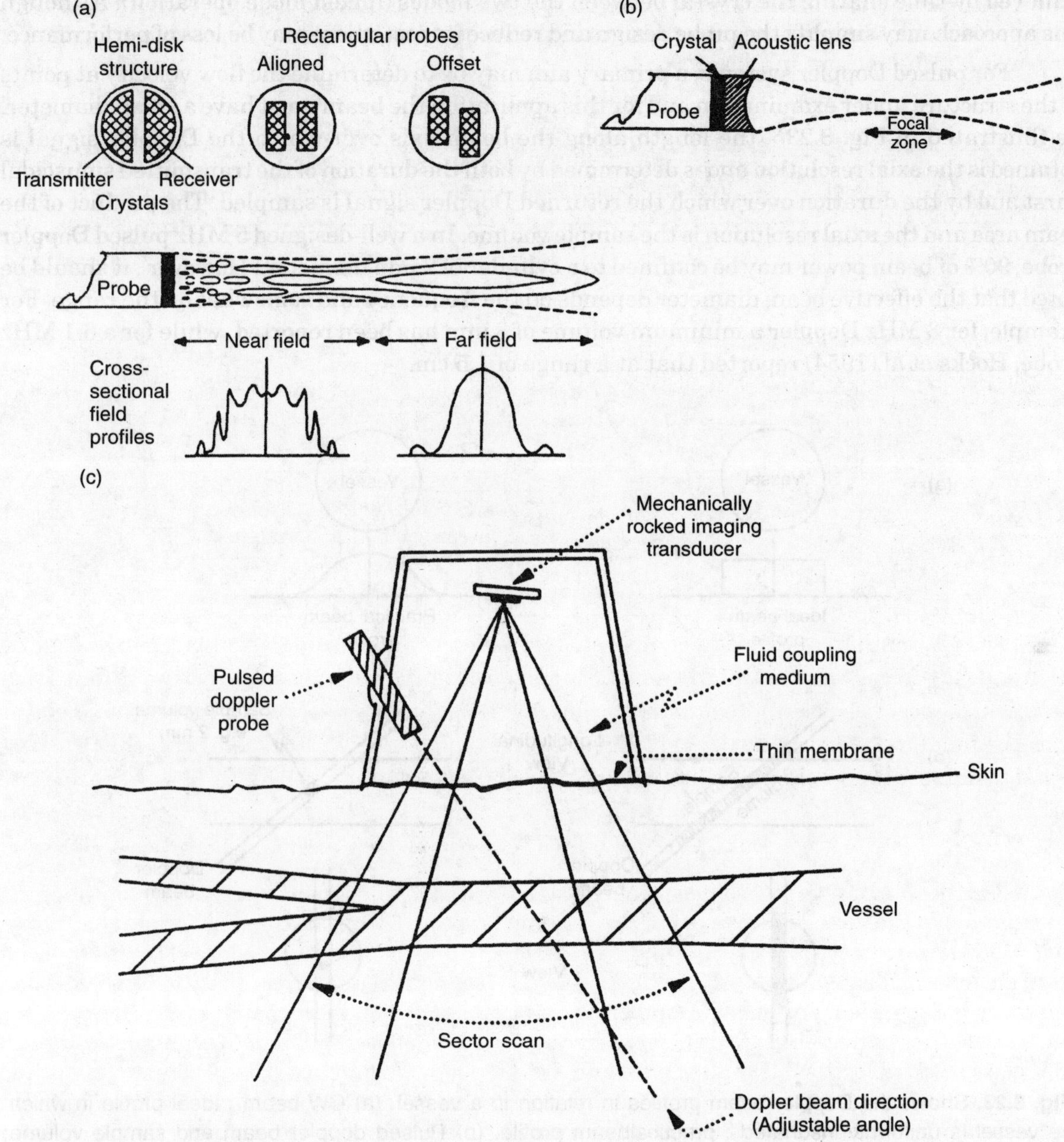

Fig. 8.22. Example of doppler transducers. (a) End view of different CW probes using separate transmit and receive crystals. The crystals may be mounted at a small angle to one another to provide some degree of focusing. Beam profiles are shown for a simple disk transducer element similar to that used in some pulsed doppler systems. (b) Disk transducer probe with an acoustic lens. (c) Example of duplex transducer that uses separate imaging and doppler transducer crystals.

For pulsed Doppler, since the functions of transmission and reception are separated in time, a single crystal is normally used to perform both functions. Generally, the crystal consists of a disc of say, 5 mm in diameter as shown in Fig. 8.22*b*, a simple acoustic lens may be bonded to the front surface in order to reduce the beam diameter in the focal zone. In some duplex systems, the same transducer is used both for imaging and Doppler measurements. This is achieved by time sharing the crystal between the two modes (mixed mode operation). Although this approach may simplify the probe design and reduce its cost, there may be loss of performance.

For pulsed Doppler systems, a primary aim may be to determine the flow velocity at points in the structure under examination and for this application the beam must have a small diameter. As illustrated in Fig. 8.23*b*, the length along the beam axis over which the Doppler signal is obtained is the axial resolution and is determined by both the duration of the transmitted sinusoidal burst and by the duration over which the returned Doppler signal is sampled. The product of the beam area and the axial resolution is the sample volume. In a well-designed 5 MHz pulsed Doppler probe, 90% of beam power may be confined to a cylinder of 2 mm diameter . However , it should be noted that the effective beam diameter depends on the frequency and somewhat on the range. For example, for 3 MHz Doppler a minimum volume of 3 mm has been reported, while for a 6.1 MHz probe, Hocks et al (1954) reported that at a range of 1.5 cm.

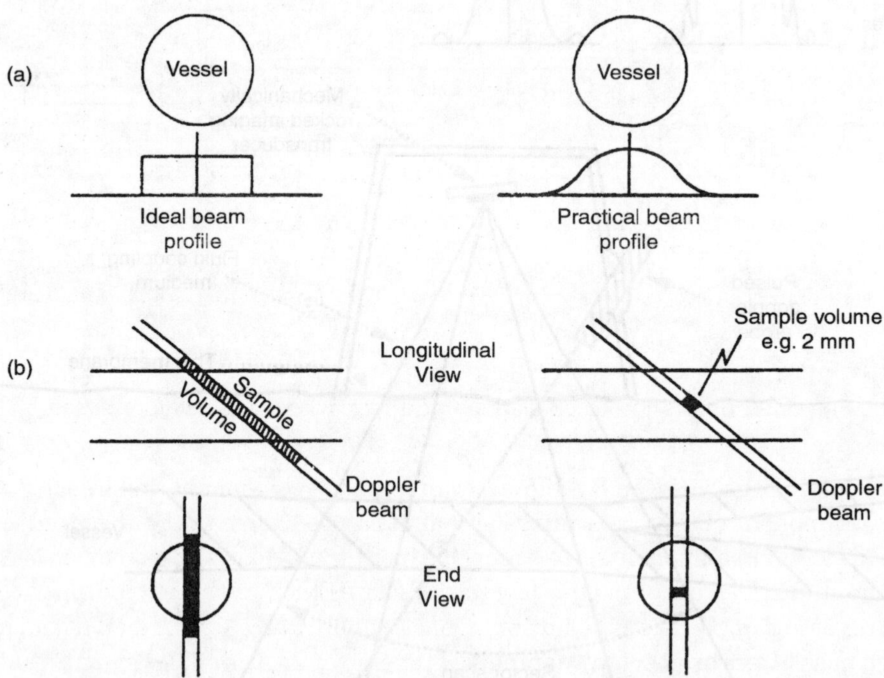

Fig. 8.23. Shows the Doppler beam profiles in relation to a vessel. (a) CW beam : ideal profile in which the vessel is uniformly insonated ; practicalbeam profile. (b) Pulsed doppler beam and sample volume; long pulse sample volume in which the doppler signal is derived from a pencil-like intersection with the vessel; arrangement in which the doppler signal is obtained from a small volume within the vessel.

DEMODULATION METHODS

For both pulsed and CW Doppler systems, it is necessary to extract the Doppler signal from the amplified RF signal. This is normally achieved in directional-sensitive systems by an analog based phase-quadrature demodulator.

A simple demodulator consists of a means of multiplying the RF signal at the transmission frequency, and then, by means of a filter, removing the RF components.

For economy, simple hand held Doppler 'flow-meters' often use this scheme. Such a simple Doppler probe system is described later in this chapter.

To separate the forward and reverse flow Doppler signal components, the phase-quadrature scheme shown in Fig. 8.24 is generally employed.

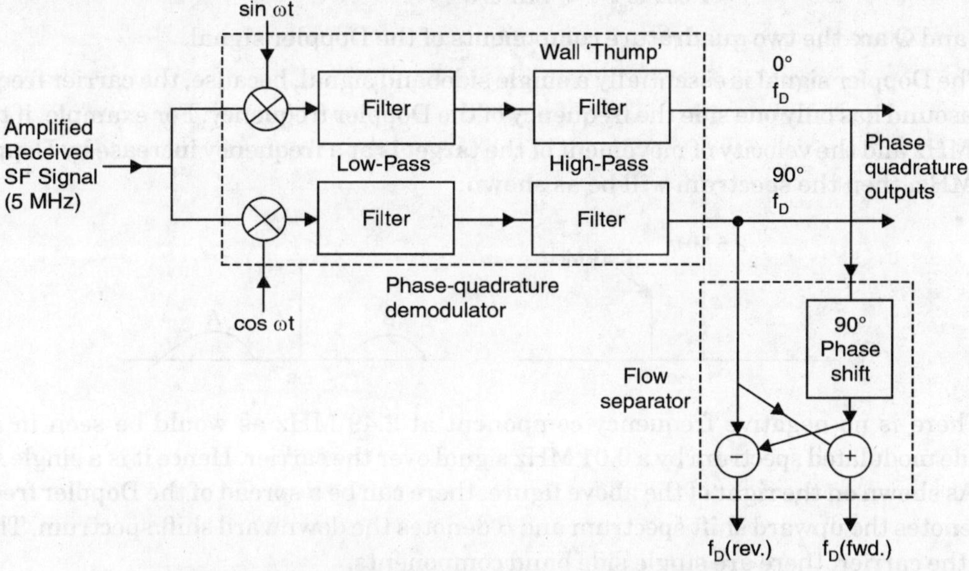

Fig. 8.24. Shows the block diagram of a typical phase-quadrature sound frequency demodulator and flow separator subsystems.

By multiplying the received RF signal by an in-phase component and by a 90° out of phase (quadrature) component of the transmitted signal, it can be shown that two outputs contain the two directional Doppler components in a separable form. Specifically, by removing the RF components from the multiplier outputs (the low pass filters), each of the two outputs contains the forward and reverse Doppler signals, but in a phase - quadrature form. In addition, as shown in Fig. 8.24, high pass filters are normally employed to remove those Doppler signals that arise from a low velocity interfaces, such as vessel walls. Typically, the cut-off frequency of such a filter is in the range of 100-400 Hz. To obtain separate forward and reverse Doppler output signals, it is necessary to perform a 90° phase shift (Hilbert transform) and then perform an addition and subtraction.

The Doppler signals can be extracted through the use of straightforward digital processing methods, such as complex Fourier transform .

In modern Doppler systems, signal processing may be performed directly on the phase quadrature output; consequently, the flow separator is likely to be used just as a means of providing stereo audio feedback to the system operator. Recording of the Doppler signal is best achieved by recording the phase-quadrature output.

THEORY OF DOPPLER SIGNAL TRANSFORMATION

If the carrier ultrasound frequency is ωc and the Doppler Shift frequency is ωd, then the shift frequency is (ωc + ω*d*) and so if it is a cosine signal

$$u = \cos(\omega c + \omega d)t$$

$$= \cos \omega_c t \cos \omega_d t - \sin \omega_c t \sin \omega_d dt$$

$$= \mathrm{I} \cos \omega_c t - \mathrm{Q} \sin \omega_c t \qquad \ldots(3)$$

where I and Q are the two quadrature components of the Doppler signal.

The Doppler signal is essentially a single sideband signal, because, the carrier frequency of the ultrasound has only one side the frequency of the Doppler frequency. For example, if the probe is at 2.5MHz and the velocity of movement of the target is at a frequency increase by Doppler shift to 2.51 MHz, then the spectrum will be as shown:

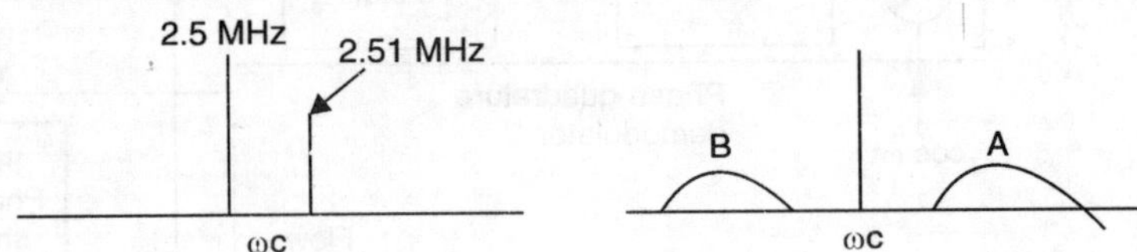

There is no negative frequency component at 2.49 MHz as would be seen in a simple amplitude modulated spectrum by a 0.01 MHz signal over the carrier. Hence it is a single sideband signal. As shown on the right of the above figure, there can be a spread of the Doppler frequencies and *A* denotes the upward shift spectrum and *B* denotes the downward shift spectrum. Thus, both sides of the carrier, there are single side band components.

After we get the synchronously detected signals in phase and quadrature to the carrier frequency as I + *j* Q, we can use it for finding the complex Fourier transform.

The complex F.T. will give the two components *A* and *B* at the negative and positive frequency parts accordingly, as shown below.

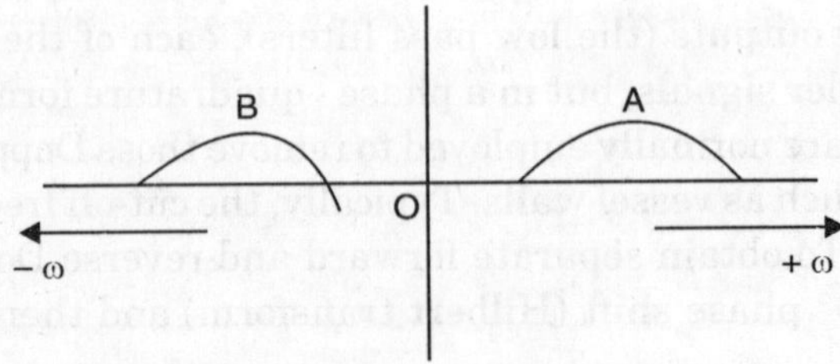

Each of these will have both real and imaginary parts, corresponding to the Cosine and Sine part of the Doppler frequencies (phase information).

PULSED DOPPLER SYSTEM

A simple pulsed Doppler system contains a number of elements that are similar if not identical to those of the CW system (Fig. 8.25) just described. The transducer is driven by a brief pulse consisting of several sinusoidal cycles. Since it is important to ensure that successive excitation pulses are identical, this driving signal is derived from a master oscillator that also determines the pulse repetition frequency (PRF). The received signal consists of signals from stationary interfaces as well as scattered signal from blood cells lying along the beam path. Since the signal amplitude is very dependent on the depth, the RF amplifier will either have a manual gain control, or the gain will be automatically increased with time (time gain control, TGC) in such a way that the signal attenuation is approximately compensated for.

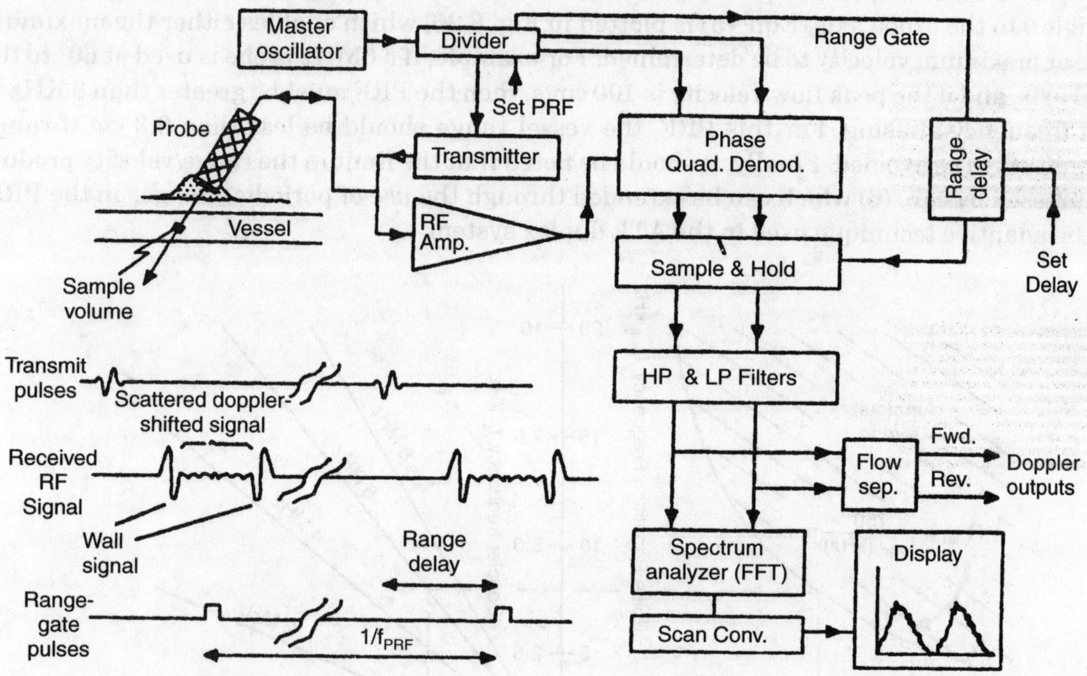

Fig. 8.25. Pulsed Doppler Modulus–Schematic Diagram.

Depth discrimination is achieved by sampling the outputs at the phase quadrature demodulators at a point in time from the start of the transmitted pulse that corresponds to twice the transit time (there and back) from the probe to the sample position. Since the range delay can be adjusted, the Doppler signal from any given point can be obtained. Furthermore, in some systems the duration of the sample can also be adjusted so that the volume sampled can be varied from a long cylindrical region along the axis, down to the minimum sample volume.

The proper choice of the PRF is of major importance since this frequency determines the maximum velocity (Vmax) that can be determined without causing ambiguity as to their positional origin. Since the time between transmitted pulses must be sufficiently long to allow an ultrasound pulse to reach the target and the resultant echo to return back to the transducer, it is necessary that

$$\frac{1}{f_{prf}} > \frac{2R_{\max}\cos\theta}{c} \qquad \ldots(4)$$

where the pulse repetition frequency (PRF) is denoted by f_{prf} and c is the velocity of sound in the medium (typically, 1500 m/s). Now, to avoid ambiguity in the Doppler signal spectrum due to frequency aliasing, it is well-known result of communications theory (the Nyquist theorem) that the signal must be sampled at a rate equal to at least twice the maximum frequency present. Failure to meet this criterion causes a 'wrap around' of the Doppler spectrum. This is the same phenomenon observed in a western movie where spokes of the wagon wheel appear to go backwards when the wagon goes sufficiently fast. Thus, since it is required that fopt > 2(f_D)max and noting the maximum frequency (Doppler frequency) and the maximum velocity related by the Doppler equation, then from eqn (4),

$$2V_{max}/c = f_D/f_s \quad \text{and} \quad f_D/f_{prf} = 1/2 \qquad \text{...(5)}$$

$$R_{max} V_{max} = c^2/(8f_s \cos \theta) \qquad \text{...(6)}$$

where f_s is the transmitted frequency and the direction of the moving target is assumed to be at an angle θ to the probe axis. Eqn. (5) is plotted in Fig. 8.26, which enables either the maximum range or maximum velocity to be determined. For example, if a 6MHz probe is used at 60° to the vessel axis, and if the peak flow velocity is 100 cm/s, then the PRF must be greater than 8 KHz to avoid frequency aliasing. For this PRF, the vessel range should be less than 9.3 cm if range ambiguity is to be avoided. Finally, it should be noted that the limit in the range/velocity product as expressed by eqn. (6) which can be extended through the use of periodic changes in the PRF, and the adaptive technique used in the ATL duplex system.

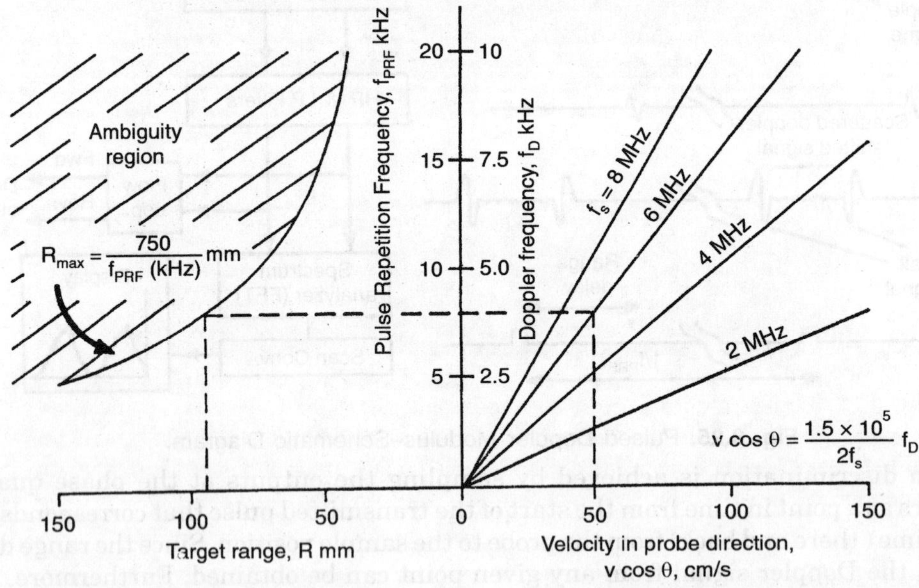

Fig. 8.26. Shows the range ambiguity and aliasing limitations of pulsed doppler system.

DUPLEX DOPPLER (B-MODE)

Systems that provide both B-mode vessel image and a Doppler signal from a specific region of a vessel are widely used in clinical practice. Such systems, which are commonly referred to as duplex Doppler systems, normally use a pulsed Doppler and provide a means whereby the beam direction and the location of the sample volume are superimposed on the B-mode display, as illustrated in the recording of Fig. 8.27. In addition, for cardiac examination, to avoid the problem of aliasing, a CW Doppler mode may also be provided. A major advantage of such systems, in spite of their increased complexity, and cost, is the ability to determine the precise location of the sample volume in relation to the vessel under examination. Furthermore, vessel abnormalities may be apparent from the image display. The B-mode imaging system may consist of mechanically rotated or rocked transducer elements, or a phased array, or a phased annular array that is rocked. The Doppler transducer can be an independently moved unit within the scan head or it may be a crystal that is time- shared with the imaging portion of the system. Through the use of an independent Doppler probe, both the imaging and Doppler subsystem designs can be optimised. In addition this arrangement also provides greater flexibility in clinical use. In the Duplex mode of operation, whereby both imaging and Doppler information are displayed, a reduction in the imaging frame rate may be required.

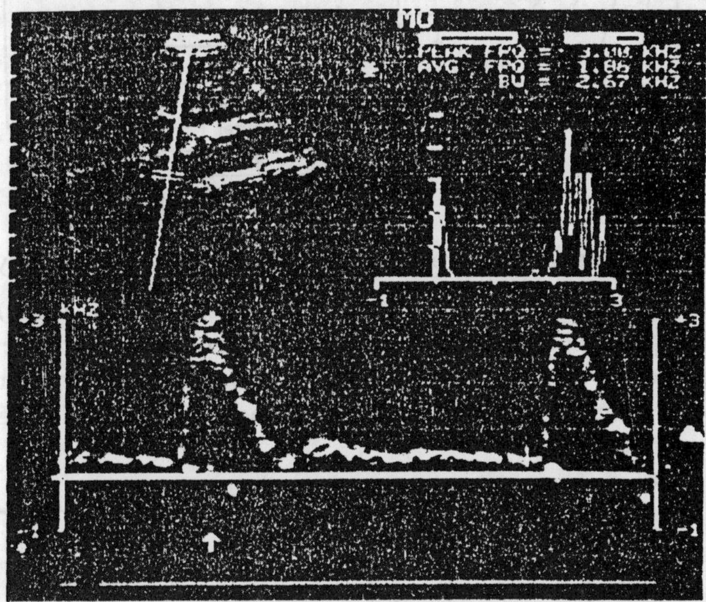

Fig. 8.27. Duplex recording from the abdominal aorta with the pulse sample volume positioned close to the vessel centre. The sample volume is 3 mm and is 6.5 cm from the transducer face (as shown by = in fig.). An individual spectrum from the spectrogram, taken at the time marked with the arrow, is also displayed.

DOPPLER FLOW IMAGING

Recently, developments in pulsed Doppler methods have made possible the presentation of real time Doppler flow images superimposed on the conventional real time B-mode (structural) images. A major difficulty in the design of such systems is the problem of processing the Doppler information sufficiency fast to extract the flow information from each scan line.

The basic principles are illustrated in Fig. 8.28, where it is assumed that the transducer produces a sector scan by means of a phased array. Each line of the sector scan is used to produce a B-mode image in the usual manner. In addition, each line is processed by comparing it to the

previous line to remove the stationary and slowly moving interface reflections (clutter removal). This leaves a signal from rapidly moving interfaces and the signals scattered from the red blood cells.

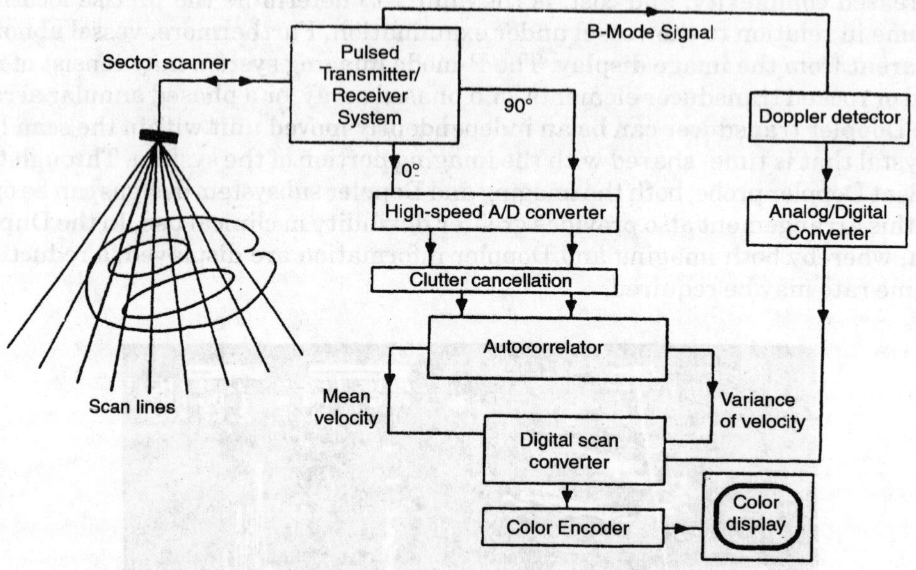

Fig. 8.28. Shows the details of real-time cardiac doppler flow imaging system.

It is necessary to integrate over several identical scan lines (*e.g.*, eight) and this reduces the frame rate. The digital scan converter and colour converter encode the velocity information as red or blue, depending on a whether the direction is towards or away from the transducer. Furthermore, the colour brightness is proportional to the velocity, while the variance in flow velocity is presented as green.

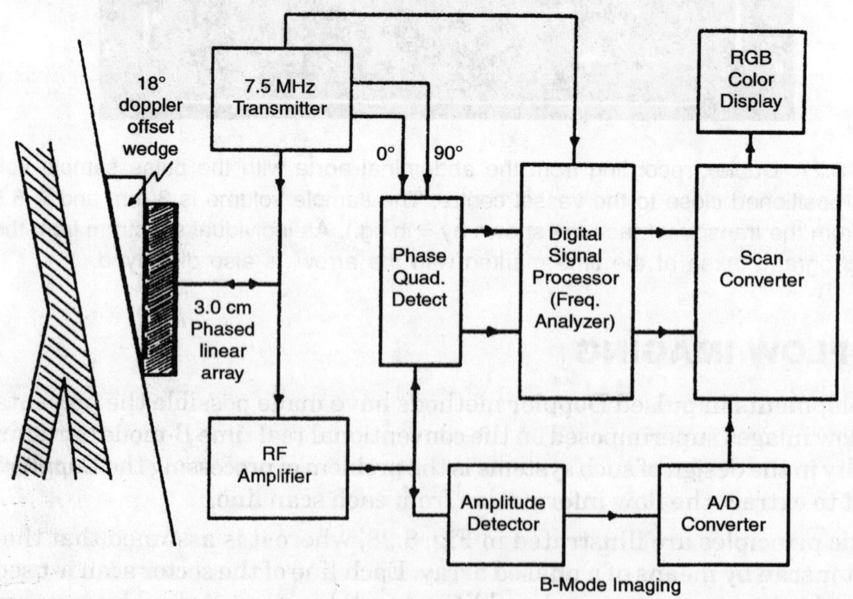

Fig. 8.29. Shows the block diagram of linear phased array Doppler imaging system.

A powerful digital signal processor determines the echo signal magnitude and phase at each point and this enables a B- mode display and Doppler display to be superimposed. In the Doppler display, red indicates slow away from and blue flow towards the transducer; higher velocities are shown by increased brightness. This image of the carotid bulb region was taken at close to peak systole, and shows a region of flow separation and reversal.

METHODS OF SPECTRAL ANALYSIS

Requirements

For both pulsed and CW Doppler systems, the special analysis requirements are generally similar. In peripheral and carotid arterial assessment, it is essential that the analysis be performed in real-time so that the clinical operator will have visual feedback of the Doppler spectral waveform to aid in optimum probe placement. In addition, for identifying venous flow artifacts, as well as for the proper presentation of spectra containing reverse flow components , it is important that forward and reverse signals be processed simultaneously. To avoid precise adjustments of the receiver gain, it is desirable that the analysis system be able to cope with a wide dynamic range: a 60 dB range.

The frequency analysis range and resolution and time resolution are governed by the nature of the Doppler signal as well as by the transmission frequency. For clinical applications, to process most Doppler signals, the anaylser must accommodate maximum forward frequencies up to 15 kHz and reverse frequencies up to 5 KHz.

A frequency resolution of approximately 100 Hz may be required. For example, for a normal carotid arterial signal, with a maximum frequency of 3 kHz at peak systole, a 100 Hz bandwidth corresponds to a division of the signal spectrum into 30 frequency bins. For real-time spectral analysis systems, the frequency resolution is the inverse of the time resolution. Thus, for a signal segment of 10ms duration, the maximum frequency resolution will be 100 Hz, while for a 5ms signal it will be 200 Hz.

It is desirable to smooth the transitions at the beginning and end by using a 'window' function that is generally of the Hanning or Hamming type.

DIGITAL METHODS

An attractive alternative to analog methods, is the use of the discrete Fourier transform (DFT). The calculations can be performed with either with the conventional DFT or the fast Fourier transform (FFT) algorithm. Suppose that the processor can perform an N-point Fourier transform (yielding N/2 positive frequency bins) in a minimum interval of T seconds. For real time operation on records of duration T, the Doppler signal must be sampled at a frequency of N/T . For this sampling frequency, aliasing will occur if the input signal spectrum contains components higher than N/2T Hz. The N/2 frequency bins will be spaced from zero frequency up to a frequency N/2T, in equal intervals, so that the bin size will be1/T. For example, if T = 0.01 s, and N/2 = 128, then the frequency at which aliasing starts to occur will be 12.8 kHz and the frequency resolution will be 100 Hz. By increasing T, the frequency resolution is improved but with a reduction in the

Nyquist frequency. While the arguments just given have considered a single-channel Doppler input signal, they can be extended to the complex input signals from a phase quadrature demodulator, i.e., for the inphase and quadrature signals.

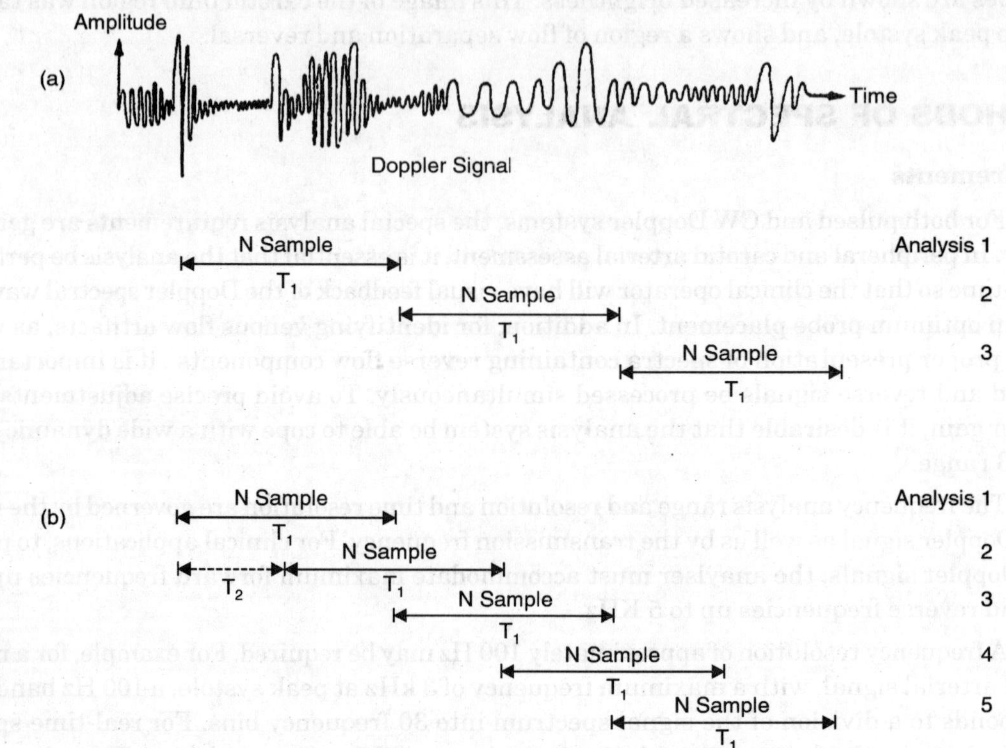

Fig. 8.30. Comparison of techniques for data sampling. (a) Conventional method : a new signal segment of duration T_1 s is used for each analysis, yielding a spectrum every T_1 s with a reolution of I/T_1 Hz. (b) Sliding method : data for each analysis contain $(T_1\text{-}T_2)$ s of old data from the previous analysis and T_2 s of a new data, creating spectra with a resolution of I/T_1 Hz but at the increased rate of one spectrum every T_2 s.

Fig. 8.30 shows the comparision of techniques for data sampling in Doppler systems.

General purpose microprocessors and microcomputers have inadequate speed to implement even the computationally efficient FFT in real-time. A s a result, high speed DSP systems have been developed which perform the analysis. The Motorola DSP56000 chip can perform a 1024-point complex FFT in 5 ms.

Spectral analysis based on the use of charge coupled devices (CCDs) is a hybrid form of signal processing which has the advantage that time and frequency information are handled digitally. The signal levels are retained in their original analog form (on a sampled basis), thereby eliminating the need for an analog to digital converter. The frequency analysis range, resolution and speed requirements for Doppler ultrasound signal analysis can all be met with available CCD-based transversal filters.

MEAN, MAXIMUM AND VOLUMETRIC FLOW WAVEFORMS

Both the maximum and the mean frequency waveforms have important applications in the quantitative assessment of vascular disease. Care must be taken to define whether it is the amplitude or the power Doppler spectrum from which the waveforms are derived. In general, the mean frequency waveform derived from the amplitude spectrum will not be the same as that derived from the power spectrum. The same is true for the maximum frequency waveform. Owing to the statistical origin of the Doppler signal, the estimates of the maximum and mean waveforms will have a statistical variability that depends on the duration over which the estimates are made.

Usually, the mean frequency waveform definition is based on the power spectrum $P(f_D)$ and this can be obtained by simply squaring the amplitude spectrum $A(f_D)$. On this basis the mean frequency waveform $f_D(t)$ is given by

$$f_D(t) = \int_{-\alpha}^{\alpha} f_D P(f_D)\, df_D \Big/ \int_{-\alpha}^{\alpha} (Pf_D)\, df_D \qquad \ldots(6)$$

where the integration extends over all frequencies, including the reverse flow frequencies, which are treated as being negative. Evidently, the above eqn.(6) is simply the first moment of the power spectrum.

An approximate analog method for estimating the mean Doppler waveform is based on the use of a circuit to count the number of zero crossings of the input signal over as short period of time and to convert this into a proportional output voltage. Of course, this same process can also be performed digitally.

It has been pointed out that even with high-resolution pulsed Doppler systems, the spectrum obtained from a sample volume positioned near a severe stenosis can have a relatively wide bandwidth. For such signals the error introduced by a zero-crossing detector may be significant.

VOLUMETRIC FLOW WAVEFORM

Three categories of method can be identified They are given as follows;

1. Velocity profile method
2. Uniform insonation method and
3. Assumed velocity profile method.

In the velocity profile method, the velocity profile across the vessel is measured using pulse Doppler techniques and then assuming semi-axisymmetirc flow, the volumetric flow can be calculated by integration across the vessel diameter, *i.e.*, by evaluating,

$$Q(t) = \int_{-R}^{+R} \pi r v(\tau, t)\, dr \qquad \ldots(7)$$

where R(*t*) is the vessel radius at a time t, and the velocity profile from – R to + R is assumed to be known. Evidently, both the instantaneous vessel diameter and the angle of incidence of the Doppler beam must also be known.

EXTREMITIES

The normal peripheral arterial waveforms have a triphasic shape with a forward, a reverse and a second forward flow component. Distal to an arterial stenosis the waveform is dampened, i.e., the peak is flattened and delayed, and the reverse flow component is reduced or absent. The waveforms can be analysed subjectively by observing the morphological changes in the shape of the waveform or they can be analysed by a variety of quantitative methods. Of fundamental importance in quantitative analysis is the dependence of the waveform frequency on the probe angle. With a CW Doppler system this angle cannot be determined with sufficient accuracy, and consequently any quantitative index derived form the Doppler waveform should be independent of the angle. Further, the maximum frequency waveform derived from the real-time spectral display is generally used since it avoids the artifacts and errors that are frequently introduced in the calculation of the main waveform as described above.

Of the reported quantitative indices, pulsatility index (PI), Laplace transform indices and principal component analysis have shown the best correlation with the results of arteriography and direct pressure measurement. Downstream from a stenosis where disturbed flow occurs, broadening of the spectrum particularly in the region of peak systole occurs. A simple quantitative measure of the degree of spectral broadening, that is approximately independent of the angle of insonation, is the spectral broadening index (SBI). This is defined in terms of the maximum and mean waveforms.

$$SBI = (\text{maximum} - \text{mean})/\text{maximum}$$

While this index varies throughout the cardiac cycle, it appears that the greatest sensitivity to disease occurs in the region of peak systole.

With a duplex scanner, the B-scan image and the Doppler spectral waveform are interpreted together.

STRUCTURE OF COLOR DOPPLER IMAGE

This is a combination of 2-D echocardiograph image and the pulsed wave Doppler signal processed pattern. Pulsed Doppler permits finding the velocity within a sample volume at a known distance from the transducer. By pulsing at a known frequency (PRF) and knowing speed of sound in the tissue, we find the depth of returning shifted frequency signal. In conventional Doppler mode, velocities are typically displayed in spectral form for a single sample volume of interest over time.

The Spectrogram is a time course of spectral data, plotted with time in the X axis and the frequency components of the signal shown in intensity modulated form in the Y axis. Thus, each vertical line can have, for instance, 128 points which correspond to frequency shifts from 0 to 8 KHz in a typical cardiac chamber blood velocity pattern by insonation. (Fig. 8.31). There are 128 points positive and 128 points negative, which corresponds to positive frequency shifts (particles moving towards the transducer) and negative frequency shifts (particles moving away from transducer).

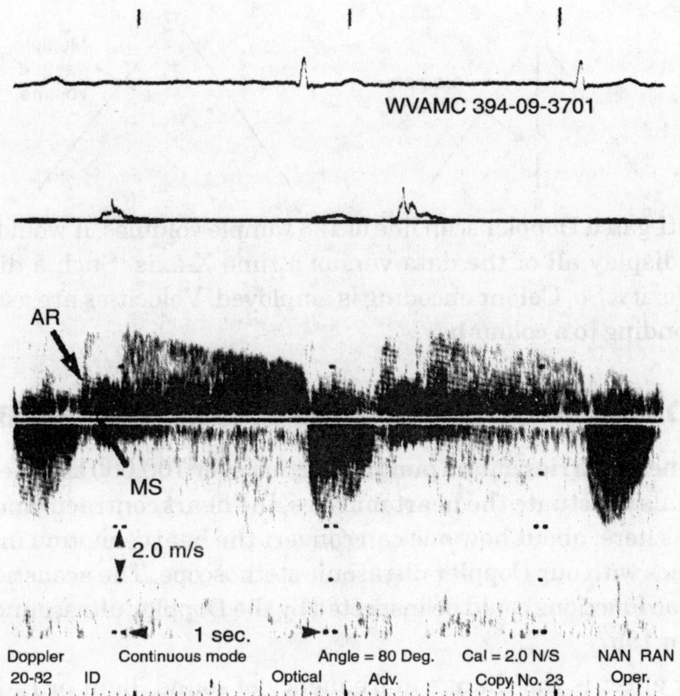

Fig. 8.31. In this continuous-wave doppler spectral tracing, the diastolic slope of the waveform is shallow, implying mild aortic regurgitation. AR = aortic regurgitation ; MS = mitral stenosis.

The simplest scheme is a greyscale display in which either the amplitude or the power of the Doppler spectra is converted into a proportional change in the CRT intensity. In practice it is found that approximately 10 greyscale levels can be discriminated.

Different spectral amplitudes can also be represented by different colour hues. It is not clear that there are any advantages to this form of real time spectral displays. However, for Doppler flow imaging systems, a colour display is vital .

A fairly high-resolution display (700 × 400 pixels) for real time display has considerably enhanced computational power.

To plot the magnitude at any frequency, intensity modulation is employed, by choosing several levels of grey, from dark representing that the amplitude of that frequency is large and white representing a zero value at that frequency bin. The spectrogram plot is shown in present machines as a real time display, because it is possible to evaluate the spectrum of the Doppler signal fast, since the time scale of X axis movement is relatively slow only in a cardiac cycle of action.

Fig. 8.31 shows the Spectrogram of the Doppler signal as a real time signal display.

MULTI-GATED DOPPLER DISPLAY

The difference between simple pulsed Doppler and the Colour Doppler is shown in the illustration below.

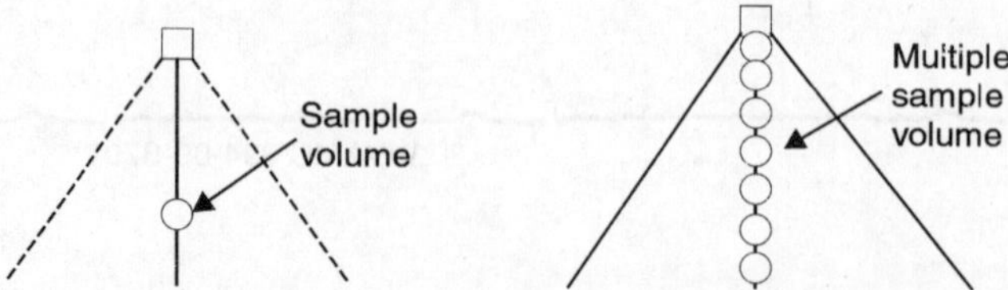

With the multi-gated Doppler scan line of 128 sample volumes, it would require 128 different velocity spectra to display all of the data versus a time X-axis. Such a display is not possible because of its complexity. So, Colour encoding is employed. Velocities are assigned varying colour intensities corresponding to a colour bar.

A TYPICAL DOPPLER-ULTRASOUND BASED HEART BEAT MONITOR

The normal human heart carries out its pumping action over 100,000 times every day. Generating its own electric signals to actuate the heart muscles, the heart contracts and relaxes during each beat. We will discuss here, about how one can convert the heart's motion into audio sound using ultrasound electronics with our Doppler ultrasonic stethoscope. The acoustical society of America described how cardiac functions could be inspected by the Doppler ultrasound using a frequency of about 2 MHz even in 1957.

The Doppler effect is the change in frequency of sound, light or radio waves that occurs when a transmitter or receiver are in motion relative to each other. When a transducer sends an ultrasonic beam into the body, a portion of the energy is reflected back by internal body structures. If the structure moves, the frequency of the reflected bam is also changed in proportion to the velocity of the movement.

This technology was developed about forty years ago. This technique is most valuable and completely harmless tool for n**on-invasive examination of movements inside the body** by the medical profession. Experiments have shown that beaming of very low energy high frequency sound into the body is not harmful. The technique is used all in the universe fɔr listening the heart beat of unborn babies in a mother's womb. It is possible to listen to the characteristic Doppler sounds from your own heart which can be heard with an easily built Doppler ultrasonic stethoscope. In this unit, Piezo electric crystals have been used for measuring the heart rate.

THE DOPPLER STETHOSCOPE

The basic component of the stethoscope is the transducer. This transducer contains two lead zirconate - titanate piezoelectric crystals. One of the crystals is energized by the output of 2.25 MHz oscillator/amplifier so that it expands and contracts at that frequency, setting up pressure or sound waves that are transmitted into the body. When that wave, which is directional, passes form one medium to another medium in the body, a portion is reflected back to the second crystal which generates a voltage. If the reflecting surface is stationary, the voltage generated by the receiving crystal has the same frequency as the transmitted wave. If the reflecting surface is moving away from the transducer, the reflected frequency is lower than the transmitted wave. Similarly, if the reflecting surface is moving towards the transducer, the reflected frequency is higher. By mixing a portion of the transmited frequency with the received frequency, the received frequency is modulated in both frequency and amplitude. Using an amplitude modulated (AM) detector, one can obtain an audio signal whose frequency is proportional to the velocity of the moving structure within the body.

WORKING PRINCIPLE OF THE CIRCUIT DIAGRAM

TRANSMITTER CIRCUIT

The transmitter circuit is shown in Fig. 8.32. An RF oscillator which is built around Q1 operates at about 2.25MHz. Positive feedback is provided for the secondary tap in T1 to the emitter of Q1. The frequency is determined by C4 and the inductive tuning of T1. The oscillator output is coupled through C5 to Q2, an inductively tuned RF amplifier. A secondary tap on T2 provides a low- impedance output to drive the transmitter crystal XTAL1 in the transducer. The ultrasonic power generated is less that 15 milliwatts per square centimeter of transducer surface.

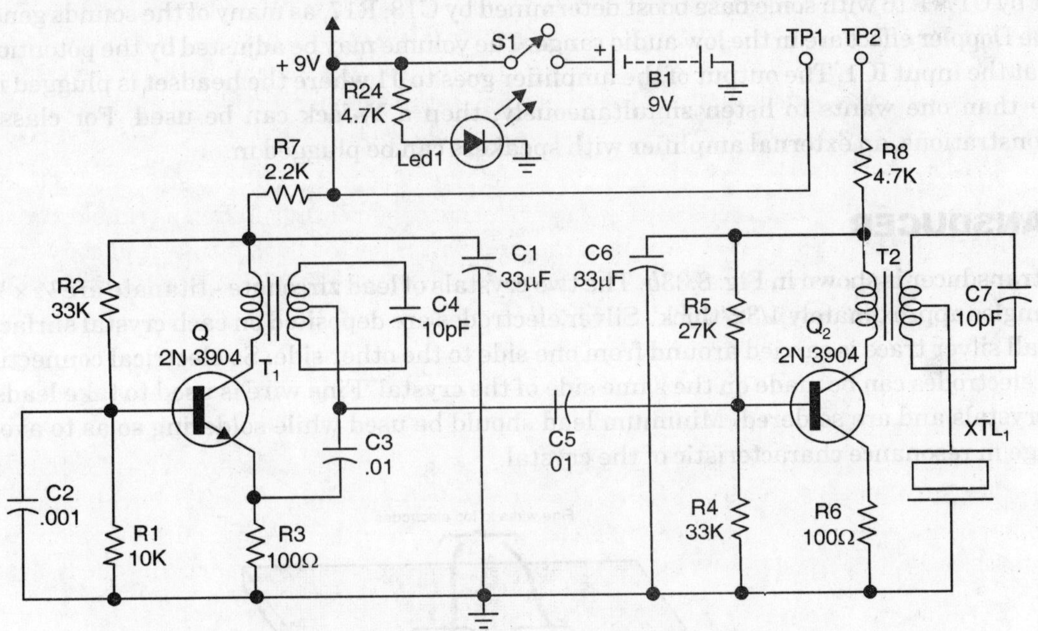

Fig. 8.32. Shows the transmitter circuit. Q1 is an RF oscillator whose 2.25 MHz frequency is determined by C4 and T1. A secondary tap on T2 provides a low-impedance output to drive XTAL1 in the transducer.

RECEIVER AND AUDIO CIRCUIT

The receiver and audio circuits are shown in Fig. 8.33*a*. The receiver uses two identical stages of inductively-tuned RF amplification. The voltage generated in the receiving crystal Xtal-2 is coupled to Q3 through C8. The output of Q3 is coupled to Q4 through C11. The combined RF gain for the two stages is about 2000. The modulated Doppler signal is detected by D1 to produce audio frequencies in the 50–2000 Hz range.

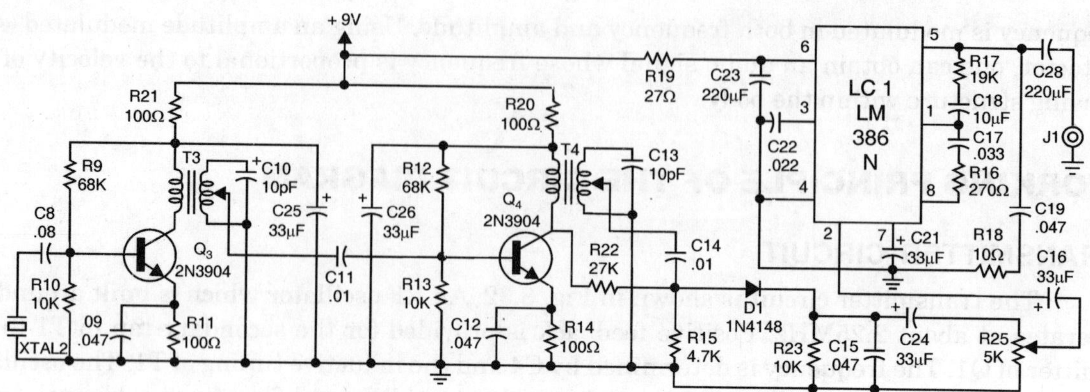

Fig. 8.33a. Shows the receiver and audio amplifier.

A low power audio amplifier, IC1, can drive one or two head sets. It has a gain of 100, which is set by C17- R16 with some base boost determined by C18, R17, as many of the sounds generated by the Doppler effect are in the low audio range. The volume may be adjusted by the potentiometer R25 at the input IC1. The output of the amplifier goes to J1 where the headset is plugged into. If more than one wants to listen simultaneously, then a Y-Jack can be used. For class room demonstrations, an external amplifier with speakers can be plugged in.

TRANSDUCER

The transducer is shown in Fig. 8.33*b*. The two crystals of lead zirconate - titanate are ½ × ¼ inch rectangles approximately 1/32 'thick'. Silver electrodes are deposited on each crystal surface, and a small silver trace is carried around from one side to the other side. So electrical connections to both electrodes can be made on the same side of the crystal. Fine wire is used to take leads from the crystals and are soldered. Minimum lead should be used while soldering so as to avoid the change in resonance characteristic of the crystal.

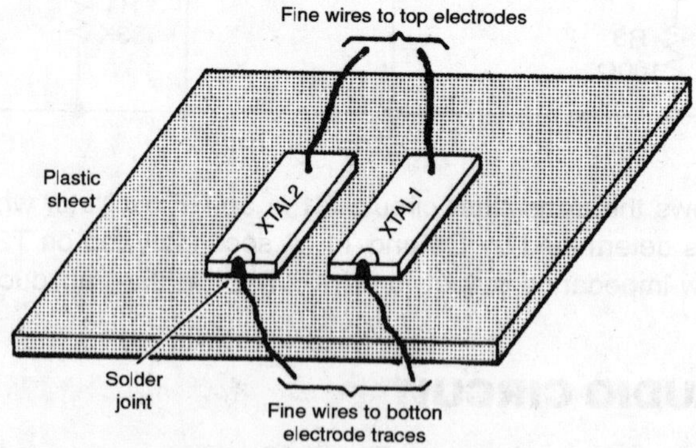

Fig. 8.33b. Transducer construction. Silver-bearing solder is used to avoid lifting the silver electrode from the ceramic crystal surface. Energy conversion is most efficient when crystals are "air-backed" resulting in energy being radiated from the front of the crystal.

ACOUSTIC IMPEDANCE

When dealing with ultrasound, the quantity of characteristic acoustic impedance is used in solving various problems dealing with waveform generation, propagation, and detection. Characteristic acoustic impedance Z is defined as

$$Z = \rho c$$

where ρ = the density of the medium in kg/m^3 and

c = the velocity of sound in m/s.

The characteristic acoustic impedance is therefore expressed as

$$\text{kg/m}^3 \times \text{m/s} = \text{kg/m}^2\text{s}.$$

To obtain the maximum energy conversion efficiency, the crystals should be acoustically matched with the plastic panel. When two mediums are closely matched, most of the energy will be transmitted through the materials. When an ultrasonic beam meets an interface of dissimilar materials, most of the energy is reflected where there is a large difference in acoustic impedance between the two materials.

The acoustic impedance of the crystals is about 30 million and that of the body is 1.5 million, with air being less than 50, all in units of kg/m2s. Because the density of air is so much lower than that of the crystal, and the velocity of sound in air is much slower than of the crystal, almost all the energy is reflected at that interface when the back side of the crystals are in contact with air. That difference in impedance results in most of the energy being radiated from the front of the crystal, and improved sensitivity of the receiving crystal. Since we want most of the energy to be reflected at the rear side of the crystal, it is desirable that most of the energy be transmitted at the front surface of the crystal and into the body. Because the crystals are too fragile to be placed in direct contact with the body, they are cemented with epoxy to a sheet of plastic about 1/16" thickness which should have an acoustic impedance between the crystal and the body. This results in more energy being transmitted in the body instead of being reflected at the skin surface. When gluing the crystals to the plastic , be sure to exclude any air from the interface and use a minimum amount of glue. Sheet acrylic of fiberglass such as that used for PC boards or a rigid vinyl sheet all have suitable acoustic impedance and provide the required protection for the crystals.

When more sensitivity is required, a dab of ultrasound gel is placed on the transducer face to improve the impedance match and exclude any air that may be trapped between the transducer face and the skin. Water or mineral oil will also work.

Fig. 8.34 shows the prototype unit of Doppler-ultrasound heart beat monitor. The transducer is mounted on the end plate of the enclosure with its leads close to their solder pads. The end plates are inserted at the end and then into the slot on the top half of the enclosure. Soldering of leads from the transducers is done at the appropriate terminals. 9V battery may be used. The stethoscope is now ready for use.

Frequency counter is connected from the emitter of Q1 to ground. Then DMM is connected with a settings at 10 mA range, between TP1 and Tp2 and turn the instrument on. Current meter should read less than 10 mA. Tune T1 to 2.3 MHz, then alternatively tune T2 and T1 to reduce the current to a minimum. After the tuning is over, the DMM is removed and solder the leads Tp1 and Tp2 together.

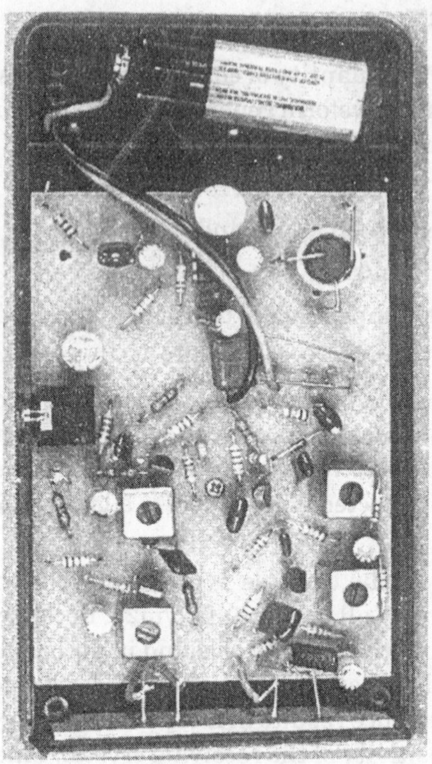

Fig. 8.34. Prototype Doppler stethoscope.

DMM is connected to the cathode of D1 and ground. Using 5 or 10 volt Range settings, alternatively tune T3 and T4 for a maximum voltage which will between 1 and 2 volts.

If you do not have the DMM, you can directly tune stethoscope while listening to your heart. With the transducer and headphones connected to the circuit board, put a little mineral oil or ultrasound gel on the face of the transducer and place the transducer firmly on your chest near your heart. The transducer may be placed between a pair of ribs rather than directly over a rib. Turn the volume up until you hear some Doppler sounds which will probably be low, as well as a hissing noise. Alternatively tune T1-T4 to increase the volume and for decreasing the hissing.

TESTING AND USE

As discussed earlier, maximum sensitivity is obtained when there is good impedance match between the transducer face and the skin with no air is trapped between them. A liquid gel such as aquasonic is specifically made for this purpose and is available at medical supply stores.

Apply a small amount of liquid gel to the transducer surface and place the transducer firmly against the bare chest, several inches to the left of the center and about 10 inches below the shoulder. Place the transducer so that ultrasonic beam passes between two ribs for best transmission. You will hear the sounds associated with movement of heart. Keeping the transducer firmly against the chest and changing the direction of the ultrasonic beam you will hear deterrent sounds depending on what surfaces are in the path of the ultrasonic beam. When you take a deep breath, the sounds may disappear because the lungs fill with air, covering aportion of the heart. As previously noted, air is a poor conductor of high frequency sound.

There are many aspects of heart action. First returning blood from the venous system fills the right atrium. A valve connecting this atrium to the right ventricle then opens and contraction of the atrium forces the blood into the ventricle. Likewise the cardiac cycle continues. Each of the four chambers of the heart contract and relax at different times of the heart cycle. Their associated valves open and close synchronously.

The movement of all those structures and the movement of blood through them provide the Doppler sounds which we can hear with the Doppler ultrasonic stethoscope.

When listening to the heart with Doppler ultrasound, a number of different sounds are heard, one after another in each rapid succession as the heart chambers and valves move and blood flows.

Blood flow sounds may also be heard form the brachial artery in the arm on the inside of the elbow. That is the location where the physician places stethoscope when measuring blood pressure.

DISPLAY SYSTEMS

The various modes of display on the ultrasound machine are:

1. Typical B scan image over the sector scanned

This is based on the pixels representing the values of the reflected signals at the points shown on the scan. The grey scale representation is enough to show the image of the area. The variations which take place with time (as in the moving heart walls) will be clearly seen. For viewing the heart, there are two or three positions of the probe. (Plate I.4)

A two chamber view from the supra sternal notch can give either the left or right side of the heart.

An apical view of the four chambers can be seen by keeping the probe at the apex of the heart position (below).

A long axis view placing the transducer at the left sternal border (between 3-5 intercoastal space, as convenient) and sliding or rotating the probe to get the view as shown in Fig. 8.34.

2. M-Mode View

This is a motion of any one chosen line as recorded with time on the X axis, in a slow time scale display.

This just plots the echo signals with time on the points of the chosen line marked by the operator on the B scan sector view.

A typical M mode view of the heart along with the views of long axis and four chamber colour Doppler pattern superimposed in shown in Plate I.5.

3. Spectrogram time display

The spectrogram is shown on the Doppler sample volume or Doppler sample direction as a time plot with the spectral bin amplitudes shown in grey scale, as for example in the Fig. 8.35.

The E and A wave indicate the Peak early velocity and peak atrial velocity and the E/A ratio is significant in clinical diagnosis. When the E and A waves merge together, and when the amplitudes indicate high velocities, it is indicative of a narrow valve.

The spectrogram can be calculated either for CW mode over the sampling line on the scan or for a typical sample volume in pulse Doppler mode.

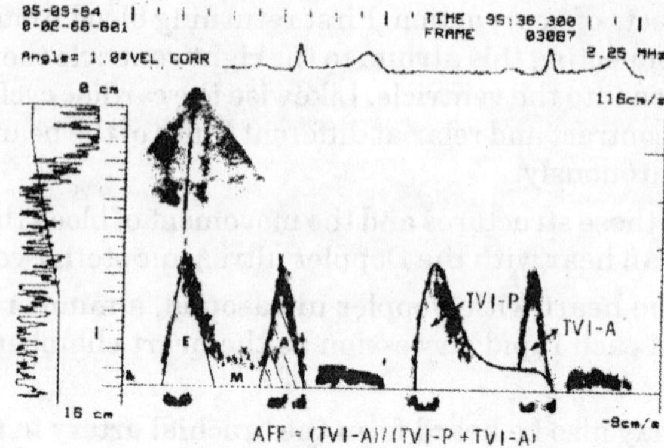

Fig. 8.35. Mitral inflow velocity recorded at the mitral annulus with superimposed diagrams illustrating the separation of the time velocity integral into early (E), mid (M), and atrial (A) segments.

DIRECT DIGITAL COMPUTER INTERFACE TO DOPPLER MACHINE

Finally, it should be remarked that it is possible to record the flow-separated Doppler signal (i.e., the forward and reverse flow components) directly form some demodulator units. This may be especially convenient for direct digital computer storage since the forward and reverse flow signals can be acquired separately so that only one anti-aliasing filter is required. However, it should be kept in mind that the analog circuitry which produces the flow separated components in the demodulator may not be precisely controlled. The separate flow components can generally be computed from the phase quadrature signal with greater precision on a digital spectrum analyser or on a computer. (Chapter 13)

Fig. 8.36 shows the system set up for this

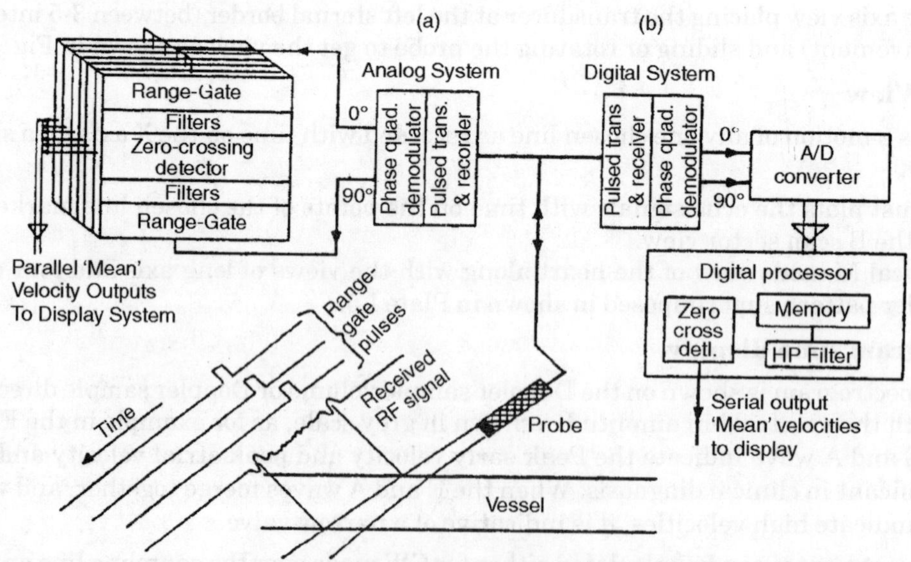

Fig. 8.36. Showing the principle of serial data signal processing technique.

This is convenient for doing considerable research work on stored samples of data on typical pathological conditions. (Chapter 13)

Chapter 9

X-Rays Instruments

X-RAY MACHINES FOR DIAGNOSIS

X-ray machines, discovered nearly a century ago, are still in use in hospitals. From the basic and simple X-ray imager for bone structures and lung observation, there are very many advanced applications of X-rays in which angiography and cine color imaging and Fluoroscopy are some recent ones. The use of X-rays for destruction of tumors has now been replaced by Radio isotope therapy.

Similar to other discoveries, X-rays were discovered by Roentgen in 1895 when he was investigating the cathode rays of a vacuum tube. What Roentgen did not discover, however and what it took scientists about 50 years to fully appreciate is that X-rays can be dangerous when they are not properly used and may cause cancer. Major engineering objectives for improving X-ray equipment are:

1. Minimize the dose of X-rays used on the patient.
2. Heighten the contrast between different tissues.
3. Improve size resolution
4. Improve the quality of the image.

The X-ray tube

The X-ray tube is simply a glass enclosed vacuum tube diode consisting of a cathode that thermally emits electrons and an anode that attracts these electrons. A functional diagram of an X-ray tube is given in Fig. 9.1 which shows a filament heated cathode, an anode, and a glass vacuum enclosure. The filament source voltage V_F caused a current I_F to flow through the filament coil, heating the cathode metal. The electrons in the cathode are boiled off the metal into the vacuum. The anode voltage V_A is the high enough that these electrons are swept across the anode and form the beam current I_B. V_A is of the order of 100 kV. This high voltage impels the electrons to a very high velocity. Approximately 1% of the electron upon entering the anode collide with atoms and produce X-rays which then pass through the tube into space. Electrons are boiled off the heated cathode because thermal agitation gives them enough energy to escape from the bonding forces into tube vacuum. The value of that energy, called the work function Ew differs among metals.

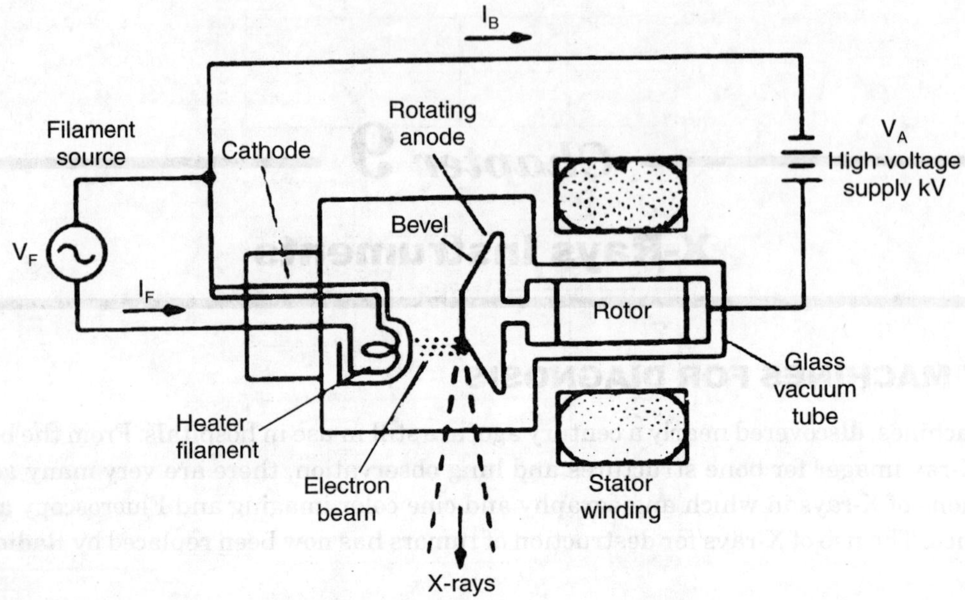

Fig. 9.1. A rotating anode X-ray generator.

Fig. 9.1. Shows an X-ray tube using a rotating anode.

Table 1: X-Ray Tube Cathode Material Coefficients and Work Functions.

Cathode	C_o ($A/m^2 K^2$)	E_w (eV)
Tungsten	$60*10^4$	4.52
Thoriated tungsten	$3*10^4$	2.63
Oxide coated	$0.01*10^4$	1

The value of the current in amperes due to thermal agitation

$$I_B = C_o A_c T^2 e^{-11600E\,w/T}$$

where A_c is the cathode area in square meters and C_o is the cathode material coefficient. Values of several materials used in cathodes are given in Table1. The equation for beam current holds good only when the anode voltage is very large to sweep all the electrons emitted. The current is limited by the temperature T and is therefore called thermally limited current. If VA is not enough, however, a space charge of electron will form around the cathode. Then the current would be depending on anode voltage and is called electronic current I_{BE}. Fig. 9.2 shows that beam current can be controlled with the temperature of the cathode. In X-ray tubes this method is used. This is done by keeping the anode voltage high enough to prevent a space charge region around the cathode. To control the cathode temperature, the operator normally varies the filament voltage. This allows the operator to change the beam current while holding the anode voltage constant.

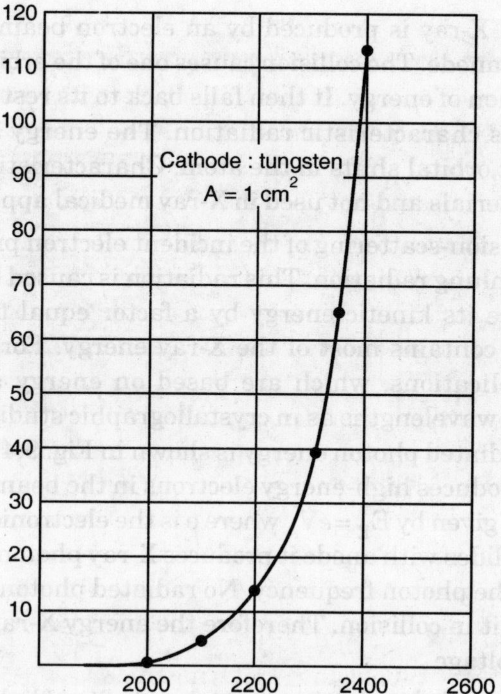

Fig. 9.2. Shows the thermally limited beam current versus cathode temperature of a tungsten cathode. (Y-axis in mA)

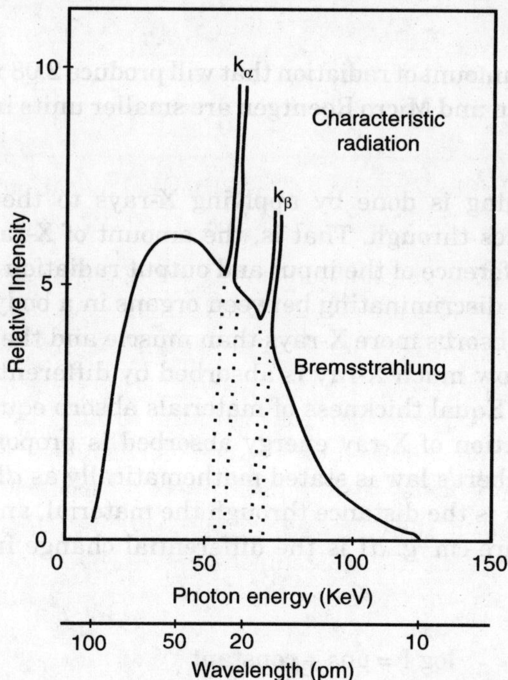

Fig. 9.3. Shows the X-ray spectrum emitted by a tungsten anode at 130 kV.

Type of X-rays. An X-ray is produced by an electron beam when one of the electrons collides with an atom in the anode. The collision causes one of the orbiting electrons of the atom to shift to higher orbital position of energy. It then falls back to its rest state and emits a photon of X-ray. This is called the as characteristic radiation. The energy shifts K_α and K_β shown in Fig. 9.3 represent different orbital shifts in the atom. Characteristic radiation is used to study the atomic structure of materials and not used in X-ray medical applications.

A second type of collision-scattering of the incident electron produces a spectrum of X-ray radiation called Bremsstrahlung radiation. This radiation is caused by changes in velocity of the beam electrons that reduce its kinetic energy by a factor equal to the energy in the X-ray. Bremsstrahlung radiation contains most of the X-ray energy. For this reason, it is the most important in medical applications, which are based on energy absorption rather than on measurement of particular wavelengths as in crystallographic studies using X-ray. The effect of the anode voltage on the radiated photon energy is shown in Fig. 9.4. Increased anode voltage at a constant beam current produces high-energy electrons in the beam. The energy of the electron when it strikes the anode is given by $E_E = eV_A$ where e is the electronic charge and E_E is measured in eV. When an electron collides with anode it produces X-ray photon of energy E_p = hf where h is Planck's constant and f is the photon frequency. No radiated photon can have more energy than the electron that produces it in collision. Therefore the energy X-ray photon cannot exceed eV_A and are limited by anode voltage.

The frequency of X-ray photon f = c/λ where c is velocity of light and λ is the wavelength of radiation emitted.

The X-rays in medical diagnostics use wavelength of X-rays between 0.1 to 1° Angstrom.

Units of X-rays

One Roentgen is the amount of radiation that will produce 2.08×10^9 ion pairs per milliliter of air at STP. Milli-Roentgen and Micro Roentgen are smaller units in application.

X-ray Absorption

Medical X-ray imaging is done by applying X-rays to the surface of the body and measuring how much passes through. That is, the amount of X-ray absorbed by the body is measured by taking the difference of the input and output radiation energies. X-ray absorption is the basic mechanism for discriminating between organs in a body under X-ray observation. Bone tissue, for example, absorbs more X-rays than muscle and therefore can be easily distinguished from it. Exactly how much X-ray is absorbed by different tissues is determined by Lambert's law for X-rays. Equal thickness of materials absorb equal proportions of radiation *I*. In other words, the fraction of X-ray energy absorbed is proportional to thickness of the material absorbing it. Lambert's law is stated mathematically as $dI/I = -\mu \rho ds$ where ρ is the medium density (g/cm^3), *ds* is the distance through the material, and μ is the mass attenuation coefficient. The units of μ are cm^2/g. *d*I is the differential change in intensity I in a distance *ds*.

Integrating,

$$\log I = \mu\rho s + \text{constant}$$

When $s = 0$, the intensity of incident radiation is I_o

$$\text{Log } I_o = \text{constant}$$

$$K \log I = -\mu\rho s + \log I_o$$

$$\text{Log}(I/I_o) = -\mu\rho s;$$

$$I/I_o = e^{-\mu\rho s};\ \mathbf{I = I_o\, e^{-\mu\rho s}}$$

Fig. 9.4 shows the effect of the anode voltage on the emission spectrum, from an X-ray tube.

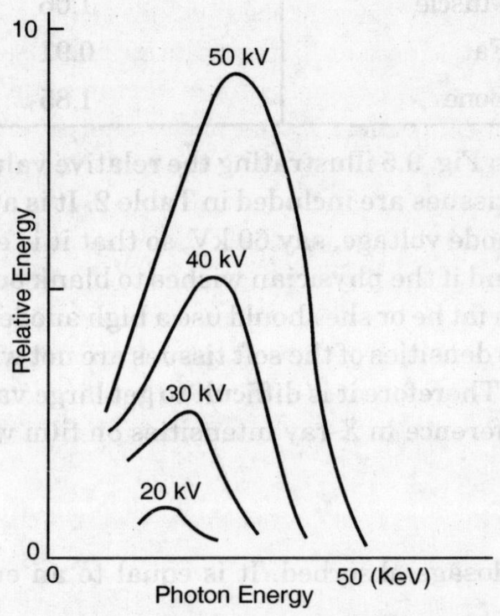

Fig. 9.4. Anode volts vs emission energy.

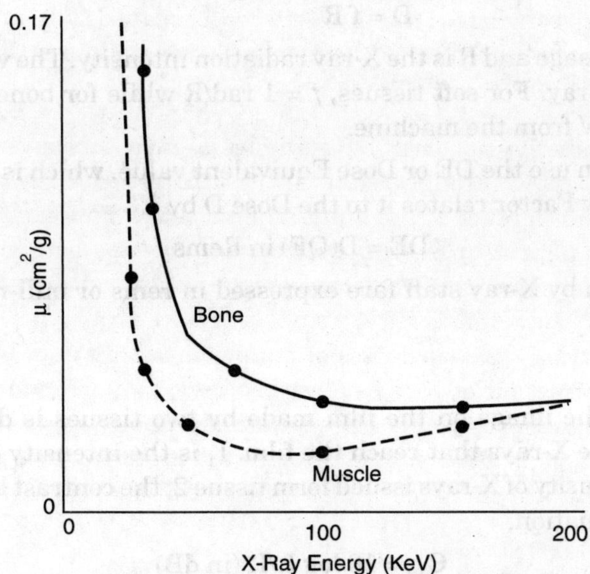

Fig. 9.5. X-ray energy keV versus attenuation.

Fig. 9.5 shows the mass attenuation coefficient versus the X-ray photon energy.

Table 2 : Density of common biological materials.

Material	Density (g/cm²)
Air	0.0013
Water	1.0
Muscle	1.06
Fat	0.91
Bone	1.85

Values for μ are given in Fig. 9.5 illustrating the relative values for bone and muscle. Also typical densities of biological tissues are included in Table 2. It is apparent that to study bone, a physician should use a low anode voltage, say 60 kV, so that it is easy to distinguish the under lying muscle. On the other hand if the physician wishes to blank out the bone to distinguish the under lying muscle tissue from fat he or she should use a high anode voltage, say 200 kV. It is also clear from the table 2, that the densities of the soft tissues are not widely different. Furthermore, the μ values are nearly equal. Therefore it is difficult to get large values of contrast between soft tissues using X-rays. This difference in X-ray intensities on film will produce an image having good contrast properties.

Dosage

'RAD" is the unit of dosage absorbed. It is equal to an energy amount of .01 J/Kg of irradiated matter.

The Roentgen and Rad D are related by

$$D = f R$$

Where D is the Dosage and R is the X-ray radiation intensity. The value of f is based on the matter absorbing the X-ray. For soft tissues, $f = 1$ rad/R while for bone, f is larger. f however decreases with higher kV from the machine.

Another concept in use the DE or Dose Equivalent value, which is based on the biological effect. The QF or Quality Factor relates it to the Dose D by

$$DE = D(QF) \text{ in Rems.}$$

Film badges worn by X-ray staff fare expressed in rems or mill-rems, where rem is the biological effect unit.

Tissue contrast

The contrast in the image on the film made by two tissues is defined in terms of the relative intensities of the X-rays that reach the film. I_1 is the intensity of X-rays emitted from tissue 1 and I_2 is the intensity of X-rays issued form tissue 2; the contrast between the two tissues is then defined by the equation.

$$C_{12} = 10 \log I_1/I_2 \text{ (in dB)}$$

Here the multiplier 10 is used because the ratio I_1 to I_2 is a power ratio.

$$C_{12} = 10 \log \frac{I_0 e^{-\mu 1 \rho 1 s 1}}{I_0 e^{-\mu 2 \rho 2 s 2}}$$

$$C_{12} = 10 (\log_e) (\mu_2 \rho_2 s_2 - \mu_1 \rho_1 s_1) \text{ or}$$

$$C_{12} = 4.3429 (\mu_2 \rho_2 s_2 - \mu_1 \rho_1 s_1) \text{ dB}$$

From this equation we conclude that the contrast between two tissues depends on their mass attenuation coefficient density and thickness. In fact C_{12} increases with difference between these parameters. To visualize soft tissues it is often necessary to administer a contrast medium. There are several media which can give positive or negative contrast. If gas is administered (CO_2, air, O_2) a negative contrast results because of high density of surrounding tissues. If contrast media consisting of elements with high atomic numbers are administered, usually Barium, a positive contrast is obtained because of the higher mass attenuation coefficient and higher density of these elements. Thus a barium meal enema is given for observations with X-rays on the lower intestine regions. These X-ray procedures are now replaced by Ultrasound scanning methods, however.

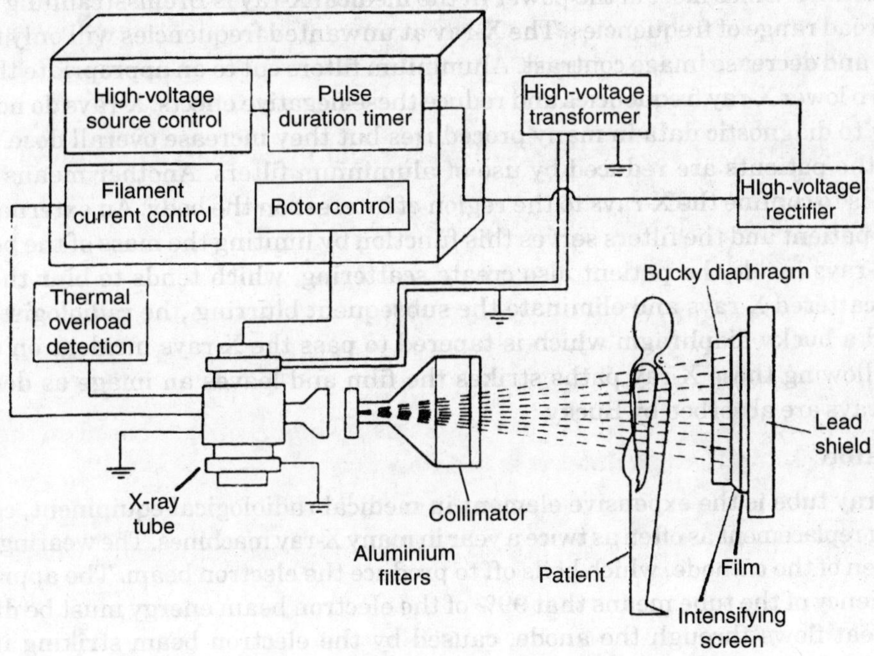

Fig. 9.6. Shows a block diagram of an X-ray machine.

X-RAY DIAGNOSTIC MACHINES

The basic components that must be part of any medical diagnostic X-ray unit are shown in Fig. 9.6. In general, the purpose of these components is to create an X-ray image of high density, high contrast and high sharpness on film or other imaging device. This must be done while minimizing the dose of ionizing radiation given to the patient. The *density* or darkness of the image is proportional to the amount of X-ray tube beam current. *Contrast* is measure of darkness of a desired image compared to its surroundings and it is basically determined by the relative attenuation by the object. This factor is often directly affected by X-ray beam voltage. Sharpness of clarity of the edges is reduced in an image by blurring due to distortions in the X-ray beam as it passes from the X-ray tube to the patient. A high voltage source from 20 to 200 kV is necessary in order to produce X-ray at the X-ray tube anode. However, the duration of the time the high voltage is applied to the tube must be carefully limited, in order that the patient does receive an excessive dose, the film does not become over-exposed and the X-ray tube does not over heat. Since the X-ray tube is operated in its thermally limited mode, X-ray intensity in Watts per square metre is adjusted by the X-ray tube filament current. As a protection against overheating, the temperature of the tube's anode is monitored with a temperature detector. If it exceeds a specified value, a thermal overload will be detected and the high voltage supply will be turned of automatically. This will eliminate source of heat and cause the X-ray tube to turn off. Most X-ray tube anodes are rotated by induction motor action in order to limit the beam at anyone spot and to help cool the anode. The voltage level from the high-voltage source is set by taps on the high voltage transformer stepped up to the 200 kV level. It is then rectified and passed through the X-ray tube, which acts as also the rectifier. Since most of the power in the medical X-ray is Bremsstrahlung radiation, it contains a broad range of frequencies. The X-ray at unwanted frequencies will only increase the patient dose and decrease image contrast. Aluminium filters cut to an appropriate thickness are used to absorb lower X-ray frequencies and reduce these negative effects. X-rays do not contribute significantly to diagnostic data in many procedures but they increase overall dose. Soft X-rays incident on the patients are reduced by use of aluminium filters. Another means of reducing patient dose is to confine the X-rays to the region of interest on the body. An external collimator between the patient and the filters serves this function by limiting the mass of the body exposed to X-rays. X-rays inside the patient also create scattering, which tends to blur the image. To absorb the scattered X-rays and eliminate the subsequent blurring ,the radiologist uses a lead screen called a bucky diaphragm which is tapered to pass the X-rays incident on the patient. Radiation following these X-ray paths strikes the film and leaves an image as desired, while scattered X-rays are absorbed by Bucky

The X-ray tube

An X-ray tube is the expensive element in medical radiological equipment, costing more and requiring replacement as often as twice a year in many X-ray machines. The wearing mechanism is the tungsten of the cathode, which boils off to produce the electron beam. The approximately 1 percent efficiency of the tube means that 99% of the electron beam energy must be dissipated as heat. This heat flows through the anode, caused by the electron beam striking it, raises its temperature to destructive levels if it is not limited. Rotating the anode at speeds ranging from 3600 to 10,000 rpm, the heat is spread over larger mass and allows its dissipation by radiation. For any tube the amount of heat that can be dissipated is fixed. Since the energy absorbed by the anode is proportional to the product of the anode voltage V_A, the beam current I_B and exposure time T_D, a set of curves called the X-ray tube rating charts must be consulted to find the maximum exposure time for a given tube V_A and I_B. An example curve is given in Fig. 9.7. The efficiency of the X-ray tube is equal to the ratio of the power emitted in the X-ray beam P_X, to the applied power at voltage V_A and is proportional to $V_A{}^2$. Also large values of both I_B and the atomic number of the material Z increase the probability of a collision of the beam electron with an atom of the anode material. Therefore the power P_X in the X-ray beam is proportional to all of these factors as

$$P_X = K\, I_B\, Z\, V_A^2$$

where K is a proportionality constant. The power in the electron beam is just $V_A\, I_B$. The tube efficiency, is defined as the ratio of P_X to the power in the electron beam.

i.e.
$$= \frac{K\, I_B\, Z V_A^2}{I_B\, V_A} = KZ\, V_A$$

Empirically the constant K is determined to be $K = 1.4 \times 10^{-9}\, V^{-1}$. The anode is shown as beveled. The bevel directs the X-rays at the side of the tube. The desired X-rays pass through a slot into a collimator and some of the X-rays fi om the anode scatter about in the tube and are absorbed by lead shielding.

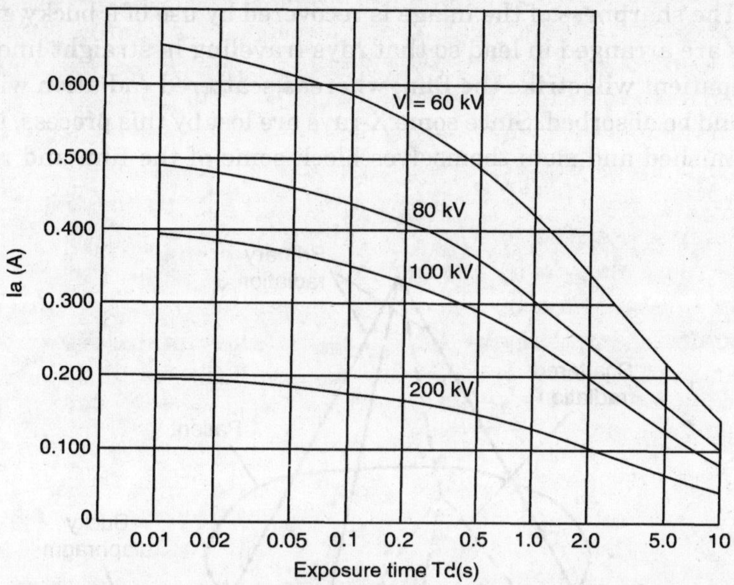

Fig. 9.7. Shows the tube exposure time limit at given current and anode voltage levels.

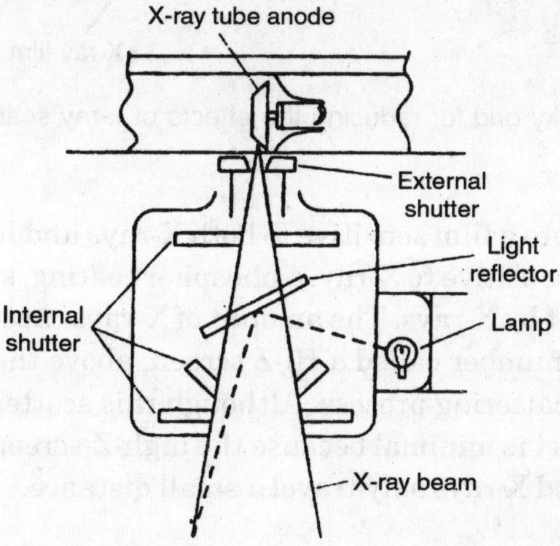

Fig. 9.8. Shows a collimator for directing X-rays at the patient.

The collimator

In order to reduce the dose of X-rays to the patient the beam should not strike any more of the body than necessary. The necessary shaping of the X-ray beam is done with a collimator as shown in Fig. 9.8. The shutters consist of heavy metal to absorb unwanted X-rays. A lamp and reflective mirror that makes a visible pattern on the patient, so that the attendant can tell where the X-rays will strike, can be used to align the beam.

The Bucky grid

After X-rays enter a patient, some rays are deflected off their straight-line course by close encounters with atoms. This scattering causes smearing of the image at the edges and deteriorates image sharpness. The sharpness of the image is recovered by use of a bucky grid illustrated in Fig. 9.9. Here slots are arranged in lead so that rays traveling in straight lines from the X-ray tubes through the patient will strike the film, whereas scattered radiation will strike the lead lining of the slots and be absorbed. Since some X-rays are lost by this process, the density of the image will be diminished and slots themselves block some of the film and reduce the image resolution.

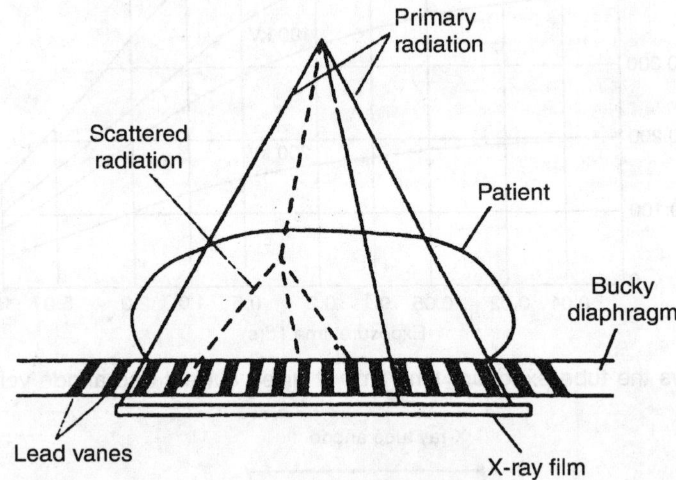

Fig. 9.9. Shows a bucky grid for reducing the effects of x-ray scattering in the patient.

The X-ray detector

The X-rays now pass into a film sensitive to both X-rays and light, such as silver bromide. Since the film is relatively insensitive to X-ray, a phosphor coating, such as shown in Fig. 9.10, is used to produce light when hit by X-rays. The amount of X-rays captured is increased by placing a material with high atomic number called a Hi-Z screen, above the phosphor. This introduces secondary radiation by the scattering process. Although this scattering would tend to decrease the image sharpness, the effect is minimal because the high-Z-screen is immediately adjacent to the phosphor and the deflected X-rays only travel a small distance.

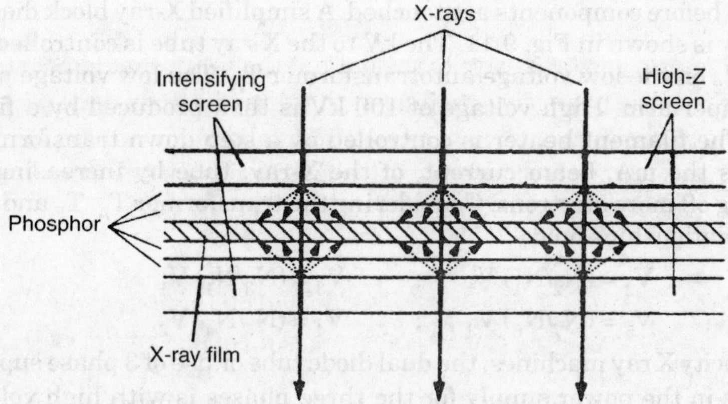

Fig. 9.10. Shows an image-intensifying film.

The Power Supply

The power supply for an X-ray machine plays a crucial and active role in X-ray production. The radiation is turned on and off in the power supply. It is used to control the X-ray energy and

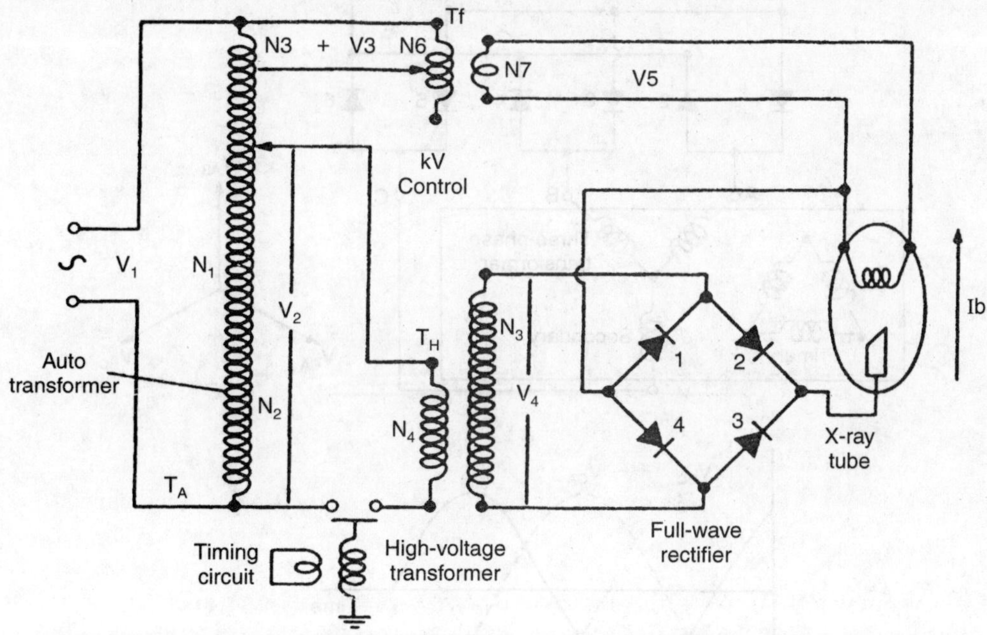

Fig. 9.11. Shows a single-phase high-voltage power supply.

consequently image contrast as well as the beam current and consequently image density. Thermal overload from X-ray tube anode creates signals that turn the power supply off as appropriate. The power supply must be large to handle several kW of power and several 100 kV levels. At such high voltages, safety precautions are necessary. The voltage breakdown of air at sea level is 30 kV/cm. Therefore, at X-ray voltages, a conductor as such as a technician's hand, within several inches of a high voltage terminal can draw a deadly arc of voltage. As a safety precaution, when working on X-ray power supplies, a technician should turn off all power supplies, if possible and the capacitors must be discharged before components are touched. A simplified X-ray block diagram for a single-phase power supply is shown in Fig. 9.11. The kV to the X-ray tube is controlled by adjusting the number of Turns N_2 on the low voltage autotransformer T_A. The low voltage prevents arcing of the transformer wiper arm. High voltage of 100 kV is then produced by a fixed high voltage transformer, T_H. The filament heater is controlled by a step down transformer T_F. Adjusting turns ratio N_6 sets the mA, beam current, of the X-ray. tube by increasing the heat to the filament and boiling off more electrons. Considering the transformer T_A, T_F and T_H to be ideal the following voltage relationships hold:

$$V_2 = (N_2/N_1)\,V_1 \quad ; \quad V_3 = (N_3/N_1)\,V_1$$

$$V_5 = (N_7/N_6)\,V_3 \quad ; \quad V_4 = (N_5/N_4)\,V_2$$

In large capacity X ray machines, the dual diode tube or use of 3 phase supply are employed. The crucial change in the power supply for the three phases is with high voltage transformer illustrated in the Fig. 9.12. In three phases voltage system V_{AB} V_{BC} and V_{CA} are the same magnitude and are displaced in phases by 120 from each other as shown in the Fig. 9.12.

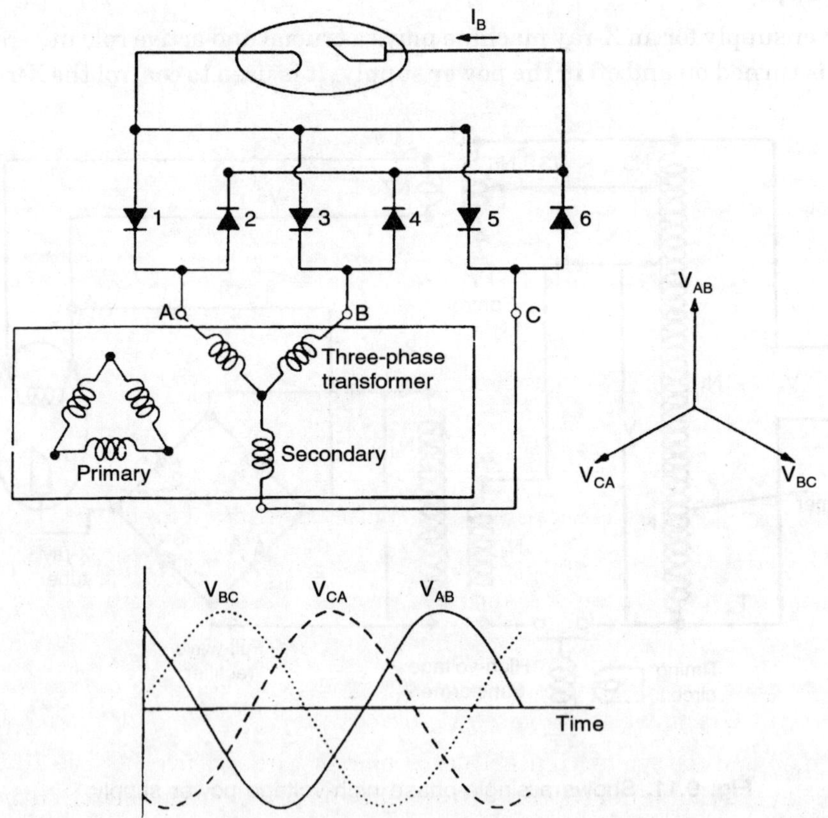

Fig. 9.12. Shows a three-phase X-ray tube power supply.

Fluoroscopic System

In various medical procedures, the physician views an X-ray image instantly, so they can monitor movements of organs and other objects put into the body. In a cardiac catherization procedure the physician may wish to watch the catheter as it is moved through the veins into the heart ventricle or when a kidney stone is being pulverized with ultrasonic waves, it may be monitored using X-rays. Such instantaneous fluoroscopic pictures are called real time images, such as we see on live television broadcasts. The basics components of the fluoroscopic unit as shown in the Fig. 9.13

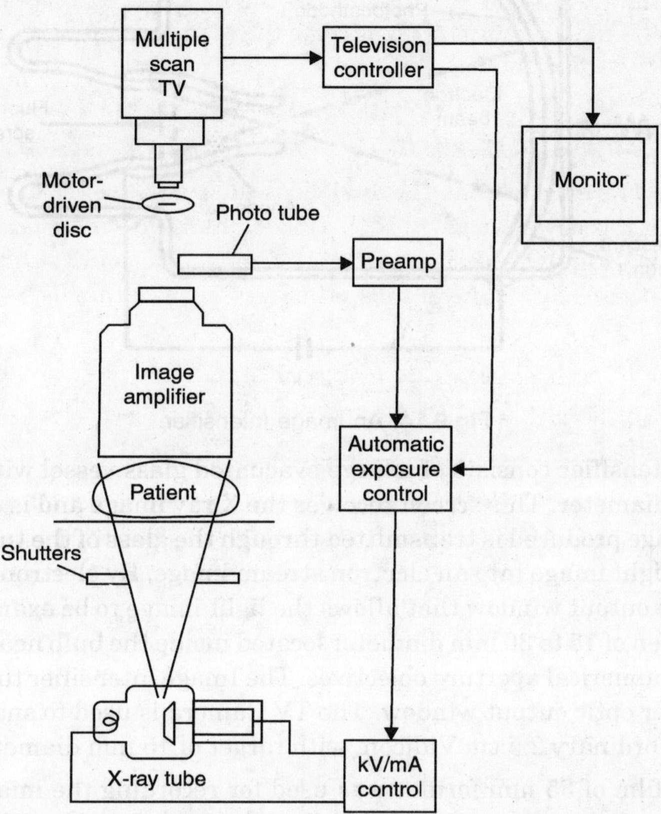

Fig. 9.13. Shows a typical digital fluoroscopic system.

1. X-ray tube fed by a high voltage supply and the control unit under the table. The patient is placed on the table top. A lead shield protects the operator from radiation.
2. An image intensifier amplifies the image and converts the X-ray into light.
3. A television camera picks up the image and transfers it to a television monitor for viewing by a radiologist or operator.

A block diagram of a typical digital fluoroscopic system appears in Fig. 9.13. In this system, information about the image density is fed to an automatic exposure control, so that if the image begins to fade, the beam current on the X-ray tube will automatically increase. The unique component of fluoroscopic system is the image intensifier, shown in Fig. 9.14. The X-rays strike a fluorescent screen, producing light. The light then strikes photocathode which produces electrons. The electrons are accelerated by 25 kV potential and are focused on the fluorescent screen which produces increased light and a denser image. This light image can be photographed or picked up with a television camera. The fluorescent screen consists of many 2–3 μm phosphor crystals that emit light when bombarded by high energy particles. For example a medium-short persistence of blue color is produced by ZnS : Ag(Ni) crystals. If light photons with sufficient energy strike a photo cathode, electrons are emitted known as photo electrons. Common photo cathode materials consist of alloys of cesium and tin.

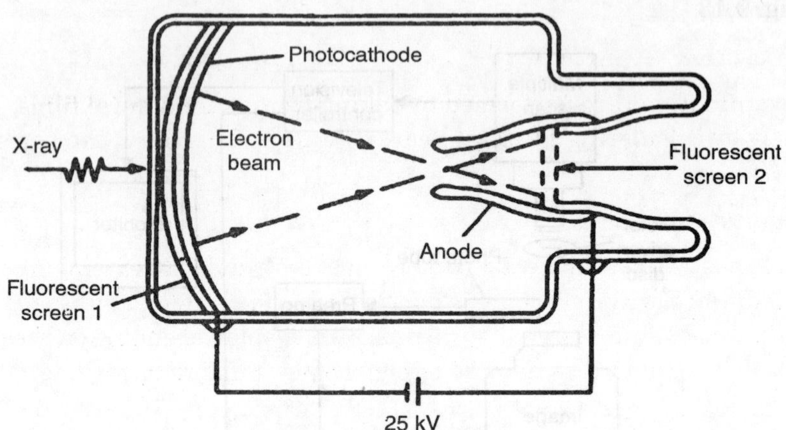

Fig.9.14. An image intensifier.

The Image intensifier consists of a large evacuated glass vessel with the input having a screen of 15–32 cm diameter. This screen receives the X ray image and is converted into a light image. The light image produced is transmitted through the glass of the tube to a photo-cathode which converts the light image into an electron stream image. By electron amplification, image gets intensified. The output window that allows the light image to be examined, is presented to the output view screen of 15 to 30 mm diameter located inside the bulb near the window. Lenses are used with large numerical aperture objectives. The Image intensifier tube by Thompson CSF Company uses a fiber optic output window. The TV Camera is used to snap the image. The TV tube pick is just the ordinary 2.5 cm Vidicon, with target of 15 mm diameter.

Earlier Cine film of 35 mm format was used for recording the image intensifier output image as useful for cardiology investigations. Today, this is replaced by CD recording, through a video input card on the PC or Computer. Video digitize cards of high resolution in colour are available from Matrox Inc., USA for this purpose.

X-ray examination of the Organs

The skeletal structures are easy to visualize since there is no need to administer a contrast medium into the body. In fracture examinations, two exposures taken in perpendicular directions are required for reliable determination of the positions of the fracture.

Respiratory Organs

Chest radiographs are taken mainly for examination of the lungs and heart. In order to reduce interfering skeletal shadows in lung examination, high tube voltages, 150 kV are chosen. Because the air is enclosed in the respiratory tract, the longer bronchi are seen as negative contrast and the pulmonary vessels are seen as positive contrast against the air filled lung tissue. Lung tumors may be primary or secondary in type.

Bronchial Carcinoma

It occurs as primary growth in the lungs and is difficult to diagnose at an early stage. A special method of examination used in cases of suspected tumor is Bronchography. A viscous water soluble contrast medium containing iodine is injected into the bronchi of one lung. Then the X-ray image is taken.

Circulatory Organs

Heart examinations are performed by taking frontal and lateral films. The evaluation is performed partly by calculating the total heart volume and partly on the basis of any change in shape.

Digestive Organs

The whole gastrointestinal tract can be imaged by using an emulsion of barium sulphate as a contrast medium. Barium sulphate is non-toxic due to its low solubility nature. The contrast medium is swallowed or administered by means of an enema depending on the part of the tract is to be examined. Ulcers, tumors, swallowed foreign bodies, inflammatory conditions etc. are clearly seen.

Excretory Organs

The urinary tract is examined by means of different contrast media which are administered either via urethral Ortium or via the blood stream when the contrast medium is excreted through the kidneys.

Radiology by X-Rays

X-rays are electromagnetic radiation located at the low wavelength end of the electromagnetic spectrum. The X-rays in the medical diagnostic region have wavelength in the order of 0.1 to 1°A. The speed of propagation is 3×10^{10} cm/s and are not affected by electric and magnetic fields. According to quantum theory, electromagnetic radiation consists of photons which are conceived as packets of energy. Their interaction with matter involves an energy exchange and the relation between the wavelength and the photon is given by

$$E = h\nu = h(c/\lambda)$$

Where h = plank's constant = 6.62×10^{-34} J s.

C = velocity of propagation of light (3×10^{10} cm/second)

ν = frequency of radiation

λ = wavelength

Any vibration of the particle can be characterized by its frequency or by its wavelength. In the case of x-rays, the wavelength is directly dependant on the voltage with which the radiation is produced.

It is therefore, common to characterize x-rays by the voltage which is measure of the energy of the radiation.

In seeking the technological development that has made the impact in medicine, there is no hesitation in selecting the X-ray machine. The discovery by Roentgen in 1985 of X-rays, with their property in penetrating substances opaque to light, has obvious advantage in medicine as a diagnostic tool for photographing internal structure of the body. At the beginning of this century, exposure of up to 30 minutes were often necessary to produce a picture and initial developments were in the production of the necessary high voltages. Then came the replacement of the gas tube by the hot cathode tube leading to the present rotating anode tubes, with outputs of up to 500 mA at switching periods down to 20ms. Later developments using electronic techniques brought further improvement in generation and control equipment.

The first use of X-rays was the detection and location of foreign bodies, urinary calcius and the demonstration of fractures, but there was little radiology of the gastro intestinal tract owing mainly to the long exposure time that was necessary. The insertion of fluoroscope intensifying screen behind the object and the introduction of contrast media have decreased the exposure time and increased contrast, respectively, opening up many new fields of investigation. In the modern image intensifier, an image of fluorescent screen can be transferred to a plate. This reduction in dosage allows the changing situation following a barium meal to be displayed continuously on either cine film or television.

Following the realization that could cause skin reaction, attempts were made to use them therapeutically and the first success came in skin cancers. For the selective destruction of tissues, higher radiation energies were needed. The early X-ray–therapy equipment with output of 2–5 mA at 200 kV has been improved to the modern therapy machine of 30mA at a voltage up to 2 MV.

Maintenance of X ray equipment in Hospitals

X-ray machines are designed to operate on 230 V AC or 416 V AC mains but in six valve rectified diagnostic machines, 3 phase system is used.

Modern 4 valve machines are 35 kW to 40 KVA at least.

The regulation should be noted (voltage drop on switching unit on and loading by taking X ray).

Cables must be of adequate cross section to minimize such voltage drop.

For self rectified (simpler X-ray circuit, the other half cycle voltage rises if the regulation is poor.

Supply must be free from fluctuations in voltage, say by other loads on the distribution line. So, separate feeder from distribution bus bar must be used. Further, the maker usually specifies the power requirements correctly and they must be adhered to.

Maintenance of X ray machine are dealt with by trained persons only.

1. Moving parts of tables, tube stands, screen stands should have no dust or dirt and they should be oiled.
2. Steel suspension cables are to be inspected for fraying.
3. Earth continuity check should be made.
4. Screws should be carefully tightened.
5. Shock proof cables should not bend sharply (*r >> 1.5 Diameter)*
6. Oil in transformer should be checked for level, leak and oil dielectric strength should be checked with an oil (H.V.) tester. If it is not good, the same should be reconditioned or the oil replaced.

Then the instrument should be checked for any incorrect functioning.

The indicating instruments on panel should be noted as working alright. (No needle stuck).

Mains voltage meter, tube filament meter ; or through transparent window the filament should be observed.

A second tube should be kept on hand.

The Exposure switch has a primary contactor which closes the primary circuit. This must be checked. Not closing may also be due to protective devices, interlocks, a series switch in the coil etc.

Tube protection interlock. kV, I (mA), t products exceeds rating or set values must be checked.

Tube overload interlock. Thermal due to previous exposures.

Cooling system interlock. For therapy tube, check flow and rate.

Door interlock. This is very important.

Filter interlock. While in therapy tube use.

Rotating anode interlock. Not rotating. Check for continuity in 3 core cable to tube shield.

Bucky interlock. Try non bucky mode.

If the interlocks are alright but still the machine does not produce X ray, check whether the filaments of all valves are alright.

Failure of one valve in a 2 valve unit filament would prevent any h.t. from reaching the tube.

Four valve unit: one fails means half wave rectification and the reading on mA would be halved.

Excessive secondary current

mA meter indicates excessive current and cannot be altered by mA control:

1. Gassy tube which may also be overheating
2. A breakdown in insulation of the shock-proof HT cables to tube. Check by switch over to another tube.
3. Gassy rectifier valve. (It is a virtual short circuit).

Antistatic. Explosive gases like Ethyl chloride, ether, cyclopropane mixed with air, N_2O, Oxygen are extremely inflammable.

Trichloroethylene is not to be used with surgical diathermy in the mouth.

Explosions data indicate that

60%—Electric spark

14%—Diathermy machines

8%—Elec. Spark from switches or sockets.

Materials which do not build up charge have to be used. Usually air is kept humid at >60%. Means for charge dissipation has to be provided.

Chapter 10

CT Scanning

COMPUTER TOMOGRAPHIC SCAN MACHINES

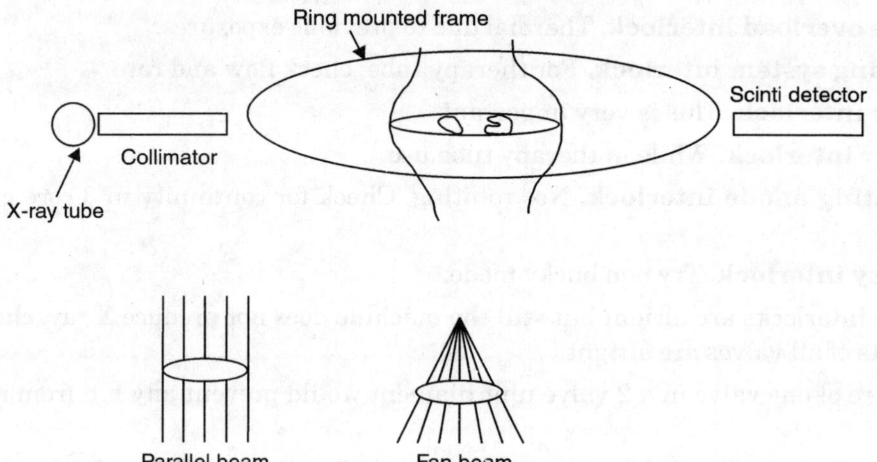

Fig.10.1. (a) Shows the schematic of the X-ray tomography b) two geometries.

The parallel beam geometry is easy to implement and the other one is useful for better image details through calculations. The fan angle is between 30 to 50°.

The patient table has provision for tilting slightly up to 15°, so that oblique sections can be taken. There is a height adjustment provision for centering by which of 84–103 cm is available for the head and 93–104 cm for the body parts.

The attenuation co-efficient μ is the ratio of the X-ray intensity obtained on the detector with the body inserted and without it.

Tissues have varying values of the co-efficient, for *e.g.*, fat (breast) has 0.19 cm^{-1}, while heart muscle has 0.212. Water has a value of 0.205 cm^{-1}.

There is another unit in the name of the inventor Hounsfield, given by the ratio

$$H = [\mu - \mu_{H_2O}] / \mu_{H_2O} \times 1000$$

Thus various tissue have a range between – 1000 (air) and + 1000 (dense matter).

As most tissue in the regions of the body lie between – 200 to + 80, it is possible to map the picture in this range for forming an image of a section.

The X-radiation from the tube is a pulsed type. During rotation of the ring, E.H.T. voltage is continuously applied to the tube. There is the grid inside the X ray tube which is used for pulsing. As the ring rotates, a timing signal generates electrical pulses each of which pulses the X ray beam. The use of pulsed recording is advantageous due to the fact that the motion artifact of the patient is less and hence the resolution does not suffer. The dosage of X rays which the body receives is to be determined by the operator in his settings.

The noise signal increases with the dosage of X ray. The Dose is dentoed by D, which is the maximum amount of absorbed skin radiation at 1.3 ± 0.1 rad (J/kg). The dose is obtained from the generator output, the length and number of X ray pulses.

Usually, about 2 to 2.5 RAD for head regions and 1–2 RAD for body region is the choice. The tube voltage can be from 100 to 125 kV. The X ray unit milliamperes, mA, as it is called is between 75 to 60 mA, and the number of projections may be from 360 to 720. The pulse time can be varied from 1.5 to 7 ms. The current mA can also be varied in some machines from 20 to 600 mA in steps.

The resolution of the image of a section is dependant on the signal to noise ratio, which is dependent on the radiation and the no. of steps.

Fluctuations in X-ray beam should be avoided by having controlled generation of X-rays with proper control circuitry to maintain the H.T. constant and by proper cooling of the target of the tube.

All the four quantities–Tube KV, Time of pulse, Intensity, and exposure time–all these contribute to signal improvement over noise.

CT is particularly done by

1. Scanning only a thin, well defined volume of interest, which serves to minimize the superimposition effects
2. minimizing scatter by collimating down to relatively thin volumes
3. using linear detectors, with computer based window functions.

The number of projections taken over the circumference decide the resolution, the larger the better, of course, at the expense of intense computation. If 240 projections are made, it will take 3 seconds, if 360 are taken it may take 5 s, and for 720 projections, it will be around 10 seconds.

The high contrast areas are resolved better with more number of projections; the low contrast tissue matter are resolved if the X radiation is adjusted to optimum.

ALGORITHM FOR TOMOGRAPHY

There are many methods of computing the image intensity (density) from the integrated value of the absorption by X ray on any path.

Thus, on the path shown, the region between pq where the object is present causes a reduction of the X ray beam intensity given by

$\int_p^q \exp[-f(x, y)]\, dl$ is the amount of attenuation when the density at a point inside is denoted by $f(x, y)$. The integral is denoted as $g(r, \theta)$. This is the observed signal at an angle θ.

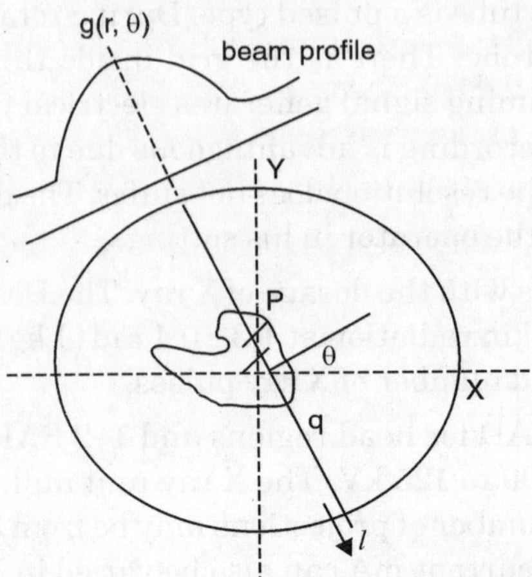

Fig.10.2. Showing the calculation of the net attenuation as an integral of the path of the object between p and q.

From the values of g at any r and θ, it is required to find the function f(x,y).

This is done by several methods.

1. Back projection technique

Out of the many machines, this is the one mostly used. The image profile at any line is resolved by the [cos θ, sin θ] transformation to give the positions of the pixels with respect the basic x, y axes. By this, each of the measured data is projected back over the area at the same angle from which it was taken. A filter function is made before the back projection.

2. The Algebraic Reconstruction Technique

This algorithm treats the pixels of the slice as a matrix of values, and the integral equations of the absorptions on the several angles are used to invert this matrix and find out the values of the density coefficients of the pixels.

3. Fourier Transform method

In this method, after convolving the shadow function with a filter so that each point in the projection has a negative value, instead of zero, the resulting profiles are transformed into the Fourier space of 2-D Fourier transform. Then, after summation, the inverse transform provides the picture. The convolution function or kernel, decides on the picture. The smoothing kernel, for instance, will reduce image noise and motion artifacts. The kernel for head calculation takes into the effect of the bones forming the skull, in order to reduce the "Cup" effect.

On CT images, the following analysis are done.

1. ROI calculation
2. 3 D reconstruction
3. histogram and image profile
4. sagittal and coronal reconstruction from axial image etc.

The reconstructed slice image is either printed on viewed on a CT monitor.

The pixel levels are divided into 2000 levels of gray scale. It is possible to expand this level scale so as to show certain regions with improved contrast, by narrowing the range to lesser numbers. Further calculations can of course be performed on the image, such as the area of an image part (organ), Histogram of the image and so on.

From multiple slices, it is also possible to show a 3-D image model of the region of the body.

With present computers, the images can be stored and distributed even on a CD for recording purposes.

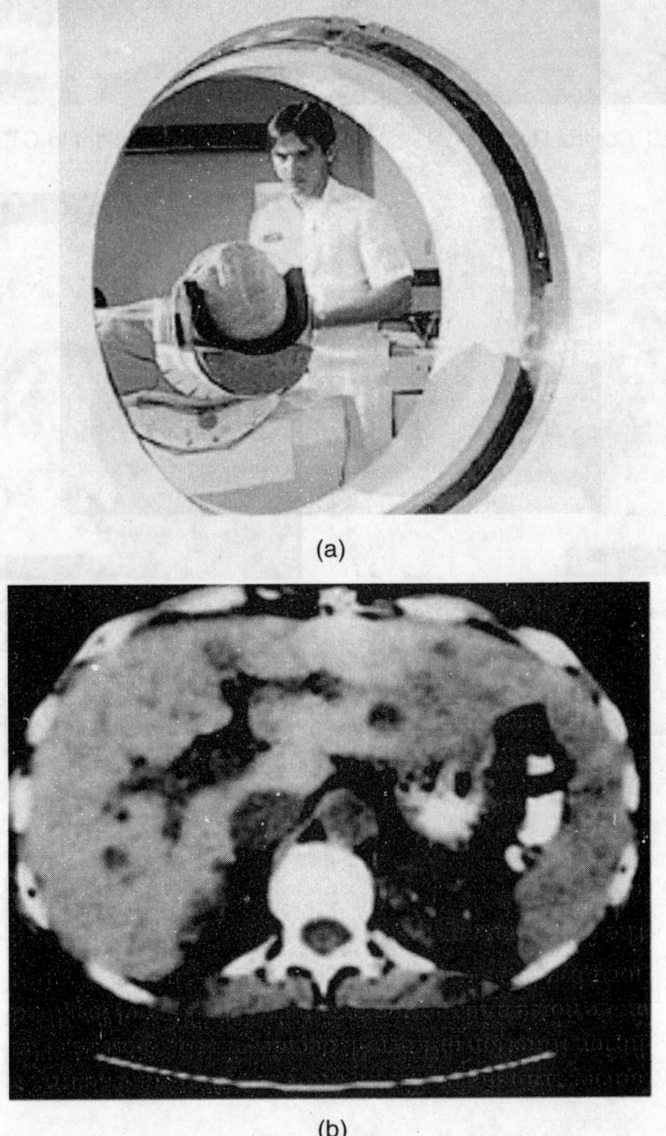

(a)

(b)

Fig. 10.3. (a) Showing the patient head being scanned Inside the ring which houses the X ray unit And the detector unit diagonally opposite. (b) Shows the CT image of liver of the body clearly inside the abdominal c.s.

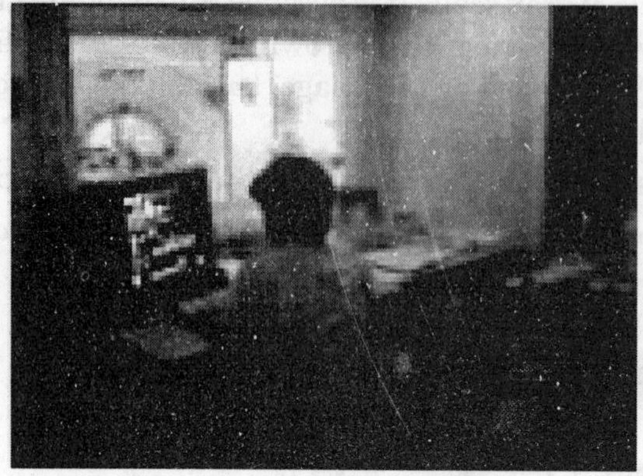

(a) CT Control Room

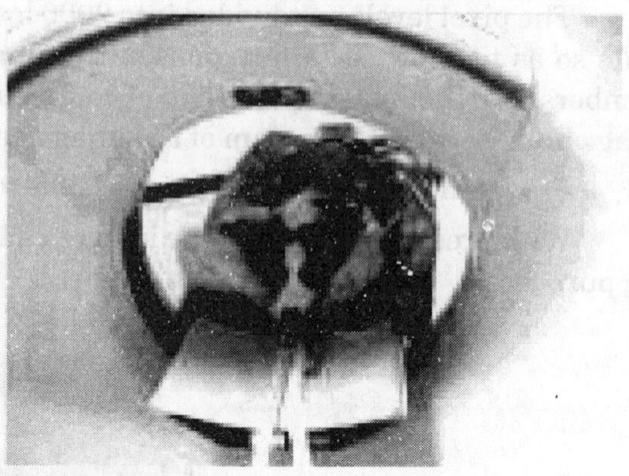

(b) Patient in CT Scanner

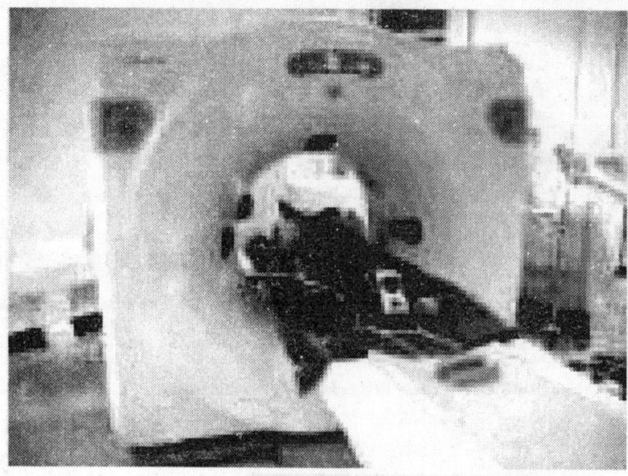

(c) Patient in CT Scanner

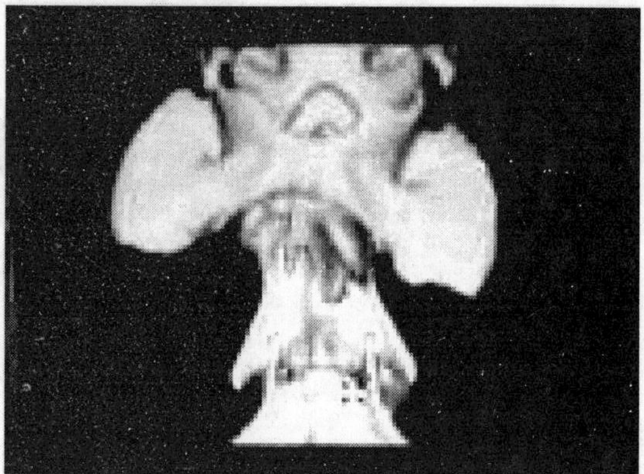

(d) 3D Reconstruction of a fracture of the 2nd cervical vertebra

Fig. 10.4. The figures show the CT room, the patient placed in the scanner and the image of fracture noted on the instrument monitor after processing of the data.

Chapter 11

Magnetic Resonance Imaging (MRI)

MAGNETIC INTENSITY

To understand how MRI works, let us start by focusing on the "magnetic" in MRI. The biggest and most important component in an MRI system is the **magnet**. The magnet in an MRI system is rated using a unit of measure known as a **tesla**. Another unit of measure commonly used with magnets is the **gauss** (1 tesla = 10,000 gauss). The magnets in use today in MRI are in the 0.5-tesla to 2.0-tesla range, or 5,000 to 20,000 gauss. Magnetic fields greater than **2 tesla** have not been approved for use in medical imaging, though much more powerful magnets—up to 60 tesla—are used in research. Compared with the Earth's 0.5 gauss magnetic field, one can see how incredibly powerful these magnets are.

Numbers like that help provide an intellectual understanding of the magnetic strength, but everyday examples are also helpful. The MRI suite can be a very dangerous place if strict precautions are not observed. **Metal objects** can become dangerous projectiles if they are taken into the scan room. For example, paperclips, pens, keys, scissors, hemostats, stethoscopes and any other small objects can be pulled out of pockets and off the body without warning, at which point they fly toward the opening of the magnet (where the patient is placed) at very high speeds, posing a threat to everyone in the room. Credit cards, bank cards and anything else with magnetic encoding will be erased by most MRI systems.

The **magnetic force** exerted on an object increases **exponentially** as it nears the magnet. Imagine standing 15 feet (4.6 m) away from the magnet with a large pipe wrench in your hand. You might feel a slight pull. Take a couple of steps closer and that pull is much stronger. When you get to within 3 feet (1 meter) of the magnet, the wrench likely is pulled from your grasp. The more mass an object has, the more dangerous it can be—the force with which it is attracted to the magnet is much stronger. Mop buckets, vacuum cleaners, oxygen tanks, patient stretchers, heart monitors and countless other objects have all been pulled into the magnetic fields of MRI machines. The largest object that is known to have been accidentally pulled into a magnet was a fully loaded pallet jack (see below). Smaller objects can usually be pulled free of the magnet by hand. Large ones may have to be pulled away with a winch, or the magnetic field may even have to be shut down.

In this photograph, one can see a fully loaded pallet jack that has been sucked into the bore of an MRI system. Prior to allowing a patient or support staff member into the scan room, he or she is thoroughly screened for metal objects. Up to this point, we have only talked about external objects. Often however, patients have implants inside them that make it very dangerous for them to be in the presence of a strong magnetic field. Metallic fragments in the eye are very dangerous because moving those fragments could cause eye damage or blindness. Man's eyes do not form scar tissue as the rest of your body does. A fragment of metal in your eye that has been there for 25 years is just as dangerous today as it was then—there is no scar tissue to hold it in place. People with **pacemakers** cannot be scanned or even go near the scanner because the magnet can cause the pacemaker to malfunction. **Aneurysm clips** in the brain can be very dangerous as the magnet can move them, causing them to tear the very artery they were placed on to repair. Some **dental implants** are magnetic. Most **orthopedic implants**, even though they may be ferromagnetic, are fine because they are firmly embedded in bone.

Even metal staples in most parts of the body are fine—once they have been in a patient for a few weeks (usually six weeks), enough scar tissue has formed to hold them in place. Each time we encounter patients with an implant or metallic object inside their body, we investigate thoroughly to make sure it is safe to scan them. Some patients are turned away because it is too dangerous. When this happens, there is usually no alternative method of imaging that can help them. There are no known biological hazards to humans from being exposed to magnetic fields of the strength used in medical imaging today. Most facilities prefer not to image **pregnant women**. This is due to the fact that there has not been much research done in the area of biological effects on a developing fetus. The first trimester in a pregnancy is the most critical because that is the time of the most rapid cellular reproduction and division. The decision of whether or not to scan a pregnant patient is made on a case-by-case basis with consultation between the MRI radiologist and the patient's obstetrician. The benefit of performing the scan must outweigh the risk, however small, to the fetus and mother. Pregnant MRI technologists can still work in the department. In most cases, they are simply kept out of the actual scan room during their pregnancy.

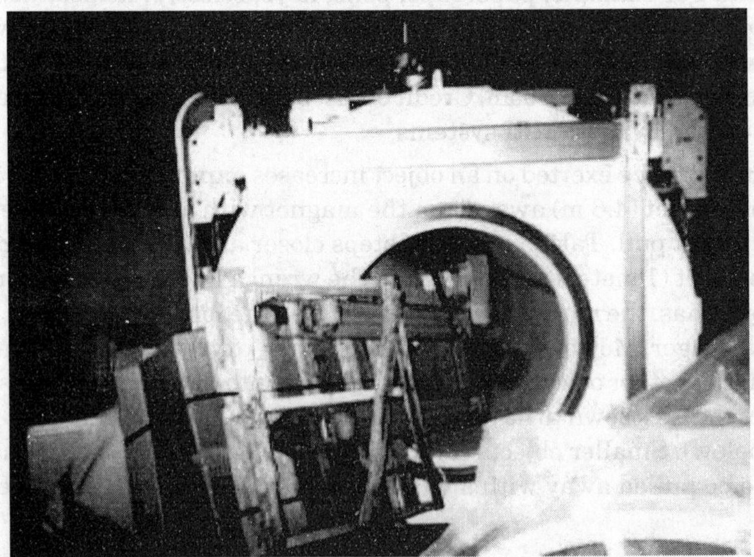

Nuclear Magnetic Resonance (NMR), as a branch of spectroscopy, has become a powerful analytical tool for investigation of the atomic nucleus and its environment that furnishes structural and dynamical information of many organic, inorganic, polymeric, and biological systems. The technique makes use of the magnetic and gyroscopic properties of atoms for studying the nature of the atomic nucleus and its interactions with its surroundings. The developments of different NMR techniques, even since its discovery on the late 1940's, are enormous with many different interests and now NMR spectroscopy has been employed extensively by biochemists, chemists and physicists. Because of the noninvasive, non-destructive nature of the NMR phenomena, the spectroscopic class of experiments is now being closely examined as a unique means to probe the biochemistry of living systems. Metabolic chemical structure, concentration and dynamics are all easily accessible through Magnetic Resonance Spectroscopy, (MRS). The result is that every animal or tissue sample can serve as its own control.

In contrast with MRS, Magnetic Resonance Imaging, (MRI) is a representation of the spatial distribution of the NMR signal intensity or other NMR parameters in heterogeneous specimens, for example, parts of the human body, which are not small, and furthermore they are placed in a deliberately nonuniform magnetic field. The purpose of this nonuniform, gradient magnetic field is to label different parts of the specimen with different field strengths, so that they represent with recongnisably different NMR frequencies, enabling the structure and internal processes of the specimen to be derived and displayed. The advantages of MRI over other medical imaging modalities using X-rays, γ-rays, positrons, etc., include absence of ionizing radiation, noninvasive, superior contrast resolution and the possibility of direct multi planar imaging. Since hydrogen is the most abundant element in all living organisms, proton MRI and MRS, lends itself particularly well as a method of investigation in medical diagnostics. Insights through relaxation parameters, which are not possible from other imaging methods are used. Let us discuss the basic principles and the application of the various NMR imaging and spectroscopic methods.

MAGNETIC RESONANCE PHENOMENA

According to quantum mechanics, every nucleus has an associated quantity called spin. This spin is quantized into units of half-integer values called the spin quantum number, with only certain precisely allowed states such as 0, 1/2, 1, 3/2 and so on. Each nucleus has its own characteristic spin quantum number. For example, all hydrogen atoms of atomic mass unity have a spin quantum number of 1/2. All carbon atoms of atomic mass number 12 and 13 have their spin quantum number 0 and 1/2 respectively. The spin quantum number dictates many of the magnetic resonance properties and as result of the spin being quantized, there is a limited number of ways a nucleus can spin, called the spin state. For a spin 1/2 nucleus, there are only two allowed spin states, + 1/2 and – 1/2 and in general, for a particle with spin I, there are 2I + 1 possible states.

From the classical point of view, the nucleus is simply a charged particle that is spinning and according to the fundamental law of physics, will induce about itself a magnetic field, called the nuclear magnetic moment, μ. This quantity μ, is related to the mass, charge, and the rate of spin of the nucleus. For any individual nucleus, the orientation of the axis of rotation, and so the direction of the nuclear magnetic moment, will be random and can be pointing in any direction. In the presence of a large external magnetic field, B_o, its axis of rotation will precess about the applied magnetic field and each spin state will have different energy at equilibrium, the lower state will have more nuclei then the higher state. Using electromagnetic radiation with an energy exactly equal to the energy difference between two nuclear energy states, one can disturb this population difference by causing some nuclei of lower energy state to absorb energy and join the higher energy nuclei. The excited nuclear spins will slowly return to its equilibrium emitting a signal that can be observed, called the NMR signal, in the very same RF coil.

The resonance frequency is just the difference in energy between the excited and ground states, $\Delta E = E_{excited} - E_{ground} = h\nu$. This relationship is readily expressed by the Zeeman/Larmor equation.

$$\omega_o = \gamma B_o \quad \text{or} \quad \upsilon_o = \gamma B_o/2\pi \qquad ...(1)$$

where υ_o is the resonance frequency expressed in Hz and γ is the nuclear gyromagnetic ratio (or) magnetogyric ratio in units of frequency/field-strength. Magnetic field strength, B_o which is usually expressed in units of Tesla (1 Tesla $=10^4$ Gauss).

The human body is made up of untold billions of atoms, the fundamental building blocks of all matter. The nucleus of an atom spins, or **precesses**, on an axis. One can think of the nucleus of an atom as a top spinning somewhere off its vertical axis.

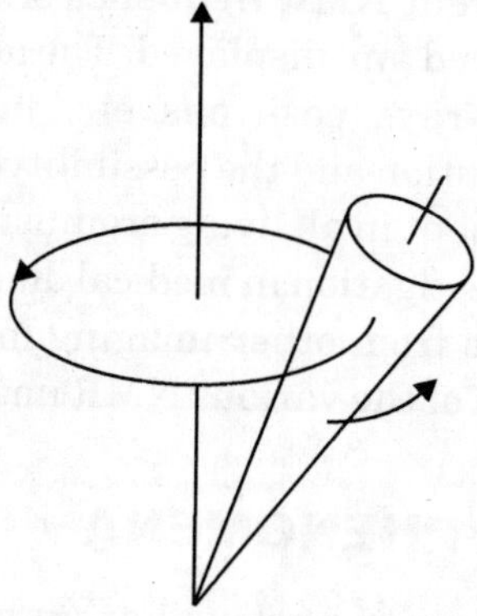

A top that is spinning slightly off the vertical axis is precessing about the vertical axis.

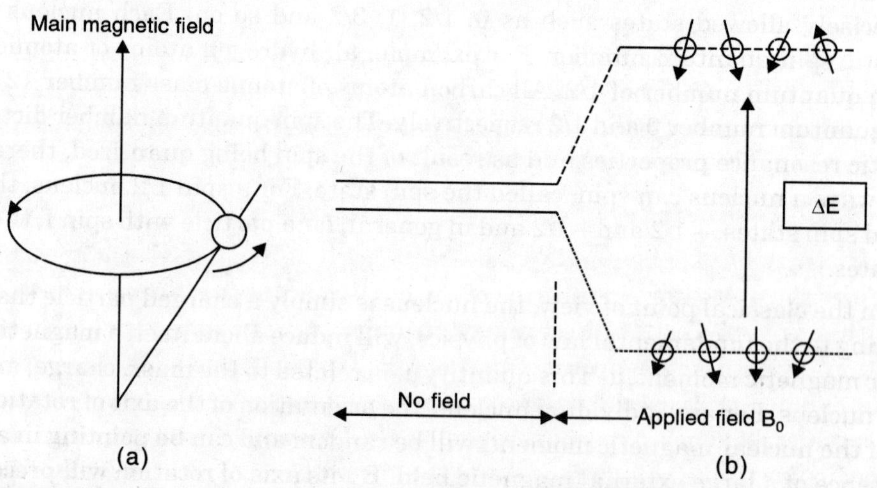

Fig. 11.1. (*a*) In the presence of an external magnetic field a spinning nucleus (proton) will precess.

(*b*) The nuclei take up discrete energy values when placed in a magnetic field. Spin transitions between these energy levels is possible by the application of electro- magnetic energy applied at the 'resonance' frequency.

A hydrogen atom precesses about a magnetic field. Imagine billions of nuclei all randomly spinning or precessing in every direction. There are many different types of atoms in the body, but for the purposes of MRI, we are only concerned with the hydrogen atom. It is an ideal atom for MRI because its nucleus has a single proton and a large magnetic moment. The large magnetic moment means that, when placed in a magnetic field, the hydrogen atom has a strong tendency to line up with the direction of the magnetic field. Inside the **bore** of the scanner, the magnetic field runs straight down the center of the tube in which we place the patient. This means that if a patient is lying on his or her back in the scanner, the hydrogen protons in his or her body will line up in the direction of either the feet or the head. The vast majority of these protons will **cancel each other out**—that is, for each one lined up toward the feet, one toward the head will cancel it out. Only a couple of protons out of every million are not canceled out. This doesn't sound like much, but the sheer number of hydrogen atoms in the body gives us what we need to create wonderful images.

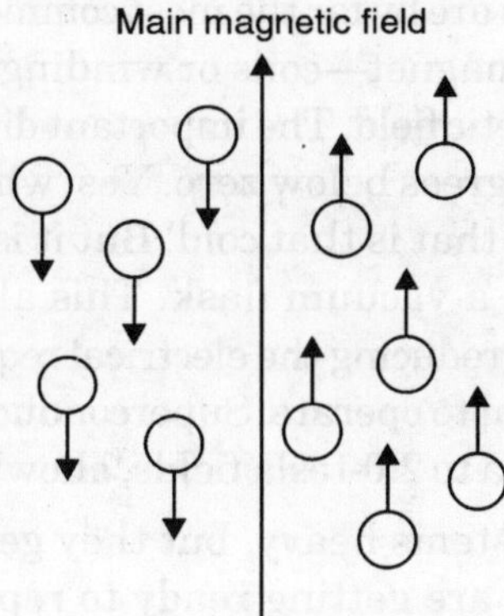

Fig. 11.1 (d)

All of the hydrogen protons will align with the magnetic field in one direction or the other. The vast majority cancel each other out, but, as shown here, in any sample there is one or two "extra" protons. Inside the magnetic field, these billions of extra protons are lined up and ready to go.

Understanding the Technology

RF The MRI machine applies an RF (radio frequency) pulse that is specific only to hydrogen. The system directs the pulse toward the area of the body we want to examine. The pulse causes the protons in that area to **absorb the energy** required to make them spin, or **precess**, in a different direction. This is the "**resonance**" part of MRI. The RF pulse forces them (only the one or two extra unmatched protons per million) to spin at a particular frequency, in a particular direction. The specific frequency of resonance is called the **Larmour frequency** and is calculated based on the particular tissue being imaged and the strength of the main magnetic field. These RF pulses are usually applied through a **coil**. MRI machines come with many different coils designed for different parts of the body: knees, shoulders, wrists, heads, necks and so on. These coils usually conform to the contour of the body part being imaged, or at least reside very close to it during the exam.

THE MAGNETS

There are three basic types of magnets used in MRI systems.

Resistive magnets consist of many windings or coils of wire wrapped around a cylinder or bore through which an electric current is passed. This causes a magnetic field to be generated. If the electricity is turned off, the magnetic field dies out. These magnets are lower in cost to construct than a superconducting magnet (see below), but require huge amounts of electricity (up to 50 Kilowatts) to operate because of the natural resistance in the wire. To operate this type of magnet above about the 0.3-tesla level would be prohibitively expensive.

A permanent magnet is just that—permanent. Its magnetic field is always there and always on full strength, so it costs nothing to maintain the field. The major drawback is that these magnets are extremely heavy. They weigh many, many tons at the 0.4 tesla level. A stronger field would require a magnet so heavy it would be difficult to construct. Permanent magnets are getting smaller, but are still limited to low field strengths.

Superconducting magnets are by far the most commonly used. A superconducting magnet is somewhat similar to a resistive magnet—coils or windings of wire through which a current of electricity is passed create the magnetic field. The important difference is that the wire is continually bathed in liquid helium at 269.1 degrees below zero. Yes, when you are inside the MRI machine, you are surrounded by a substance that is that cold! But it is very well insulated by a vacuum in a manner identical to that used in a vacuum flask. This almost unimaginable cold causes the resistance in the wire to drop to zero, reducing the electrical requirement for the system dramatically and making it much more economical to operate. Superconductive systems are still very expensive, but they can easily generate 0.5-tesla to 2.0-tesla fields, allowing for much higher-quality imaging.

The magnets make MRI systems heavy, but they get lighter with each new generation. For example, at one hospital, they are getting ready to replace an eight-year-old scanner that weighs about 17,000 lbs (7,711 kg) with a new one that weighs about 9,700 lbs (4,400 kg). The new magnet will also be about 4 feet shorter (about 6 feet/1.8 m long) than our current one. This is very important to claustrophobic patients. Our current system cannot handle anyone who weighs more than 295 pounds (134 kg). The new one will be able to accommodate patients over 400 pounds (181 kg). The systems are getting more and more patient friendly. A very uniform, or **homogeneous**, magnetic field of incredible strength and stability is critical for high-quality imaging. It forms the main magnetic field. Magnets like those described above make this field possible.

Another type of magnet found in every MRI system is called a **gradient magnet**. There are three gradient magnets inside the MRI machine. These magnets are very, very low strength compared to the main magnetic field; they may range in strength from 180 gauss to 270 gauss, or 18 to 27 millitesla (thousandths of a tesla). The function of the gradient magnets will become clear later in this article. The main magnet immerses the patient in a **stable** and very intense magnetic field, and the gradient magnets create a **variable** field. The rest of an MRI system consists of a very powerful computer system, some equipment that allows us to transmit RF (radio frequency) pulses into the patient's body while they are in the scanner, and many other secondary components. Let's find out about some of the basics involved in creating an image.

At approximately the same time, the three **gradient magnets** jump into the act. They are arranged in such a manner inside the main magnet that when they are turned on and off very rapidly in a specific manner, they **alter** the main magnetic field on a very **local** level. What this means is that we can pick exactly which area we want a picture of. In MRI we speak of "**slices.**" Think of a loaf of bread with slices as thin as a few millimeters—the slices in MRI are that precise. We can "slice" any part of the body in any direction, giving us a huge advantage over any other imaging modality. That also means that we need not move the machine to get an image from a different direction—the machine can manipulate everything with the gradient magnets. When the RF pulse is turned off, the hydrogen protons begin to slowly (relatively speaking) return to their **natural alignment** within the magnetic field and **release** their excess stored energy. When they do this, they give off a signal that the coil now picks up and sends to the computer system. What the system receives is mathematical data that is converted, through the use of a **Fourier transform**, into a picture that we can put on film. That is the "imaging" part of MRI. So this image converted into a picture that reveals the specific details we are looking for.

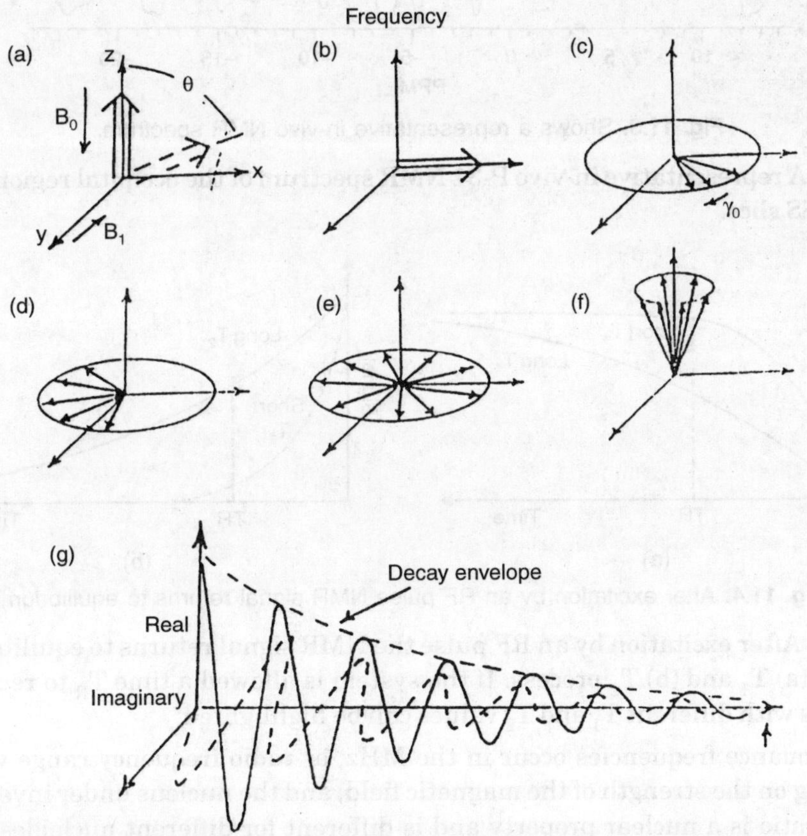

Fig. 11.2. Shows the spin magnetization tipped away from B.

Fig.11.2 spin magnetization tipped away from B (or) by application of RF field B. when the RF field is removed the spins continue to rotate in the transverse plane at different rates. (c), (d), (e) causing the resultant magnetization M_{xy} to diminish. Meanwhile spin-lattice relaxation causes the spins to realign along B_o, (f). Free induction decay (FID) or time domain signal of a nmr line, is a complex function consisting of Real and Imaginary components.

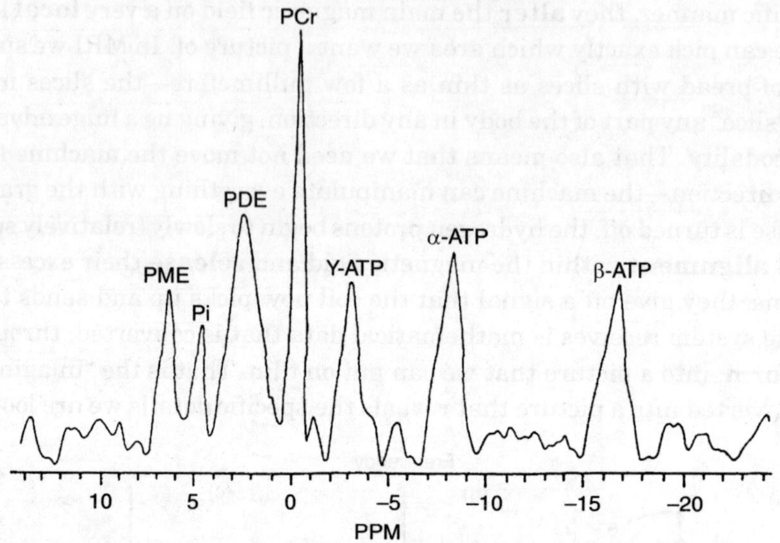

Fig. 11.3. Shows a representative in-vivo NMR spectrum.

Fig.11.3 A representative in-vivo P-31 NMR spectrum of the occipital region of the head of a subject-DRESS slice.

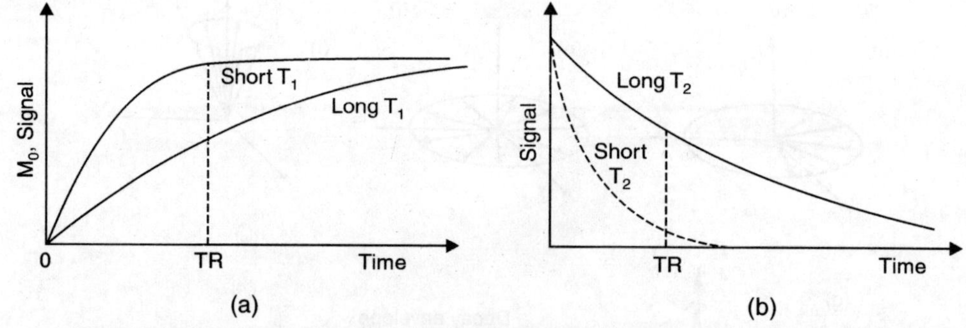

Fig. 11.4. After excitation by an RF pulse NMR signal returns to equilibrium.

Fig. 11.4 After excitation by an RF pulse the NMR signal returns to equilibrium at a rate determined by (a) T_1 and (b) T_2 process. If the system is allowed a time T_R to recover, contrast between tissues with different T_1 and T_2 values can be highlighted.

MRI resonance frequencies occur in the MHz, or radio frequency range with the exact value depending on the strength of the magnetic field, and the nucleus under investigation. The magnetogyric ratio is a nuclear property and is different for different nucleides, allowing the observation of magnetic resonance to be easily tuned to one particular nucleus. Table 1 lists some of the diagnostically important nuclei along with their gyromagnetic ratios, which also corresponds to their resonance frequencies at a field of 1 Tesla.

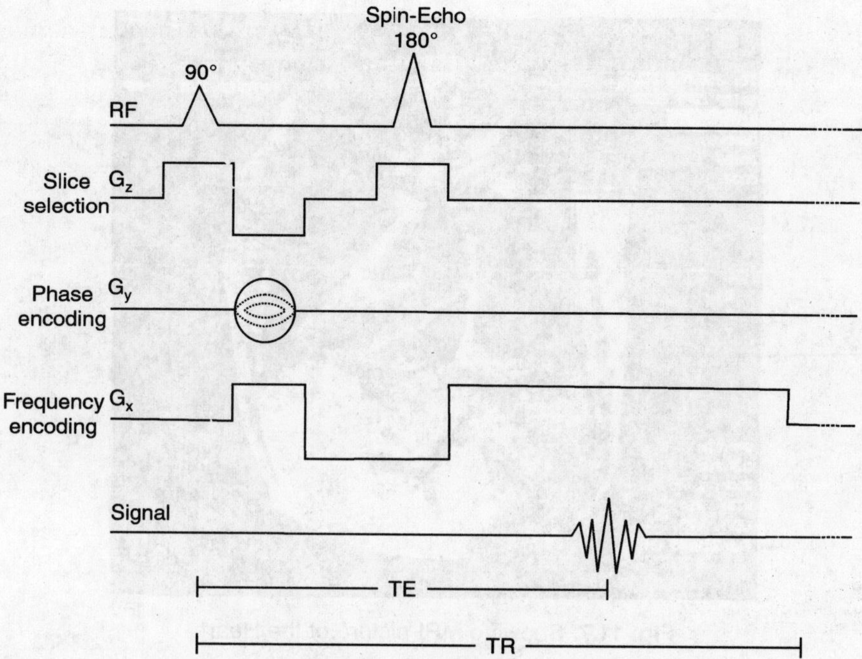

Fig. 11.5. Shows a Spin-echo pulse sequence.

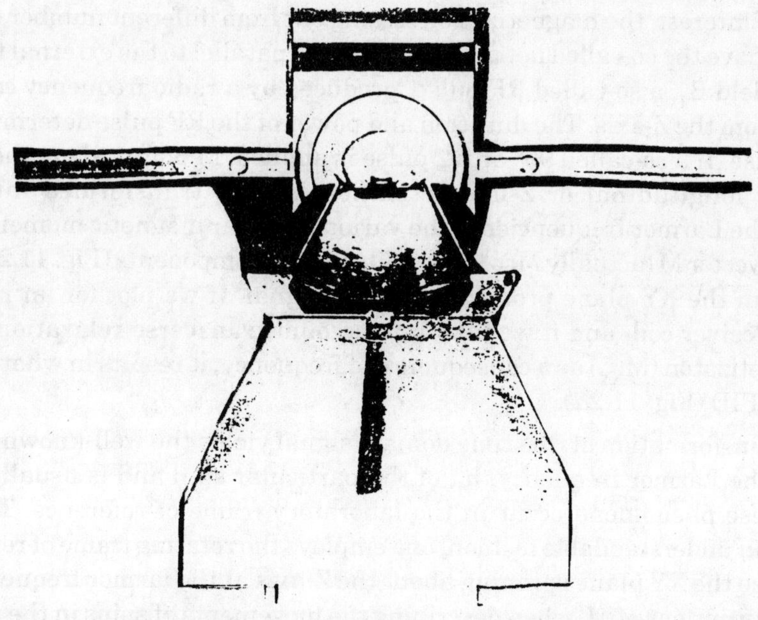

Fig. 11.6. Shows a typical MRI apparatus

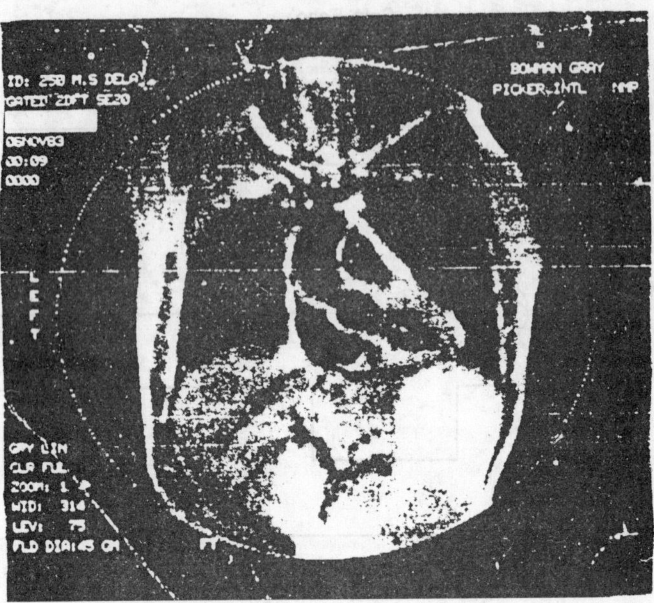

Fig. 11.7. Showing MRI picture of the Heart.

FOURIER-TRANSFORM IN NMR

For the nucleus of interest, the magnetization arising out from different number of nuclei present in the sample we have the so-called net magnetization M parallel to the external field B_o. A strong radio frequency field B_1, a so-called RF pulse, produced by a radio frequency coil on the X-axis carries M away from the Z-axis. The duration and power of the RF pulse determine the direction of M after the pulse. If a so-called 90° or $\pi/2$ pulse is applied, M points along the positive Y-axis (Fig. 11.2b), the longitudinal or Z-magnetization is thus transformed into a transverse magnetization. The Larmor frequencies of the various nuclear magnetic moments vary and as a consequence, the vector M (actually M_{XY}) now splits into its components (Fig. 11.2c). The magnetic vectors rotating in the XY plane produce a voltage signal. If we plot for an individual vector induced in the receiver coil, and if we take into account transverse relaxation, i.e., the loss of transverse magnetizaton (M_{XY}) as a consequence of frequency, it results in what is known as free induction decay, FID (Fig. 11.2*d*).

Fourier transformation of this time domain signal yields the well-known NMR signal frequency, v_o, and the Larmor frequency, u_l, of the particular spin and is usually in the order of several kHz. These phenomena occur in the laboratory frame of reference. To describe what happens to M in an understandable fashion, one employs the rotating frame of reference, in which one must visualize the XY plane spinning about the Z-axis at the larmor frequency. This simplifies the vector descriptions of M, when describing the movements of spins in the rotating frame of reference, in which one must visualize the XY plane spinning about the X-axis at the Larmor frequency. This simplifies the vector descriptions of M. When describing the movements of spins in the rotating frame, the notation of X′, Y′, Z′ is frequently used to differentiate the three axes in this frame of reference from the X, Y and Z axes of the laboratory frame.

THE CHEMICAL SHIFT

The FID obtained during an NMR experiment after Fourier transformation (FT) gives the NMR spectrum, which is a plot of signal intensity versus the frequency. The appearance of the NMR spectrum is dependent on several conditions. The resonance frequency of a particular nucleus may be altered by effects from its environment. This arises from a magnetic shielding effect of the surrounding electrons, which when placed in a magnetic field, create their own magnetic field which may reduce or add to the Bo field seen by the nucleus. The relative change in the field strength depends on the electronic million (ppm) and is defined as

$$\delta = \frac{(v_s - v_{ref}) \times 10^6}{v_{ref}} \quad ...(2)$$

where v_s is the spin frequency of the sample of interest and vref is the frequency of an arbitrarily chosen reference. The accepted standard for proton and carbon NMR is the resonance frequency of the Hydrogen in tetramethylsilane (TMS). Observation of chemical shift differences provides the basis for the use of NMR as a method for spectroscopic chemical analysis, which is one of the most powerful applications of NMR and is useful for identifying chemical and molecular structure. It is known that normal tissue and malignant tissue exhibit differences in their NMR spectra and it is hoped that in-vivo spectroscopy will aid in diagnosis.

MAGNETIC RESONANCE SPECTROSCOPY in-vivo

A variety of methods have been tested in the application of NMR to living systems. They include, for instance, measurement of P-31, H-1 and C-13 in portions of tissues taken from a living animal and P-31 measurement of a whole excised organ while perfusing it with a perfustrate. These methods, however, are not measurements that do not need any pretreatment such as extraction, which is characteristic of (H^1) density distributions, H^1 relaxation time distribution, and others are produced as an image. In this method each pixel of the image reflects the proton signal intensity of a small area of living system. On the other hand, this method, by measurement of living systems using surface coil and localization methods needs no pretreatments such as extraction and permits measurement of spectra of different nuclei. Hence by the application of in-vivo NMR spectroscopy, it is be possible to obtain various spectra from patients and gain information about the chemistry of life.

The nucleus that is currently receiving much attention for following metabolism is phosphorus-31 (or) P-31 which is a well behaved NMR nucleus and its natural abundance is 100%. It is found in several important metabolites particularly, adenosine tri-phosphate (ATP),the main energy carrier inside cells. It is also present in adenosine di-phosphate (ADP), a byproduct of ATP; adenosine mono-phosphate (AMP), a building block of ADP and ATP; creatin phosphate (PCr), the immediate storage form for high phosphates in many tissues and inorganic phosphates (Pi), the raw material for building the previous high-energy phosphates. These signals dominate in the in-vivo NMR spectrum for most tissues and provide a window into the energy state of the tissue. A representation P-31 spectrum is shown in Fig. 11.3, the possible applications include diagnosing metabolic disorders, assessing the damage done by a stroke or heart attack, and serving as a research tool for studying the effects of drugs and other treatments. Another well behaved NMR nucleus that is attracting attention is carbon-13 which has a spin quantum number of 1/2. Unfortunately, the relative abundance is only 1.1% and its scarcity makes it attractive for MRS, since synthetic compounds can be enriched with C-13. These compounds act as tracers and can be used to follow metabolic pathways both in research and in clinical applications. Recently, C-13 in-vivo spectra of normal and hyper plastic human and rat prostate are reported, which show great promise for monitoring the citrate levels.

Fluorine (F-19) represents a unique opportunity for spectroscopy in living systems, including patients. Fluorine has 100% natural abundance and has almost the same inherent sensitivity as hydrogen. However, it is almost entirely absent from the human body and for this reason, it is a perfect tracer for NMR studies. The only fluorine signal that will be detected comes from the fluorine that is deliberately introduced before any measurement. F-19 NMR is now being used increasingly to follow the detection of drugs in-vivo which are antipsychotic. Recent results have suggested that F-19 in-vivo NMR may be a useful tool to follow the pharmacokinetics and as well as to monitor the metabolism of fluorinated drugs in-vivo in human systems. The pharmacokinetics of lithium substrate was also recently measured using lithium (Li-7) nucleus NMR spectroscopy in the brain of humans.

Proton MRS bears the potential of providing access to a much larger number of metabolites compared to other nuclei because of their greater sensitivity and 100% natural abundance. Hence it is possible to obtain detailed biochemical information not only on the energy metabolism (e.g. lactate production), but also on free amino acids, fatty acids, and neurotransmitters. Moreover, with the recent improvements in different in-vivo localization techniques, it is possible to get a good NMR spectrum from l cc volume size of human organs. Commonly used localization techniques for in-vivo spectroscopy are STREAM, ISIS, DRESS, SPARS methods and these have been extensively applied for obtaining good proton MR spectrum from different human organs.

MAGNETIC RELAXATION AND MRI PARAMETERS

These are three principal MRI parameters: spin density, T_1 and T_2 relaxation times. Each of these is fundamentally different and independent of the others and plays a major role in pixel brightness in an MR image but not in a simple manner.

Spin density

One of the most important aspects of NMR is that the signal is proportional to the number of nuclei present, say for *e.g.* the presence or absence of hydrogen nuclei and also the signal is very sensitive to the environment of the hydrogen nuclei. For imaging, it turns out that hydrogen which is very tightly bound, creates no usable signal. Thus, the signal received should be arising from mobile hydrogens, that is, hydrogen nuclei that are loosely bound such as those in liquids. A good example is bone, which always appears black in an MR image not because there is no protons present but rather due to that rigid structure, producing no detectable signal. Hence, the measure of the concentration of mobile hydrogen nuclei available to produce an NMR signal is called the spin density (SD). Higher the concentration of mobile hydrogen nuclei, stronger will be NMR signal and hence better MR image. Table 2 reports relative values of spin density for several tissues.

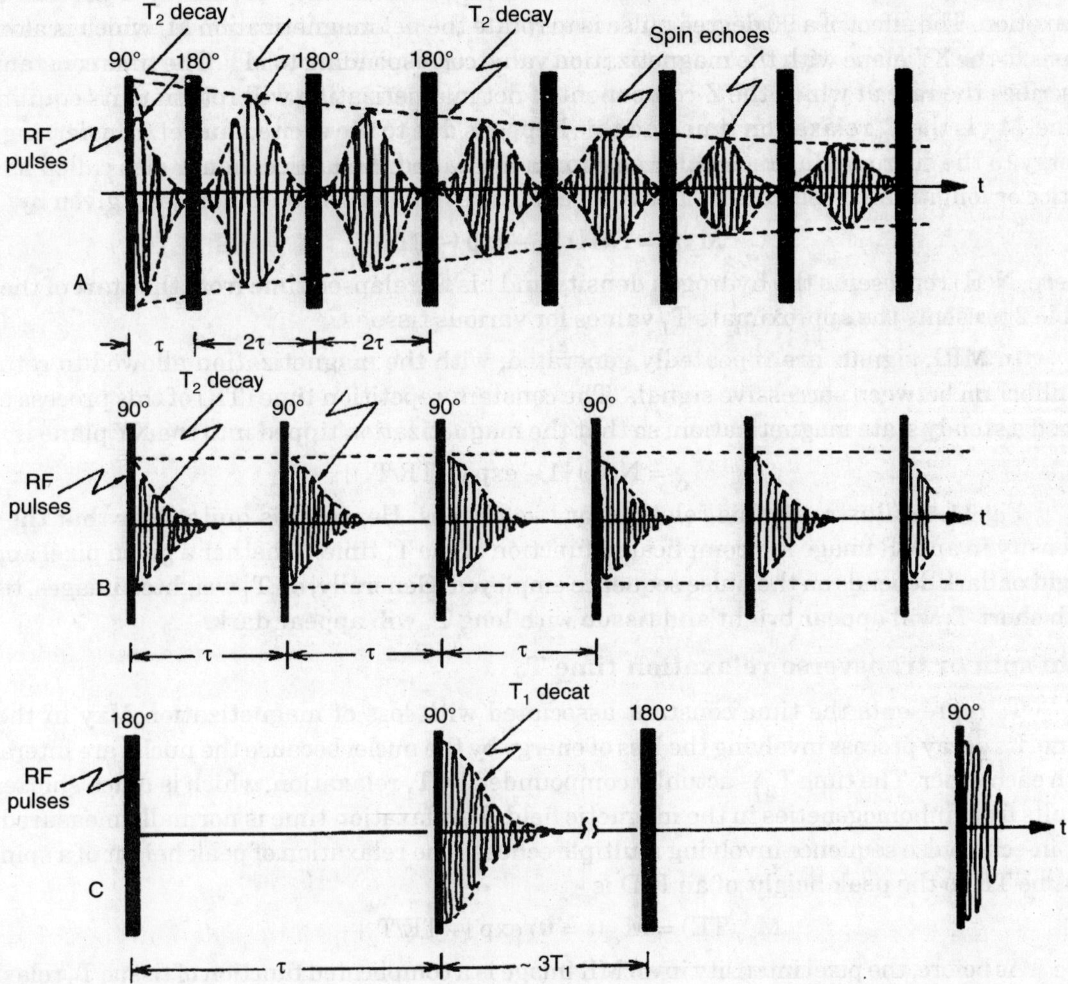

Fig. 11.8. The decay times of the MNR signal, called T_1 and T_2, are used to distinguish between diseased and healthy tissue. T_2 can be measured by a Carr-Purcell sequence of pulses as in A. In this sequence, an RF pulse rotates the magnetisation vector by 90°. The effect of inhomogeneities in the magnetic field is then reversed by a series of 180° pulses, creating a train of signals called spin-echoes. The rate of decay of these echoes is T_2. There are two techniques of measuring T_1. In partial saturation, (Fig. B), a train of 90° pulses separated by a time τ is used. The amplitude of the signal grows smaller as τ is reduced, thus giving a measure of the T_1.

In inversion recovery (Fig. C), the bulk magnetization is reversed by a 180° pulse. It then starts to grow back toward the positive *z*-axis. After time τ a 90° pulse flips the magnetization vector into the transverse plane, producing the NMR signal. Again, by plotting the signal strength against τ the decay constant T_1 can be found.

Spin-lattice (longitudinal) relaxation time T_1

Let us now return to our earlier discussions on the nuclei at equilibrium. For example, by the 90° RF pulse, they return to equilibrium with the static field, B_o, when they are completely aligned. Anytime the nuclei are disturbed from equilibrium they return by a process called relaxation. The effect of a 90 degree pulse is to rotate the net magnetization M_z which is along the Z-axis to the XY plane with the magnetization value corresponding to M_{xy}. The time constant that describes the rate at which the Z-component of net magnetization will return to its equilibrium value, M_o, is the T_1 relaxation time and this happens due to the excited nuclei transferring their energy to the surrounding molecular environment, called the lattice, hence also called as spin-lattice or longitudinal relaxation. The recovery of the magnetization is normally given by

$$M_z(t) = N(H)\,[1 - \exp(-t/T_1)] \qquad ...(3)$$

where, N(H) represents the hydrogen density and t is the elapsed time from the start of the FID. Table 2 presents the approximate T_1 values for various tissues.

In MRI, signals are repeatedly generated, with the magnetization allowed to return to equilibrium between successive signals. The constant repetition time (TR) of this process established a steady state magnetization, so that the magnetization tipped into the XY plane is

$$M_{xy} = N(H)\,[1 - \exp(-TR/T_1)] \qquad ...(4)$$

Fig.11.4a illustrates this relation for two tissues. Hence, it is quite clear that the pixel intensity in an MR image is a complicated function of the T_1 time. Whether a given pixel appears bright or dark depends on the pulse sequence employed. Generally, on T_1 weighted images, tissues with short T_1 will appear bright and tissue with long T_1 wili appear dark.

Spin-spin or transverse relaxation time T_2

T_2 represents the time constant associated with loss of magnetization Mxy in the XY-plane. Its decay process involving the loss of energy by the nuclei because the nuclei are interacting with each other. The time T_2 is actually compounded by T_1 relaxation, which is much shorter and results from inhomogeneties in the magnetic field. T_2 relaxation time is normally measured with a spin-echo pulse sequence involving multiple echoes. The relaxation of peak height of a spin echo at time TE to the peak height of an FID is

$$M_{xy}(TE) = M_{xy}(t = 0)\exp[-TE/T_2] \qquad ...(5)$$

As before, the pixel intensity in an MR image is a complicated function of tissue T_2 relaxation time and the pulse sequence employed will appear bright for tissue with long T_2. Normally, the measurements of relaxation times as well as for obtaining an MR image, one employs different pulse sequences. A pulse sequence in MR is basically a set of instructions to the magnet telling it how to make an image.

MAGNETIC FIELD STRENGTH AND GRADIENTS

MRI systems are generally characterized by the strength of magnetic field. Most imaging procedures are performed with field strengths in the range of 0.3 to 1.5 Tesla, although imaging outside this range is possible. The strength of the magnetic field determines the tissue (proton) resonant frequency. This is the frequency that is receptive to the RF pulses applied to the tissue and is also the frequency of the RF signals emitted during the imaging process. Prior to the actual image acquisition process, the magnetic field is same at all points throughout the region say, a patient's body. However, during the acquisition, the gradient coils within the body resonate at different frequencies. The purpose of these magnetic field in-homogeneities (gradient coils) is two-fold: slice selection and pixel localization within the slice. The combination of field gradient in-homogeneity and excitation by a specific frequency permits slice selection. The presence of a gradient field during relaxation helps to localize protons within the slice that was selected during excitation.

The steeper the gradient field, the thinner will be the slice. The narrower the RF pulse, the thinner will be slice. The gradient coils consist of three pairs :

X-gradients,

Y-gradients and

Z-gradients.

Z-gradients coils change the gradient magnetic field along the Z-axis thereby allowing a slice of the patient to be selected for imaging. X-gradients coils produce a magnetic gradient across the patient, thus providing spatial localization along the X-axis of the patient. This technique is usually called as frequency encoding. On the other hand, the Y-gradient coils produce magnetic gradient through the patient from front to back and by convention, the Y-axis is the vertical axis through the patient used for phase encoding gradient in the NMR signal. Together, the Y and X-gradients allow precise determination of where within the imaging plane the contribution to the NMR signal from each voxel or pixel originates. The Z-gradients is always used for selection of a trans axial plane to be imaged and is called slice selection. To select either the axial, sagittal or coronal plane for imaging, only the Z, X or Y-gradients, respectively, will be energised as magnetic fields and vectorially added. When all the three gradients are energized at the same time, an oblique plane is defined.

PULSE SEQUENCES

As discussed briefly earlier, a pulse sequence is a set of instructions that accomplishes two tasks. First, it tells the imager how to collect data in an orderly fashion so that the origin of the signals can be determined for the requisite-pixel position and this is the function of the gradient magnetic fields outlined earlier. Second, it influences image contrast-pixel character by specifying the timing and power of the RF pulses. Many of the parameters that have to be specified in a pulse sequence, such as the timing and magnitude of gradient magnetic fields (normally denoted as G_x or G_y or Gz), are included in the computer software.

Number of pulse sequences are in use for obtaining an image: partial saturation, inversion recovery, spin echo, FLASH (fast low angle shot), GRASS (gradient recalled acquisition in the steady state), and others. Multi-slice and multi-echo techniques help to decrease total scan time. The spin-echo pulse sequence shown in Fig. 11.5 is probably the most commonly used pulse sequence in clinical diagnosis. To get a spin echo, one starts with a 90° RF (sinc) pulse to tip the magnetization vectors into the XY plane. After a small period of time T, this is followed by a 180° RF pulse which refocuses the spin vectors in the XY plane exactly after an equal amount of time T to give an echo at a time 2T with respect to the initial 90° with pulse. The NMR signals from the echo are acquired to make an image. Z gradient is on during the 90° RF pulse for slice

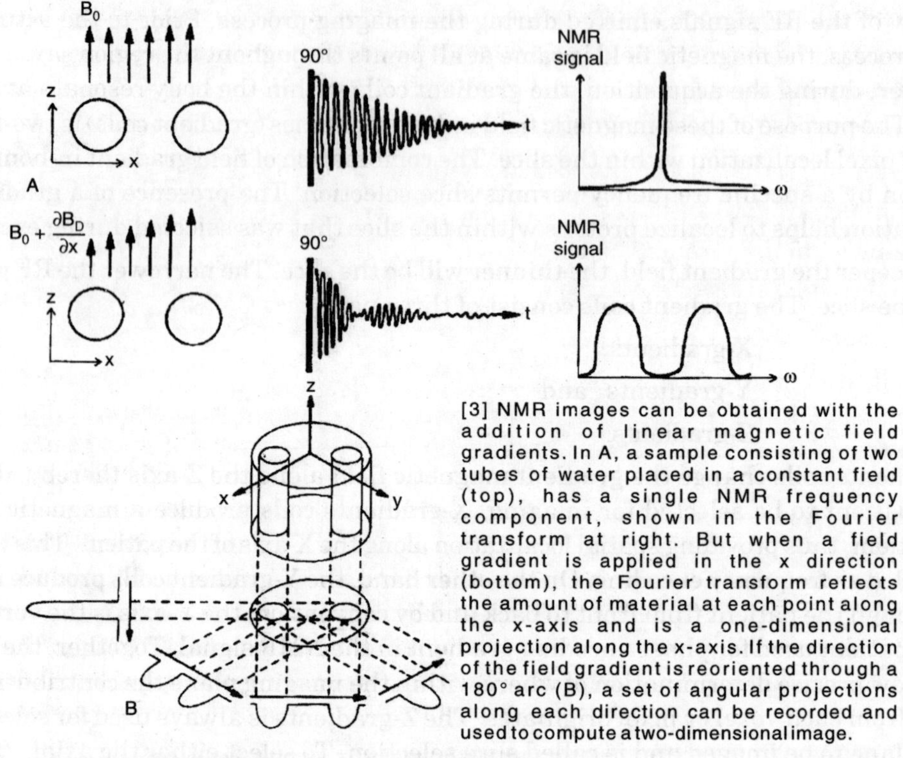

Fig. 11.9. Showing the use of gradient fields in reconstruction of the image.

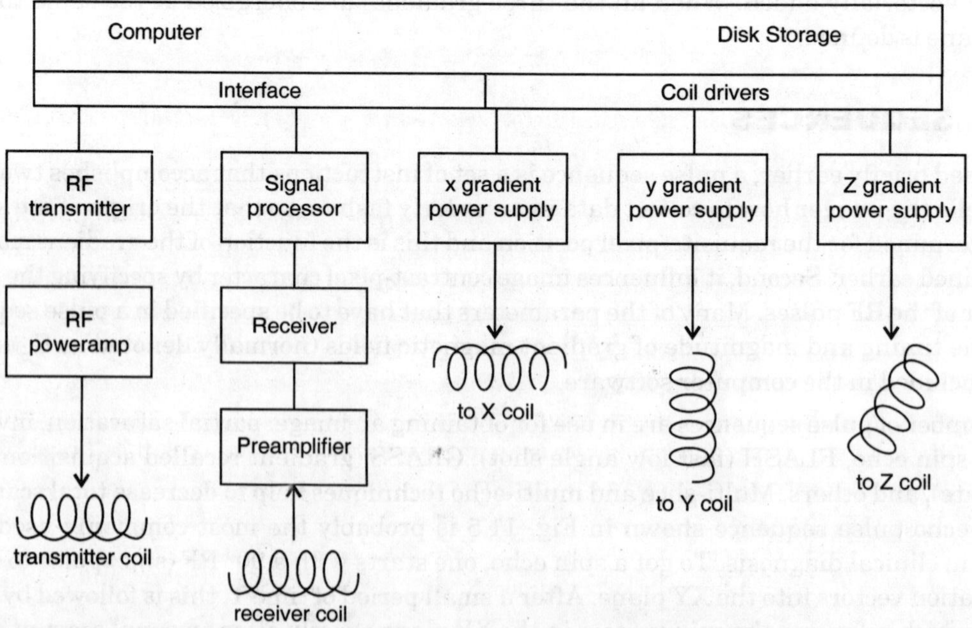

Fig. 11.10 (a). The main hardware elements of an NMR machine are shown in this simplified block diagram. A computer controls the RF excitation pulses and the gradient magnetic fields. Detected signals from the RF receiver are fed to a signal averager and back to the computer for processing into image sections, which are then displayed on the monitor.

selection. The various timings and the pulses of gradients are as shown in Fig. 11.5. In order to get images with good contrast and quality one need to specify:

(a) type of pulse sequence,

(b) time intervals such as TR, TE, TI etc.,

(c) matrix size, that is, the number of signal acquisitions,

(d) number of signal averages,

(e) plane of image, (f) slice thickness and

(f) spatial separation of the slices.

Imaging Process

The NMR signal that is produced through the use of above pulse sequences cannot be directly translated into an image. It is necessary to convert from a frequency representation to a location representation. A digital computer, with sufficient memory and storage place, performs the mathematics of this conversion or transformation. In the presence of a magnetic field gradient, the NMR signal yields one-dimensional distribution of information. The various techniques of MRI are different schemes for using this one-dimensional measurement to sample the two, dimensional image plane. Of the two techniques, projection reconstruction imaging and 2D-Fourier transforms (FT) imaging, the 2D-FT has become the method of choice because of fast computational facility. Two dimensional FT imaging samples a line at a time in only one direction of the frequency representation. The direction of sampling is determined by the direction of the phase-encoding gradient. The information along this line is determined by using the frequency encoding gradient. When the entire frequency representation of the image has been sampled by repeated cycles of the 2D FT process using different phase-encoding gradient strengths, the sampled frequency representation is converted to an image in the computer by using a two-dimensional Fourier transform.

Visualization

Most imaging modalities use **injectable contrast**, or dyes, for certain procedures. MRI is no different. What is different is the type of contrast we use, how it works and why we use it. The contrast or dye materials used in X-Ray and CT scan work in the same way because both areas use X-rays (**ionizing radiation**). These agents work by **blocking** the X-ray photons from passing through the area where they are located and reaching the X-ray film. This results in differing levels of **density** on the X-ray/CT film. These dyes have no direct physiologic impact on the tissue in the body. The contrast used in MRI is fundamentally different. MRI contrast works by altering the local magnetic field in the tissue being examined. Normal and abnormal tissue will respond differently to this slight alteration, giving us differing signals. These **varied signals** are transferred to the images, allowing us to visualize many different types of tissue abnormalities and disease processes better than we could without the contrast. Now that we have explained how MRI works, let us find out what circumstances might call for an MRI scan.

Advantages and Disadvantages

Why would your doctor order an MRI? Because the only way to see inside your body any better is to cut you open. MRI is ideal for:

- Diagnosing **multiple sclerosis** (MS)
- Diagnosing **tumors** of the pituitary gland and brain

- Diagnosing **infections** in the brain, spine or joints
- Visualizing **torn ligaments** in the wrist, knee and ankle
- Visualizing **shoulder injuries**
- Diagnosing **tendonitis**
- Evaluating **masses** in the soft tissues of the body
- Evaluating **bone tumors**, **cysts** and **bulging or herniated discs** in the spine
- Diagnosing **strokes** in their earliest stages.

These are but a few of the many of reasons to perform an MRI scan. The fact that MRI systems do not use ionizing radiation is a comfort to many patients, as is the fact that MRI contrast materials have a very low incidence of **side effects**. Another major advantage of MRI is its ability to image in **any plane**. CT is limited to one plane, the axial plane (in the loaf-of-bread analogy, the axial plane would be how a loaf of bread is normally sliced). An MRI system can create **axial images** as well as images in the **sagittal plane** (slicing the bread side-to-side lengthwise) and **coronally** (think of the layers of a layer cake) or any degree in between, without the patient ever moving. In the case of X-ray, it is well known that every time they take a different picture, patient has to move. The three gradient magnets discussed earlier allow the MRI system to choose exactly where in the body to acquire an image and how the slices are oriented.

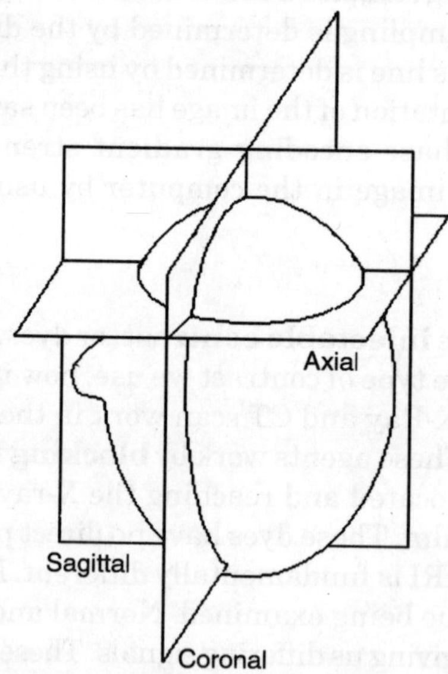

Fig. 11.10 (b). Planes of NMR imaging.

Axial, coronal and sagittal slices MRI does have drawbacks, however. For example:

There are many people who cannot safely be scanned with MRI (for example, because they have **pacemakers**), and also people who are **too big** to be scanned.

There are many **claustrophobic** people in the world, and being in an MRI machine can be a very disconcerting experience for them.

The machine makes a tremendous amount of **noise** during a scan. The noise sounds like a continual, rapid hammering. Patients are given earplugs or stereo headphones to muffle the

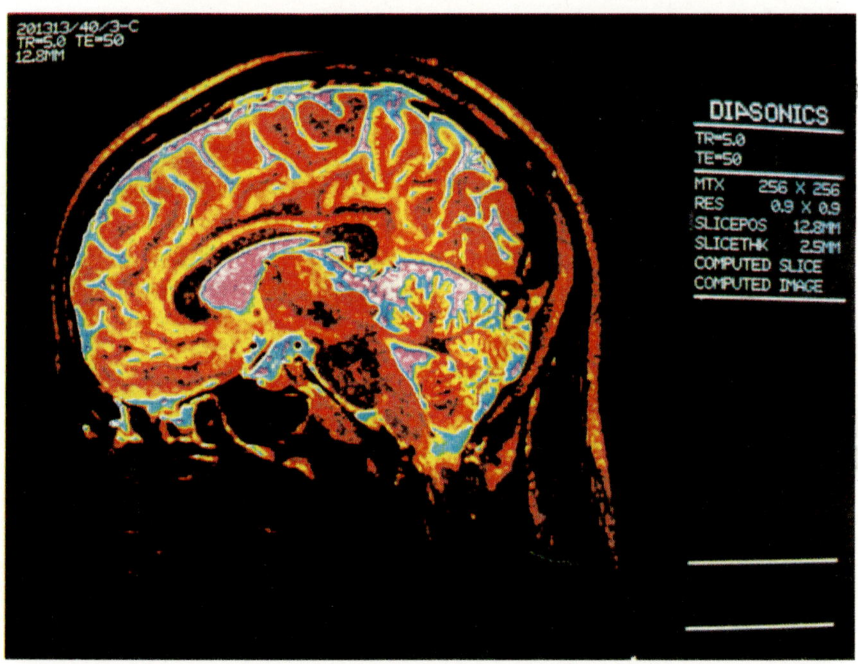

Plate II.1. Shows a typical image obtained by magnetic resonance imaging.

noise (in most MRI centers you can even bring your own cassette or CD to listen to). The noise is due to the rising electrical current in the wires of the gradient magnets being opposed by the main magnetic field. The stronger the main field, the louder the gradient noise.

MRI scans require patients to **hold very still** for extended periods of time. MRI exams can range in length from 20 minutes to 90 minutes or more. Even very slight movement of the part being scanned can cause very distorted images that will have to be repeated.

Orthopedic hardware (screws, plates, artificial joints) in the area of a scan can cause severe **artifacts** (distortions) on the images. The hardware causes a significant alteration in the main magnetic field. Remember, a uniform field is critical to good imaging.

MRI systems are very, very **expensive** to purchase, and therefore the exams are also very expensive. The almost limitless benefits of MRI for most patients far outweigh the few drawbacks.

The Future of MRI The future of MRI seems limited only by our imagination. This technology is still in its infancy, comparatively speaking. It has been in widespread use for less than 20 years (compared with over 100 years for X-rays). Very **small scanners** for imaging specific body parts are being developed. For instance, a scanner that you simply place your arm, knee or foot in are currently in use in some areas. Our ability to visualize the arterial and venous system is improving all the time. Functional **brain mapping** (scanning a person's brain while he or she is performing a certain physical task such as squeezing a ball, or looking at a particular type of picture) is helping researchers better understand how brain works. Research is under way in a few institutions to image the ventilation dynamics of the Lungs through the use of hyperpolarized helium-3 gas. The development of new, improved ways to image strokes in their earliest stages is ongoing. Predicting the future of MRI is speculative at best, but I have no doubt it will be exciting for those of us in the field, and very beneficial to the patients.. MRI is a field with a virtually limitless future.

The future of MRI and MRS looks very promising in the area of medicine. Multinuclear applications will undoubtedly be forthcoming with improvements in field strength and sensitivity, three and four-dimensional extensions to chemical shift imaging, and examination of dynamic processes will occur rapidly. Combination of MRI, MRS and other techniques will open entirely new approaches to a wide variety of problems in the medical field. Numerous manuscripts, articles and books have appeared on the basic principles and application of MRI and MRS.

Table 1: NMR Properties of Medically Important Nuclei

Nucleus	Spin-quantum Number	Magnetogyric ratio (MHz/Tesla)	Relative abundance (%)	Relative sensitivity
H-1	½	42.58	99.98	1
Li-7	3/2	16.54	92.58	0.27
C-13	½	10.71	1.11	0.0096
F-19	½	40.05	100.00	0.83
Na-23	3/2	11.26	100.00	0.093
P-31	½	17.23	100.00	0.066

Table 2: Approximate relaxation times, T_1 and T_2 at a field strength of 1.0 Tesla for various of mobile hydrogen nuclei (spin density).

Tissue	T_1 (ms)	T_2 (ms)	Relative spin density (%)
Fat	180	90	98
Liver	270	50	91
White matter	390	90	100
Gray matter	520	100	94
Spleen	480	80	92
Muscle	600	40	100
Blood	800	180	90
CSF	2000	300	96
Water	2500	2500	100

MAGNETIC RESONANCE IMAGING IN MEDICINE

It is now established that ^1H spectroscopy has given a technique called magnetic imaging or MRI. One great advantage of MRI is that unlike X-rays, it does not use dangerous ionizing radiation, and it does not require the injection of potentially harmful chemicals in order to produce contrasts in the image. In MRI, a portion of the patient's body is placed in a powerful magnetic field and irradiated with RF energy, but he is not aware of it and hence it is non invasive.

A typical image is given in Plate II.1. The instruments used in producing images like this one use the pulse method to excite the protons in the tissue under observation and use a Fourier transform calculation to translate the information into an image. The brightness of various regions of the image are related to two aspects. The first factor is the number of protons in the tissue at that particular place. The second factor arises from what are called the **relaxation times** of the protons. When photons are excited to a higher energy to return to the lower energy spin state before they can be excited again by a second pulse, the process by which the nuclei lose this energy is called **relaxation**, and the time it takes to occur is the relaxation time. There are two basic modes of relaxation available to protons . In one, called **spin-lattice relaxation,** the extra energy is transferred to neighboring molecules in the surrounding (or lattice) . The time required for this to happen is called T_1 and is characteristic of the time required for the spin system to return to thermal equilibrium with its surroundings. In solids, T_1 can be hours long,. For protons in pure liquid water, T_1 is only few seconds. In the other type of relaxation, called **spin-spin relaxation**, the extra energy is dissipated by being transferred to nuclei of nearby atoms. The time required for this is called T_2. In liquids the magnitude of T_2 is approximately equal to T_1. In solids, however, the T_1 is very much larger.

Various techniques based on the time between pulses of RF radiation have been developed to utilize the differences in relaxation times in order to produce contrasts between regions of soft tissues. The soft tissue contrast is inherently higher than that produced with X-ray techniques.

Magnetic resonance imaging is being used to great effect in locating tumors, lesions, and edemas. Improvements in this technique are occurring rapidly, and the method is not restricted to observation of proton signals.

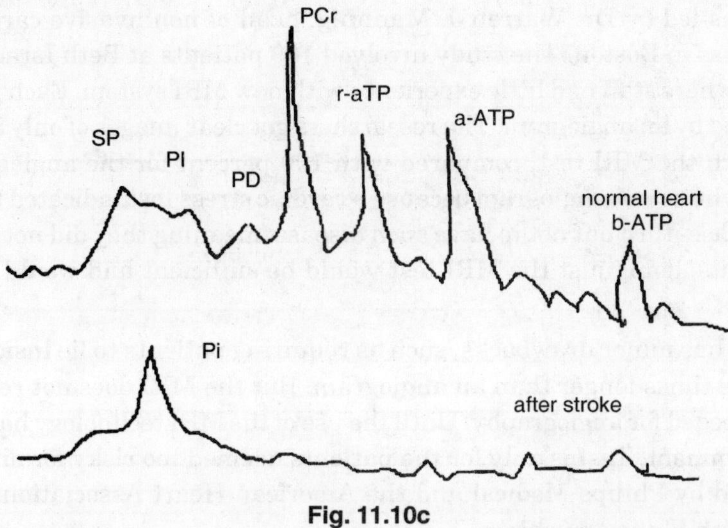

Fig. 11.10c

One important area of medical research is based on the observation of signals 31P. Compounds that contain phosphorus as Phosphate esters such as adenosine triphosphate (ATP) and adenosine diphosphate (ADP) are involved in most metabolic processes. By using techniques on NMR, researchers now have a noninvasive way to follow cellular metabolism.

Typical imaging techniques yield the best results. (Fig. 11.9). There are several software that are available for processing. Better than the Fourier Transform, there is now interest in Gabor transforms, which gives better time frequency relationships. Hence, the field is prospective for research at any time.

Cardiac MRI Advanced New Non-Invasive Alternative to Catheterization

This MRI test for diseased arteries could replace angiograms. The study involved 109 patients at Beth Israel and six other US and European sites where staff had experience with the new MRI system. Each patient first and the MRI test, followed by an angiogram. Still, the MRI test has drawbacks, such as requiring patients to lie inside the device for an hour, about three times longer than an angiogram takes. But the MRI does not require the eight hour hospital stay needed for angiography. The study was sponsored by Philips medical Services, which makes MRI equipment, and by the American heart Association. The technique tested works only with Philips machine.

The new technique is still not as thorough as the more invasive angiogram, but the findings raise hope that for some patients with relatively mild symptums, there could soon be a safer way to detect the disease. MRI is excellent at delivering pictures of soft tissue, but has had trouble getting a clear view of arteries, which are blurred by the constant motion of the heart and lungs. This new technique gets around theat problem by special proprietary software. In an angiogram, a catheter is threaded form groin or arm artery up to the heart. The catheter then injects a dye that can be seen on a cine *x*-ray, helping doctors spot blockages. Angiograms produce very clear pictures but cause complications in about 1% of the 1.2 million patients getting the test each year, inclucing a slight chance of artery damage or a heart attack. Cardiac MRI has the potential to get similar results without the risks or other drawbacks.

The study was led by Dr. Warren J. Manning, head of noninvasive cardiac imaging at Beth Israel Deaconess in Boston. The study involved 109 patients at Beth Israel six other U.S. and European sites where staff had little experience with new MRI system. Each patient first had the MRI test, followed by an angiogram. The researchers got clear images of only 84 percent of the artery segments with the MRI test, compared with 100 percent for the angiograms, about 40 percent of patients who got an angiogram because a cardiac stress test indicated they might have coronary artery disease–turn out not to have such disease, meaning they did not need the $5,000 test. In those patients, doing just the MRI test would be sufficient and would cost only about $1000.

The MRI test has minor drawbacks, such as requiring patients to lie inside the device for an hour, about three times longer than an angiogram. But the MRI does not require the eight-hour hospital stay needed for angiography. Until the use of the MRI technology has been approved by the Fedral Government. Test is only for the patients deemed too risky for angiography. The study was sponsored by Philips Medical and the American Heart Association. The technique tested works only with Philips machines.

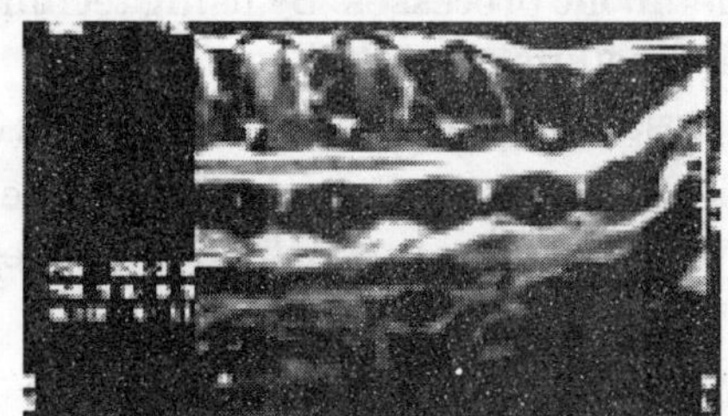

A theacal cyst at the base of the spine compressing lower spinal nerve

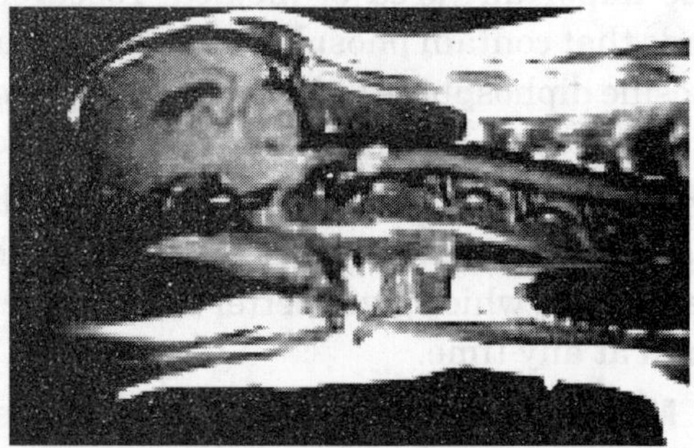

A spinal tumour just behind the brain stem

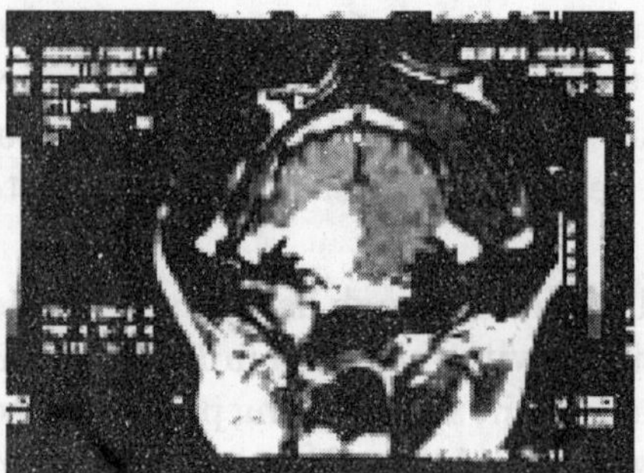

Fig. 11.11. Typical imaging techniques based on MRI.

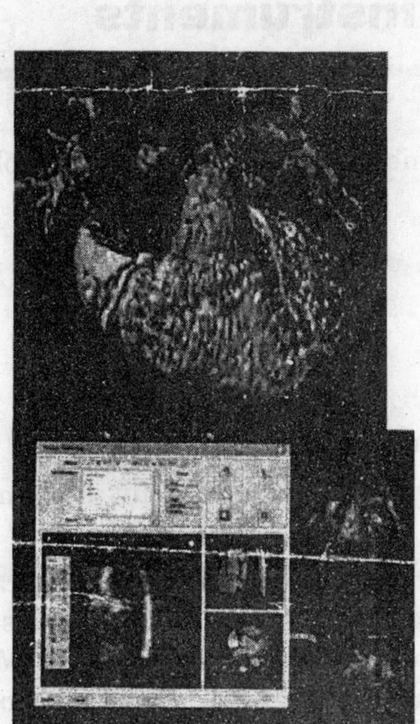

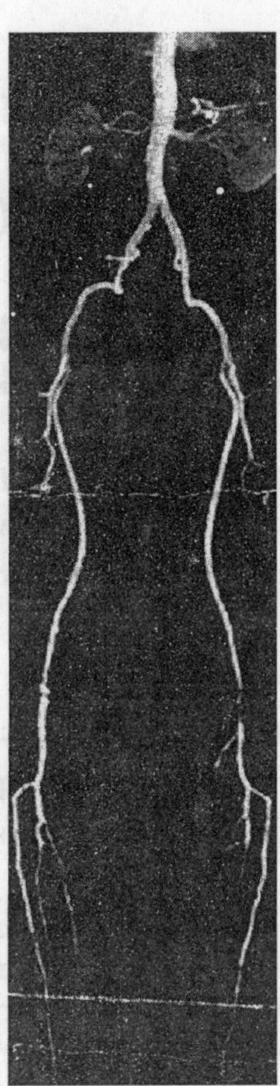

Fig. 11.12. MRI based "Angiogram" arteries of the heart (Philips).

Chapter 12

Surgical Instruments

This is going to deal with the use of electronic aided surgery based and physiotherapy related equipment, as for instance the following:

1. Diathermy Units for Physiotherapy
2. Pacemakers
3. Defibrillators
4. Modern electro surgical equipment
5. Lasers for Ophthalmology applications

Diathermy tissue heating uses tissue as part of a tank circuit. Maximum power is 500W to 1000 W only.

Therapeutic diathermy units are widely used in departments of Physical Medicine to provide heat treatment for affected joints and other areas, lumbago and abscesses (Zeirter 1950). They operate mainly at 27MHz with maximum output power of some 300 W. Microwave diathermy units are employed when a preferential heating of superficial tissue layers of good conductivity is required, with only slight heating of fatty tissues. A typical maximum output power would be 200W at 2425 MHz.

HEAT THERAPY

While it was recognized several thousand years ago that hot baths were therapeutic, it was not until the mid 1980's that the pain relieving properties of heat were somewhat understood. Two primary therapeutic effects take place in the heated area; there is an increase in metabolism resulting in relaxation of the capillary system (vasodilatation), and there is an increase of blood flow, which moves in to cool the heated area. The relaxation and increased blood flow are beneficial to damaged tissue, although the details of the therapeutic action are not well understood. In this section, we will briefly discuss about the physical method of producing heat in the body. This is achieved by the following methods. They are:

1. Conductive heating
2. Infrared (IR) radiation heating
3. Radiowave heating (Diathermy) and
4. The ultrasonic wave heating

The conductive method is based on the physical fact that if two objects of different temperatures are placed in contact, heat will transfer by conduction from the warmer object to the cooler one. The total heat transferred will depend upon the area of contact, the temperature difference, the time of contact and the thermal conductivity of the materials. Hot baths, hot packs, electric heating pads, and occasionally hot paraffin applied to the skin heat the body by conduction. Conductive heat transfer lead to local surface heating since the circulating blood effectively removes the heat that penetrates deep into the tissue.

Applications

Conductive heating is used in treating conditions such arthritis, neuritis, sprains and strain, contusions, sinusitis and back pain.

Radiant heat is (IR) is also used for surface heating of the body. This is the same form of heat we feel from the sun or from an open flame. Man-made sources of radiant heat are glowing wire coils and 250 W incandescent lamps. The IR wave lengths are between 800 nm and 40000 nm (1 nm = 10^{-9} m). The waves penetrate the skin about 3mm and increase the surface temperature. Excessive exposure cause reddening (erythema) and sometime swelling (edema). Very prolonged exposure causes browning or hardening of the skin. Radiative heating is generally used for the same conditions of the conductive heating, but it is considered to be more effective because the heat penetrates a bit deeper.

When alternating electric current passes through the body, various effects such as heating and electric shock take place. The amount of heat that can be transferred to the body by electrical diathermy increases as the frequency of the current increases. Short wave diathermy utilizes electromagnetic waves in the radio range (wavelength–10m); and microwave diathermy uses in the radar range (wavelength–12 cm).

DIATHERMY

The use of frequencies near 30 MHz for heating is called short-wave diathermy. Long wave diathermy, at frequencies near 10 KHz was used, but this has become obsolete. In 1951, a mode of diathermy that use microwaves of a frequency of 2450 MHz was introduced. Microwaves are used in radar and in microwave ovens.

Heat from diathermy penetrates deeper into the body than radiant and conductive heat. It is thus useful for internal heating and has been used in the treatment of inflammation of the skeleton, bursitis, and neuralgia.

SHORT WAVE DIATHERMY

Short wave diathermy heats the deep tissues of the body. It has been used in relieving muscle spasms; pain from protruded inter vertebral discs, degenerative joint disease, and bursitis, and as a deep heating agent for joints with minimal soft tissue coverage such as knee, elbow, and ankle.

In short-wave diathermy, two methods are used to get the electromagnetic energy into the body; the **capacitance coupling method** and **inductance coupling method.**

Capacitance Coupling Method

In both methods, the body part to be heated becomes a part of a resonant electrical circuit. A simple resonant circuit consists of a capacitor and an inductor. Electrical energy from a power supply flows back and forth between the capacitor and the inductor, thus providing an alternating electric field (or current).

In the capacitance coupling method of short wave diathermy, the tissue to be heated is placed between two capacitor plates that have an oscillating electric field across them (Fig. 12.1*a*) The changing electric field forces the ions in the tissue to move back and forth; they thus acquire kinetic energy, part of which is dissipated when the ions collide with molecules in the tissue. The heat produced when the energy is dissipated depends approximately on the square of the current times a constant determined by the tissue properties. This type of energy loss is called *joule (resistive) heating.*

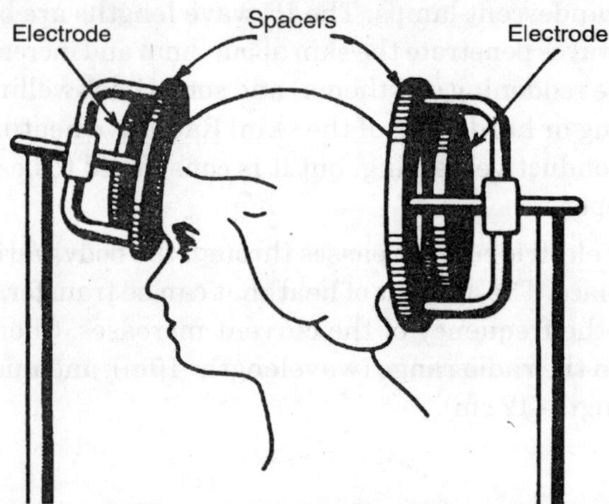

Fig. 12.1a. Location of capacitive coupling electrodes for S.W. diathermy of the head.

Inductance coupling Method

In inductive diathermy, the portion of the body to be heated is placed within or near the inductor (Fig. 12.1*b*). A 30 MHz current in the coil produces an alternating magnetic field in the tissue that produces eddy current in it. The energy lost by eddy currents appears as heat in the tissue.

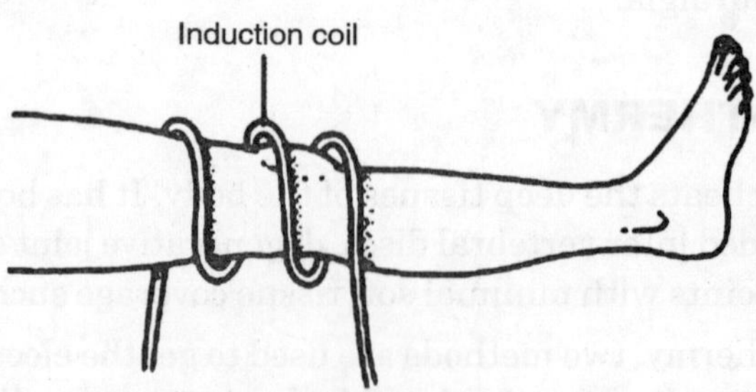

Fig. 12.1b. Location of inductive coupling coil for short wave diathermy of the leg.

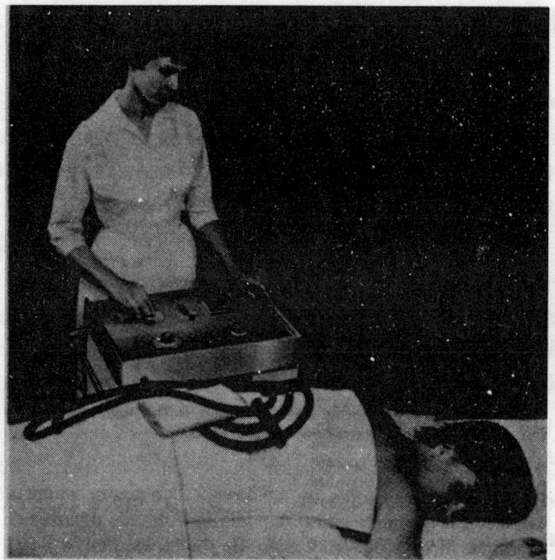

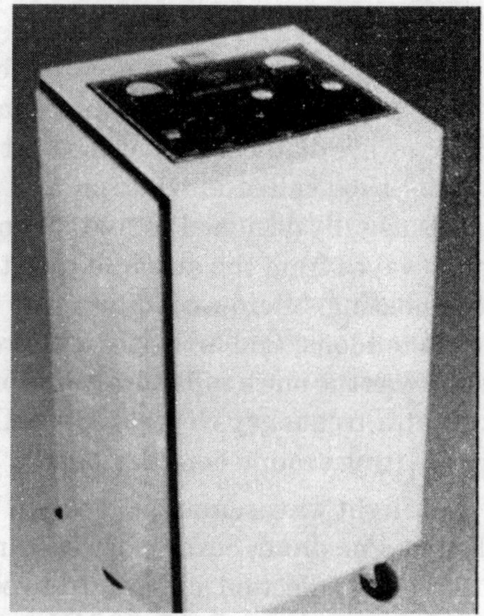

Fig. 12.1c. Photo showing inductive physiotherapy application and a machine.

Applications of Short wave Diathermy

Short -wave diathermy is used in the treatment of bursitis, arthritis, traumatic injuries, strains, and sprains. However, it does have a limitation, when short-wave diathermy is used on muscle tissue surrounded by a fatty layer, a disproportionate amount of energy is lost in the fat. While short- wave diathermy is a much better heater of deep tissue than the hot packs, or infra-red lights, it is far from ideal because of the large amount of energy deposited in surface fatty layers. For this reason microwave diathermy is frequently employed.

Pad Electrodes have great current density in the superficial tissues with spread of current in the deeper tissues.

Cuff Electrodes cause deeper heating but they are applicable only for limbs and not for body region.

Electrodes separated from tissue by an insulting ring is to transfer the R.F.energy through the air-gap. The air - gap acts as a coupling capacitance.

Cable Wrap A few turns wrapped causes inductive heating.

Pancake coil is used for flat body parts.

Fig. 12.1*d* shows various types of electrodes used in diathermy Units.

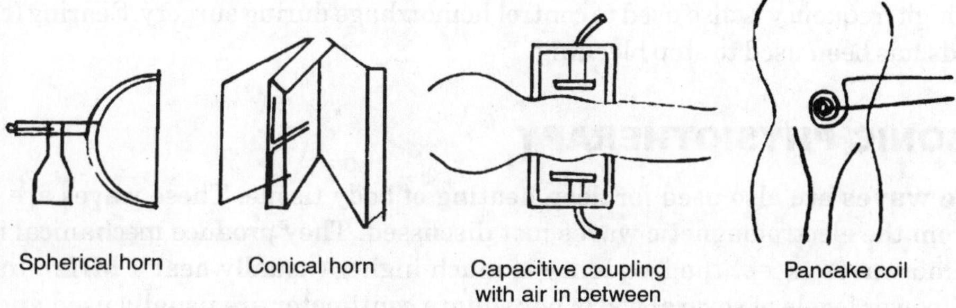

Fig. 12.1d. Various methods of application of physiotherapy in diathermy.

Microwave diathermy

Microwave diathermy, is another form of electromagnetic energy, is usually easier to apply than short wave diathermy. We are all aware of the tissue heating ability of microwave home ovens; microwave diathermy developed out of radar research in 1940s. The microwaves are produced in a special tube called magnetron and are then emitted from the applicator (antenna). The antenna is usually designed so that it can be placed several inches from the region to be treated. The microwaves from the antenna penetrate deep into the tissues, causing a temperature rise and deep heating. Microwave diathermy is used in the treatment of fractures, sprains, bursitis, injuries to tendons, and arthritis. The frequency used in microwave is 2450 MHz because this frequency was the one available after World War II. This is unfortunate since later research has shown that a frequency closer to 900 MHz would be more effective in therapy, causing more uniform heating around bony regions.

Like light waves, microwaves can be transmitted, reflected or refracted at a surface, and absorbed by a medium. Several of the standard antenna arrangements for microwave diathermy make use of the reflection property to direct the radiation to the tissue, where part of it is reflected and part is transmitted. For 2450 MHz radiation, the energy reflected form the skin may be over 50%. A good impedance match between the antenna and the tissue increases the amount of radiation that is transmitted. The transmitted radiation is absorbed by the body and produces heat. For homogeneous tissue, the absorption can be described by an exponential equation. The radiation intensity I at a depth x in the tissue is given as

$$I = I_o \, e^{-x/D}$$

where I_o is the radiation intensity at the surface and D is the tissue thickness that absorbs 63% of the beam, that is, where I is 37% of I_o.

Experiments have shown that the absorption is linked to the amount of water in the tissue and that the heat producing interaction occurs between the electric field in the microwave radiation and the electric dipole moment of the water molecules in the body. The water molecule has a permanent electric dipole, because the center of the net positive charges in the nuclei of the three atoms that make up the molecule is not at the same place as the center of the negative charge.

The slight displacement of the centers of the charge in the molecule results in a permanent electric dipole in the water molecule. The electric field from the microwaves tries to align the dipole of the water molecule with it. In the alignment process, work is done and energy absorbed by the tissue, thus producing heat. The amount of heat of energy absorbed depends upon the frequency of the microwaves. The energy is absorbed best at frequencies near 20 GHz, and poorly at lower frequencies near 1200 MHz and at higher frequencies around 1000 GHz.

The high frequency is also used to control hemorrhage during surgery. Searing (cauterizing) open wounds has been used to stop bleeding.

ULTRASONIC PHYSIOTHERAPY

Ultrasonic waves are also used for deep heating of body tissue. These waves are completely different from the electromagnetic waves just discussed. They produce mechanical motion like audible sound waves except the frequency is much higher (usually near 1 MHz). In ultrasonic diathermy, power levels of several watts per square centimeter are usually used and the sound source is directly in contact with the body. As the ultrasonic waves move through the body, particles in the tissues move back and forth. The movement is similar to a micro-massage and results in heating of the tissues. Ultrasonic heating has been found useful in relieving the tightness and scarring that often occur in joint disease. It greatly aids joints that have limited motion. It is useful for depositing heat in bones because they absorb ultrasound energy more effectively than does soft tissue. Because ultrasound has so many diagnostic uses, it is given more importance in the medical field.

Cancer studies in the early 1970's have indicated that heat therapy may be beneficial in the treatment of cancer when it is combined with radiation therapy. The tumor is heated by diathermy to about 42°C for 20 to 30 minutes and the radiation treatment is given after the heat treatment. Long -term studies under controlled conditions are necessary to evaluate this treatment.

The Ultrasound is applied with piezoelectric crystal transducer with a radiating surface of approximately 10 cm^2. A gel or mineral oil is used between the transducer and the skin for impedance matching. The probe should be calibrated and tuned in water before the treatment to determine the average intensity and total power output. A treatment plan may be several watts per square centimeter for periods of 3 to 120 min from once or twice a day to three times a week. Many a time, the applicator is moved slowly in a back and forth stroking motion to avoid forming "hot spots" in the tissue. When a joint is being treated, the applicator may be moved over the entire external surface of the joint.

Ultrasound deposits its energy in the deeper muscles and tissues of the body while causing little temperature rise in the soft surface tissue layers. Research suggests that ultrasound is the most effective deep heater of bones and joints. Figure shows a change in temperature inside a hip joint as a function of time for ultrasound and microwave diathermy.

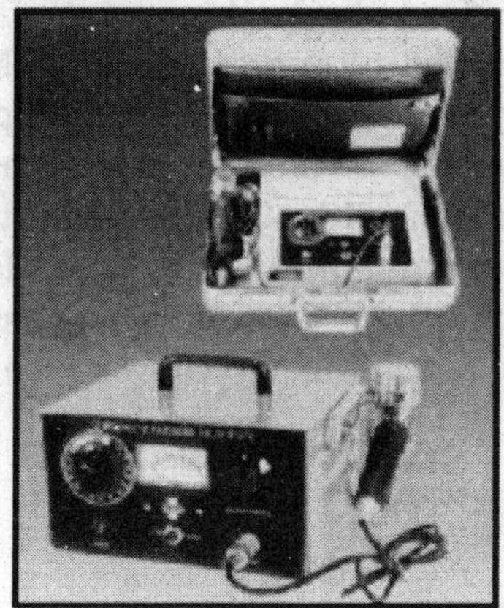

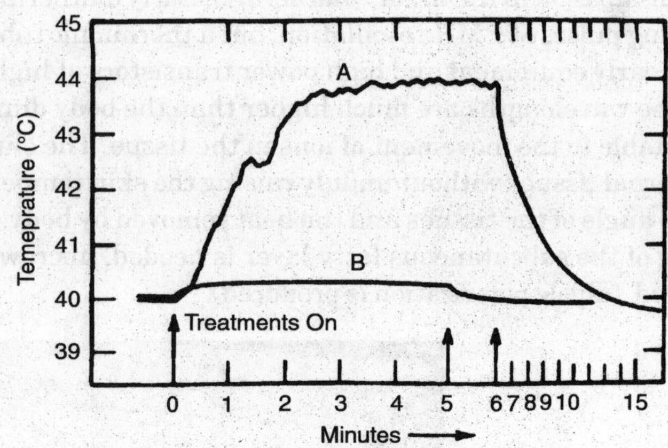

Fig. 12.1e. Figure shows hip joint temperature rise a) for Ultrasound heating b) for microwave heating. The arrows indicate that the first was stopped at 5 min and second in 6 minutes of treatment. The unit is 15 W output.

Ultrasound diathermy is helpful in the treatment of joint disease and joint stiffness. It has also been used on joints that have calcium deposits; there are some indications that it aids in the removal of the deposits. It is not used on regions on the body such as the eyes and gonads where increased temperatures can cause damage.

At power levels of 10^3 W/cm^2, it is possible to selectively destroy tissue at a desired depth by using a focused ultrasound beam. Work on the brains of cats indicates that the mechanism for the destruction of tissue appears to be biochemical and not merely due to local heating.

One might conclude that an intense ultrasound wave would be an ideal agent for destroying cancer tissue. Some studies with ultrasound have shown that cancer cell destruction does occur in some regions of treated tumor; however, other cancer cells in these tumors sometimes show stimulated growth.

Ultrasound was at once used successfully on patients suffering from Parkinson's disease. However, it was found that directing the focused sound to the correct region of the brain was difficult. Because of the possibility of complications due to improper aim, the ultrasound treatment is currently not being used for Parkinson disease.

Meniere's disease, a condition involving 'dizziness' and hearing loss, has been treated with intense ultrasound with nearly 95% success. The ultrasound destroys tissues near the middle ear.

DIATHERMY FOR PHYSIOTHERAPY

The term diathermy was first given by C.F. Nagel Schmidt.

The FCC has allotted 27.32 MHz, 40.98 MHz and 12.68 MHz for short wave (S.W) diathermy. 2450 MHz (12.24 cm) is generally employed for microwave diathermy.

At frequencies approaching 10 kHz, the muscle response was insignificant. It was thus possible at higher frequencies to pass much larger currents through the body, and at frequencies above 100kHz, neither nerves nor muscles are stimulated , but the current does produce heat by ohmic dissipation in the tissue (diathermy). Early diathermy (h.f.) used a spark-gap and induction coil giving pulses of 1 MHz oscillation, but a thermionic tube oscillating approximately 30 MHz is used in early equipment and high power transistors at high frequency in the present equipment. Since the wavelengths are much higher than the body dimensions, the mechanism of heating is attributable to the movement of ions in the tissue. The clinical objective of diathermy is to heat the internal tissues without unduly raising the skin temperature and this heating depends upon the loss angle of the tissues and the heat removed by body circulation. Where a greater localized heating of the subcutaneous fatty layer is needed, microwave diathermy (10 cm wavelength) is employed. (dipole polarization is produced).

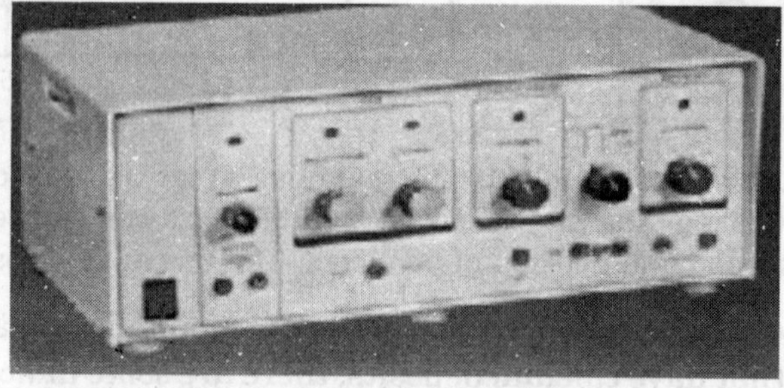

Showing a portable diathermy H.F.apparatus.

The circuit diagram of a 27 MHz h.f. diathermy unit is given in Fig. 12.2*a* and that of typical microwave diathermy unit in Fig. 12.2*b*. The use of tubes is because of the high voltages involved, since transistors for high voltages are not reliable. The taps in the transformer winding permit variation of the power output over a range.

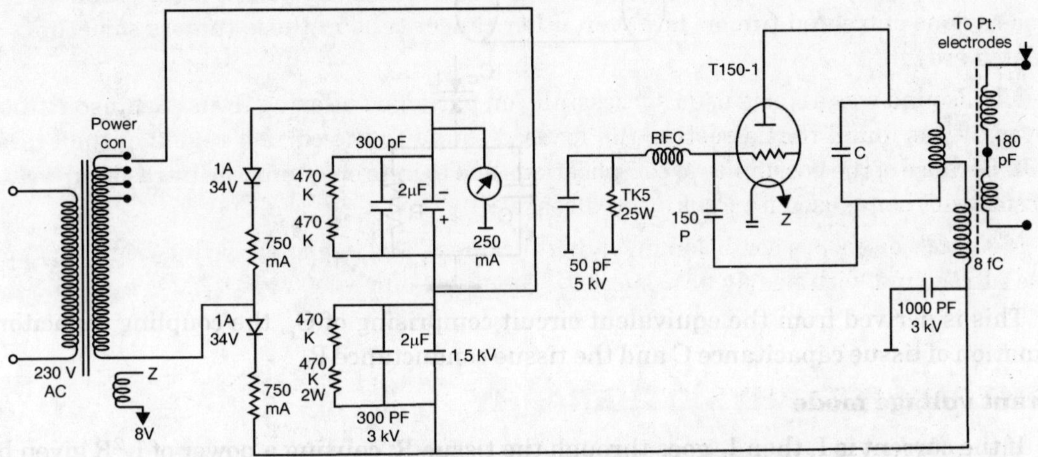

Fig. 12.2a. Circuit diagram of the Diathermy physiotherapy unit.

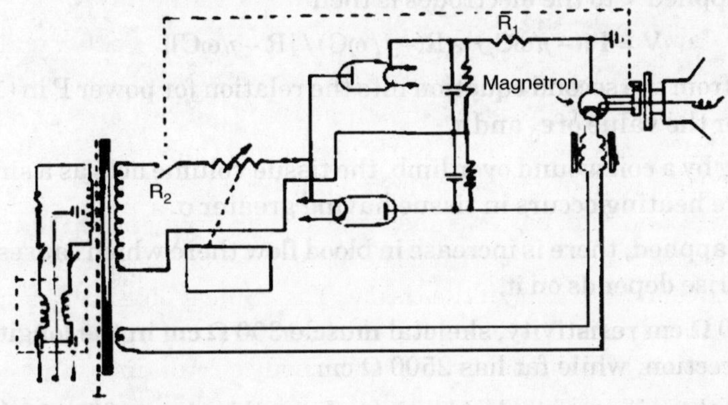

Fig. 12.2b. Circuit diagram of microwave diathermy unit using magnetron.

Power calculations in Physiotherapy

For a tissue volume of length L and cross section A, the power P dissipated through R.F. coupling is to be calculated. Here,

ε = ionic polarization component of dielectric constant

Direct electrodes

$$P = 4I^2 \cdot (L/A) \ (\sigma/(f^2 \varepsilon^2 + 4\sigma^2))$$

The above formulae can be used when electrodes are directly applied.

Here, when P is maximum, $\sigma = f\varepsilon/2$. Then $P_{max} = I^2 l/2A\sigma$.

Air gap method

When one electrode is applied via a small air-gap L_0, with a coupling C_c,

$$P = V^2(L/Lo^2) . A . (f^2 \sigma) / (f^2 (\varepsilon_r + L/Lo)^2 + c . \sigma^2)$$

where c is the constant arrived through ε_o and π as 324×10^{22} for σ given in mho/m.

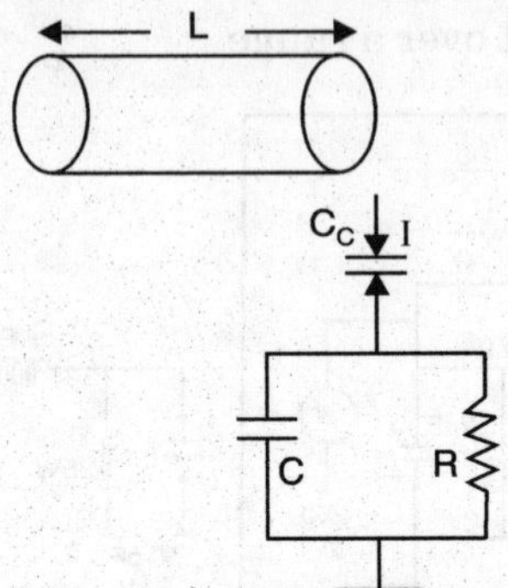

This is derived from the equivalent circuit comprising of C_c, the coupling capacitor, the combination of tissue capacitance C and the tissue conductance R.

Constant voltage mode

If the current is I, then I_1 goes through the tissue R, causing a power of I_1^2R given by

$$P = I^2R(-j/\omega C)^2 / [R - j/\omega C]^2$$

The voltage applied V to the electrodes is then

$$V = I \{(-j/\omega C_c) + R(-j/\omega C) / [R - j/\omega C]\}$$

Expressing I from the second equation into the relation for power P in (1), we get the result after substitution for the value of ε_0 and π.

When heating by a coil wound over limb, the tissue volume acts as a single shorted turn of a secondary. So more heating occurs in tissue having greater σ.

When heat is applied, there is increase in blood flow there which causes cooling, and so the actual temperature rise depends on it.

Blood has 150 Ω cm resistivity, skeletal muscle 300 Ω cm in the longitudinal and 1500 Ω cm in transverse direction, while fat has 2500 Ω cm.

Problem. In the air gap mode, the tissue heated had a σ of 1×10^{-4} and Area was 100 s.cm. The voltage is 2000 V Freqeuncy 10 MHz. ε_r could be taken as 80.

The length is 10 cm and L_0 is 2 cm.

$$P = (2 \times 10^3)^2 \times \{10/2^2\} \times 100 \times (10 \times 10^6)^2 \times 1 \times 10^{-4} / [\{10 \times 10^6\{80 + 10/2)\}^2 + 324 \times 10^{22} \times \{1 \times 10^{-4}\}^2]$$

$$= 13.25 \text{ W}.$$

Problem. In the direct contact method, a mass of tissue on leg 500 gms over 10 cm long and area 6 × 6 cm², at 13 MHz diathermy was heated by 4°C and the value of resistivity of skeletal muscle is 300 ohm-cm. Find the heat in Joules required and the voltage and power required. Assume specific heat 0.9.

$$\sigma = 1/(300 \times 10^{-2}) \text{ mho/m}$$

$$\varepsilon_0 = 8.854 \times 10^{-12}$$

$$Q = ms\ d\theta = \text{heat required} = \text{mass} \times \text{specific heat} \times \text{temperature rise}$$

$$= 500 \times 0.9 \times 4$$

$$1800 \text{ cal} = 1800 \times 4.18 \text{ Joules.}$$

Assume that the heat loss is 50% during the time applied,

The required heat is 3600 × 4.18 J.

This is given by (using metre units) $L = 0.1$, $\sigma = 0.33$

$$\frac{4I^2\{L/A\}\sigma}{f^2\varepsilon^2 + 4\sigma^2}$$

$$\frac{4 \times I^2 \times 0.1 \times 0.33}{36 \times 10^{-4} \times \{2x\pi \times 13 \times 10^6 \times 8.854 \times 10^{-12}\}^2 + 4 \times 0.33^2} \times 5 \times 60 \text{ seconds}$$

$$= 24000\ I^2 \text{ Joules}$$

Equating, and taking root,

$$I = 710 \times 10^{-3} \text{ or } 710 \text{ mA.}$$

$$\text{Voltage} = 0.710 \times \{L/A\sigma\} = 0.71 \times 0.1/[36 \times 10^{-4} \times 0.33] = 60 \text{ and } W = 42 \text{ Watts.}$$

DIATHERMY IN SURGICAL APPLICATIONS

In modern surgery, the use of high frequency surgery currents offer a number of important advantages. The simplified method of hemostatis saves valuable time since bleeding can be arrested immediately by touching the spot briefly with the blade of a lancet or coagulation electrode. Blood vessels with a lumen of up to 1 mm can be quickly and efficiently sealed by grasping the vessel with hemostatic forceps and then touching the forceps with an electrode. As the forceps are removed immediately after this procedure, the operating field is kept clear. With high frequency coagulation a homogeneous coagulation zone is formed that gradually merges into the adjacent tissue, thus avoiding the danger of hemorrhage.

Electric cutting permits particularly elegant and effortless surgery. The electrode virtually melts through the tissue, instantaneously sealing capillary and lymphatic vessels to prevent contamination by bacteria and resorption of toxic tissue products. Moreover, "cutting" or "tearing" surgery is possible with the cutting electrode, depending upon whether the high frequency is switched "on" or "off". The degree of coagulation of the cut surface can be varied by selecting a suitable current intensity and cutting speed from a smooth and fine incision to a separation of tissue with coagulated edges.

Now a days therefore, a high frequency (H.F.) equipment is regarded as standard in a theatre.

In addition to its use as therapeutic procedure, diathermy is also an established surgical tool and then it works as 1.5 – 3 MHz. Insertion of pointed electrode, energizing produces high local current densities. As blood vessels, using surgical diathermy units, are cut, they may be sealed by passing diathermy currents through an electrode or forceps to the ends of the vessel. By using a surgical scalpel as the active electrode, the various tissues can be sealed as they are cut, to allow for 'bloodless surgery'. Current methods by treatment for 'Parkinson's disease' necessitate the destruction of localized sections of brain tissue which may be accomplished by a controlled amount of heating or cooling (cryogenic probes). Laser beams are also used for precise coagulation of the brain surface and other tissues.

Surgical Diathermy units in the operating room for tissue and coagulation consist basically of a power radio-frequency oscillator. Typically, assuming a patient tissue load of 150 Ω, a maximum power output of 200 to 500W would be available at some 1.75 Mc/s.

MODERN ELECTROSURGERY

As discussed earlier, electric devices to assist in surgical procedures for cutting and hemostatis (for stopping bleeding) are being employed in the operation theatre. These devices are known as electrocautery apparatus. Cutting and coagulation by h-f currents are used in the following fields:

1. Urology
2. Neurology
3. Ophthalmology and
4. Carcinoma surgery.

This technique is generally called electro surgery, electrotomy or cold cautery.

The spark gap unit originally in use was to suffer from a number of disadvantageous, such as burning down of electrodes, varying output, noise, interference with TV and radio, high cost, etc., which could be eliminated by using an electronic tube as high-frequency generator.

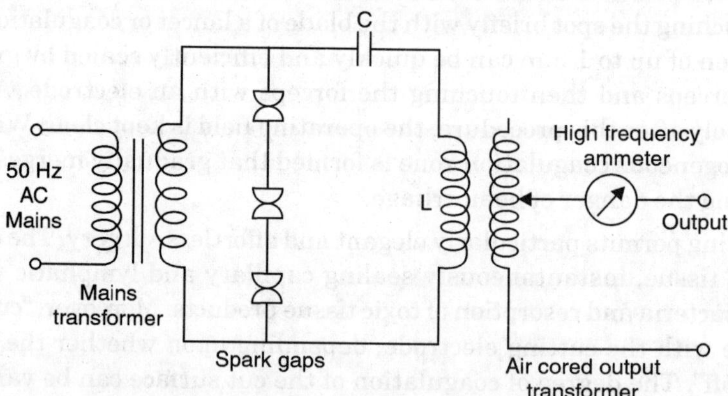

Fig. 12.3. Circuit schematic of the Spark gap diathermy unit.

The current obtained from tubes produces an almost smooth cut similar to that made by a scalpel, which heals well. However, it lacks two properties of spark gap currents, to which the surgeon has become used and which are very valuable.

1. Effective control of bleeding and
2. Good fulguration due to the fact that the spark gap current is composed of individual pulses. This typically pulsed current of spark gaps consisting of pulses of steep front, high amplitude and exponential tail, can also be achieved by electronic means, the ordinary tube current being subjected to pulse modulation. The modulated pulse current obtained

in this way is fully equivalent to the effect achieved by spark gap current, as far as stopping bleeding, the degree of fulguration and depth and width of action are concerned.

Another important feature is that these tube circuits based are protected against explosions in the operating theatre caused by ignitable gases used for anesthesia (mostly ether). Other anesthetics which recently have come into use and are less sensitive in this respect cannot replace ether in every case. It is therefore general practice not to use equipment in the operating theatre, parts of which tend to spark ; otherwise to use equipment with protected parts.

This process involves the application RF spark between a probe and tissue to cause for localized heating and damage to that tissue.

The basic electrosurgical unit consists of the following:

1. High frequency power needed to produce the spark using high frequency generation circuit.
2. Modulator circuit controls the output which is controlled by the surgeon through the control circuit provide . The output of energy from the high frequency needs to be at various levels for the various actions.
3. A coupling circuit is involved between the generator output and the electrodes to control the energy.

CIRCUIT DIAGRAM OF ELECTROSURGERY UNIT

The circuit diagram for a portable surgical diathermy unit shown in Fig. 12.3. This unit is small and a portable one. The power output from this unit is about 80-W. A half wave rectifier power supply feeds a shunt fed Hartley oscillator. The output is derived from a secondary winding. The output current is adjusted by the tuning capacitor, and by varying the coupling between the primary and secondary of the radio-frequency transformer. In larger diathermy units, a power output stage is used to generate the required level of output power.

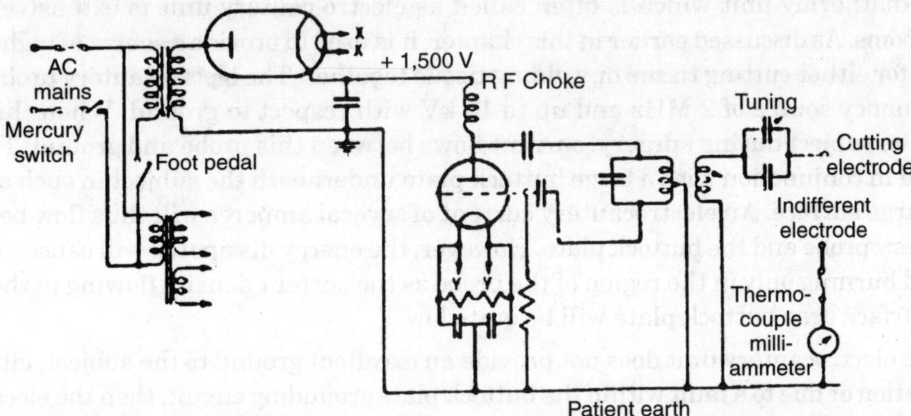

Fig. 12.4a. Continuous Wave tube generator diathermy circuit.

For cutting and coagulation 500 W, 150 ohms load, 1.75 MHz for cutting and 1.75 MHz with 60 KHz burst for coagulation. For cutting in water 20 W is enough with 1.75 MHz modulated with 50 Hz.

For smooth cutting, a sine wave output is used. For cutting and coagulation, bursts of 1.75 kHz R.F. are used, the repetition rate being of the order of 20 to 60 kHz.

Fig. 12.4*a* and 4*b* show some surgical diathermy circuitry used in machines in which the R.F. generator can be placed outside the operating room, and the R.F.. leads and cutting electrode continuously purged within nitrogen. In this way, explosion risks when using anesthetic agents such as cyclopropane are minimized.

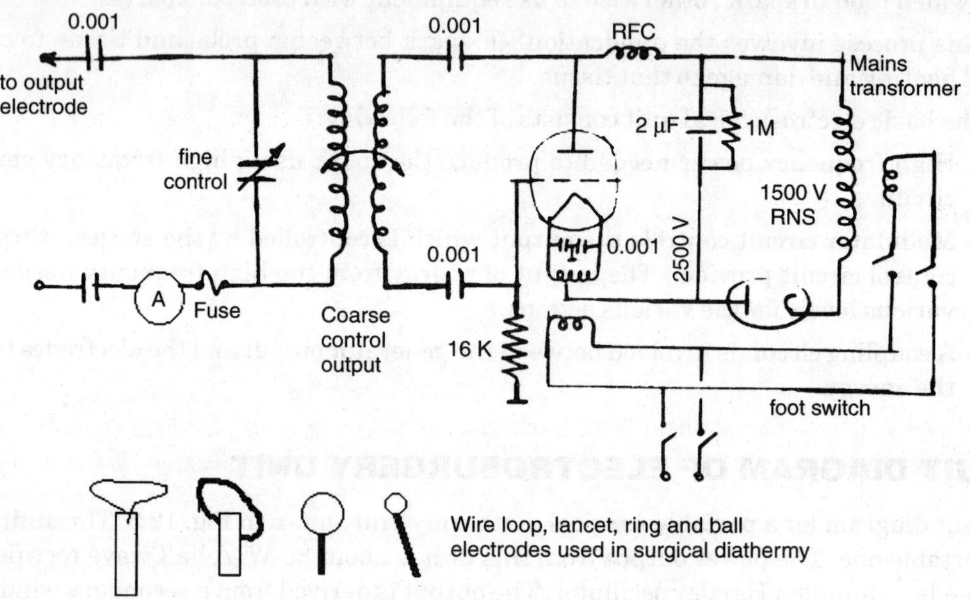

Fig. 12.4b. Shows another circuit for diathermy using tube.

Diathermy Units

The diathermy unit which is often called as electro-cautery unit is extensively used in operating rooms. As discussed earlier in this chapter, it is used to provide a source of high frequency RF current for either cutting tissue or welding tissue together. The electrocautery probe provides a high frequency source of 2 MHz and up to 15 kV with respect to ground. When this probe is applied to the subject during surgery, current flows between this probe and ground. This unit is always used in conjunction with a large buttock plate underneath the subject in such a way as to provide a large surface. An electrocautery current of several amperes will thus flow between the electrocautery probe and the buttock plate. However, the energy dissipated will cause appreciable heating and burning only in the region of the probe as the current density flowing in the region of the large surface area buttock plate will be quite low.

If the electrocautery unit does not provide an excellent ground to the subject, either due to poor application or due to a fault within the buttock plate grounding circuit, then the electrocautery current will be diverted to other grounded points on the subject. It is not common for ECG electrodes to provide this alternative grounding point as all ECG monitoring equipment essentially provide a low impedance for the path to this high voltage, high frequency current. Unfortunately, the ECG electrode does not behave in the same manner as the buttock plate as the contact area involved is

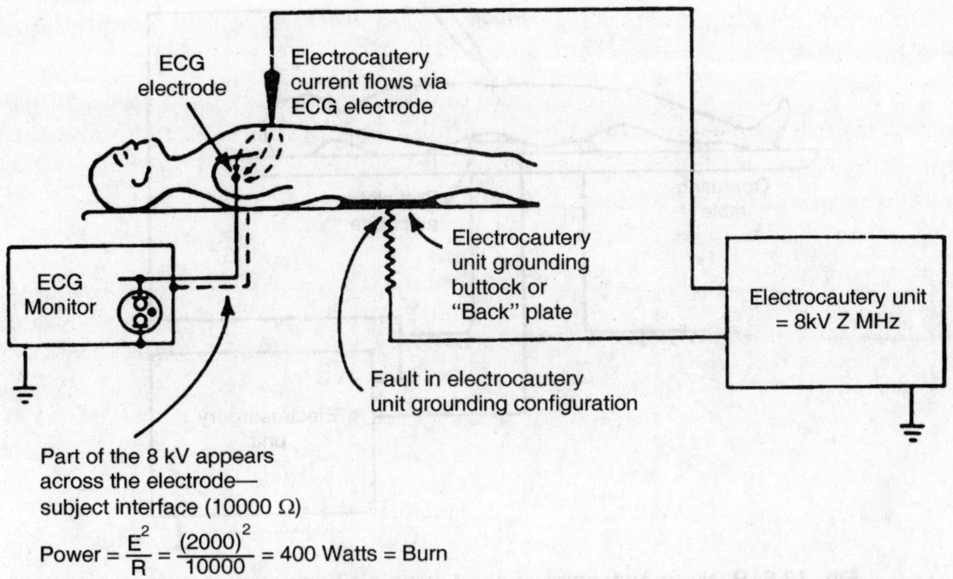

Fig. 12.5. Shows how the electrocautery diathermy unit causes burns at electrode site.

smaller by a factor of at least 100, perhaps 1000. The current density is thus increased by a corresponding factor and will almost certainly cause heating and burns at the ECG sites. The high frequency current used in electrocautery is at higher frequency and will not cause ventricular fibrillation. In practice, if a surgeon suspects that the electrocautery unit " is not cutting too well" he should be suspicious of the electrocautery ground circuitry and should have the electrocautery unit adequately checked before continuing to use it.

"SPARK-GAP" BASED DIATHERMY UNIT

As explained earlier, older types of surgical diathermy work on the "spark gap" principle. Fig. 12.3 gave the circuit diagram of a simple spark-gap type diathermy unit. The AC mains supply voltage is stepped up to several thousand volts by the mains transformer and applied to several spark gaps in series. Twice per cycle of the mains (on the + and - half cycles) sparks are produced. The capacitor is discharged through the gaps is an oscillatory fashion, the combination of L and C being chosen to oscillate at some 800 kHz. The output of the diathermy thus consists of bursts of damped radio-frequency waves at intervals of 10ms (one complete mains cycle takes 20 m sec at 50 Hz). A tapping on the output transformer allows the output current to be adjusted. A typical maximum power output would be 250 W. The basic surgery arrangement is shown below in Fig. 12.6.

Spark-gap generators are very robust, but anesthetic explosion risks are greater with them, and they do generate a substantial proportion of harmonic frequencies. These can cause interference with communications and monitoring equipment. Valve and transistor oscillators seem to be preferred by surgeons, and any interfering radiation from them can be more easily suppressed by filter circuits because of the greater purity.

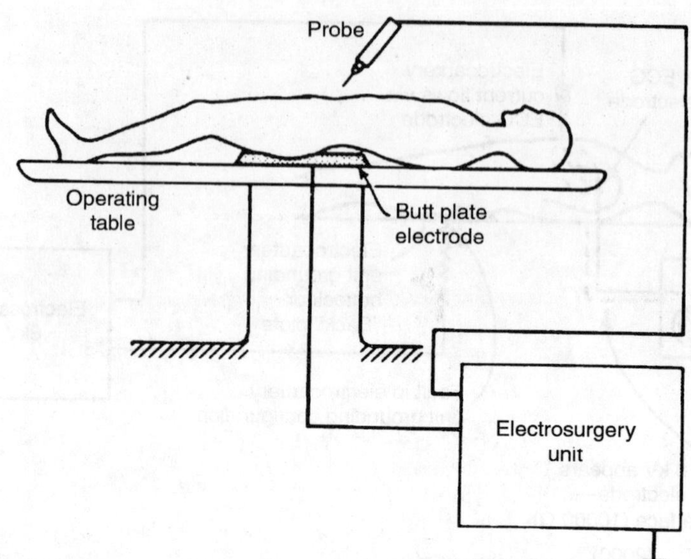

Fig. 12.6. Basic arrangement of short wave diathermy unit in surgery.

CARDIAC PACEMAKERS

As discussed in Chapter 2 when dealing with the heart and the circulatory system, the steady rhythm of the heart is maintained by a biological "pacemaker" within the sinoartrial node of the heart. Failure of this pacemaker will cause the pumping action of the heart to be interfered with, causing a seizure and possible death. Emergency resuscitation from a seizure might be accomplished by external electrical stimulation or cardiac massage of the heart by trained medical personnel. Since in many subjects seizures are unpredictable, continuous stimulation is required to ensure continuous reliable function of the heart. Long term stimulation from an external electrical source requires a considerable level of stimulating current to ensure that a sufficient level of current passes directly through the heart, thus causing considerable pain to the subject. This pain may be avoided by using external electrical stimulation using internal electrodes placed directly on the heart; however, tissue irritation and rejection present a problem that is difficult to overcome.

The modern cardiac pacemaker concept avoids tissue irritation and rejection by surgically implanting a pacemaker within the subject's abdomen and connecting it to the heart via internal electrodes. Modern internal pacemakers use mercury batteries which can operate the pacemaker continuously for a year or more. Since the pacemaker is placed in the subject's abdomen rather in the heart, a relatively unsophisticated surgical procedure is necessary on a routine basis to replace the pacemaker with one having a fresh battery. The problem of determining just when an internal pacemaker's battery is nearly discharged, and thus, when the pacemaker must be replaced, has not yet been completely solved; however, many researchers have proposed various techniques, for determining pacemaker-end-of life by analyzing the pacemaker output pulse as recorded on the surface of the body. At this stage there does not appear to be sufficient evidence in favor of any one for it to be universally accepted.

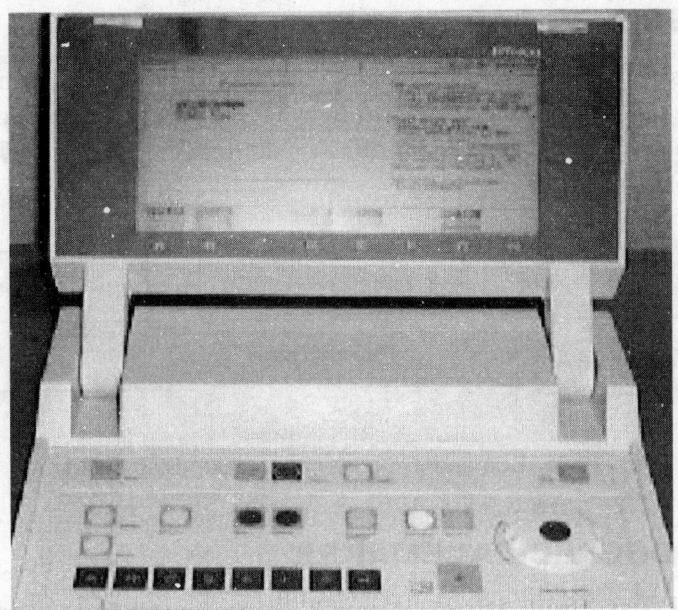

The internal cardiac pacemaker consists of a transistorized blocking oscillator producing pulses of approximately 10V in amplitude level, a few (2 or 2.5) milliseconds in width and at an approximate 60 per minute rate. The equivalent circuit for a pacemaker and the subject together with a photograph of a commercial pacemaker, is shown in Fig. 12.7*b*, while a typical early day external variable rate pacemaker is shown in Fig. 12.7*a*. Today, typical circuits like the one using cmos gate IC building block oscillator are used. This circuit given uses two gates and R1, R2, C to produce a pulse once a second, and another similar gate pair would produce a 2.5 ms square wave, both when gated will give a 2.5 ms pulse once every second. The latter time can be made variable with an external resistor so as to vary the pacemaker rate from 60 to 120. Such a combination of gates can now be had in a very tiny SMD (surface mount device VLSI module. The cmos circuitry draw very little power and can work from 3 V supply onwards.

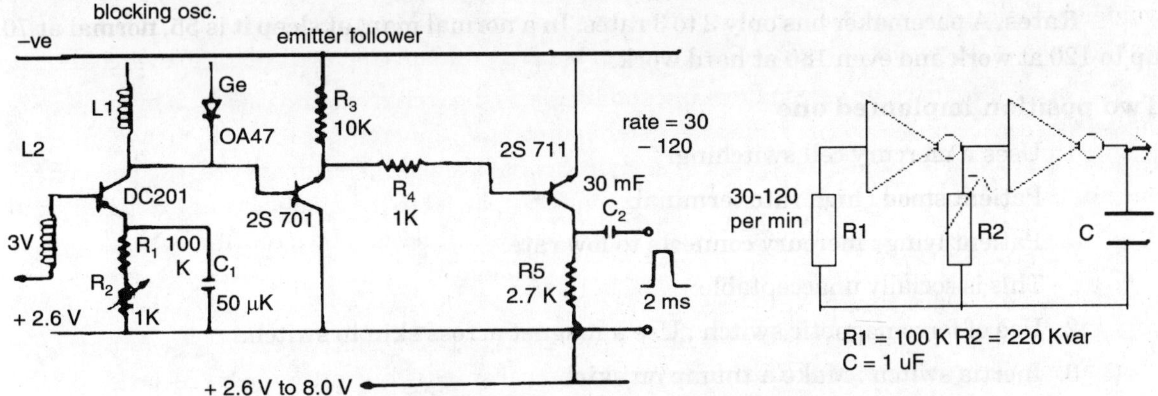

Fig. 12.7. Circuit of one type of variable rate pacemaker. The right half shows a CMOS 4069 based oscillator.

DEMAND TRIGGERED PACEMAKER

This is also an implantable pacemaker. This delivers a fixed rate pacing stimulus only when the normal QRS waves fail to follow the natural P-wave stimulus. It can therefore never trigger ventricular fibrillation by delivering a stimulus to relaxing heart muscle. This relaxing period is known as the "vulnerable period".

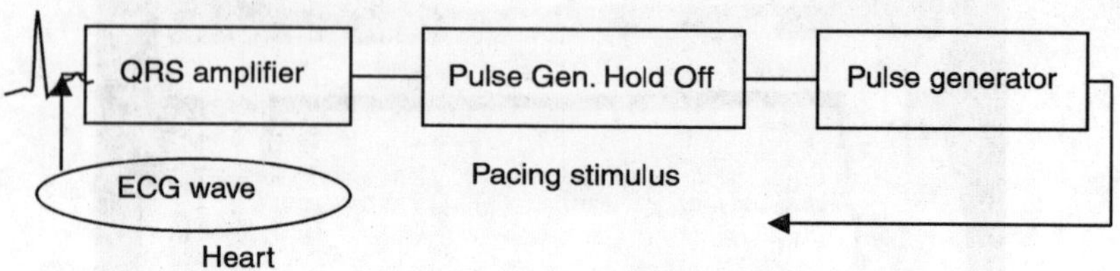

Fig. 12.8a. Demand Triggered pacemaker-Block diagram.

ATRIALLY TRIGGERED PACEMAKER

Natural excitation P-wave from atrium is somehow prevented from reaching the ventricles. Pacemaker amplifies this wave, delays it for an appropriate interval, then fires a pulse into the ventricular muscle.

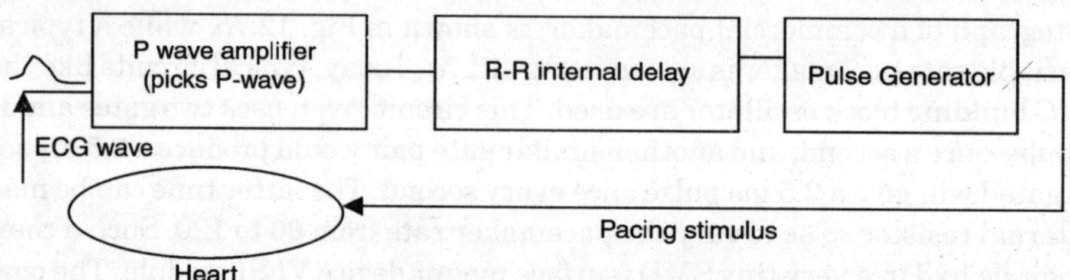

Fig. 12.8b. Shows the block diagram for the artificially triggered Pacemaker unit.

Rates. A pacemaker has only 2 to 3 rates. In a normal man, at sleep it is 55, normal at 70, up to 120 at work and even 180 at hard work.

Two position implanted one

1. Uses a mercury cell switching.

   Patient stood : high rate terminal.

   Patient lying : mercury connects to low rate.

   This is socially unacceptable.

2. Use of ferromagnetic switch : Use a magnet across skin to switch.
3. Inertia switch : Make a thump on skin.

An early version of the implantable pacemaker is given in Fig. 12.8c.

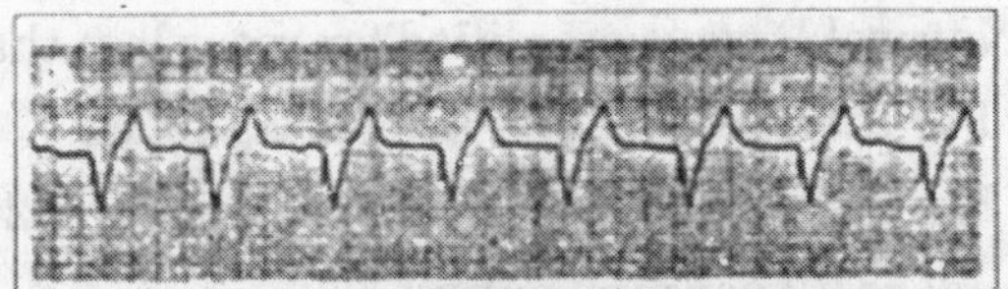

Typical ECG from a subject with an implanted cardiac pacemaker

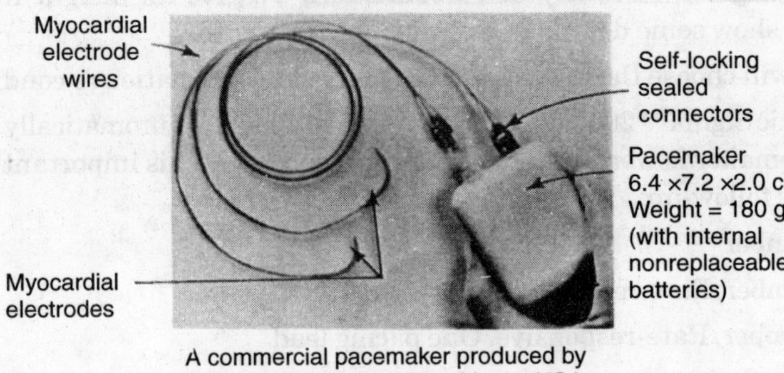

A commercial pacemaker produced by elecrodyne company Inc., Mass., USA

Fig. 12.8c. Shows an early version of a Demand pacemaker of implantable type.

It was in 1966 that the Demand pacemaker came into being. In many, heart block is intermittent and it is dangerous to stimulate at a fixed rate pulse, which may coincide with a point in the cardiac cycle where it is likely to trigger a ventricular fibrillation.

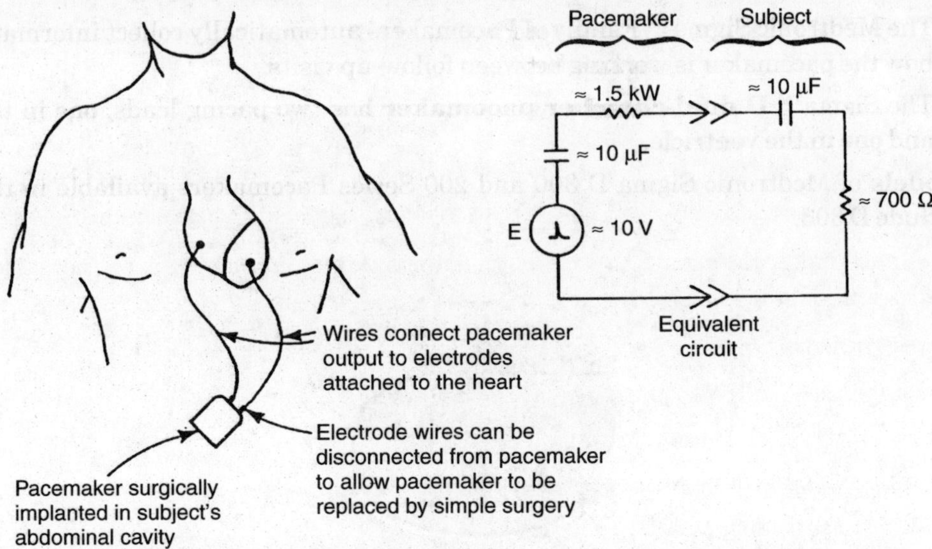

Fig. 12.8d. Shows an early version of a Demand pacemaker of implantable type.

The equivalent circuit of pacemaker to heart interface is shown in Fig. 12.8*d*. The demand pacemaker works at 72 beats a minute. Most satisfactory pacemaker is the atrial triggered type. The three modes of its operation are :

1. **Standard mode :** Natural P wave amplified for rates less than 150
2. (*a*) **Block mode 1 :** For rates over 250, it inserts 2:1 block

   (*b*) **Block mode 2 :** Inserts a 3:1 block for rate greater than 240.
3. **P-wave fails:** Standard 72 per min. output.

A typical advanced Pacemaker from Medtronic Sigma™ and its uses are given below.

Medtronic Sigma™ Family of Pacemakers To give an insight into actual units of pacemakers, let us show some details from Medtronic Sigma Inc.

The Doctor will choose the pacemaker that is best for the patient's condition.

The Medtronic Sigma™ 200 and 300 Family of Pacemakers automatically collect information about how the pacemaker is working between follow-up visits. This important information helps the clinician during follow-up.

- Dual-chamber
- Dual-chamber, Rate-responsive
- Dual-chamber, Rate-responsive, One pacing lead
- Single-chamber
- Single-chamber, Rate-responsive

MEDTRONIC SIGMA™ DUAL-CHAMBER MODELS

The pacemaker is chosen that is best for the patient's exact condition.

- The Medtronic Sigma™ Family of Pacemakers automatically collect information about how the pacemaker is working between follow-up visits.
- The Sigma™ **D dual-chamber pacemaker** has two pacing leads, one in the atrium and one in the ventricle.

Models of Medtronic Sigma D 300 and 200 Series Pacemakers available in the United States include D 303.

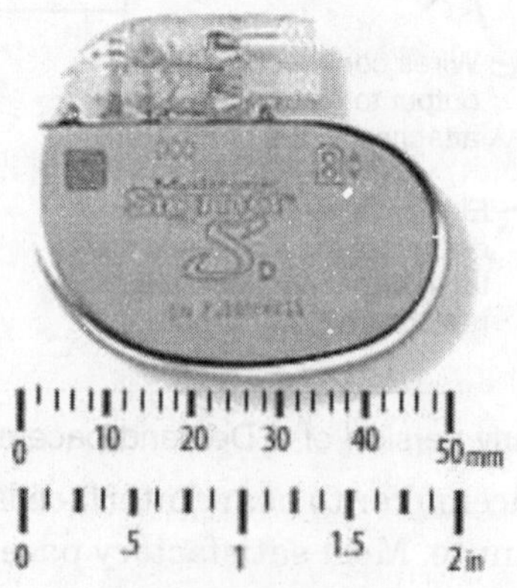

Fig. 12.8c

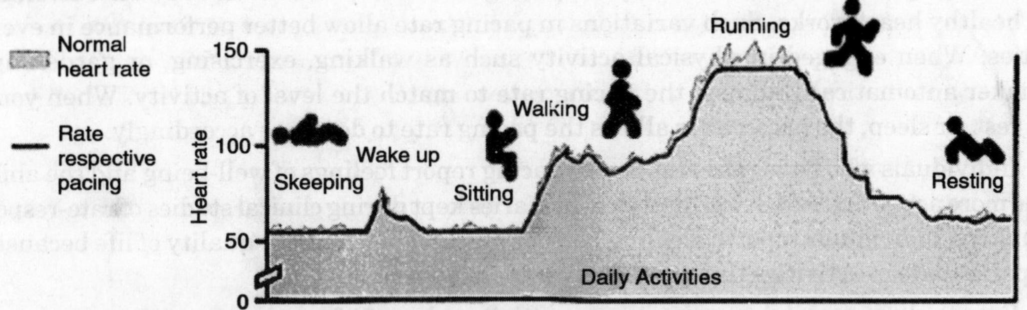

Fig. 12.8e. shows a typical Pacemaker units and the activities of the heart-Medtronic Sigma™ 200 make

Approximate dimensions. Height: 1 3/4 inches (45 mm) Length : 2 inches (51 mm), Width : 1/3 inch (7 mm)

How long this pacemaker battery lasts depends upon the patient's medical condition, how often a pacing pulse is emitted, and the amount of energy for each pacing pulse. Based on general conditions, the estimate is 7 to 9 years. The Doctor can tell a more accurate estimate based on the patient's exact condition.

Type : Rate-responsive Pacing Systems

A normal heart rhythm slows down or speeds up many times during the day. The heart beats slower while resting or sleeping. Exercise or emotional excitement makes a heart beat faster because, in an excited state, a body requires greater amounts of oxygen. And, oxygen is brought to all parts of the body through the blood. When a heart is unable to adjust its pumping rate, a rate-responsive pacemaker is used.

A rate-responsive pacemaker mimics the heart's natural function to adjust the heart rate. A rate-responsive pacemaker uses one or more special sensors to recognize changes in how much blood and oxygen are needed by the body. Based on this information, the heart rate is adjusted to meet the body's changing needs for blood flow.

How Rate-responsive Pacemakers Function?

A rate-responsive pacemaker uses one or more special sensors to detect changes in the body that indicate more oxygen is needed. Some sensors may detect motion or how often you breathe. When a change is detected, the pacing rate is increased according to how the doctor programmed the pacemaker.

A pacemaker may have one or more sensors . The two most common sensors are an **activity sensor** and a **minute ventilation sensor.**

Benefits of Rate-responsive Pacing

For people whose heart rate does not increase when needed, rate-responsive pacing:

- Provides people with a more appropriate heartbeat for their current activity.
- Allows people to perform ordinary, daily activities more effectively.
- Allows people to perform more vigorous exercise.
- Gives people a greater sense of well-being in their day-to-day lives.

Rate-responsive pacemakers vary the pacing rate in response to the body's needs, similar to how a healthy heart works. Such variations in pacing rate allow better performance in everyday activities. When engaged in physical activity such as walking, exercising, or gardening, the pacemaker automatically adjusts the pacing rate to match the level of activity. When you slow down, rest, or sleep, the pacemaker allows the pacing rate to decrease accordingly.

Individuals who have rate-responsive pacing report feelings of well-being and the ability to resume more active and satisfying lifestyles. In diaries kept during clinical studies of rate-responsive pacemakers, individuals reported feeling better and enjoying a higher quality of life because they could participate in activities that previously were not possible.

One need not engage in very strenuous activity to benefit from a rate-responsive pacemaker. For example, the simple act of walking may require a rate of more than 100 beats per minute.

Rate-responsive pacing can be done with a dual- or single-chamber pacing system.

CARDIAC STIMULATION IN I.C.U. by internal means uses the following four types of apparatus. They are:

1. By means of wires attached to the heart and brought and to an external pacemaker.
2. By an electrode catheter passed along a vein and terminating in the right ventricle.
3. An implanted unit which receives its power from an external source.
4. A completely self-contained implanted unit.

Lead wire can be of braided stainless steel and insulated, the space filled with anti biotic enforced silicone grains.

Pulse 2 m sec, 30–120 variable

External Pacemakers

Temperature range – 0 to 50°C

Implanted-external powered-receiver coil implanted within the rectus sheath and the transmitting coil around the waist of the patient.

Effect of waist movement = ± 4 inches (10 cm)

Transmitter coil is in endless loop 42″, around belt, no plugs and sockets.

Internal Stimulation by Pacemakers

(1 to 5Volts only) (but external stimulus requiring 200V which is very painful).

One electrode sited at the heart. Other electrode is buried in tissues or placed on body surface. Any one of the above types may be employed.

Such pacemakers should ensure least infection hazard for I.C.U. emergency pacing.

A Blocking oscillator circuit is shown in figure 12.7 for use in external pacemaker with internal electrodes in emergency pacing at the ICU.

CARDIAC DEFIBRILLATORS

Ventricular Defibrillators

Resuscitation from either from a heart seizure or from ventricular fibrillation can be accomplished by external electrical stimulation. Ventricular fibrillation is produced within the

human heart due to a variety of reasons, including accidental electrocution. When the heart is in ventricular fibrillation, individual portions of the ventricular muscle contract independently instead of synchronously and effective output of blood ceases. External stimulation can be achieved with a cardiac defibrillator which essentially consists of a capacitor charged to several thousand volts which then discharged though the subject via a large surface area—"paddle" electrodes as shown in Fig. 12.9. The energy produced within a cardiac defibrillator is typically 200 joules given by 0.5 CE^2, where C = is the value of the storage capacitor and E is the voltage level to which it is charged.

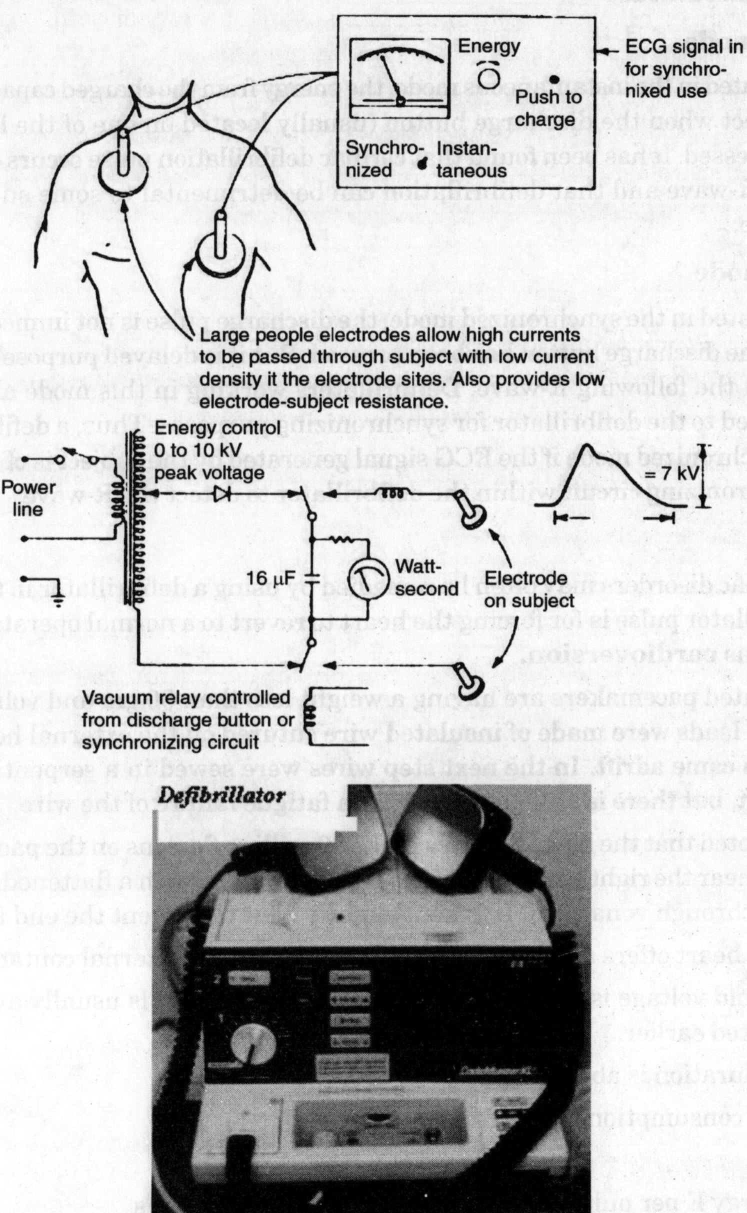

Fig. 12.9. Application of defibrillator and a typical DC defibrillator.

Defibrillation shocks from 200 watts- second to 400 watts- second are normally required to get satisfactory cardiac defibrillation. Not all the energy will be available for dissipation at the subject as the efficiency of discharge will be considerably less than 100%; typically 20% to 70% is noteworthy.

The cardiac defibrillators may be operated in one of the two modes; they are:

1. Instantaneous mode and
2. Synchronized mode

Instantaneous mode

When operated in the instantaneous mode, the energy from the charged capacitor is discharged through the subject when the discharge button (usually located on one of the hand held paddle electrodes) is depressed. It has been found that cardiac defibrillation pulse occurs during the falling part of the ECG R-wave and that defibrillation can be detrimental to some subjects if it occurs during the T-wave.

Synchronized mode

When operated in the synchronized mode, the discharge pulse is not immediately applied to the subject after the discharge button has been pressed. But it is delayed purposely to occur during the falling edge of the following R-wave. Defibrillators working in this mode also need an ECG signal being applied to the defibrillator for synchronizing purposes. Thus, a defibrillator can only be used in the synchronized mode if the ECG signal generated by the subject is of sufficient quality to allow the synchronizing circuit within the defibrillator to detect the R-wave.

Cardioversion

Many cardiac disorders may often be remedied by using a defibrillator in the synchronized mode. The defibrillator pulse is for forcing the heart to revert to a normal operating rhythm. This process is known as cardioversion.

The implanted pacemakers are having a weight less than 80 gm and volume less than 70 ml. Originally the leads were made of insulated wire sutured on the external heart muscle. Frequently, the wires came adrift. In the next step wires were sewed in a serpentine fashion. This anchored it alright, but there is still possibility for a fatigue failure of the wire.

It may be noted that the heart muscles make 80 million flexions on the pacemaker wire. So, the wire is placed near the right ventricle via the tricuspid valve, with a flattened beaded end, sent via the neck vein through vena cava. It is kept slightly bent to prevent the end from slipping.

The typical heart offers a resistance of 100 to 300 ohm for external contact.

The threshold voltage is only 1 to 2 Volt, but higher voltage is usually available from the pacemaker, as stated earlier.

The pulse duration is about 2 ms.

The energy consumption can be calculated now.

$$E = V^2/R \times t$$

So, the energy E per pulse will be $= (1 - 2)^2/(100 - 300) \times 2$ ms

$= 20 - 80$ micro Joules.

For internal contact the resistance rises from 500 to 1000 ohm and the threshold drops to 0.8V to 1V and hence the power is reduced to 3 micro J per pulse.

Consumption of battery is reckoned as

$$3\ \mu J/\text{pulse} \times 60\ \text{pulse/min} \times 60 \times 365 \times 24$$

This itself is noted to be less than 120 J. So, the batteries have long shelf life as used in the pacemaker. Up to 7 years these present batteries are lasting.

Defibrillators

Ventricular fibrillation is not spontaneously reversible in man; one has to quickly take corrective measures.

Pottasium Chloride into circulatory system stops it. Sudden cold abolishes fibrillation , but slow or localized cooling increases fibrillation (Brooks).

A sufficiently large electric shock abolishes fibrillation.

Early A.C. fibrillators – 2 Amps on exposed heart

5 Amps on closed heart.

(50, 90 ohms), 60 Hz current, 100–300 V.

Recommended duration ¼ second only.

Energy delivered = 500 watts per second.

Capacitor discharge system is more effective and less damaging to the heart.

But a.c defibrillator can be used instead of waiting for the capacitor - discharge defibrillator to be rolled in.

Energy limits

A.C. defibrillator

$$0.25\ \text{sec} \times 230\ \text{volts} \times (I\ \text{Amps}) = 450\ \text{watts-sec.}$$

Required required

$$I = 7.5\text{Amps.}$$

But preferable 0.01 sec. Pulses.

Then $I = 450/(230 \times 0.01) = 175$ A.

This is too much to be supplied by household mains.

Capacitor discharge

16 μF capacitor = 400 Watts-sec.

This capacitor can store this energy **in a few seconds** without drawing more than 5 Amps form the mains.

But stored voltage is **(for 16 μF, 400 W-Sec.)** high

$$\tfrac{1}{2} CV^2 = 400$$

$$V = \sqrt{(400 \times 2) / 16} = 7000\ \text{V}$$

This peak voltage will be applied at the instant of application. So, reduce it by inductive damping. Peleska tried and used inductive damping, because it causes myocardial damage.

AC Defibrillator. (Fig. 10)

Internal defibrillators = 80–100 V for 0.1 sec

External Defibrillators = 800 V

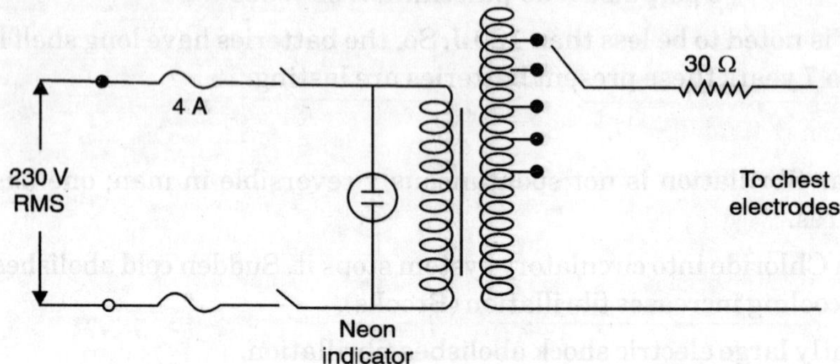

Fig. 12.10a. AC defibrillator.

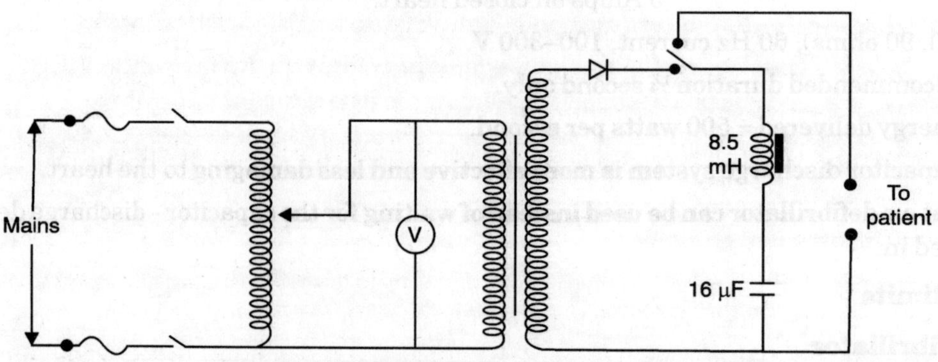

Fig. 12.10b. DC defibrillator.

DC Defibrillators

5000–10,000V, 3–4 seconds time between successive pulses.

Discharge adjustable in 5 steps. In the range 60-400W/s.

Charging time = 3 sec for 90% of full charge.

Open chest 50 Ω–75 Ω large spoon shaped electrodes

85–500 V can be selected (4 to 6Amps r.m.s through heart)

closed chest 5000 V, 100 Ω and more (5A flow)

Time .25 sec is enough

Foot switch. A timing circuit allows 5–10 cycles of the mains on, then cuts out till switch is pressed again. Electrodes are housed in well insulated handles with a finger switch.

Output secondary winding must be free from earth so that there is no risk of shock. ECG machines are provided with limiting circuits in their input stage and a high degree of isolation from earth so that defibrillation voltages will not permanently damage the recorder. (protection circuit operates between 5 mV to 60 mV).

DC Defibrillation (Fig. 12.10b)

1. Safety housings for electrodes–capacitor discharges only when the electrodes are making firm contact with the heart or chest wall.
2. Two set of electrodes - not interchangeable sockets
   1. Internal 50–72 J (5–3 kV)
3. Meter indicates Joules
   1. External 400J (7 kV).
4. Charging time constant of 4 seconds
   1. 0.25 M $\Omega \times 16\ \mu$F
   2. (charging resistor)

   Takes about 16 secs. to charge to 4 kV.

Synchronous Defibrillator

Ventricular Fibrillation: use DC defibrillators

Atrial fibrillation and Arrhythmia use Synchronous DC defibrillator

(i) Discharge the capacitor during the down stroke of the R-wave of the ECG.

(ii) Discharge must not occur during T-wave.

It picks up R wave of ECG and uses it to trigger a 30 ms delay and then there is a capacitor discharge time.

Kugelberg/Double-Pulse system

Conventional fibrillation produces myocardial injury with a diminished ventricular function for a period of approximately 30 minute following the delivery of the shock.

8–60 volts only needed compared to the 800–1500 V employed in DC capacitor discharge defibrillators.

Some cells get depolarized.

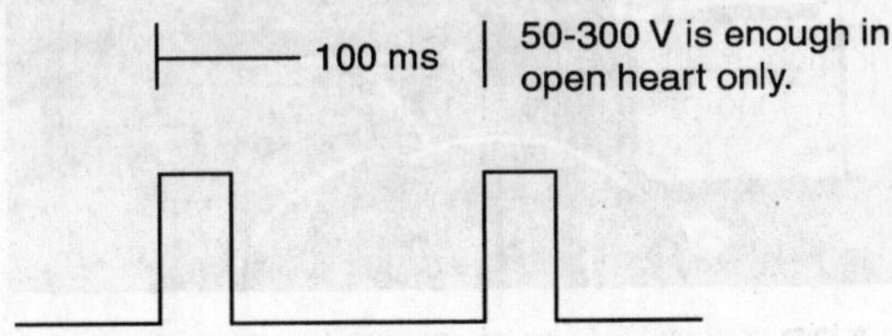

Fig. 12.11. KugelBerg Double Pulse system

Monitor for ECG cum Defibrillator

In intensive care units for patient monitoring, the E.C.G. is continuously seen on a monitor. As soon as the need for defibrillation arises in an emergency when the heart beat stops or goes into fibrillation state, the alarm on the monitor sounds and then the Doctor has to rush to provide the emergency defibrillation. Such units have provision for defibrillation as well. The Fig. 12.12b shows one such unit.

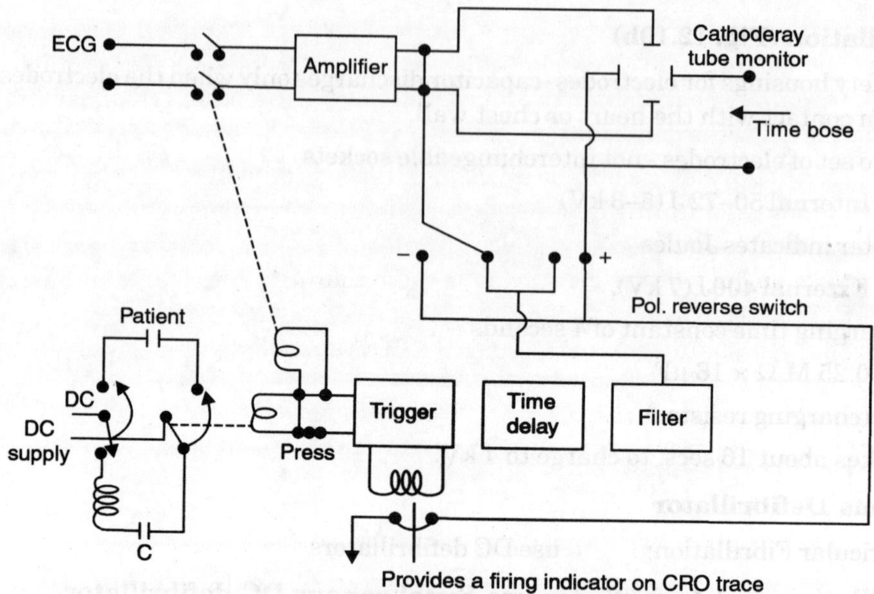

Fig. 12.12a. Shows the block Diagram of a synchronous pacemaker unit.

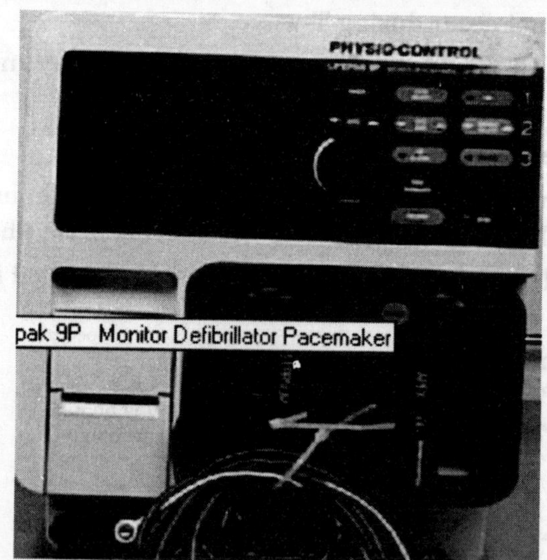

Fig. 12.12b. ECG monitor cum Defibrillator. The black looking screen on the top left is the CRT monitor display.

Problems with Defibrillators for the patient' s safety

The defibrillator is another high voltage device commonly used in patient care units. The defibrillator provides a single short duration pulse of up to 10 kV between two large electrodes. These electrodes are normally applied for a patient's chest in cases where the heart got into ventricular fibrillation or has stopped completely. The high energy defibrillation pulse is transmitted between the electrodes and a great portion of the energy is dissipated in the heart. Defibrillation hopefully either re-starts the heart or reverts it from ventricular fibrillation to a normal beating action. Defibrillators should have both electrodes isolated from ground. Even when the high voltage pulse is applied, it can normally be expected to provide safe operation if other personnel are not in contact with the subject during the defibrillation process.

Although a defibrillator's output is isolated, this output will be unbalanced capacitively to ground. Thus, unless monitoring devices, such as an ECG instrument, incorporate input circuit protection they may be damaged by the defibrillator pulse. If a subject's heart has not stopped beating altogether but is beating erratically, a defibrillator may be operated in a synchronized mode to revert the heart to a normal rhythm. This is referred to as cardioversion. The defibrillator synchronizing pulse is obtained from the subject's ECG R-wave, the defibrillation pulse occurring sometime after the ECG R-wave but avoiding the vulnerable period during the upswing of the ECG T-wave.

What happens after defibrillator is applied ?

Subsequent to the application of the defibrillator on the heart which went into fibrillation with an electric shock, (12V 50Hz through an internal electrode between heart and right leg (dog), what happens to the ECG during recovery is shown in Fig.12.12. The heart goes into the full diastolic phase immediately after the impulse is given. Then, fast and forcible contractions follow. Figs.12.12 (1) to (3) show samples of the records of ECG during the post defibrillation period. It may be noted that (1) the ECG is initially showing only oscillations without any sharp qrs and has no T wave of the usual nature. The rate is fast because the action potential swings negatively and there is quicker re-triggering for the cell (2) With lapse of time, the ECG shows increasingly sharper QRS and develops T waves, the ST interval increasing little by little. There is an ST depression which becomes iso-electric only slowly because of partially damaged tissue.

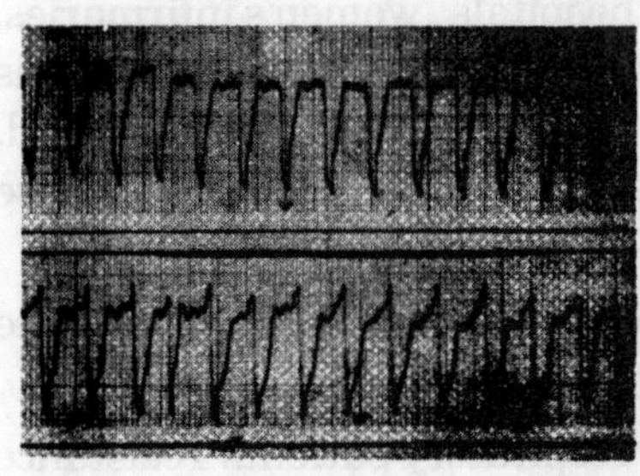

1.

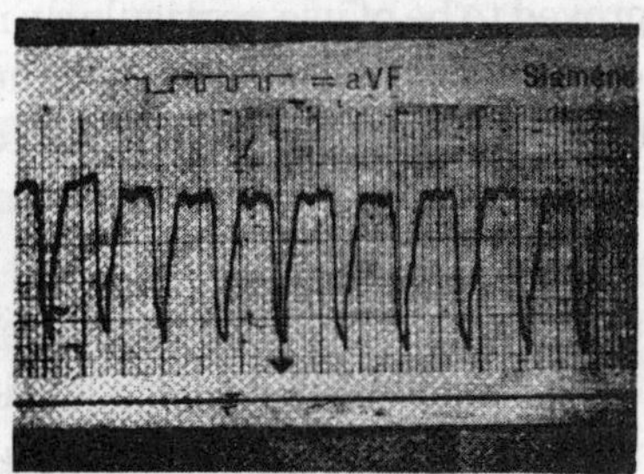

2.

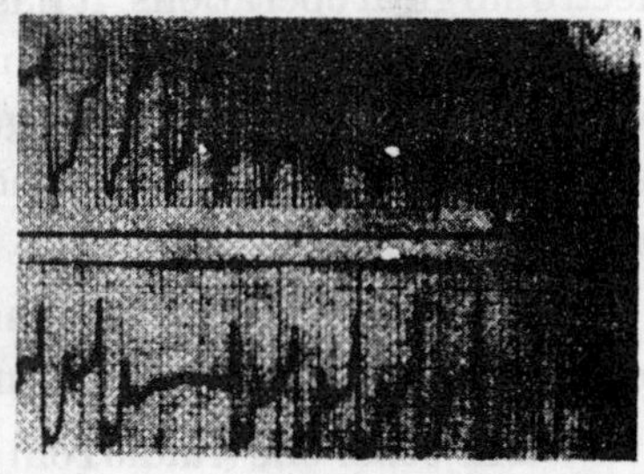

3.

Fig. 12.12b. Shows the progressive changing after defibrillation on heart after it went into fibrillation (Dog). (Dr. K. Padmanbhan and N. Pitchai, 1975)

Records of ECG obtained during the post defibrillation period were studied to examine the role of defibrillation in general and of the membrane recovery process. Initial results of this study are given as above.

TYPICAL SURGICAL DIATHERMY UNITS STANDARD RADIO TOM 612

Portable high frequency generator (Tube and transistor circuits based) for use in general electrosurgery is discussed here.

Sl No.	Type	Application
1.	Rugged tube generator	Meeting all demands generates electro-surgery currents
2.	Automatic adaptation of high frequency unit	Makes it unnecessary readjustment of pre-set mA to different tissue structure
3.	Parallel connection of 2 electrode handles	There is no electrical change during operation (switch not needed)
4.	Safety device for the dispersive electrode	Allows "cutting/coagulation" only if properly connected. (contact resistance low).
5.	Endoscopy connection facilities	For special operation.(Urology)

The RadioTom-612 has adaptation of the high -frequency surgery output to the electrode being used which facilitates operation, since in most cases, no readjustment is necessary when exchanging the electrode or when using two electrodes alternately.

The apparatus may be switched with the aid of relay connection from the operation handle or by pedal switch. The connections of ten power stages placed independently of each other and visible to a physician or the nurse allow a simultaneous connection of 10 handles prepared with electrodes. This eliminates the replacing of electrodes during the operation. For stable cuts as for instance in dermatology and diseases of the throat, nose or ear, a separate (stage less) fine adjustment is installed. By means of a set up regulating transformer, efficient service is being provided even if voltage conditions are found to be unsatisfactory. The apparatus has been furnished with an automatic safety device for neutral electrode.

The apparatus DUO-SECAREX is a smaller unit, especially adaptable for small and medium electro surgical operations. It has proved to be of use particularly in hospitals , women's infirmaries, clinics, rural ambulances and in dental surgery. As per statement of surgeons, the apparatus is being successfully applied in general surgery. For example, for skin cuts, stanching of blood, resection cuts, at the stomach and so on, for gynecological and dermatological operation and likewise in the jaw surgery.

The DUO-SECAREX has two separate regulations one of it being stage less and more accurately adjustable to perform even the finest cuts, coagulation etc.

The other one (RadioTom 612) has 9 stages adjustable to the respiratory patients' resistance and permitting, in case of larger coagulations, a maximum of power.

The SECAREX-special is the valve equipment electro-surgical apparatus for the ophthalmology It is chiefly used for detachment of the retina. To assure a precise dosage of operation-current, device is applied (measuring range up to 150mA), adjusting itself more rapidly to the measuring value and which is much less sensible to short-time overload than by thermal measurements used up to now. Therefore, and by employment of a valve, it generates not only a most possible reliability of service but also in the case of the detachment of the retina, an exceedingly easy penetration of the operating needle though the cut is precisely adjustable.

This is also well suited for the minor electro surgical operations. It is suitable for small knife and sling cuts, coagulation and piercing such as usually are being performed at dermatologists, general practitioners and dental surgeons.

The operation current is to be switched by foot contact in order to eliminate any changes of position of the dedicated electrodes.

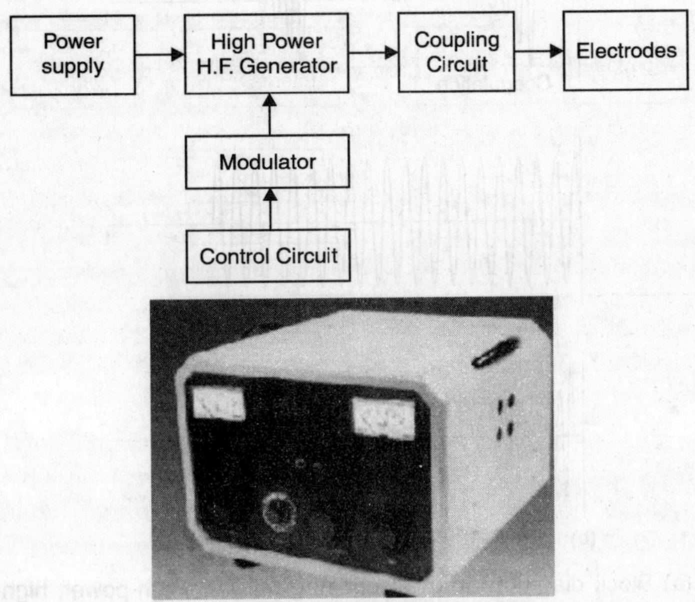

Fig. 12.13. Shows the internal block diagram of a modern electro surgical Unit.

Three different electric waveforms are generated by the above unit as shown in Fig. 12.13 for different actions to be performed such as coagulation, cutting and for blending purposes.

For coagulation, (Fig. 12.14*a*) sinusoidal waveform with frequency of 250 to 200 kHz and are usually pulsed at a rate of 120 per second is employed. Open circuit voltage ranges from 300 to 2000V with a power of 80 to 200W for a load of 500 W.is available in the unit. The magnitude and power may be controlled depending on the particular application.

Cutting is done with RF power source as shown in figure-14b. Cutting is done at higher frequency in the range of 500 kHz to 2.5 MHz. Since the intense heat is required, higher power is involved say 100 to 750 W. That is for cutting , a high frequency, high power is involved because the intense heat at the spark destroys tissue rather than just dissecting it as in the case with coagulation. The unit is provided with an open circuit voltage of 9 kV, with a power level of 100 to 750 W, is selectable for different applications.

The cutting current results in bleeding at the site of incision. But usually surgeon prefers to have bloodless cutting. These electrosurgical units can achieve this by combining the waveforms shown in Fig. 12.14*c*. The frequency of blended waveform is generally same as the cutting current waveform. For best results, surgeons prefer to operate at higher voltage and power when they want to have bloodless cutting, and hence they use the blended waveform.

Modern electro-surgical units use solid-state electronic circuits for generating high frequency and the necessary modulation coupling and in the controlling circuitry.

The high voltage needed for the sparking at the surgeon's electrode is obtained by stepping up through the ferrite core coupling transformer.

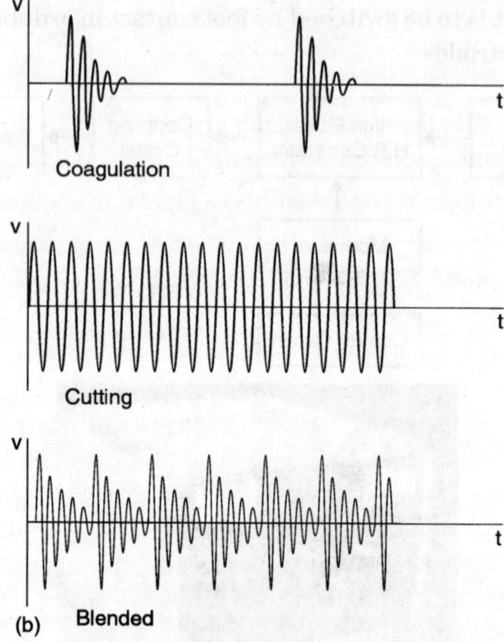

Fig. 12.14. (a) Block diagram for an electrosurgical unit. High-power, high-frequency oscillating currents are generated and coupled to electrodes to incise and coagulate tissue. (b) Three different electric voltage waveforms available at the output of electrosurgical units for carrying out different functions.

The Torch (Russian) make unit has the following Specifications

It provides three different types of current, the modulator can be changed over or switched off.

Two channels with separate adjustment and pre selection of strength and type of current.

Utilization of the advantages presented by the two channel system also for single electrode technique, by means of a double foot switch.

Simultaneous connection of up to 4 electrodes to the equipment.

Automatic adaptation of current strength to the electrode connected to the unit. Explosion proof model without restriction as regards mobility.

Safety circuit for the indifferent electrodes. Handy holder for the electrodes where they are kept ready for use.

Sterilizable electrode handles.

Sockets for endoscopy providing variable voltage.

Design

To meet clinical requirements, so as to be easily movable and take up less space. In another model, the standard control cabinet can be set-up outside the operating theater and the remote control which is suspended from the theatre ceiling. Thus there will be more free space around the operating table for setting up narcosis equipment, circulation monitors, cardiac stimulators, instrument table etc. Provision is made in the remote control unit for the connection of any equipment including foot switch and endoscopy lamp (urology).

The average height of 1.5 m above floor level ensures protection of the switches and contacts in the remote control unit from explosion since explosive ether and air mixtures are, as is generally known, heavier than air and rest at the floor level..

The anti-explosion system is a suction tube projecting from the top; this tube is also used as stand for the rotate table and displaceable arm holding electrode handles.

The heavy high voltage generator assembly is placed in the lower third so that the entire equipment is very stable.

For relatively long life, components, printed circuits are used and arranged neatly for easy maintenance.

The anti-explosion system is effective in the case of all explosive gases heavier than air (ether). In order to prevent these gases from entering the control cabinet or replace entered gases by fresh air before the unit is put into operation, a fan sucks in air free from explosive gases into the interior of the unit through a tube, the upper end of which is 1.5 m above floor level. This clean air scavenges the interior of the equipment and leaving it through an air -flap on the sides when the pressure exceeds 0.4 mm Hg above atmospheric. This overpressure effectively prevents ingress of explosive gases which are heavier than air. Electric interlocks permit operation only after it is scavenged for one minute with the air at inlet and outlet, apparatus is wide open and the casing and properly closed thereafter.

TYPICAL PHYSIOTHERAPY DIATHERMY UNIT

Therapy Neuroton 627. An all transistor electro-stimulation unit for exponential current and diadynamic currents.

For Therapy

1.	Selective stimulation with exponentially progressive current (faradic current)	Treatment of paralysis with totally or partially degenerated muscles.
2.	Stimulation and analysis with dia-dynamic currents	Treatment of painful inflammatory diseases of the muscular, ligament and skeletal systems and the peripheral nerves. Improvement of circulation, rapid absorption of bacteria
3.	Electric muscle exercise with reproducible non faradic current	With disuse atrophy and muscle weakness after lengthy immobilization
4.	Aimed stimulation with special exponentially progressive current	Treatment of chronic constipation and peripheral circulatory disturbances.
5.	Achievement of intensive hyperemia with galvanic current	With pain and muscular spasm.

For Diagnosis

1.	Stimulation with measurable and reproducible galvanic and neofaradic currents	For qualitative and quantitative determination of the galvanic and faradic excitability.
2.	Stimulation with defined measurable and reproducible rectangular and triangular current pulses.	For testing the accommodation

All transistor electro-stimulation pulse unit for the entire fields of modern electro-therapy and for simple methods of electro diagnosis are presently available.

Output

Exponentially progressive current pulses with continuously adjustable pulse duration of 0.1 to 1000 milliseconds and the interval pulse duration of 0.1 to 1000 milliseconds and internal durations in steps of 20/500 μs.

LASERS IN SURGERY—OPTHALMOLOGY

The introduction of lasers in Ophthalmology has had a major impact on several of the most important disorders encountered by ophthalmologists.

In 1940's, a young Ophthalmologist Myer. Schwickerath considered the idea of using light to produce a thermal reaction in the retina to produce a coagulation. Thus originated the word photocoagulation.

The interaction of a specific laser emission wavelength with various ocular tissues can be divided into six different tissue changes which are given as follows:

1. Photocoagulation therapy
2. Photodynamic therapy
3. Photo vaporization therapy
4. Photo disruption therapy
5. Photo ablative therapy and
6. Photo therapy

We will discuss briefly about each of the above categories.

PHOTCOAGULATION THERAPY

The first category of the ophthalmic tissue interaction with the laser is photocoagulation. In this, temperature of the tissue is increased from 37°C to 50°C, producing denaturation of protein (coagulation) in the region of the absorbent tissue element.

The lasers most commonly employed are:

1. Argon (488–Blue, 514.5 nm–Green)
2. Krypton (630 nm) and
3. Tunable Dye laser (488–630 nm).

Photocoagulation is used to treat Diabetic retinopathy, weak areas in the retina, new blood vessels on the retina and tumors of the eye.

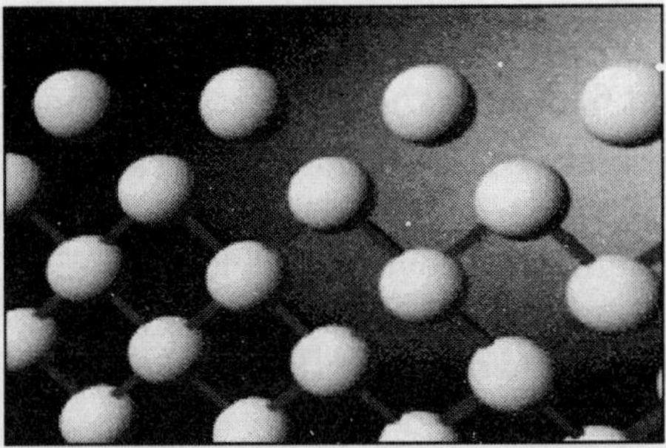

The Excimer laser produces a "cool" light beam that does not damage surrounding tissue. High-energy photons from the laser break the molecular bonds a few layers a time.

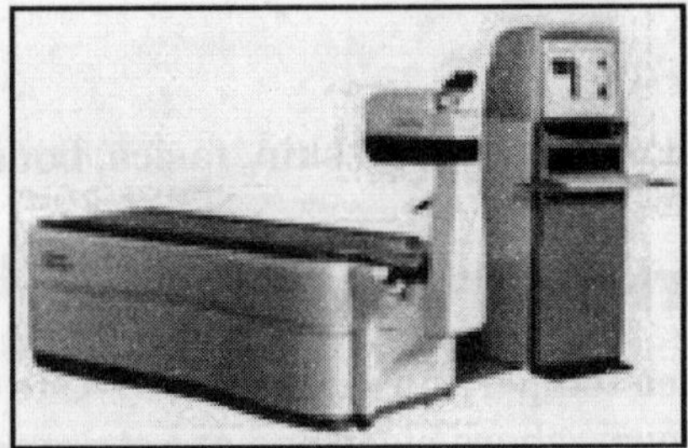

LADARVision®s unique small-spot laser beam (less than one millimeter in diameter) offers micron size reshaping of the cornea resulting in an extremely smooth surface. LADARVision's ability to use a larger optical zone for treatments minimizes potential nighttime side effects of glare, halos, and starbursts. This feature is most important for patients with large pupils.

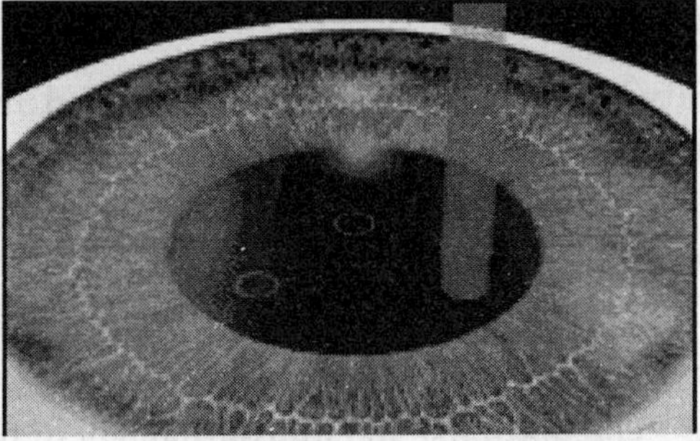

Fig. 12.15-1. The use of Excimer laser-Illustrations from actual products.

PHOTODYNAMIC THERAPY

In this, the temperature rise is only about 1°C . The main lasers are the

1. the Dye laser at 630nm and
2. the Gold vapor laser at 628nm in the red portion of the spectrum.

A haematoporphyrin derivative is first injected intravenously and allowed to concentrate in the tumor inside an eye. In the next 72 hours the drug washed away from normal tissue. The tumour is then treated with the laser, providing a photochemical reaction with the haemato-porphyrin derivative which by now is closely approximated with the malignant cell. In the process, single oxygen molecule is liberated and destroys the cancerous cell immediately.

PHOTOVAPORISATION THERAPY

In this process, the tissue absorbs the laser beam almost totally within 75–100 microns of space raising the temperature from 37°C to well above 100°C and photovaporisation takes place. The typical laser used is

1. The carbondioxide laser (CO_2).

The CO_2 laser can be used to cut through skin, fasica, bone etc., without loss of blood.

PHOTODISTURPTION THERAPY

Leads to a microscopically localized temperature rise from 37°C to over 15000°C. The action of the laser depends on optical breakdown where electrons are stripped from the atoms of the target tissue and a plasma field and bubble are established , leading to a hydrodynamic and acoustic shock wave and mechanical stress factors that tear the impact tissue apart on a microscopic level.

The commonly used laser is the **Nd-Yag Laser.** Its main application in Opthalmology is to cut through the remnant of a Cataract that has been surgically removed .

PHOTOABLATIVE THERAPY

There is no change in temperature in this method, and lasers used are all of shorter wavelengths of the UV spectrum. The lasers used are :

1. Excimer Laser (157 to 351 nm) and
2. The frequency quadrupled Nd-Yag (266nm)

The high energy photons of the excimer laser enable the laser beam to disrupt and break the intra-molecular bonds of tissue, which then disappear from the area of impact without the production of heat or charring. The main use in Ophthalmology in photo refractive Keratotomy where the cornea is reshipped to reduce the myopia of a short sighted eye.

PHOTOTHERAPY

Photo therapy is an ill understood process. Fibroblasts, endothelial cells and Collagen can all be stimulated to proliferate but the mechanism is obscure.

Normal healing , vascular growth and asepsis of surfaces are all enhanced. Further work is needed before this becomes clinically acceptable.

COMPONENTS OF A TYPICAL LASER SYSTEM IN OPTHALMOLOGY

The following are the four major Components of a typical Laser system in Ophthalmology. They are:

1. the laser system
2. the delivery system
3. the operator room
4. the patient

The laser system is the one which is in use depends upon the particular type of laser for particular application. The type of lasers and their uses are given below:

Sl No.	Type of Laser	Application
1.	Argon, Krypton Dye lasers	Photocoagulation
2.	The Carbon dioxide laser	Cutting
3.	Nd-Yag Laser	Photo disruption
4.	Excimer Laser	Photo ablation

Most Opthalmic lasers (except carbon dioxide laser) are delivered through an optical magnification device. The Argon, Krypton, Dye and Nd-Yag are delivered through a lamp microscope which require no anesthesia by themselves. However for photocoagulation , a contact lens may need to be placed on the front of the eye and for this anesthetizing eye drops may have to be used.

In the case of the Excimer laser it is delivered through an operating microscope and requires the use of anesthetizing drops.

In addition, the Argon Laser, Diode etc., can be delivered by fiber optic cables within the eye during surgery in a procedure called Endo-photocoagulation.

In all the above cases of larger usage in Ophthalmology, it is important to protect the operator from the reflection of laser coming off lenses used in this procedure

Photo-phako-fragmentation is being studied as possible treatment of Cataracts.

Flourescein Antibody laser asepsis is a procedure in which a known organism infecting the Cornea is allowed to conjugate with topical drops that contain an antibody to the organism, that has been tagged with Florescien. The antibodies with the Flourescien tag attach themselves to the organism and with a non focused Argon beam is directed on the lesion for two minutes. The flourescein absorbs the laser energy raising the temperature of the Flourescien antibody organism complex to a temperature above its thermal death point.

THE EXCIMER LASER

The most common type of excimer laser uses molecularly diatomic rare-gas halides such as ArF, KrF, XeF, XeCl, as the active species from which the laser light is produced. In their common, unexcited form, atoms of the rare gases Ne, Ar, Kr, and Xe are unreactive or inert and do not readily form molecules.

Rare gas halide molecules are held together by electrostatic forces similar to the way alkali halides (salt) molecules are formed.

Rare gas halide molecules cannot be bought in bottle, but must be created in the laser vessel in-situ. It is usually done by high voltage electrical discharges in gas mixture of halogen-bearing molecules and rare gas atoms.

TABLE

Name of the Gas Mixture	Wave length (nm)	Energy/pulse (mJ)
F_z	157	40
ArF	193	500
KrF	249	1000
XeF	351 353	500
KrCl	222	100
XeCl	308	500

The above table shows the wavelength of light produced by an excimer laser depends upon the type of molecule created. It can be selected simply by changing the gas mixture originally added to the laser tube as in the left hand column. The pulsed energies of the light obtainable from typical commercial excimer lasers are given (Col. 3) in the above table.

Nearly all the rare gas halide molecules in the vessel are excited and have energy available for extraction as ultraviolet laser photons. The wavelength of the laser light is determined by the type of molecules created and can be selected simply by changing the gas mixture originally added to the laser tube as shown in the table.

Such devices can produce pulsed burst of light lasting approximately 2×10^{-8} sec at up to 500 times a second.

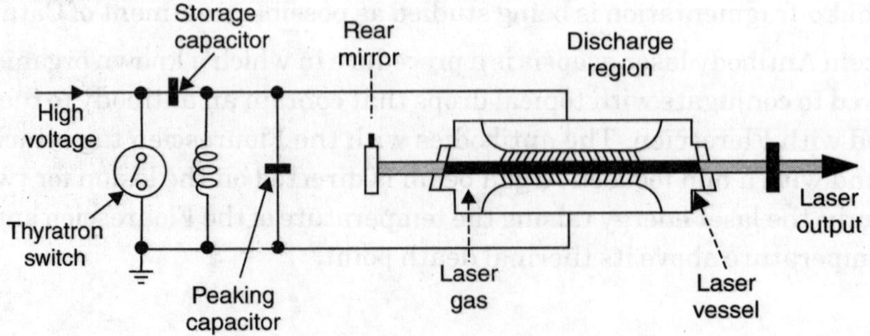

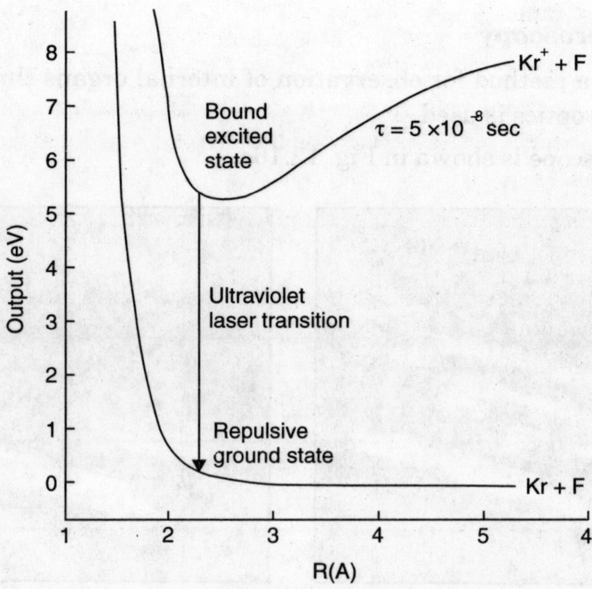

Fig. 12.15.2. (a) shows a simplified energy potential curve for KF excimer molecule, showing energies plotted against the internuclear separation R. and b). shows the features of an excimer laser.

BALLOON ANGIOPLASTY

Research work is also going on to investigate the use of the excimer laser to unblock arteries, a procedure known as angioplasty. Blockage near the heart by accumulation of plaque, the condition known as atherosclerosis, eventually leads to a heart attack. Most widespread of surgical methods now used to alleviate this condition is extremely invasive open - heart surgery in which surgeons bypass the blockage by grafting a new artery around it. Less invasive is a recently developed technique called balloon angioplasty, in which a fiber is threaded through the arteries to the blockage and a balloon on the end is inflated to open it out; the patient remains conscious throughout. But the techniques can also damage arterial tissue. An alternative method might be to use light from an excimer laser, passed down through an optical fiber in the artery., to burn through the blockage cleanly. Initial studies have shown that for soft, non calcified plaque the excimer laser can remove the constriction efficiently and cleanly. Calcified blockage are much more difficult to remove.

Among other medical applications being studied are very precise neurological cutting in the brain and spinal column. While most applications of high power visible and infrared lasers use the laser merely as a sophisticated cutting and welding torch, the most exciting potential applications of excimer lasers make use of the high powers which they are capable of producing and the ability of the ultraviolet photons to induce changes in the chemical state of matter in a most efficient way.

Endoscopes and Laperoscopy

An Endoscope is a method for observation of internal organs through a light tube with optics, now a days, fiber optics is used.

A simple laryngoscope is shown in Fig. 12.16*a*.

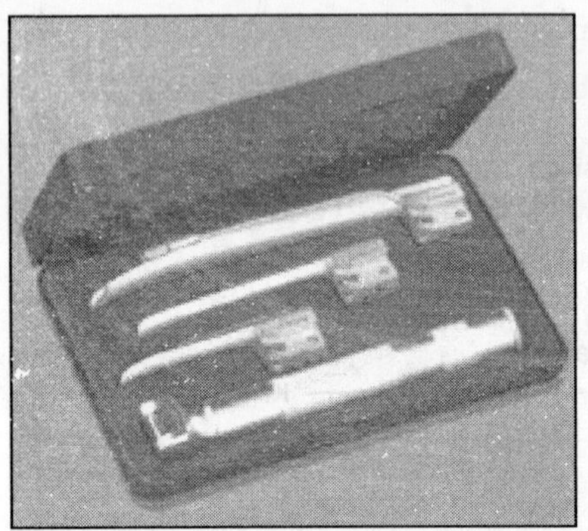

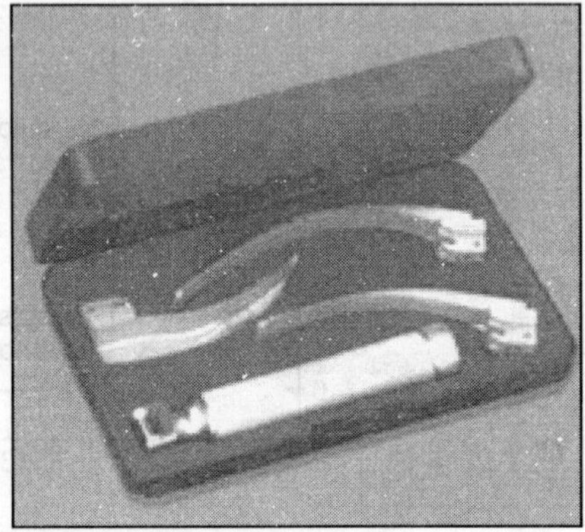

LARYNGOSCOPES - CONVENTIONAL
Stubby Handle, Oxiport Macintosh/Miller & S.V. (Superior View)
Macintosh blades, Available in Paediatric & Adult Sizes
with the choice of 0, 1, 2, 3, 4 blades.

Fig. 12.16a. A simple laringoscope.

Standard Flexible Gastroscope

This is an instrument having a rubber finger tip and a 12 mm diameter through the flexible portion and 8.5mm diameter in upper rigid portion as shown in figure (7.7 cm long).

This rubber tip is a conical rubber finger of 4.6 cm long. Special light bulb in a removable light housing which also holds the rubber ; screwed.

8 V, 0.3 A or 9.6 V, 0.33 A can be used.

For replacing the lamp or finger tip, the entire unit is to be replaced.

Lamp or finger tip needing replacement means entire unit is replaced.

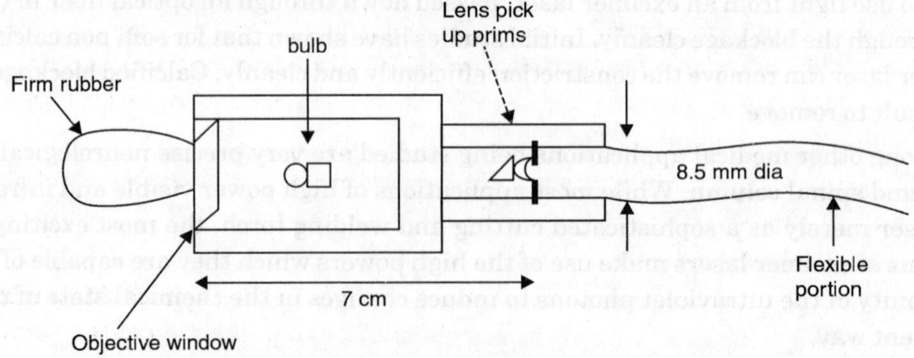

Fig 12.16b. Shows the standard flexible Gastroscope.

Prism 90°, gable prism of Amici is used. Angle of vision is 45° and 50–90° for Wolf make gastroscope.

Objective windows are provided in sideways.

Objects lens will be having short depth of focus.

A number of lenses (46, 42) transmit the images to the rigid portion on top.

Cylindrical hollow spacers - special hoiders are provided.

Image passes through optical system reaches the ocular which is only a plain window.

Flexible portion spiral sheath of stainless steel is used here.

The metal spiral is tapered to assure uniform bending-proximal and distal portion of spiral are thicker.

Spiral is covered with rubber tubing. Then paratubing.

A lacquered double insulated electrical wire is laid in the spirals of the tubing and covered with liquid rubber and vulcanized.

Rubber tube or sheath covers entire unit, anchored at both ends.

Air inflate the stomach- from hand bulb at ocular end through air channel up to the junction of rigid and flexible parts- a group of holes

- air goes between inner and outer rubber tubing.

3 or 4 perforations at distal end.

Proximal part–eye piece

Terminals

Handle points meridian of objective.

German Instrument–Infinite depth of focus small lens.

American make Wider objective–less depth of focus.

German : Flexible part of Phosphor–Bronze and has uniform diameter

2 rubber tubes–3 small specks of rubber seen as block spots.

American

Rubberising the inner spiral is done and only one tube is used.

All parts of stomach cannot be visualized satisfactorily.

Taylor : Special rubber sheath fitted over entire scope down to the level of objective with air channel, balloon like arrangement at distal end.

'Blister'-separates mucosa adjustment to objectives so that is could be brought into visual field.

Taylor–Instrument :

30 inches long, flexible part has two tubes left - right handed spirals . Movement controlled by means of two longitudinal wires between them. A push pull action of the wires control the bending. Controlled by a differential Rack and pinion.

Cameron Omniangle

Instead of the Prism, it is replaced by tilting mirror and fixing.

45° angle of vision can be thrown 20° forward electromagnet coil placed under-side of mirror - Rotating the control button.

Uses reversing prism at the ocular with 47 elements.

Cystoscope: tube with a reflective mirror was used in early days and that enables the bladder to be seen.

Modern Endoscopes

Modern endoscopes make use of flexible part in fiber optic light guide. The objective and the eyepiece are similar. The eyepiece is also replaced by fixing into a camera, for recording, Since the camera is reflex type, one can view and take snaps.

Laparoscopes

Many applications are now available in this field.

In an endoscope, the surgeon gets a view of an internal organ. The laparoscope enables simple surgical procedures to be done through a hole in the unit with a cannula.

For e.g., prolapse of the uterus in old women can be made good by surgical procedure of this type. Figs. 12.18, 12.19 and 12.20, show the laparoscopes and their functions. The camera attachments for photography is also shown.

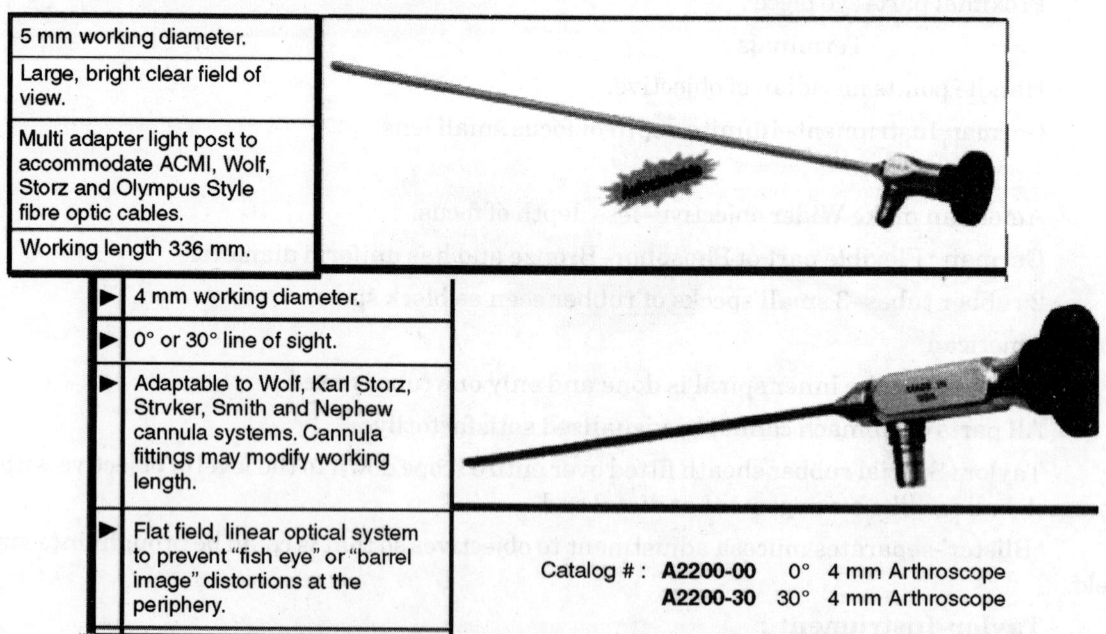

Fig. 12.17. Shows a Laparoscope and the Arthroscope.

Precision Optics Corporation provides numerous adapters and can custom design adapters to integrate B-style eyecups with your still camera, digital or video cameras.

Catalog #:
DSC Sony P1
Digital Still Camera
adapter tripod mount

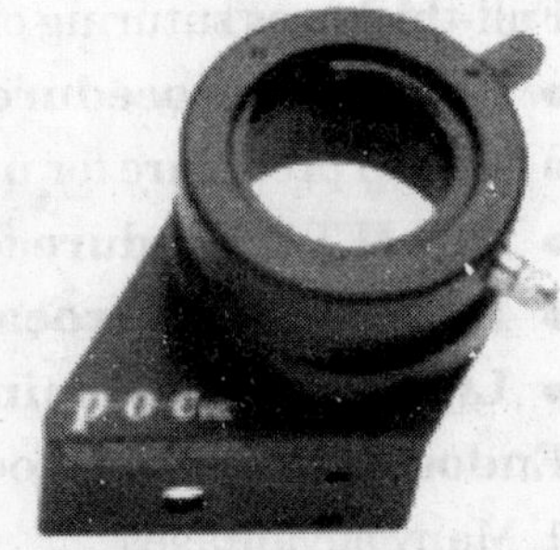

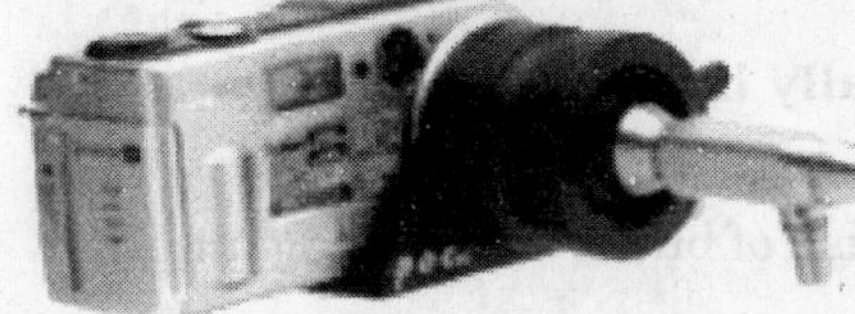

Sony DSC-PI Digital Camera with DSC Sony PI adapter holding a POC 2200-30

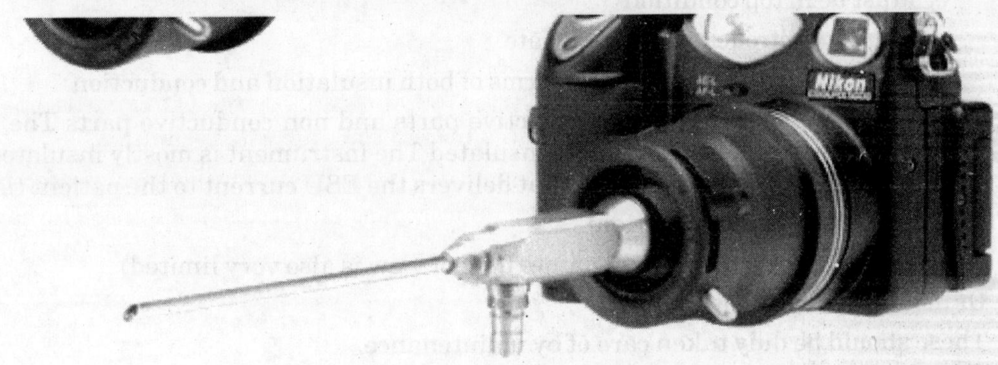

Nikon 5000 Digital Camera with **DSC Nikon 5000** adapter holding a Pro Vision 636 flexible scope

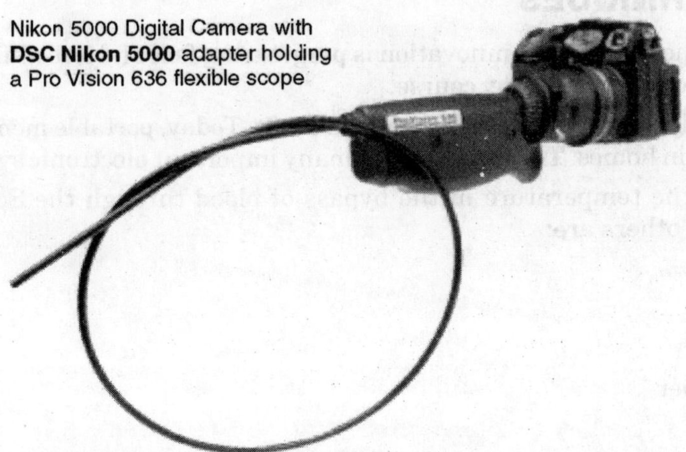

Fig. 12.18. Showing some laparoscope view adapters through digital or film camera.

Innovative therapies and procedure kits are available for:

- **Repairing uterine prolapse without hysterectomy.**
- **Preventing vaginal vault prolapse after hysterectomy.**
- **Treating collision dyspareunia and dysmenorrhea related to a retroverted uterus.**
- **Preventing adhesions after endometriosis surgery.**

Full-thickness suturing of all trocar wounds-including 5 mm sites. **Surgical Procedures**

- **ELEVEST procedure** for laparoscopic uterine prolapse repair.
- Avesta procedure for uterosacral support after hysterectomy.
- **UPLIFT procedure** for uterine suspension.
- **Full-thickness trocar wound closure**
- **Ligation of abdominal wall bleeders**

Endoscopic (ESU) procedures are minimally invasive

1. Many advantages
2. One of the disadvantages is that there is a risk of burns when using an ESU.

- **ESU** Can cut

  Can Coagulate

  Must be in top condition

  Return electrode to be appropriate

  Lead integrity is essential in terms of both insulation and conduction

- ESU instruments consist of conductive parts and non conductive parts The surgeon holds the instrument part that is insulated The instrument is mostly insulated except for the exposed conductive part that delivers the ESU current to the patient tissue

ESU burn is a risk to the patient

Can be due to poor surgical technique (field of view is also very limited)

Or insulation breakdown.

These should be duly taken care of by maintenance.

OTHER SURGICAL TECHNIQUES

The techniques of surgical equipment and their innovation is progressing fast and it is difficult to define present day instruments completely in any course.

For instance, the urine dialysis unit is a complex surgical outfit. Today, portable membrane dialysis unit are used by patients in homes. These have quite many important electronic systems.

For instance, measuring the temperature in the bypass of blood through the Scribner shunt to the machine is one. The others are:

Blood pH

Blood PCO_2

Rate of flow

Level in membrane chamber

Detection of blood leak

and many other aspects, depending on the type and usage time.

Stimulators for bladder for urination is another surgical procedure, dependant on electric shock.

Like this, in the years to come, one can find new developments in the surgical area very much more than in the diagnostic area.

The safety aspects of each and every instrument is to be analysed carefully.

Chapter 13

Some New Development in Medical Instruments

GENERAL ULTRASOUND IMAGING RESOLUTION IMPROVEMENT TECHNIQUES

Even with the best of transducers the poor lateral resolution of ultrasound echoes cannot be compensated. The point spread function of the transducer may be determined by direct measurement using a point reflector at various 'y' values. This is possible only for the usual general imaging transducer (2.5 MHz), but for dermatological scanners using > 10 MHz Ultrasound, they cannot be realized (depths in < 1 mm).

Hoess and Ermert have dealt with a mathematical evaluation of the Point Spread Function (PSF) using Diffraction theory. For a curvilinear transducer of radius R, the Fig. 13.1*a*, *b* and *c* show the variations at different depths. They stored the different scattered positions and the results in a computer, which was used in the process of deconvolution.

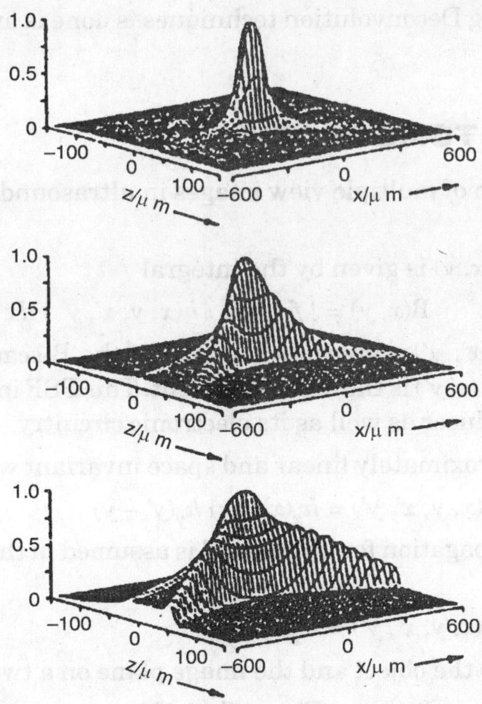

Fig. 13.1. Envelope of point spread function for different values of y.

DECONVOLUTION

This is the standard principle of finding the actual image from the observed image by using the pattern of the PSF function by the relation

$$g = h ** F + n \text{ and}$$

$$G(u, v) = H(u, v).\ F(u, v) + N(u, v)$$

where u and v are the two dimension variables.
where g is the observed image function

h is point spread function of transducer

F or f denotes the actual picture data function i.e. echoes

n is the noise and $**$ denotes convolution

In the frequency domain

$$F(u, v) = G(u, v) / H(u, v) + N(u, v) / H(u, v)$$

provided N is clearly known.

Since the properties of noise are rather known only statistically it is required to use the methods involving noise properties in actual finding of the F function or image that is real.

In the actual method the constrained minimization of the difference between the image and the actual, *i.e.*, $g - Hf$ which is the unknown quantity, (noise n), can be performed by using a Lagrange multiplier and using a modified Wiener filter.

No such method using Deconvolution techniques is done is any of the practical machines, however.

LIMITED ANGULAR TOMOGRAPHY

Tomographic reconstruction of multiple view images in ultrasound has been first referred to by Hiller and Ermert.

The B-scan image $B(x, y)$ is given by the integral

$$B(x, y) = \int f(x, y)\ .\ h(x, y, x', y')\ dx\ dy$$

The quantity $h(x, y, x', y')$ represents the PSF of the B-scanner instrument for a point scatterer at the location x, y. $(x' y')$ is the observing point. This PSF includes the wave propagation characteristics of the transducer as well as its electronic circuitry.

Since the PSF is approximately linear and space invariant we can write the function into

$$h(x, y, x', y') = h_x(x' - x)\ h_y(y' - y)$$

If the direction of propagation for ultrasound is assumed in the x direction, using the space invariant property,

$$h(x, y, x', y') = h_x(x)\ h_y(y)$$

Using this, it leads to the object and the image plane on a two dimensional convolution:

$$B(x, y) = F(x, y) * h_x(x) * h_y(y)$$

In the frequency domain the same becomes

$$B(u, v) = F(u, v) . H(u) . H(v)$$

where $u = 2\pi / x$ and $v = 2\pi / y$

$H_x(u) . H_y(u)$ represent the Point Spread frequency function. Using this, system analysis for the resolution with tomographic reconstruction has been dealt with by Roherlein and Ermert.

A conventional B-scan image $B(r, \theta)$ is approximated by the linear transform of the two functions of reflectivity at the point $a(r, \theta)$ and $h(r, \theta)$ or the Point Spread function for the B-scan image taken by the sector scanner as

$$B(r, \theta) = \int a\ (r, \theta)\ h\ (r' - r, \theta' - \theta)\ r'\ dr'\ d\theta$$

From which the convolution relation in the frequency domain results as

$$B(\omega_r, \omega_\theta) = A(\omega_r, \omega_\theta) * H\ (\omega_r, \omega_\theta)$$

The value of the H function can be split into $H(\omega r)$ and $H(\omega q)$ and their maximum values noted as $Hm(\omega_r)$ and $H_m(\omega_\theta)$. As the lateral resolution is less than the axial resolution which varies with depths, the object function is low-pass filtered by the B-scan image. While making the reconstruction using the rotating co-ordinates the point (x, y) transform into or as x_1, y_1.

$$\begin{vmatrix} \cos\theta & \sin\theta \\ -\sin\theta & \cos\theta \end{vmatrix} \begin{vmatrix} x \\ y \end{vmatrix}$$

In frequency domain the point transfer function rotates with respect to $A(\omega_r\ \omega_\theta)$. On the reconstruction summation, the image is represented by the convolution of the object and the summed PSF $H(\omega_r, \omega_\theta)$. If the object frequencies are greater than H_m, then reconstruction does not provide them in the final picture. With the integration performed over a smaller angle, the same is true. If the object function is band limited by a window function then the final picture is well resolved even for a limited angular set of views.

Summation of the B-scan image from the conventional B-scan image $B(r, \theta)$ for limited angular view from 0 *to* γ_{max} is given by

$$S(r, \omega) = \int B(r, \omega)\ d\omega$$

And this becomes

$$S(\omega_r, \omega_\theta) = A\ (\omega_r, \omega_\theta)\ H_s(\omega_r, \omega_\theta)$$ in the frequency domain.

In principle, the resolution in the frequency domain plane shows as an ellipse with a small mirror axis (lateral resolution << axial resolution). The image has the frequency transform shown as $S(r, \theta)$ but when we rotate over all angles (γ), the resolution ellipse fills the entire area and hence the resolutions are equalized in both directions in a tomographic reconstruction from multiple angular views Fig. 13.2.

The problem of anisotropic resolution as improved by the Limited angular reconstruction technique is reported in the next section and the improvement is estimated. The ratio of contrast is shown from plain B-scan to a complete tomogram (where feasible) in Fig. 13.3. (Padmanathan and Sunder, 1993)

As a practical application, the imaging of the Pancreas obtained by such summing up of the multiple views and by tomographic reconstruction was shown to be much improved and giving details of the Head, body and tail of the organ.

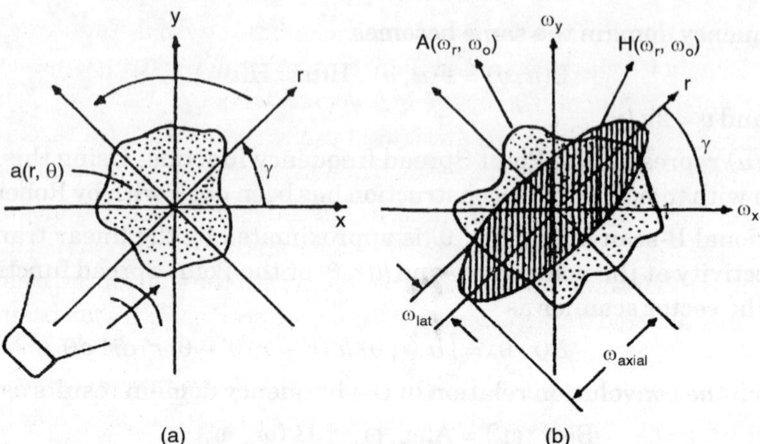

Fig. 13.2. (a) Shows a region of the object and a particular view of a (r, θ) representing density function (b) Shows the object frequency and the odd shaped figure and the ellipse shows the point spread function in the *r* and θ directions.

Fig. 13.2 (a) Shows a region of the object and a particular view of a(r, θ) representing density function (b) Shows the object frequency and the odd shaped figure and the ellipse show the point spread function in the r and θ directions.

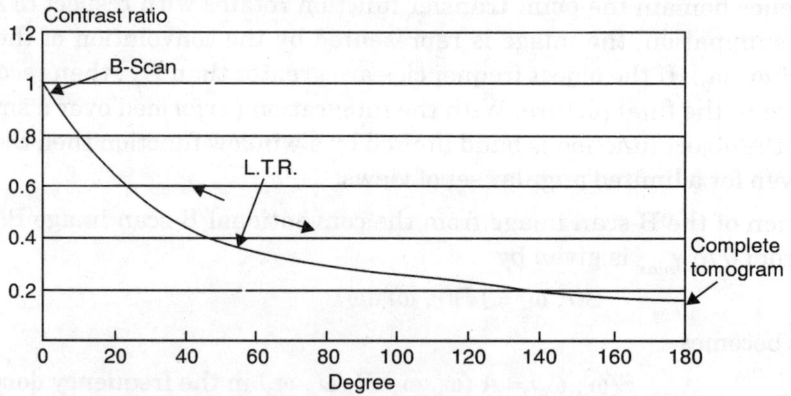

Fig. 13.3. Contrast ratio evaluated for varying angles of limited tomographic reconstructed images.

Fig. 13.3 shows the contrast ration evaluated for varying angles of limited tomographic reconstructed images. (LTR) from one B scan to complete 360° tomogram.

TOMOGRAPHIC RECONSTRUCTION OF SECTOR-SCAN B-SCAN ULTRASONOGRAMS GIVE MORE DETAILS EVEN WITH LIMITED ANGULAR MOVEMENTS

A method of improving the B-scan ultrasonograms by the Limited Angle Tomography Reconstruction (LTR) is presented. By this method, the image gives more anatomical details with increased resolution. The method of implementation is explained with principles and results of views of the Kidney and Pancreas. (Padmanabham and Sunder, 1993), Ananth in 1998.

Tomography with B-scan views: B-scan ultrasonography is a standard clinical diagnostic procedure today. Even with the best transducers optimally chosen by frequency, power and type - Sector scan, curvilinear or linear, the image lacks clarity of detail, especially where fine details of anatomy are required. Generally, this is attributed to the reduced lateral resolution of the B-scan reflected signals. Ultrasound tomographic reconstruction is being experimented to improve the same.

However, the scan over a full semi-circle, as needed for a complete tomogram, is impractical even with the use of suitably formed water-bath attachments. A sector scan transducer provides sector views in its plane of insonation depending on the type of the transducer, over a 60° to 110°. The scan paths are radially directed from the center of the transducer, as with a fan beam. If the transducer can be moved over an arc of a circle and several views taken, then, it is possible to do a combined reconstruction of these views. For this, a full 180° movement or over a semi-circle is ideal, though not essential. Such a limited angular reconstructed image and its features are described here.

Among the possible methods of making a set of angular views for tomography, the following are noteworthy:

1. For limbs such as neck (Thyroid) and legs (veins), the transducer is moved over a water-bath of thin rubber annular ring placed encircling the organ. The several angular positions are viewed by moving the transducer over the circular outer profile of the water-bath ring. For females, observations by a rotation of the transvaginal probe can provide such angular views.
2. For abdominal area, a spherically shaped cap type water- bath can be employed, which has a circle of radius sufficiently large for viewing up to 10cm deep of tissue.
3. For most regions of the abdomen and other areas as well, it is possible to manipulate the transducer over the fleshy surface of the body by indenting or pressing in such a way that a fixed anatomical location deep within the area of observation always lies at the

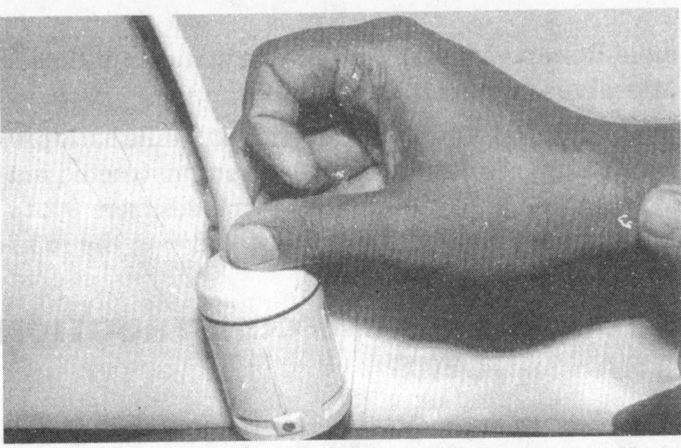

Fig. 13.5a. Showing US Probe positioning of various angles for L.T.R. Imaging.

same distance from the transducer, as the transducer is moved over the angles. The B-scan view with depth marking makes this easy. As the transducer is moved over a chosen marked path on the surface of the body with its angular position varying from straight vertical to ± 30° either side, if such an anatomical location is manipulated to be always at the same depth, then, the path of the transducer becomes a circle, with that location as its center. By pressing on the surfaces to a small depth, this is convenient to handle for abdomen, kidney, neck and also some parts of the chest.(Fig. 13.5)

PRINCIPLES OF LIMITED ANGULAR TOMOGRAPHY

It was Roehrlein and Ermert [1] who have described the system analysis of B-scan image formation, with reference to resolutions in the two perpendicular directions, axial and transverse. The reflectivity function $a(x, y)$, the point spread function $h(x, y)$ and the B-scan image function $b(x, y)$ are related by

$$b(x, y) = \int_0^{\infty}\int_0^{\infty} a(x', y' . h(x' - x, y' - y) . dx' \, dy' \qquad ...(1)$$

A 2-D Fourier transform of this leads to the expression in frequency domain as

$$B(u,v) = A(u, v) . H(u, v) \qquad ...(2a)$$

Here u,v are the spatial frequency variables along x,y.

For sector scan geometry, we need relations along r and θ, which gives

$$B(\omega_r, \omega_\theta) = A(\omega_r, \omega_\theta). H(\omega_r, \omega_\theta) \qquad ...(2b)$$

where $B(\omega_r, \omega_\theta)$ is the B-scan image function, and it can be shown similar to eqn.(1) that

$$H(\omega_r, \omega_\theta) = H(\omega_r) . H(\omega_\theta) \qquad ...(2c)$$

These two H functions are low-pass filter functions, the first one relating to axial and the second to lateral direction. For every transducer under identical instrument setting (power-level, frequency, etc.), the point spread function is invariant, where multiple tomographic views are taken. As different from the parallel beam geometry of earlier day transducers, the presently popular sector-scanners have better uniformity of the PSF function and hence the approximate splitting of $H(\omega_r, \omega_\theta)$ into two functions $H(\omega_r)$ and $H(\omega_\theta)$ is even more accurate for these sector-scan transducers.

Usually, for simple B-scan views, the cut-off frequencies of these filters are in the ratio 5 : 1, meaning a poor lateral resolution of the plain B-scan.

The process of inverse filtering improves a given view, while back-projection and summation provide improved lateral to axial resolution ratio in the reconstructed image. The ratio between the resolutions in the two perpendicular directions increases from 0.2 to 1.0, as the number of views summed is increased from a single B-scan view to all over the semi-circle. (Fig. 13.5*b*)

LIMITED ANGLE TOMOGRAPHIC RECONSTRUCTION (LTR) FROM SECTOR SCAN TRANSDUCERS

With sector scan probes, let us try to estimate the PSF $h(r', \theta', r, \theta)$. Here, r denotes the depth along the beam in the sector and θ, the angular position with respect to the central axis of the transducer. Taking $r'\theta'$ at (0,0), the variation of $h(r, \theta)$ with depth r is mainly caused by the ray divergence. It is easily noted the lateral resolution in a sector beam decreases as depth increases. A tomogram taken over a full semicircular movement will quite compensate this one. Quantitatively, it is worked out as below:

Consider a strip of object of width x at a depth (R-a) below the top of the scanning point (Fig. 13.5a). The angle-θ is subtended by this strip at the point of the transducer and hence this

determines the rays which define this pixel; it is dependent on the transducer's piezo-elements and therefore determines the resolution

$$\propto_0 = \delta x \,/\, (R - a) \; (\propto_0 \text{ in radians}) \qquad ...(3)$$

For a view from transducer position 1 at an angle γ, the angle subtended becomes

$$\propto_1 = \delta x \cos \beta \,/\, (R - a \cos \gamma) \qquad ...(4)$$

where $\tan \beta = [a \sin \gamma / (R - a \cos \gamma)]$.

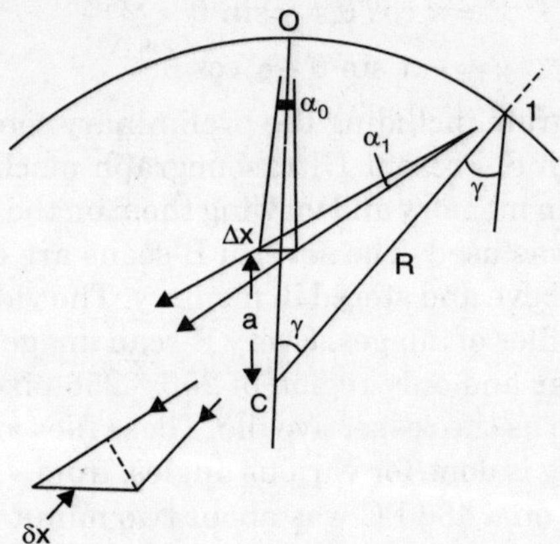

Fig. 13.4. Estimation of resolution at various depths for different soan angles.

Substituting the depth ratio as $d = a/R$, we get the ray density of pixels of any angle γ w.r.t. the straight view as given by

$$\text{Ray intensity} = \cos \beta / (1 - d \cos \gamma) \qquad ...(5)$$

After evaluating the ray densities at all depths from various angular views, we can estimate the resolution of the point at any depth by taking the reciprocals of the ray densities and summing up over all angles upto which the tomograph LTR is done. This is presented as a normalized graph of percentage increase in resolution for various depths, versus the angle of LTR, in Fig 13.5. This shows how the resolution increases as we include more and more projections of views, and how even limited angular tomographic procedures can improve the picture. (Fig. 13.5*a*)

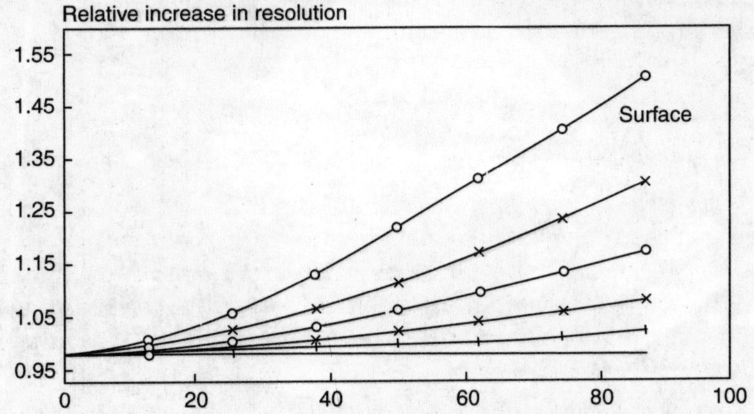

Fig. 13.5b. Resolution for various depths vs. the angle of LTR.

Practical applications and results: The program for tomographic reconstruction consisted of 1) preliminary discrete convolution with a set of coefficients extending to two points on either side of the grid, based on a Sheep-Logan type of filter function, with the co-efficients altering with depth 2) Back-projection by the usual methods, and 3) summation. In the first step, each B-scan image is convoluted individually with the filter and saved in a file. The file was 256 * 256 pixels and each occupying one byte as its intensity value. The picture file at an angle θ is back projected by using the relationship between the two co-ordinate systems, one at zero and another at θ.

$$x' = x \cos \theta + y \sin \theta$$

$$y' = -x \sin \theta + y \cos \theta \qquad \ldots(6)$$

The reconstruction program including the preliminary convolution of the B-scan images was done by a computer, off-line. Present Ultrasonograph machines have got the features of storing several B-scan images in memory and viewing them on the screen one after another. A 3.5 MHz sector-scan transducer was used. The several B-scans are obtained as per any the of the methods (1) to (3) mentioned above and stored in memory. The video is taken to a video digitiser of the Computer and stored as files of images. Every B-scan image was digitized with a 640 * 442 resolution in the frame grabber and only region of 256 * 256 pixels, surrounding the region of interest, was clipped and saved as the respective file. These files are operated by these programs developed for the PC. Summing is done for various angles, from – 10° to + 10°, – 20° to + 20° and – 30° to + 30°. The time taken on a 486 PC was about two minutes.

After reconstruction, the file was again transferred through an analog to video output card available on the PC to generate the video, which was directed to the same monitor. All these operations could be done within a few minutes with a fast Computer. The video prints of reconstructed views are useful for documentation and reports.

The results of two different anatomical placements for the limited angular reconstructed images are given herewith.

Fig. 13.6 shows the cross sectional view of the normal Pancreas and the aorta. Usually, the Pancreas is described with its head, body and tail. In the simple B-scan view (a), the tail

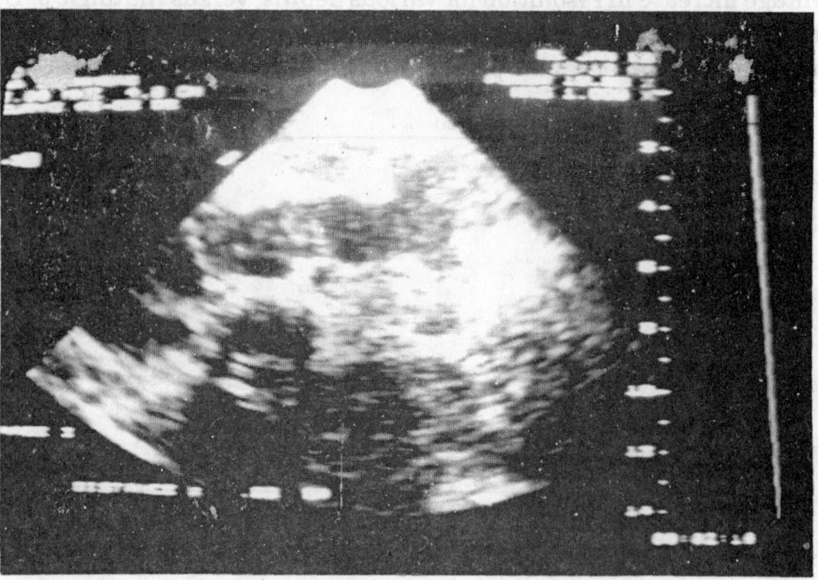

Fig. 13.6a

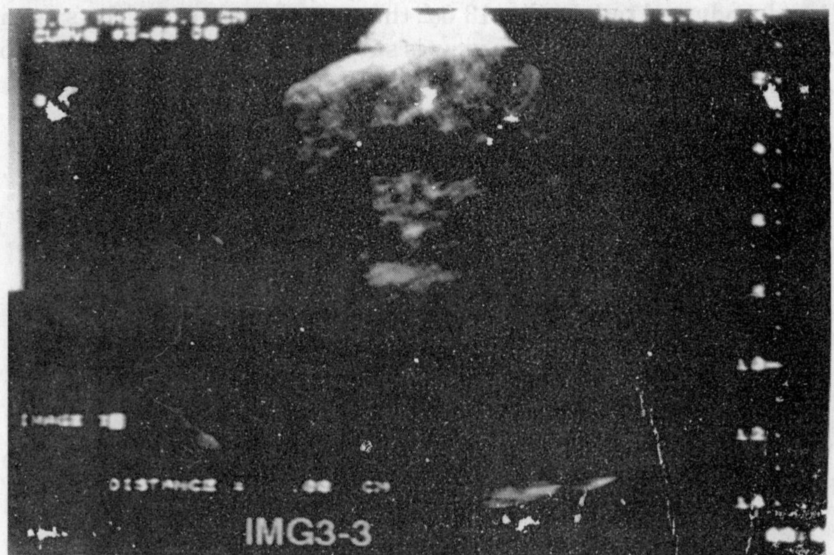

Fig. 13.6b

portion is not seen. This view has considerably improved with the reconstruction. For locating the center of the circle of transducer movement, an echogenic region was identified near the aorta (pancreas) and this point was maintained at the same depth while taking the angular views, so as to constrait the transducer movement on the circular arc. In order to eliminate the transducer movements in other planes, a line mark made on the surface helped to maintain the orientation manually. In Fig. 13.6*b*, the reconstruction is done with B-scans over the angles – 10° to + 10°. There is not appreciable additional information in this. However, in Fig. 13.6*c*, the Pancreas is

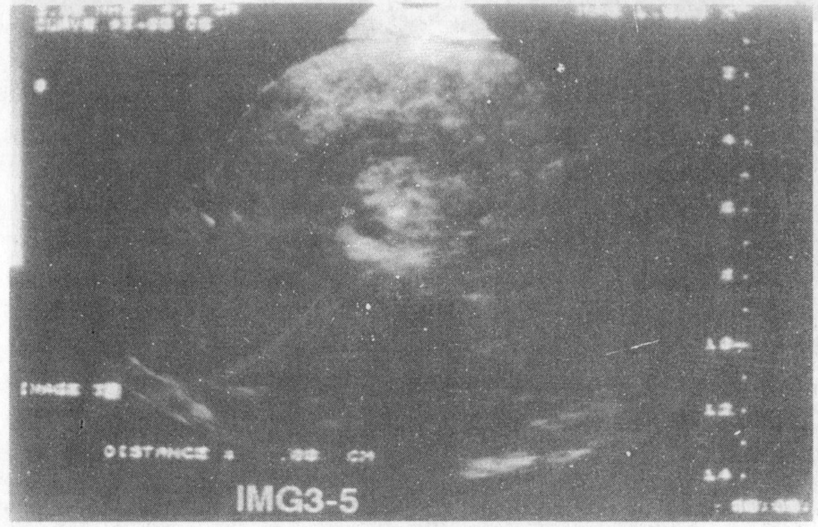

Fig. 13.6c

seen fully with head, body and tail. In Fig. 13.6*d*, the curved structure of the same is completely visible and is better than in Fig. 13.6*c*. This view is stated to be useful for the study of anatomical relationship of tumors if present in the Pancreas.

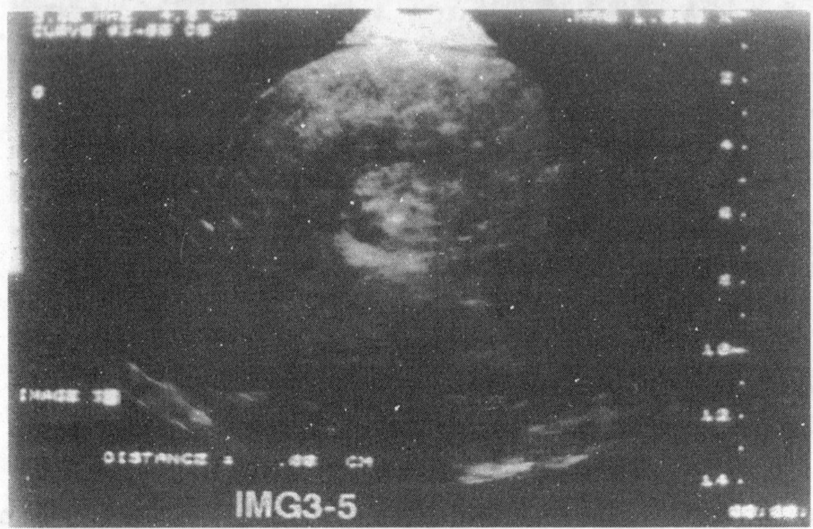

Fig. 13.6d

Fig. 13.7a shows the cross-section of the lower pole of the kidney, the renal cortex and central Calyceallical echo complex. The center of the tomogram was manipulated as the renal sinus. In the simple B-scan view (Fig. 13.7*a*), the central Calyceal complex is seen as collection of

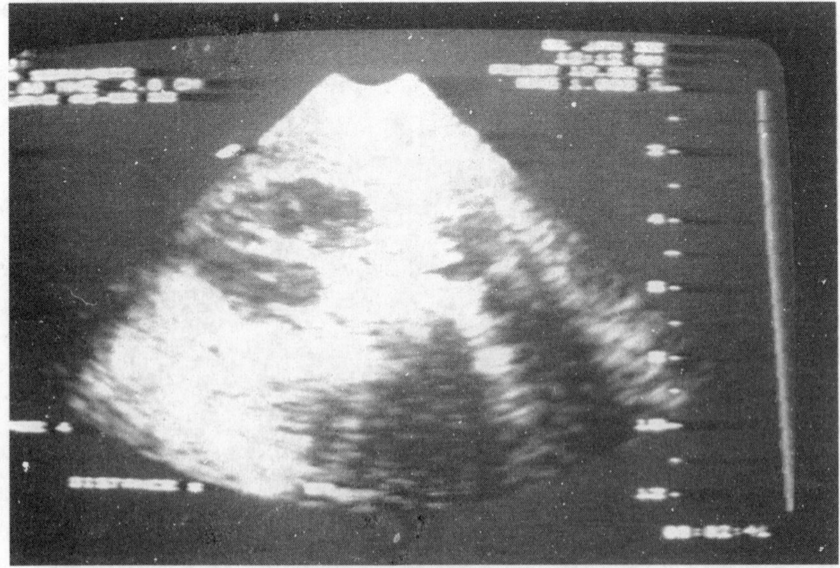

Fig. 13.7a

relatively bright echoes. In the reconstructed image Fig. 13.7(*b*), the branching of at least two calyceas are seen. In the 7(c), two more calyceas in addition to that of Fig. 13.7(*b*) are seen. This reconstructed image is helpful for localizing small stones if present in them. In Fig. 13.7(*d*), the image of Calyceas is not shown any better than in Fig. 13.7(*c*), but the medullar portion of the kidney is resolved better.

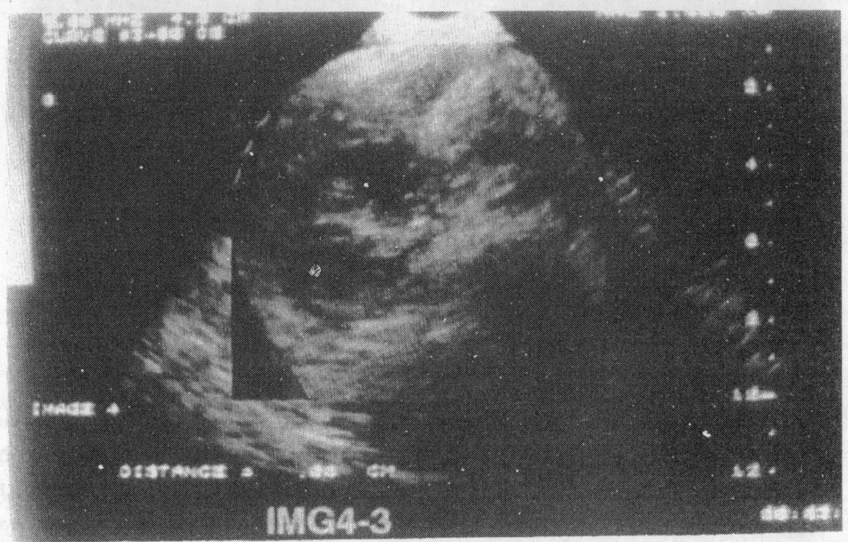

Fig. 13.7b

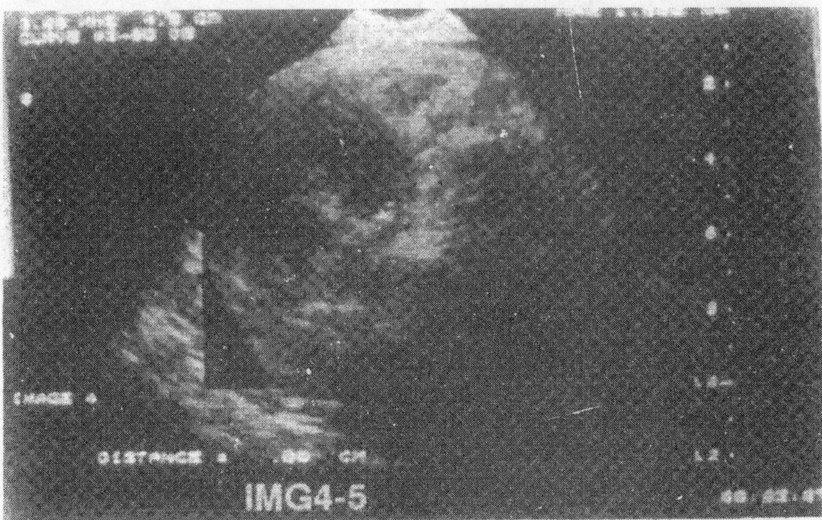

Fig. 17c

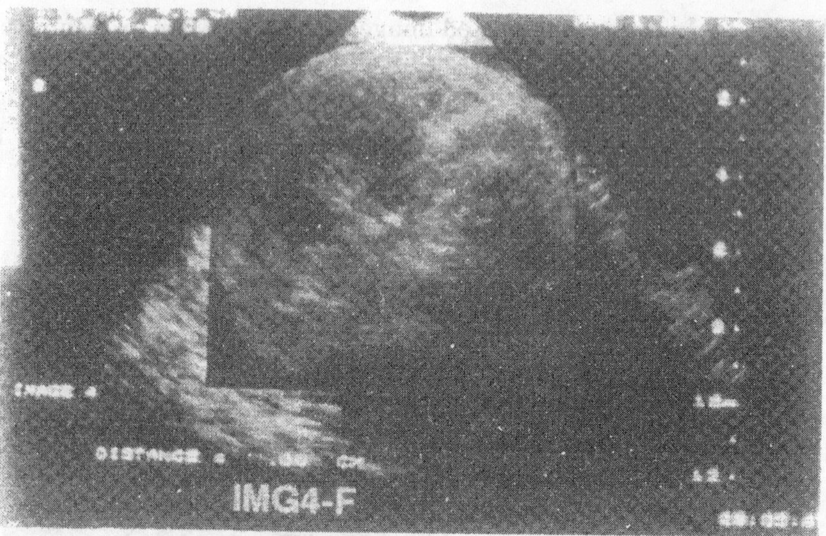

Fig. 13.7d

The above clearly brings out the simplicity of the techniques which can be easily adapted with present machines to provide improved information. Additionally, it was found that the usual artifacts such as shadow and enhancements are almost eliminated with these limited angular summed-up images. As a sonologist could infer from the figures, they appear to give not merely a resolution improvement but increased perceptual details, resulting in good dimensional accuracy as needed for reporting the pathology, wherever present.

MODULATION METHOD FOR RESOLUTION ENHANCEMENT

Ikegmi has given a method for improving resolution and Signal to noise ratio. In normal B- scan imaging techniques of that day, with a plain transducer and mechanical movements bursts of ultrasound are transmitted and the echoes collected. In this method encoded waves with Chirp signals were used. They showed that the range resolution and S/N ratio had improvements. They took image views at several angles over an arc length L. In their system these ultrasound signals were modulated signals.

$$S(t) = \exp(j\omega_0 t + \tfrac{1}{2} kt^2) \qquad (\text{for } t <= T/2)$$
$$= 0 \qquad (\text{for } t > T/2)$$

where ω_0 denotes the angular frequency of the center of the chirp signal, k denotes the chirp rate and T is the pulse duration time. The received signal has a carrier and an modulated part.

The reflected signals

$$r_1(t) = \int \exp\{j\omega_0(t - 2(x + L)/v\}.\ \exp\{(jk/2)(t - 2(x + L)/v\}.f(x)\, dx$$

where x represents the distance between the transducer and the center of the object. L represents radius of the circular scan. The carrier component is eliminated, because it does not contain any information by multiplying with $\exp(-j\omega_0 t)$. The phases term is proportional to t^2 is also eliminated by multiplying another factor of $r_1(t)\exp(-j\omega_0 t)$ for $x = 0$. Finally

$$r_2(t) = \int f(x) \exp(k(x) \,.\, \exp(-jk\,\{2x/v\})\,t)\,dx$$

where $k(x) = (-j\omega_0 2\,(x + L)/v + jk2x(x + 2L)/v^2)$

The above is the Fourier transform of *f(x) exp k(x)*. From the above steps, *f(x)* can be calculated. The spatial resolution of the system depends on the Band width B of the chirp signal as under.

$$\delta x = v\pi/B$$

SPECKLE REDUCTION IN ULTRASOUND PULSE IMAGING

Healey and Leeman have discussed methods of speckle reduction in the echoes. Speckle may be defined by the difference between the ideal image and the actual image. They use second moment of amplitude distribution M2 for an image. M2 = 1.27 to 3 for a particular image chosen by them. M2 parameter is just a measure of relative image smoothness, yielding unity for a uniform nonzero image segment. They use an adaptive unsharp mask filter at different local spots (each of 11 × 11 pixels) and show improvement.

USE OF WAVELET TRANSFORMS

An ultrasound imaging device that uses a wavelet transformation as the image reconstruction algorithm has been described by Letcher who describe a digital filtering technique which improves the practicality of the device by easing the constraints on ultrasound generation allowing the use of simple and inexpensive sound transducer and drives. The extent to which filtering can compensate for poor control of the generated ultrasound was investigated by simulation and experiment.

DEVELOPMENTS IN REAL TIME IMAGER INSTRUMENTS

The high end instruments employ latest Digital signal processing devices for general digital image storage, scan conversion and even 3-D views are made available virtually in real time. Using this Ving-Med Company has produced an echocardiac machine with 3D views of reconstructed slices of the cardiac chambers in addition to the Colour Doppler 3D images. Availability of high-speed cache memory enables such applications while DSP devices presently available up to 200 MHz clock speed can work out two MAC (multiply accumulate) instructions in 5ns. Also floating point 32 bit DSP devices are available for such applications.

Already even in the general-purpose machines hardware for processing metric calculations obstetric image calculations etc are provided. For fetus examinations, evaluation of gestational age from head perimeter measurements etc. are some of them. In Doppler machines the provision for evaluations of valve area by the Hatle relation using the pressure half time measurement made on the Spectrogram is a routine feature. Quantification in Colour Doppler images may also been soon available using Doppler colour flow mapping since manufacturers are now permitting the user to access the digital information used to create the colour flow image. Fetal colour Doppler echocardiography and trans-esophageal echocardiography are also recently developed applications, with the prospects of 3-D and 4-D views of the heart being investigated.

DOPPLER SIGNALS FROM PROBE

Today's machines have built-up Doppler processing of the echo signals. When an ultrasound signal strikes a moving target, the reflected echoes have a change of frequency (or Phase) corresponding the motion of the target given by the Doppler frequency shift.

$$f_D = f_0 \, 2v \cos \theta / c \qquad \text{...(1)}$$

where f_0 is the ultrasound frequency, v is the velocity of the target and θ the inclination and c is the tissue sound velocity (usw. 1540 m/s) (Fig. 13.8).

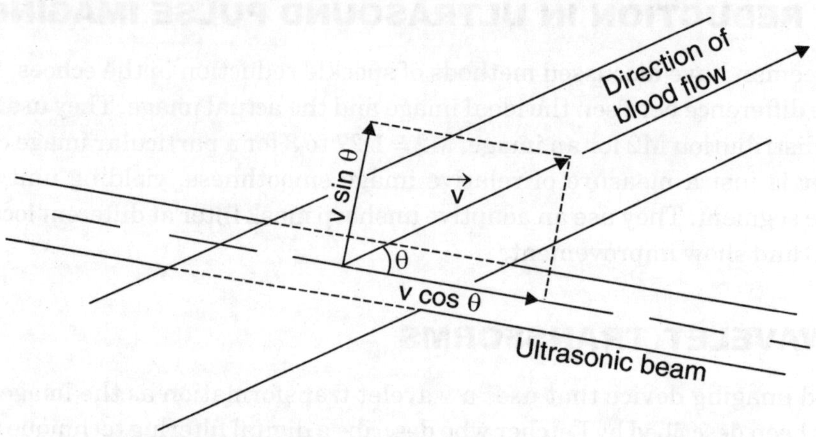

Fig. 13.8. Doppler relation for ultrasound signal in a blood vessel.

While scanning takes place over a region by the linear or sector transducer, typical paths of the beam could be chosen to process the Doppler sampled volume inside the region. The velocity information in that region can be processed by using the shift of frequency and plotting the spectrogram. The received signal generally comprises of reflections from blood vessels, walls and signal from the blood flow in arteries. The former two are low frequency shifts, while the latter is attributed to Raleigh scattering of the beam by the moving particles of blood. It is of a higher frequency, varying from 2 to 16 KHz depending on the nature of blood flow, laminar or turbulent or jet.

Echo cardiography analyses the pathology of valves and their narrowness in diseased or abnormal conditions by noting the velocity patterns during the systole and diastole in the heart beat cycle which is usually accompanied with ECG waveform display also. Plate III.1*a* shows the usual spectrogram display given by a machine for a region of insonation under the mitral valve flow, giving forward high velocity flow patterns due to narrowed (stenosed) valve. In some other pathologies, there may be regurgitation also observable (negative frequencies), which would show high velocities in the spectrogram during the period when the valve closes. Plate III.1*a* shows a colour Doppler view of the ventricular jet of blood flow. Plate III.1*b* shows the spectrogram. The valve area is calculated by noting the time to reach the half of the peak pressure (shown by the cursor line from E-wave towards A-wave), called pressure half-time. Hatles's empirical relation then yields valve area as

$$A = 200/(\text{P.H.T.}) \text{ in S. cm.}$$

Doppler attachment in many machines provides additional circuits. The choice of sample volume for which the Doppler signals are collected is related to the scan time course. Hence, it is possible to pick up the pulse echoes during that scan angle and do the Doppler processing for a lesser angle than for imaging. The RF demodulators separate the two components of the signals using phase sensitive demodulators using typical high frequency integrated circuits meant for the purpose. These two I and Q signals are in the audio frequency range (f_0 and f_{90}).

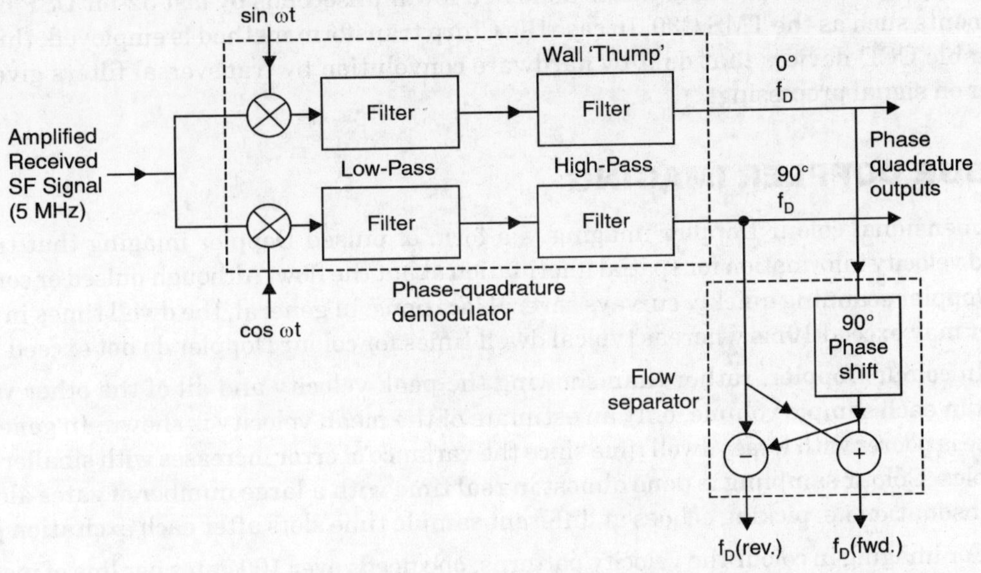

Fig. 13.9. Shows the phase quadrature scheme of doppler signal extraction.

Doppler processing is done usually with DSP hardware. Chirp-z transform is performed using dedicated integrated circuits on the signals after demodulation. They can also be done by DSP hardware so that the spectrogram display can follow the speed of the ecg signal along with it.

In order to give an insight into this Doppler processing which is a typical signal processing step in these instruments, let us consider the complex signal $I + jQ$ and see how the spectrogram giving the separated forward and reverse flow velocities can be generated.

Suppose two frequencies (w_a) and (w_b) are present in the forward and reverse directions in the Doppler Echo signal, so that

$$x(t) = x_a(t) + x_b(t) \qquad \ldots(2)$$

$$= \text{A} \cos w_a(t) + \text{B} \sin w_b(t) + j(\text{A} \sin w_a t + \text{B} \cos w_b t)$$

The Fourier Transform of the complex time function is

$$\text{X}(\omega) = \int x(t) \exp(-j\omega t)\, dt = \int \{x_a(t) + j\, x_b(t)\} \exp(-j\omega t)\, dt \qquad \ldots(3)$$

were the integral limits are $-\infty$ to $+\infty$.

$$\text{X}(\omega) = \int \text{A} \cos \omega_a t \exp(-j\omega t)\, dt + \int \text{B} \sin \omega_b t \exp(-j\omega t)\, dt$$

$$+ j \int \text{A} \sin \omega_a t \exp(-j\omega t)\, dt + j \int \text{B} \sin \omega_b t \exp(-j\omega t)\, dt$$

Writing $\cos\theta \pm \sin\theta$ as $\exp(\pm j\theta)$, we get,

$$\text{X}(\omega) = \text{A}\delta(\omega - \omega_a) + j\, \text{B}\delta(\omega + \omega_b)$$; the δ function is unity only at its argument = 0.

The result substantiates the above statement that the CFFT separates the two components of forward and reverse velocities in the positive and negative frequency spectra.

A spectrogram display which is of particular importance in showing the Doppler flow in blood vessels and cardiac chambers appears as in Plate III.1*b*. The display is managed to be shown almost in real time along with the ECG by the fast processing that is performed in the machine either by the CFFT method or the Chirp z-transform method. The former method is done for typical 8K samples and this is done in a few milliseconds by fast 32-bit DSP hardware components such as the TMS C30. In case the Chirp transform method is employed, this is done by suitable CCD devices that do it by hardware convolution by transversal filters given in the chapter on signal processing.

COLOUR DOPPLER IMAGING

Two dimensional colour Doppler imaging is a form of pulsed Doppler imaging that trades off detailed velocity information for spatial information about the flow. Although pulsed or continuous wave Doppler scanning quickly surveys several locations, in general, the dwell times in spectral Doppler may exceed 10ms whereas typical dwell times for colour Doppler do not exceed 1-2 ms.

In colour Doppler, rather than showing the peak velocity and all of the other velocities present in each sample volume, only an estimate of the mean velocity is shown. In general, this estimate is poorer with lesser dwell time since the variance of error increases with smaller number of samples. Colour sampling is done almost in real time with a large number of gates along each line of insonation i.e. picking echoes at different sample time slots after each excitation pulse.

For imaging in colour the velocity patterns, one needs over 100 gates per line of insonation. Because of the brief interrogation times and the limited number of pulses per line (6-12 usually) no Complex Fourier analysis can be performed. Instead, most manufacturers of machines use auto-correlation technique. In this, the entire signal from all depths is stored in memory and then compared or correlated with the Doppler returns from successive pulses or samples. The larger the memory size used for storing the samples the more gates along each line are there for the analysis. Ten samples would produce nine correlations times 100 gates for a total of 900 mean estimate computations in 1 ms. An average is taken for the cluster of estimated mean values for each gate and then assigned a colour for the display. A variance of the means is also evaluated from the samples and can be related to the turbulence in flow.

Within a 90° color sector a minimum of 64 lines is required and each line of sight or vector must be sampled a least six to twelve times though more would be desirable. For this reason, frame rates for colour are very much slow. The area of interest should be limited to the points at which a minimum of ten frames per second can be achieved to preserve the fluid like motion for the blood. Fig. 13.10 (Table) shows the interaction of the key variables that can affect the quality of the Colour Doppler display. Plate III.1*a* shows the typical colour Doppler view of the Left ventricular jet and the Colour Doppler angle is only a small region of the total scan angle.

3-D PLOTS OF DOPPLER SPECTRA

When the Doppler signal is shown in a spectrogram, that pertains to a certain time variation called the time window of observation.

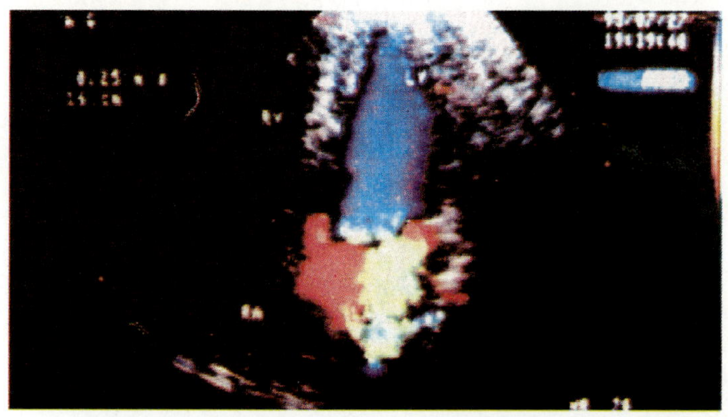

Plate III.1a. Shows the typical colour doppler view of the left ventricular jet and the colour doppler angle is only a small region of the total scan angle.

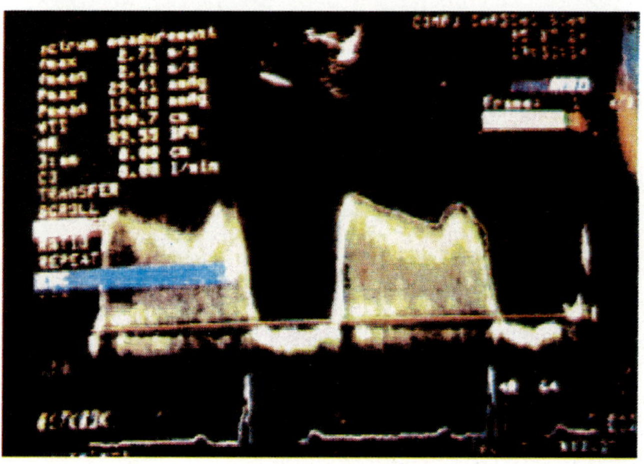

Plate III.1b. Shows the usual spectrogram display for a mitral valve insonation. The curves are drawn by operator to evaluate pressure halftime and thence valve area.

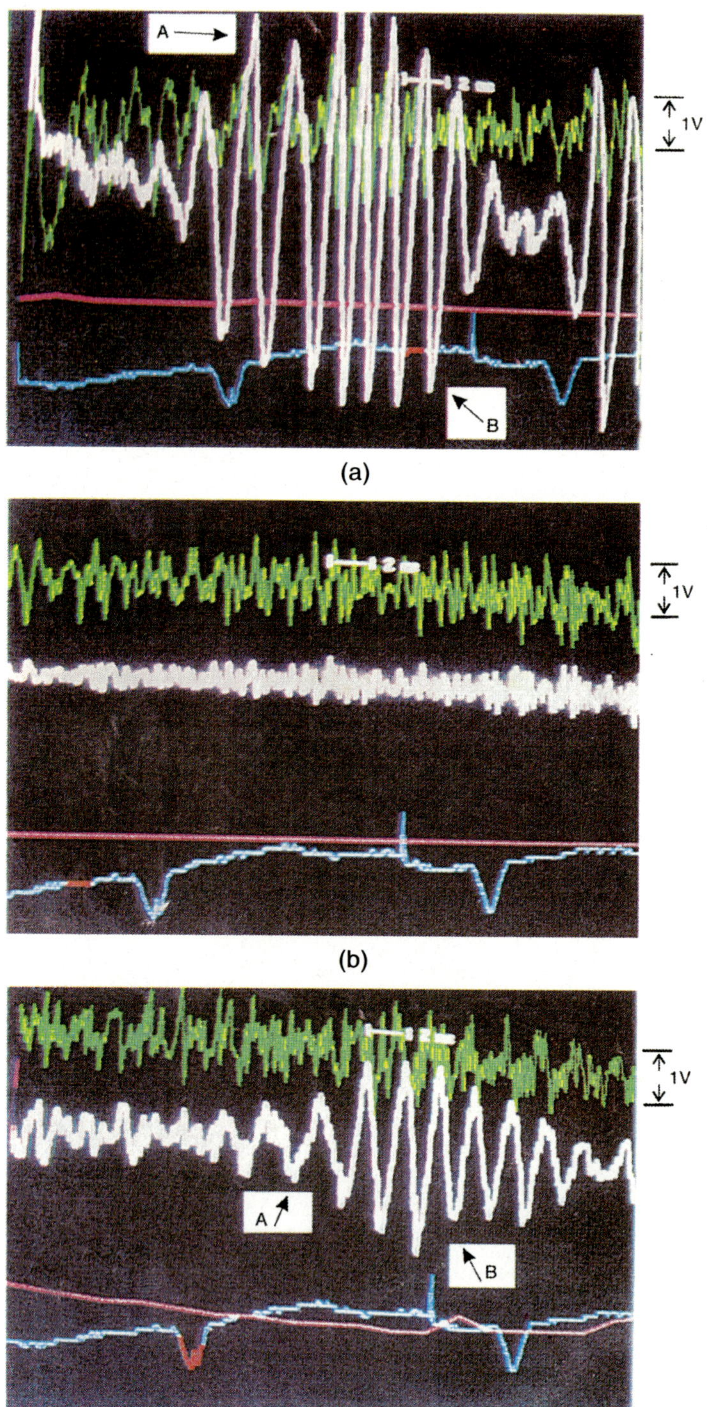

Plate III.2. (*a*) Mitral opening valve oscillations at T-wave end; top trace shows flow. A and B indicate two different leaflet vibration frequencies. (*b*) Flow through an opened mitral valve. (*c*) Closing oscillations of the mitral valve. [Padmanabhan et al., July 2000, *IEEE Med. Biol. Journal*].

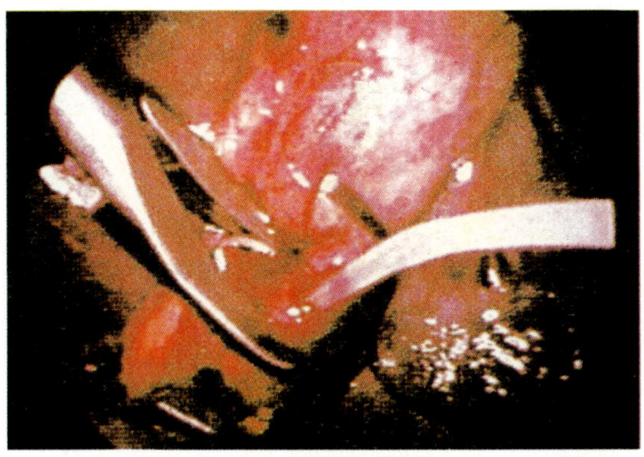

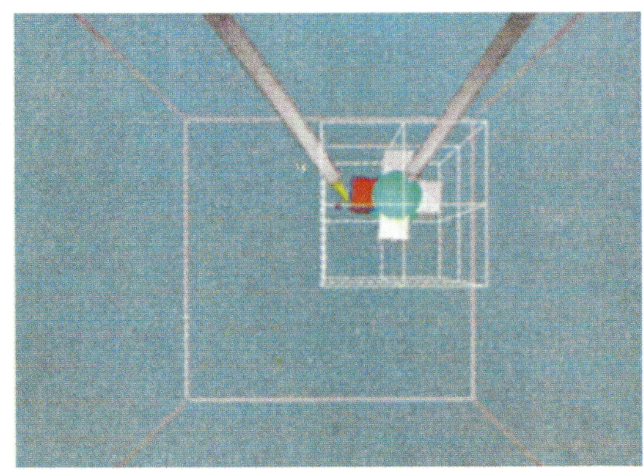

MUSE TECHNOLOGIES LTD.

Medical schools have begun using virtual reality "games" to test students' surgical aptitude.
Among the most popular surgical trainers is the MIST VR system, from MUSE Technologies Ltd., Albuquerque, of the actual tools used for laparoscopy on the gall bladder or ovaries.
"It's not attempting to be a simulator [of what] you would see during surgery," explains Christopher Sutton, project manager for MIST.

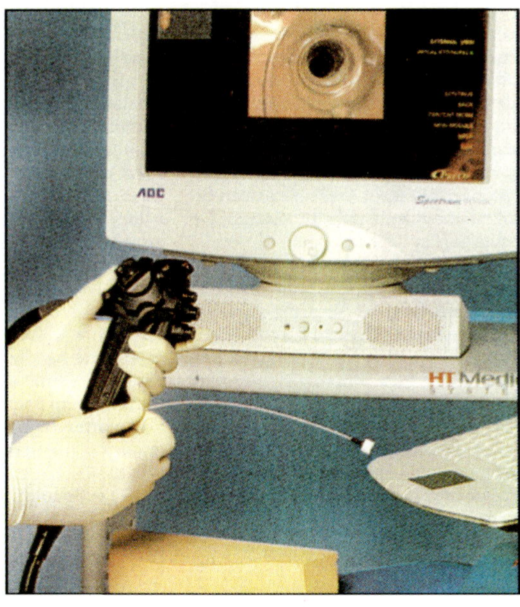

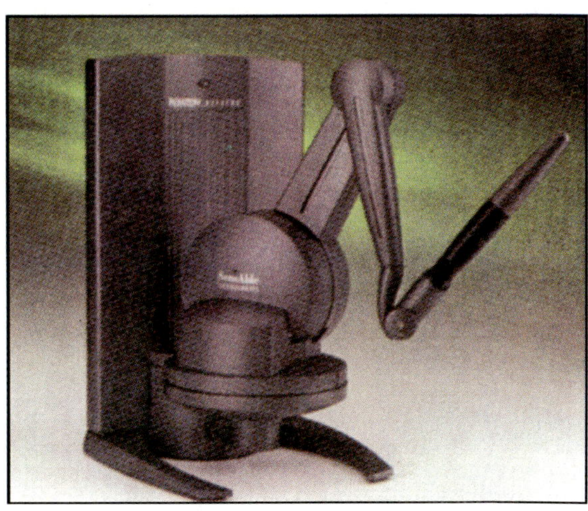

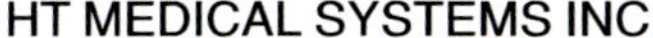

HT MEDICAL SYSTEMS INC.

A virtual sigmo doscope from HT Medical Systems Inc. trains doctors to maneuver the flexible probes used to view the colon, shown on the computer display. The system incorporates haptic feedback and video imaging synchronized to the position of the probe. The simulation software warns the user when injury to the "patient" is imminent, and it can also rate the user's performance.

SENSABLE TECHNOLOGIES INC.

The Phantom haptic interface from SensAble Technologies Inc. is popular in virtual reality surgical simulators. The device has three or six degrees of feedom and users actuators to relay resistance at about 1000 Hz.

Plate III.3. Virtual Surgery.

...ctrogram represents the Doppler signal in the frequency domain when it is observed ...me window. In real life the Doppler signal is observed continuously (over successive ...ws) resulting in sequentially observed frequency spectrums. These different spectrums reflec... variations in the Doppler frequency shift as a function of time.

Plotting a single-frequency spectrum requires two axes, the frequency axis and the amplitude axis. To plot sequential spectrum, a third axis (time) is required. Therefore plots depicting successive frequency spectrums as functions of time are known as 3-D spectrograms. Since they may also be looked on as representing sequentially obtained frequency spectrums in successive planes they are sometimes also called multiplane plots (Fig. 13.11).

Number of lines in degrees Fig.13.10 (Table)

PRF	# SAMPLES	20	30	40
4 KHz	5	40	26.6	20
	10	20	13.3	10
6 KHz	5	60	40	30
	10	30	20	15
8 KHz	5	80	53.3	40
	10	40	26.6	20

Fig. 13.10. (Table) Shows the interaction of the key variables that can affect the quality of the Colour Doppler display.

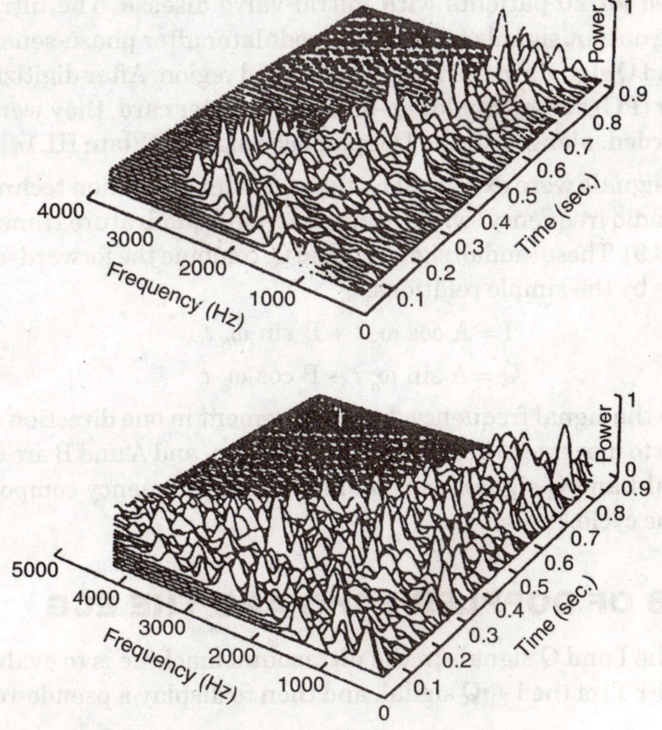

Fig. 13.11. Shows 3-D Spectrogram plot pattern.

II. DOPPLER ULTRASOUND OBSERVATION OF PATHOLOGICAL HEART VALVES

A simple, Noninvasive Technique Based on Hilbert Transform Time-Signal Displays :

Current diagnostic techniques using two-dimensional (2-D) B-Scan ultra-sound imaging are only able to determine whether the anterior or posterior mitral-valve leaflets are thickened: accurate quantitative measurements are not possible. Approximate measurements from the 2-D B-scan images have an uncertainty of plus or minus 25% due to the poor lateral resolution of ultrasound images, even with the best positioning of the probe. Actual thickness cannot be measured in vivo.

A theoretical formula for thickness can be modeled on the basis of general mechanics of vibration of a cantilevered beam. Nonlinear and stress-relaxation properties of the valve tissue are not included in this model. An empirical formula that can estimate valve thickness using results obtained from Doppler echocardiography would suffice.

In this section, methods of showing forward- flow and reverse-flow Doppler echocardiograph signals as a time course of events relating to valve stenosis and regurgitation are considered for providing additional cardiac insonation diagnostic information. The Doppler ultrasound demodulated signals are separated using the Hilbert transform (HT) technique and then shown as segments of waveforms along with the corresponding electrocardiogram. This allows us to relate cardiac activity events, to assess valve leaflet thickness in severe mitral-valve stenosis cases, and to examine the opening and closing of valve leaflets for diagnosis.

The ultrasound Doppler echo machine can be used both to examine cardiac chamber blood flow velocity and for anatomical imaging. Four-chamber Doppler views of the mitral valve flow region were recorded for 20 patients with mitral-valve disease. The ultrasound machine has provisions for taking output signals from the demodulator after phase-sensitive detection, which are the so-called I and Q signals in the Doppler-sampled region. After digitizing these signals with a personal computer (PC) add-on analog-to-digital converter card, they were analyzed. The ECG signal was also recorded, along with the Doppler echo signals (Plate III.1*a*).

The Doppler signals were extracted by the usual demodulation technique; multiplying the ultrasound signal (radio frequency) with the in-phase and quadrature transmitter frequency and then filtering (Fig. 13.9). These (audio) signals, I and Q, combine the forward- and reverse-frequency Doppler components by the simple relations:

$$I = A \cos \omega_a t + B \sin \omega_b t$$

$$Q = A \sin \omega_a t + B \cos \omega_b t$$

where ω_a represents the signal frequency due to movement in one direction and ω_b represents the signal frequency due to movement in the opposite direction, and A and B are their peak intensities. Of course, the actual I and Q signals contain many such frequency components that vary with time over the cardiac cycle.

TIME SIGNALS OF DOPPLER ECHO AND THE ECG

The current use of the I and Q signals in the ultrasound machine is to evaluate the complex fast Fourier transform (FFT) of the I + *j*Q signal, and then to display a pseudo-real-time spectrogram plot along with the ECG. Clinical evaluation is done using the (frozen) Doppler spectrogram plot. For mitral-flow imaging, measurement of peak velocity of valvular flow (PFV) in the E-wave of the spectrogram and the increase of flow velocity following atrial contraction (A-wave) are notable (Fig. 13.12). This figure shows the difference between the adult and neonate. For velocities greater than 0.9 m/sec, Hatle, et al., related the valve area to the pressure half-time (PHT) by an empirical formula (rather than by a mathematical Bernoulli orifice equation):

$$\text{Valve Area} = 220/\text{PHT cm}^2$$

The PHT is determined from the display screen of the machine by drawing a line along the E-A slope and calculating the time at which the velocity falls to 0.707 of the maximum value. If the I and Q signals are digitized, and similar spectrogram plots made on the PC by suitably fast-running programs, the display can show the ECG, the spectrogram and the cursor based measurements of PHT, valve area, etc. Additionally, a Gabor-type spectrogrm was made that showed some additional fine streaks of signal at low frequencies (around 300–1000 Hz) at valve opening and closing times. It was thus considered worthwhile to separate the I and Q signals into the forward and reverse components. In order to do this, and HT operation was performed on the quadrature signal. Using the relations.

$$V_f = [1 + \text{Hilbert transform (Q)}] / 2$$
$$V_r = [1 - \text{Hilbert transform (Q)}] / 2 \qquad ...(1)$$

the two components are clearly separated.

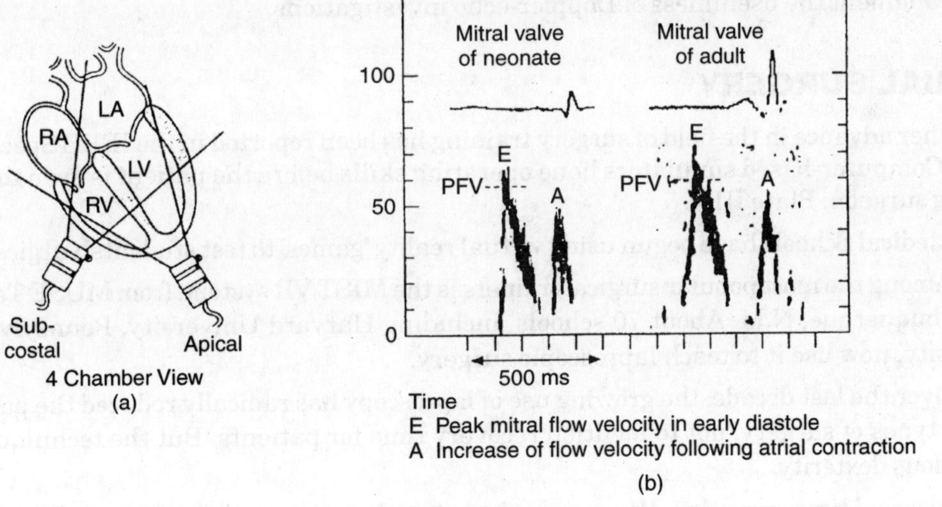

Fig. 13.12

The method employed for finding the HT of the stored data points (32K points corresponding to one or more cardiac cycles) will be considered in the chapter on "Signal Processing".

After the HT-based separation of the actual forward and reverse signals, the signals were displayed as short segments of 40 m sec, one after another, over the ECG cycle, so to observe their patterns at different points of cardiac activity (Plate III.2). Since 640 data samples of signal were shown at a time on a PC screen, the total data of one ECG cycle would appear on several screens, one by one, each for 40 m sec. While showing the forward and reverse time signals, the whole

ECG of that cardiac event was also displayed as a third trace with that (40 m sec) segment highlighted (in red). Such a display presentation would facilitate clinical observations and inferences.

MITRAL-VALVE PATHOLOGY USING THE TIME SIGNALS

In cases of mitral-valve disease with leaflet thickening, there were notable vibrations at the exact onsets of opening and closure of the valve. The severity of the condition could be related to signal peak amplitude and damping. Valve leaflet thickness could be assessed by vibration frequency. The 2-D echo images do not ordinarily permit any precise measurement of valve thickness, which this method indirectly provides by use of the theory of cantilever vibration. The damping is indicative of stenosis and possible regurgitation. For a typical case of mitral stenosis, Plate III.2 shows these vibrations at the start of the ECG P-wave, when the mitral valve opens.

The importance of such time signals is that they also provide better indications of the durations of the valve opening and closing in the cardiac cycle.

In all case studies, which involved 20 patients with similar rheumatic or related mitral-valve disease, the observations of the time signal based on the HT method are noted to provide additional information about the condition of the valve leaflets. The results supplement the usual techniques of the M-mode echocardiogram, the 2-D echo image, and the color Doppler, giving additional detailed information about the leaflets and their thickening. (Padmanathan et al., July 2000).

Commercial ultrasound machines may incorporate this time waveform display technique so as to augment the usefulness of Doppler-echo investigations.

VIRTUAL SURGERY

An another advance in the field of surgery training has been reported in the IEEE Spectrum 2002. Today. Computer-based simulators hone operating skills before the patient is even touched by a budding surgeon. Plate III.3.

Medical Schools have begun using virtual reality 'games' to test students' surgical aptitude.

Among the most popular surgical trainers is the MIST VR system, from MUSE Technologies Ltd., Albuquerque, N.M. About 70 schools, including Harvard University, Pennsylvania State University, now use it to teach laproscopic surgery.

Over the last decade, the growing use of laproscopy has radically reduced the pain and cost of some types of surgery, not to mention recovery time for patients. But the technique requires tremendous dexterity.

In a real time operation, the surgeon inserts a tiny camera through a small incision in the patient's body and then watches the internal organs on a video monitor; surgical instruments are fed and manipulated through several more tiny holes.

At first instance, MIST (short for minimally invasive surgery training) looks nothing like a surgical set up. The colour monitor displays simple geometric shapes, not simulated body parts. An interface device hooked to the Computer has the handles of the actual tools for laproscopy in the gall bladder or ovaries.

It does not appear to be a simulator, you would see yourself during surgery; explains Christopher Sutton, Project Manager.

The student grasps the principle through repeated practice and close observation of the video.

REFERENCES

1. Hoess A., Ermert, " adaptive wiener filtering for B-mode Image enhancement, IEEE Symp. On Ultrasonic, 1992.
2. Hiller D. & Ermet H., "Tomographic Reconstruction of B-scan Images", Acoustical Imaging Journal, vol.10, 1982, p. 347-64.
3. K. Padmanathan and K. Sunder, Limited angular ultrasound tomography...', I.E.E. Symp on Med. Imaging, 1993, London (ASI-93).
4. Padmanabhan K., Sunder K., Ananthi S., "Improvements in B-scan Image-some new methods, Jl. of Pure and applied ultrasonics, July-Dec.-1998, Vol. 20 (3&4), pp. 45-56.
5. Ikamin M., Yama Mota T. and Aoki Y., " Back Projection with an efficient computation for reflection Tomography", Acoustic Imaging, vol. 15, 1987, pp. 35-45.
6. Hatle A.J and Leeman S., "Speckle reduction methods in U.S. Echo imaging," IEE Conference on Acous. Imaging, publications-369, 1993.
7. Letcher J.H., "An Imaging device using Wavelet transform as reconstruction algorithm", Inst. Jl. of Image System & Tech., 1992 (4), pp. 98-108.
8. S. Navin Nanda, "Doppler Echocardiography", 2nd Edition, Lea Febiger, Phil. 1993.
9. K. Padmanabhan, S. Dhanasekaran, S. Ananthi and D. Nedumaran, "Doppler ultrasound observation of Pathological Heart valves", IEEE Engg., in Medical & Biol., July 2000, pp. 111-116.
10. K. Padmanabhan and K. Chandrasekharan, "Ultrsound medical diagnostic Instrumentation" a Review, Jl of Inst. Soc. of India, Jan. 2000.
11. K. Padmanabham and N. Pitchai, "Forced Response and Defibrillation". I.I.T. Bio Med. Soc., Delhi, 1975.

Chapter 14

Signal Processing in Medical Instrumentation

NOISE VERSUS SIGNAL

The ultimate accuracy and detection limit of an analytical method is determined by the inevitable presence of unwanted noise which is superimposed on the analytic signal causing it to fluctuate in a random way. Fig. 14.1*a*, which is a strip chart recording of a tiny DC signal (10^{-15} A), illustrates the typical appearance of noise on a physical measurement. Fig. 14.2*b* is theoretical plot showing the same current in the absence of noise. Unfortunately, at low signal strengths, a plot of the latter kind is never experimentally realizable because some types of noise arise form fundamental thermodynamic and quantum effects that can never be totally eliminated.

Ordinarily, amplification of a small noisy signal, such as shown in Fig. 14.1*a*, provides no improvement in the detection limit or precision of a measurement because both the noise and the information bearing signal are amplified to the same extent; as a matter of fact, the situation is often worsened by amplification as a consequence of added noise introduced by the amplifying device.

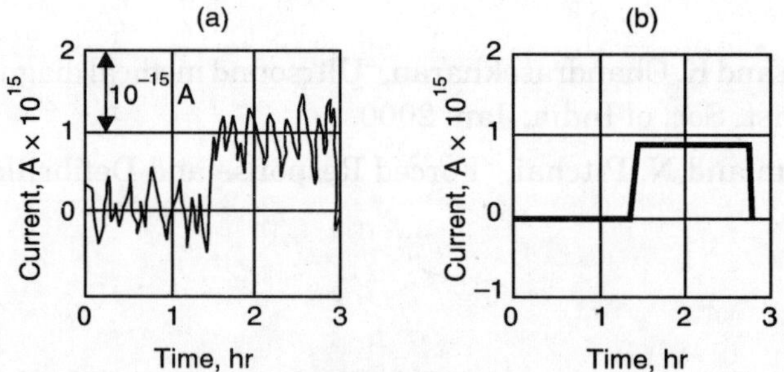

Fig. 14.1. Shows the effect of noise on a current waveform (a) Experimental strip chart recording of a 10^{-15} A direct current (b) Mean of the fluctuations.

In any biological method of analysis, both instrumental and biological noise are encountered. Example of sources of the latter include variability in the methods of application, side effects, interferences by artifact signals, and the uncontrolled effects on the rate of biological behavior as such.

Now let us discuss about the various noise generated in various components of our instruments. EEG noise which is associated with the overall behavior of cells and neurons is an example.

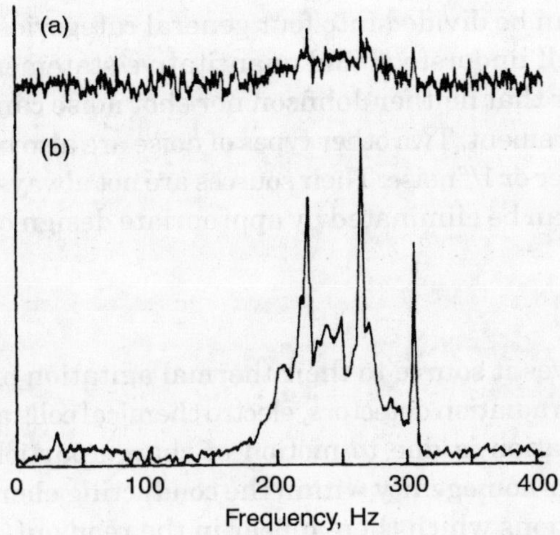

Fig. 14.2. Shows the effect of SNR on the NMR.

SIGNAL TO NOISE RATIO

It is apparent from Fig. 14.1 that the noise becomes increasingly important as its magnitude approaches that of the useful signal. Thus the signal-to-noise ratio (S/N) is a much more useful figure of merit for describing the quality of a measurement or an instrumental method than noise itself.

For a DC signal, the ultimate noise typically takes the form of the time variation of the signal about the mean as shown in Fig. 14.1*a*. Here, the noise N is conveniently defined as the standard deviation of the signal while the signal S is given by the mean. The signal to noise ratio is then reciprocal of the relative standard deviation of the measured signal. That is

$$S/N = \text{mean/ standard deviation}$$
$$= 1 / \text{relative standard deviation} \quad \ldots(1)$$

For an AC signal, the relationship between measured precision and S/N is less straight-forward. Since most AC signals are converted into DC signal before display, this relationship will not be dealt with and the above eqn. (1) then applies.

As a rule, the visual observation of a signal become impossible when S/N is smaller than perhaps 2 or 3 as the Fig. 14.2 illustrates this. The upper plot is a recorded nuclear magnetic resonance spectrum for progesterone with a signal to noise ratio of approximately 4.3; in the lower plot, the ratio is 4.3. At the lower ratio, the presence of some but not all of the peaks is apparent.

NOISE SOURCES IN INSTRUMENTS

Noise is associated with each component of an instrument-that is, with the source, the transducer, the signal processor, and the read-out. Furthermore, the noise from each of these components may be of several types and arise from several sources. Thus, the noise that is finally observed is a complex composite, which usually cannot be fully characterized. Certain types of noise are recognizable, however, and a consideration of their properties is useful.

Instrumental noise can be divided into four general categories. Two, thermal or Johnson noise and shot noise, are well understood and quantitative statements can be made about the magnitude of each. It is clear that neither Johnson nor shot noise can ever be totally eliminated from an instrumental measurement. Two other types of noise are also recognizable, environmental noise or interference and flicker or 1/*f* noise. Their sources are not always well defined or understood. In principle, however, they can be eliminated by appropriate design of circuitry.

JOHNSON NOISE

Johnson or thermal noise owes it source to their thermal agitation of electrons or other charge carriers in resistor, capacitor, radiation detectors, electro chemical cells and other resistive elements in an instrument. This agitation is due to motion of charge particles, is due to random and periodically created charge in-homogenity within the conducting element. This inhomogenity in turn creates voltage fluctuations which then appear in the read out as noise. It is important to note that Johnson noise is present even in the absence of current in a resistive element.

The magnitude of Johnson noise is readily derived from thermodynamic considerations and is given by

$$V_{rms} = \sqrt{4k\,TR\Delta f} \quad \text{...(2)}$$

where V_{rms} is the root-mean-square noise voltage lying in a frequency bandwidth of Δf Hz, k is the Boltzmann constant (1.38×10^{-23} J/deg), T is the absolute temperature and R is the resistance in ohms of the resistive element.

It is important to note that Johnson noise, while dependent upon the frequency band-width, is independent of frequency itself; thus, it is sometimes termed white noise by analogy to white light, which contains all visible frequencies. It is also noteworthy that

Johnson noise is independent of the physical size of the resistor.

Two methods are available to reduce Johnson noise in a system : narrow the band-width and lower the temperature. The former is often applied to amplifiers and other electronic components, where filters can be used to yield narrower band-widths. Thermal noise in photo multipliers and other detectors can be attentuated by cooling. For example, lowering the temperature of the detector from room to liquid Nitrogen temperature will have the Johnson noise.

SHOT NOISE

Short noise is encountered wherever a current involves the movement of electrons or other charged particles across a junction. In the typical electronic circuit, these junctions are found at *p* and *n* interfaces; In photo cell and vacuum tubes, the junction consists of the evacuated space between the anode and cathode. The currents in such devices involve a series of quantized events, namely, the transfer of individual electrons across the junction. These events are random, however, and the rate at which they occur are thus subject to statistical fluctuations, which are described by the equation

$$I_{rms} = \sqrt{2Ie\Delta f} \quad \text{...(3)}$$

where I_{rms} is the root-mean-square current fluctuation associated with the average direct current *I*, *e* is the charge of the electron (-1.6×10^{-19} Coulombs), and Δf is again the band-width of frequencies being considered. Like Johnson noise, shot noise has a "white" spectrum.

FLICKER NOISE

Flicker noise is characterized as having a magnitude that is inversely proportional to the frequency f of the signal being observed; it is sometimes termed 1/f (one-over-f) noise as a consequence. The causes of flicker noise are not well understood; its ubiquitous presence, however, is recognizable by its frequency dependence. Flicker noise becomes significant at frequencies lower than about 100 Hz. The long-term drift observed in dc amplifiers, meters, and galvanometers is a manifestation of flicker noise.

ENVIRONMENTAL NOISE

Environmental noise is a composite of noises arising from the surroundings. Fig. 14.3 suggests typical sources of environmental noise.

Software Methods

With the widespread availability of micro-processors and microcomputers, many of the signal-to-noise enhancement devices described in the previous section are being replaced or supplemented by digital computer software algorithms. Among these are programs for various types of averaging, digital filtering, Fourier transformation, and correlation techniques. Generally, these procedures are applicable to non-periodic or irregular wave forms, such as an absorption spectrum, or to signals having no synchronizing or reference wave.

Some of these common software procedures are discussed briefly here.

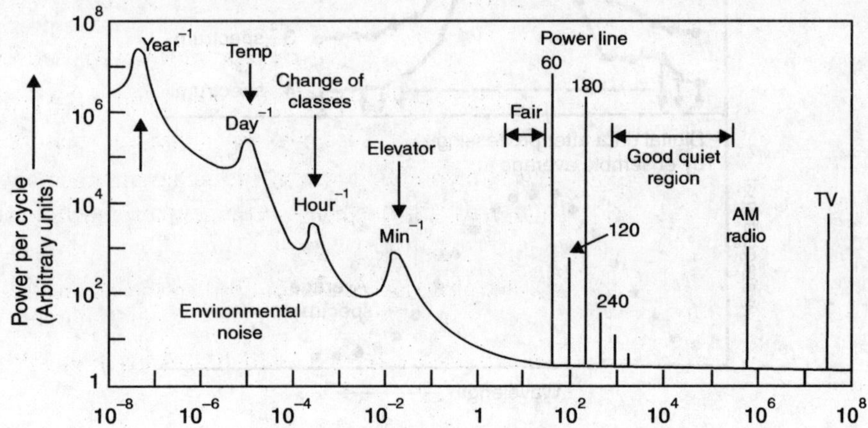

Fig. 14.3. Shows some sources of some environmental noises x-axis = frequency.

Ensemble Averaging

In ensemble averaging, successive sets of data (arrays), each of which adequately describes the signal wave form, are collected and summed point by point as an array in the memory of a computer (or in a series of capacitors for hardware averaging). After the collection and summation is complete, the data are averaged by dividing the sum for each point by the number of scans performed. Fig. 14.4 illustrates ensemble averaging of a simple absorption spectrum.

Ensemble averaging owes its effectiveness to the fact that individual noise signals N_n, insofar as they are random, tend to cancel one another. Consequently, their average N is given by a relationship,

$$N = N_n/\sqrt{n}$$

where n is the number of arrays averaged. The signal to noise ratio of the averaged array is then given by

$$S/N = (S_n/n)/(N_n/\sqrt{n})$$

$$= (S_n/N_n)/\sqrt{n} \qquad \ldots(4)$$

where Sn/n is the average signal. It should be noted that this same signal-to-noise enhancement is realized in the boxcar averaging and digital filtering, which are described in subsequent sections.

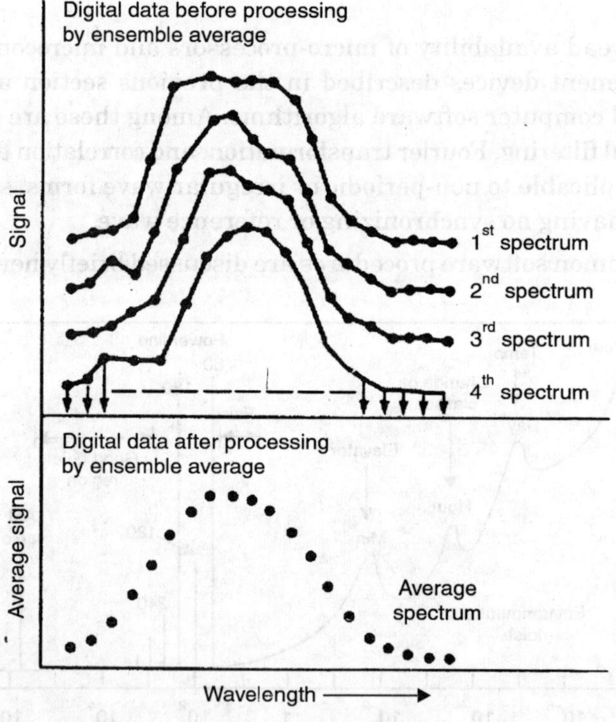

Fig. 14.4. Shows the Ensemble averaging of a Spectrum.

To realize the advantage of ensemble averaging and still extract all of the information available in any wave form, it is necessary to measure points at a frequency that is at least twice as great as the highest frequency component of the wave form. Much greater sampling frequencies, however, provide no additional information but include more noise. Furthermore, it is highly important to sample the wave-form reproducibly (that is, at the same point each time). For example, if the wave form is a section of ultrasound image echo, each scan of the beam must start at exactly the same position and the rate of transducer movement must be identical for each sweep. Generally, the former is realized by means of a synchronizing pulse, which is derived from the original carrier itself. The pulse then initiates the recording of the wave form.

Ensemble averaging can produce dramatic improvements in signal-to-noise ratios. Ensemble averaging for evoked cortical potentials was considered earlier.

Ensemble averaging can be performed by either hardware or software techniques. The latter is now the more common with the signals at various points being digitized in a computer memory for subsequent processing and display.

Boxcar Averaging

Boxcar averaging is a digital procedure for smoothing irregularities in a wave form, the assumption being made that these irregularities are the consequence of noise. That is, it is assumed that the analog analytical signal varies only slowly with time and that the average of a small number of adjacent points is a better measure of the signal than any of the individual points. Fig. 14.5*b* illustrates the effect of the technique on the data plotted in Fig. 14.5*a*. The first point on the boxcar plot is the mean of points 1, 2 and 3 on the original curve; point 2 is the average of points 4, 5 and 6, and so forth. In practice 2 to 50 points are averaged to generate a final point. Most often this averaging is performed by a computer in real time, that is, as the data is being collected (in contrast to ensemble averaging, which requires storage of the data for subsequent processing). Clearly, detail is lost by boxcar averaging, and its utility is limited for complex signals which change rapidly as a function of time. It is of considerable importance, however, for square-wave or repetitive pulsed outputs where only the average amplitude is important.

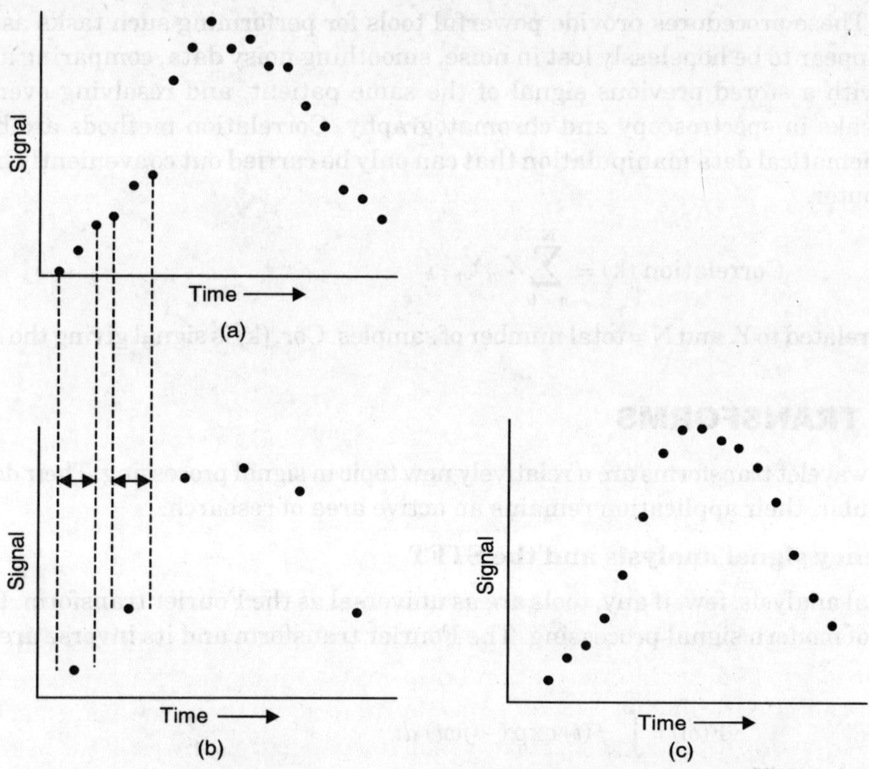

Fig. 14.5. Shows the effect of Boxcar averaging (a) Original Data (b) Data after Boxcar averaging (c) Data after moving-window boxcar averaging.

Fig. 14.5*c* shows a moving-window boxcar average of the data in Fig. 14.5*a* Here, the first point is the average of original points 1, 2 and 3; the second boxcar point is an average of points 2, 3 and 4, and so forth. Here, only the first and last points are lost. The size of the boxcar again can vary over a wide range.

Digital Filtering

The moving-window, boxcar method just described is a kind of linear filtering wherein it is assumed that an approximately linear relationship exists among the points being sampled in each boxcar. More complex polynomial relationships can, however, be assumed to derive a center point for each window.

Digital filtering can also be carried by a Fourier transform procedure (see next section). Here the original signal, which varies as a function of time (a time-domain signal), is converted to a frequency-domain signal in which the independent variable is now frequency rather than time. This transformation, is accomplished mathematically on a digital computer by a Fourier transform procedure. The frequency signal is then multiplied by the frequency response of a digital filter, which has the effect of removing a certain frequency region of the transformed signal. The filtered time-domain signal is then recovered by an inverse Fourier transform.

Correlation

Correlation methods are beginning to find application for the processing of data from medical instruments. These procedures provide powerful tools for performing such tasks as extracting signals that appear to be hopelessly lost in noise, smoothing noisy data, comparing a diagnostic (ecg signal) with a stored previous signal of the same patient, and resolving overlapping or unresolved peaks in spectroscopy and chromatography. Correlation methods are based upon complex mathematical data manipulation that can only be carried out conveniently by means of a digital computer.

$$\text{Correlation (k)} = \sum_{n=0}^{N} X_m Y_{n+k}$$

where X is correlated to Y. and N = total number of samples. Cor. (k) is signal giving the correlation.

FOURIER TRANSFORMS

Wavelets and wavelet transforms are a relatively new topic in signal processing. Their development and, in particular, their application remains an active area of research.

Time-frequency signal analysis and the STFT

In signal analysis, few, if any, tools are as universal as the Fourier transform. It is used as the keystone of modern signal processing. The Fourier transform and its inverse are defined as follows:

$$F(\omega) = \int_{-\infty}^{\infty} f(t) \exp(-j\omega t)\, dt \quad \text{...(5)}$$

$$f(t) = 1/2\pi \int_{-\infty}^{\infty} F(\omega) \exp(j\omega t)\, d\omega \quad \text{...(6)}$$

where F(ω) is the Fourier transform of the signal *f(t)*.

Using the identity.

$$\text{Exp}\,(jk\theta) = \cos k\theta + j \sin k\theta$$

the inverse transform can be described in terms of sine and cosine functions rather than complex exponentials:

$$f(t) = 1/2\pi \int_{-\infty}^{\infty} F(\omega)\,(\cos \omega t + j \sin \omega t)\, d\omega \qquad ...(7)$$

From this it can be seen that the Fourier transform F(ω) of a signal is a function describing the contribution of sines and cosines to the construction of the original time domain signal.

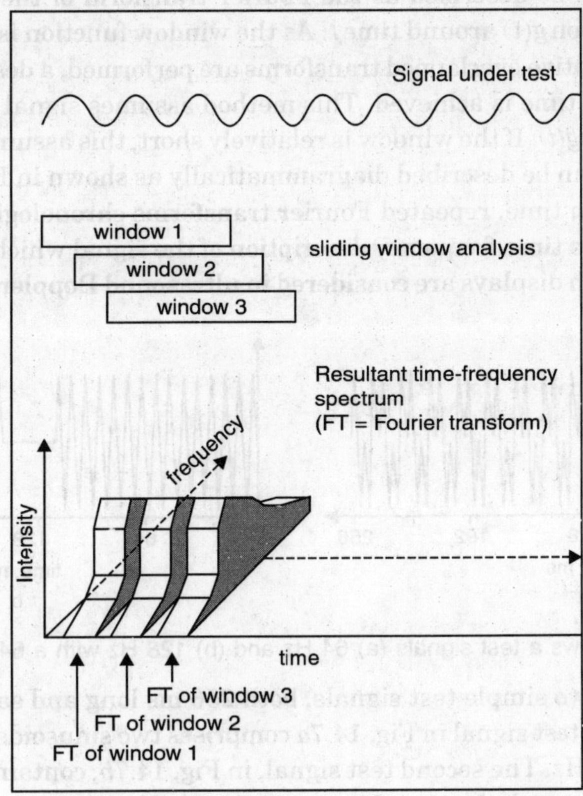

Fig. 14.6. Shows STFT sliding window analysis.

Software Methods

With the widespread availability of micro-processors and microcomputers, many of the signal-to-noise enhancement devices described in the previous section are being replaced or supplemented by digital computer software algorithms. Among these are programs for various types of averaging, digital filtering, Fourier transformation, and correlation techniques. Generally, these procedures are applicable to non-periodic or irregular wave forms, such as an absorption spectrum, or to signals having no synchronizing or reference wave.

Some of these common software procedures are discussed briefly here.

Fig. 14.6 shows the STFT sliding window analysis.

The time independence of the basis functions of the Fourier transform results in a signal description purely the frequency domain. The description of a signal as either a function of time or as a spectrum of frequency components contradicts our everyday experiences. The human auditory system relies upon both time and frequency parameters to identify and describe sounds.

For the analysis of nonstationary signals a function is required that transforms a signal into a joint time-frequency domain. Such a description can be achieved using the well known STFT, which is an extension to the classical Fourier transform as defined by Gabor:

$$\text{STFT}(\tau, \varpi) = \int s(t)\, g(t-\tau)\, e^{-j\omega t}\, dt \qquad ...(8)$$

This function can be described as the Fourier transform of the signals *s(t)*, previously windowed by- the function *g*(t) around time *t*. As the window function is shifted in time over the whole signal and consecutive overlapped transforms are performed, a description of the evolution of signal spectrum with time is achieved. This method assumes signal is stationary effectively over the limited window *g(t)*. If the window is relatively short, this assumption of local stationary is often valid. Eqn. (8) can be described diagrammatically as shown in Fig. 14.6. As the window function *g(t)* is shifted in time, repeated Fourier transforms chronologically, on a common frequency axis, it provides a time-frequency description of the signal which is commonly called the signal spectrogram. Such displays are considered in ultrasound Doppler cardiography.

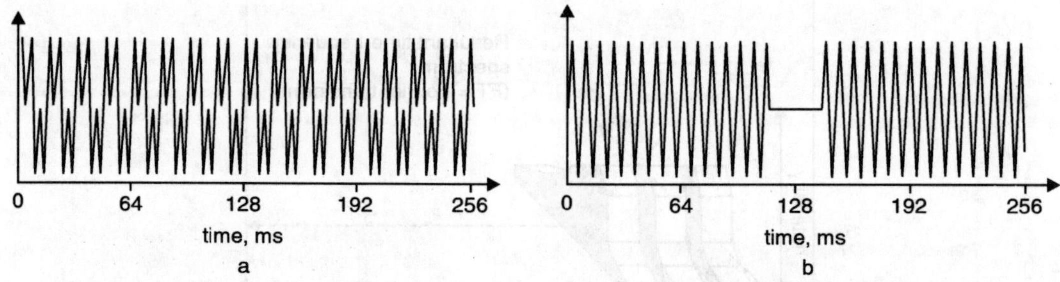

Fig. 14.7. Shows a test signals (a) 64 Hz and (b) 128 Hz with a 64 sample gate.

Fig. 14.7 shows two simple test signals, both 256 ms long and sampled at a rate of 2000 samples per second. The test signal in Fig. 14.7*a* comprises two sinusoids of equal amplitude, one at 64 Hz and one at 192 Hz. The second test signal, in Fig. 14.7*b*, contains a single sinusoid with a 64-sample gap, during which the signal is 'switched off'. Fig. 14.7*a* shows the STFT of the test signal in Fig. 14.8*a* using a relatively long window length of 128 samples and Fig. 8b shows the STFT of the same signal with a shorter 32-sample window. The longer window length results in better frequency resolution and, as can be seen in Fig. 14.8*a*, the two sinusoids are clearly resolved. The shorter window length results in reduced frequency resolution and this analysis, shown in Fig.8b, fails to resolve the two sinusoidal components. Fig. 14.9 clearly demonstrates how transform window length affects resolution in frequency.

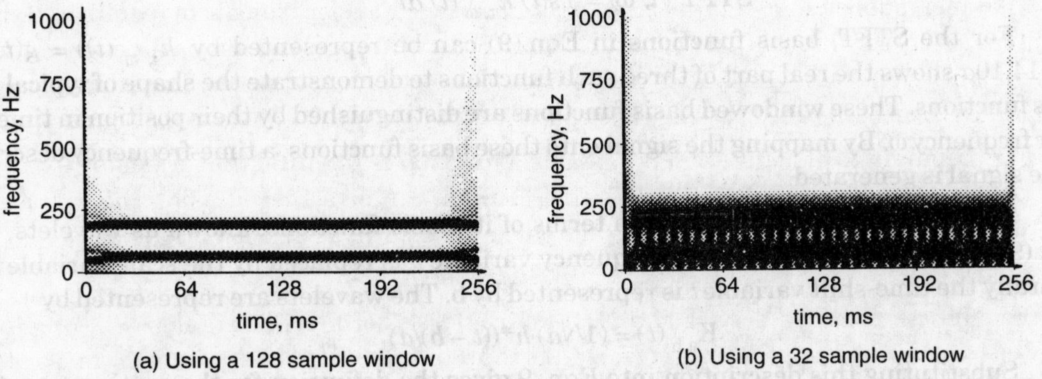

Fig. 14.8. Shows STFT of the TEST signal (a) using different windows.

Fig. 14.9 shows the results of transforming the test signal in Fig. 14.7*b*, again using a long 128-sample window and a short 32-sample window. As would be expected, applying the longer 128-sample analysis (Fig. 14.9*a*) fails to resolve the signal gap but the short 32-sample analysis (Fig. 14.9*b*) quite clearly resolves the position and length of the gap. Fig. 14.8 and Fig. 14.9 together illustrate the joint time and frequency resolution limitations of the STFT implied by the uncertainty principle.

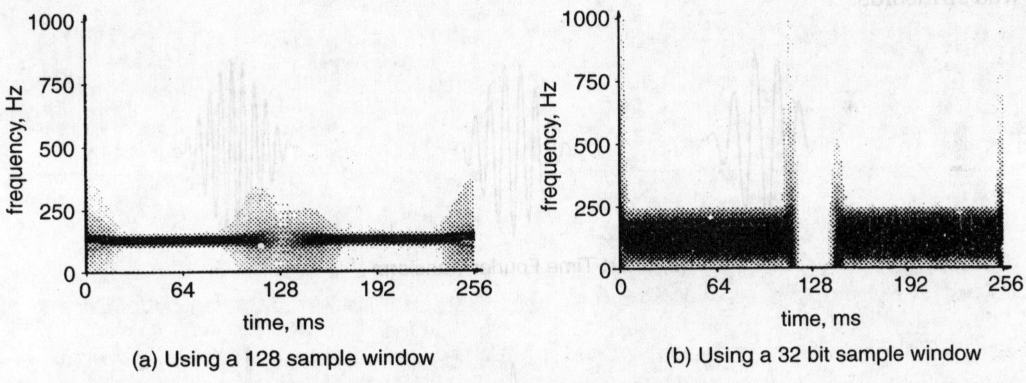

Fig. 14.9. Shows STFT of the signal (b).

In most bio signals, high frequency resolution characteristics are not required.

THE WAVELET TRANSFORM

Previously, the STFT (Eqn.8) has been analysed as the Fourier transform of the windowed signal $s(t) \cdot g(t-\tau)$, but it is just as valid to describe this function as the decomposition of the signal s(t) into the windowed basis function $g(t-\tau)\exp(-j\omega t)$. The term 'basis functions', refers to a complete set of functions that can, when combined as a weighted sum, be used to construct a given signal. In the case of the STFT these basis functions are complex sinusoids, $\exp(-j\omega t)$, windowed by the function $g(t)$ centered around t.

It is possible to write a general equation for the STFT in terms of basis functions $k_{\tau,\varpi}(t)$ and signal $s(t)$ as an inner product:

$$STFT(\tau, \omega) = \int s(t)\, k_{\tau,\omega}(t)\, dt \qquad ...(9)$$

For the STFT, basis functions in Eqn.(9) can be represented by $k_{\tau,\varpi}(t)) = g(t)\, e_{-j\omega t}$. Fig. 14.10*a* shows the real part of three such functions to demonstrate the shape of typical STFT basis functions. These windowed basis functions are distinguished by their position in time τ and their frequency ω. By mapping the signal onto these basis functions, a time-frequency description of the signal is generated.

The WT can also be described in terms of its basis functions, known as wavelets, using Eqn. (9). In the case of the WT, the frequency variable v is replaced by the scale variable a and generally the time-shift variable t is represented by b. The wavelets are represented by

$$K_{a,b}(t) = (1/\sqrt{a})\, h^*((t-b)/a)$$

Substituting this description into Eqn. 9 gives the definition for the continuous wavelet transform (CWT):

$$CWT(b,a) = (1/\sqrt{a}) \int h^*((t-b)/a) \,.\, s(t)\, dt \qquad ...(10)$$

From the above Eqn.(10), it can be seen that the WT performs a decomposition of the signal $s(t)$ into a weighted set of scaled wavelet functions $h(t)$. In general the wavelet $h(t)$ is a complex-valued function; Fig. 14.10*b* shows the real part of the Morlet wavelet at three different levels of scale. Comparing the two sets of basis functions in Fig. 14.10, it can be seen that the wavelets are all scaled versions of a common 'mother wavelet' whereas the basis functions of the STFT are windowed sinusoids.

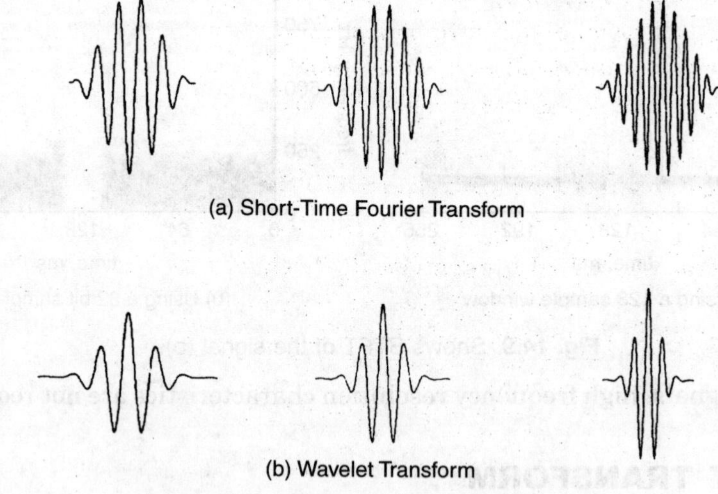

Fig. 14.10. Shows a typical basis functions

Due to the scaling shown in Fig. 14.10*b*, wavelets at high frequencies are of limited duration and wavelets at low frequencies are relatively longer in duration.

These variable window length characteristics are obviously suited to the analysis of signals containing short high-frequency components, and extended low frequency components which is often the case for signals encountered in practice.

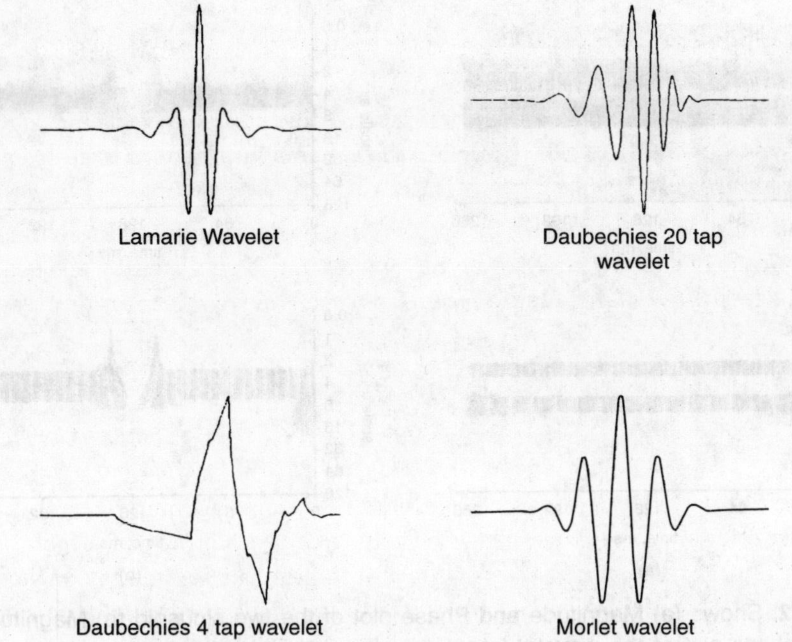

Fig. 14.11. Shows common wavelets used.

Fig. 14.11 shows a number of commonly used wavelets.

The CWT as a time-scale transform has three dimensions. The three dimensions are represented on a log (a),b half-plane. The log (a) axis (scale) faces downwards and b- axis (time-shift) faces to the right. The respective intensity of the transform at points in the log(a), b half-plane is represented by grey level intensity. These conventions allow a standard plot of time evaluation from left to right and decreasing frequency from top to bottom,

The phase is not displayed if the transform modulus drops below a predetermined cutoff value.

By employing scaled window functions, the WT does not overcome the uncertainty principle, but by employing variable window lengths, and hence variable resolution, an increase in performance may be achieved. Fig. 14.8 and Fig. 14.9 demonstrated the resolution limitations imposed upon the STFT by the uncertainty principle. Fig.14.12 shows the magnitude and phase plots generated by applying the WT to the two test signals of Fig. 14.7. It can be seen from Fig. 14.12 that in both test cases the WT has clearly separated the signal components.

Localization of signal discontinuities by the V-shape in Fig. 14.12b is an important characteristic of the WT that can be used in signal interpretation.

Many algorithms have been developed by the researchers for calculating WTs. One such algorithm is based upon the fast Fourier transform (FFT), By analyzing the CWT in the Fourier domain the basic convolution operation of the CWT can be achieved via simple multiplication operations. Writing the CWT in the Fourier domain gives

$$F\{CWT\,(b, a)\} = (1/\sqrt{a})\, H^*(\omega/a)\, S(\omega) \qquad \text{...(11)}$$

where F{$CWT(b, a)$} is the Fourier transform of the continuous wavelet transform, $H^*(w)$ is the Fourier transform of the wavelet and S(w) is the Fourier transform of the input signal. This

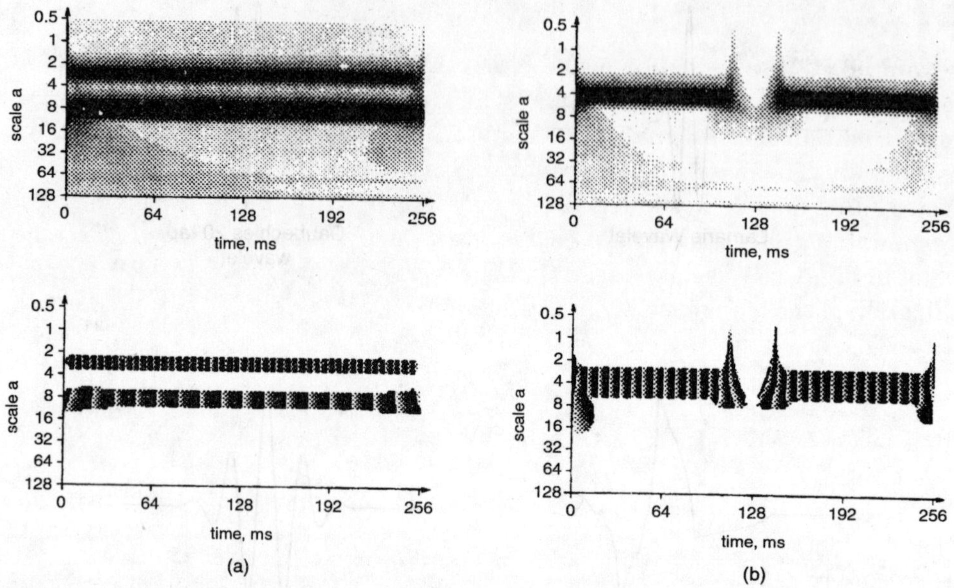

Fig. 14.12. Shows (a) Magnitude and Phase plot of the two sinusoid (b) Magnitude and phase plot of the wavelet transform of a sinusoid with gap test signal.

equation can be used as the basis of an FFT-based fast wavelet transform. Eqn. (11) can be represented graphically as shown in Fig. 14.13.

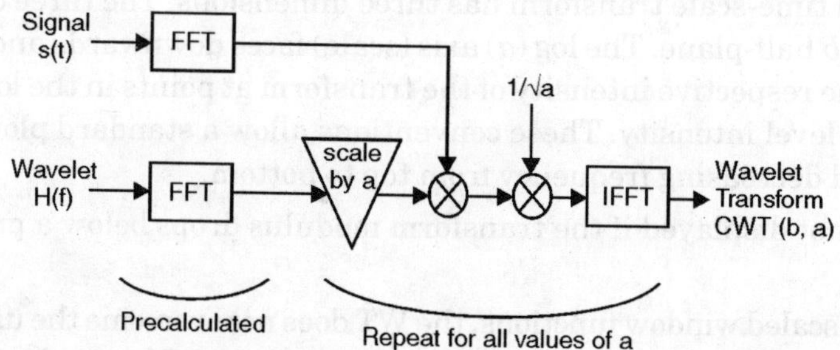

Fig. 14.13. Showing the Block Diagram of the FFT based Fast Wavelet transform.

If the **Morlet wavelet** is adopted:

$$h(t) = \exp(j\, \omega_0\, t) \cdot \exp(-t^2/2) \quad \text{...(12)}$$

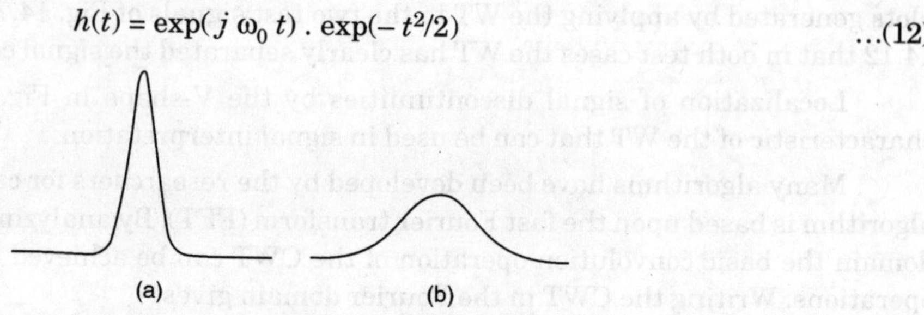

Fig. 14.14. Shows magnitude of the Morlet wavelet (a) low value (b) increased scale value.

WAVELET TRANSFORM OF A TYPICAL ECG

The example of the application of the WT is the transformation of an electrocardiograph (ECG) trace. A typical ECG trace is shown in Fig. 14.15*a*. The magnitude and phase plots resulting from the transformation of this signal, again using the Morlet wavelet, are shown in Figs. 14.15*b* and 15*c*, respectively. The magnitude plot shows a large degree of spreading over the time-scale plane. This spreading may be explained in two ways. *Localisation in the time-scale plane occurs when the signal and wavelet show a high degree of similarity*. Comparing the ECG trace and the Morlet wavelet in Fig. 14.11, it can be seen that the two waveforms show little, if any, similarity. Hence, localization of the transform is not expected.

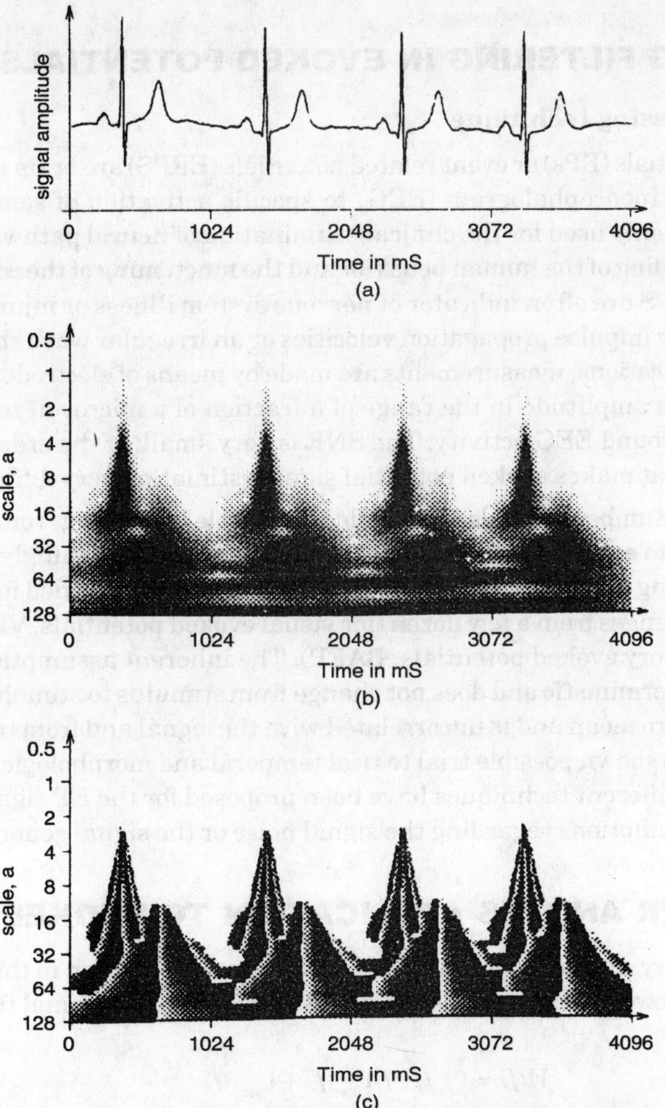

Fig. 14.15. Shows the wavelet transform of a typical ECG : (a) Input signal (b) Transform magnitude (c) Transform phase.

The WT is particularly apt at highlighting discontinuities. Due to the sudden depolarization and repolarisation of cardiac tissue, the ECG contains a number of distinct peaks. It can be seen from the WT of the ECG that these peaks are highlighted as upturned V's, which become increasingly spread in time as scale increases. Although the impulsive nature of the ECG trace results in a spread transform at high scale values, it can be seen that at low values of scale, distinct time localization occurs. This localization characteristic can be used to pinpoint the significant peaks of the ECG trace. The position of significant complexes and peaks in the ECG waveform is an important diagnostic tool in detecting pathological conditions relating to the muscular and electrical aspects of tissue of the heart. These results point to the application of the WT to the automatic identification and characterization of such pathological conditions.

TIME VARYING FILTERING IN EVOKED POTENTIALS

New Signal Processing technique

Evoked potentials (EPs) or event related potentials (ERPS) are brain responses which occur along with the electroencephalogram (EEG) to specific activation of sensory pathways. Such responses are commonly used for the clinical examination of neural pathways of perception and for better understanding of the human behavior and the functioning of the central nervous system (CNS). Abnormal EPS are often indicator of nervous system illness or injury. Abnormalities can be in the form of slow impulse propagation velocities or an irregular wave shape measured on the scalp. For most applications, measurements are made by means of electrode attached to the scalp. The ERPs having an amplitude in the range of a fraction of a microvolt to a few millivolts, are buried in the background EEG activity. The SNR is very small, of the order of – 10dB or less. It is this small SNR that makes evoked potential signal estimation very difficult.

Averaging a number of trials, also called ensemble averaging, remains one of the most popular techniques to extract the ERP signal from the ongoing, seemingly random background EEG noise. Depending on the SNR, the number of measurements needed for averaging to obtain a reliable estimate ranges from a few dozen (for visual evoked potentials, VEP) to a few thousand (for brainstem auditory evoked potentials, BAEP). The inherent assumptions in averaging are, that the signal is deterministic and does not change from stimulus to stimulus and the EEG noise is stationary with zero mean and is uncorrelated with the signal and from trial to trial. However, statistical tests have shown possible trial to trial temporal and morphological variability of event related processes. Different techniques have been proposed for the EP signal estimation on distinctly different assumptions regarding the signal noise or the signal generating processes.

WIENER FILTER AND ITS APPLICATION TO EVOKED POTENTIALS

Wiener original theory solves the problem of optimal signal estimation in the presence of additive noise, with known power density spectra of signal and noise. His optimal filter function is given by,

$$H(f) = \Gamma_{ss}(f) \,/\, \Gamma_{ss}(f) + \Gamma_{nn}(f) \qquad \ldots(13)$$

where $H(f)$ is the filter transfer function and $\Gamma ss(f)$ and $\Gamma nn(f)$ are the known power density spectra of signal and noise. This filter, when applied to the observed signal, leads to an optimal estimate of the signal in the mean square error sense. Wiener's theory assumes both the signal and the noise to be random, stationary, ergodic processes with known correlation functions. The application of the evoked potentials is done using the estimated power density spectra of signal and noise.

A POSTERIORI WIENER FILTER

Wiener theory for filtering noisy signals has been used in the study of EPs, by many researchers. De Weerd et al have done an exhaustive study of the effectiveness of Wiener filtering in improving the SNR of average evoked potentials. The idea behind a *posteriori filtering* is to improve the estimation of the real signal, as obtained after ensemble averaging, still further by a linear filtering procedure. The appropriate filter transfer function is computed form the estimates of the underlying spectra of signal and noise. A *posteriori* Wiener filtering is suggested to obtain an improved signal estimate beyond averaging in the case of evoked potentials by De Weerd et al. The central idea of a *posteriori* Wiener filtering is that an averaged signal that is still contaminated with noise could be improved using a posterior estimated power density spectra of the signal and noise. However, with decreasing signal to noise power density ratio (SNPNR), the transfer function suffers from larger bias and variance due to the variability in the spectra computed.

Considering a fixed latency evoked potential model,

$$x_i(t) = s(t) + n_i(t) \qquad i = 1, 2, 3 \ldots\ldots N; \quad 0 \le t \le \mathrm{T} \qquad \ldots(14)$$

$s(t)$ represents the signal, $n_i(t)$ noise, N is the number of stimulus presentation and T is the duration of evoked potential.

Responses which show considerable trial to trial variability may be denoted by variable latency evoked potential model,

$$z_i(t) = s(t - \tau_i) + n_i(t) \qquad \ldots(15)$$

where τ_i represents the random variable. The following matter, however assumes the fixed latency model.

If the power density spectra of signal and noise were known a priori, the optimum Wiener filter transfer function for use on the ensemble average is

$$\mathrm{H(f)} = \Gamma_{ss}(f)/(\Gamma_{ss}(f) + (1/\mathrm{N}) \,.\, \Gamma_{nn}(f)) \qquad \ldots(16)$$

where $\Gamma_{ss}(f)$ and $\Gamma_{nn}(f)$ represent known power density spectra of the signal and the noise. In practice, however, these spectra are unknown but can be estimated from the ensemble as suggested. In this, a spectrum of the ensemble average in which the noise power is reduced by a factor proportional to the number of ensemble elements is taken as the PSD of the signal and an average of the spectra of individual ensemble elements, in which the noise power is not reduced, is taken as the PSD of the noise. If the PSD of the ensemble average $\mathrm{X_N}(t)$ be denoted by $\phi_{xxn}(\omega)$, it implies that the transfer function itself becomes an estimate.

By alternate averaging, (*i.e.*) by alternate addition and subtraction of ensemble elements, the signal averages out, and the power density spectrum of the alternate average $\mathrm{X_N}(t)$ is an estimate of the power density spectrum of the noise reduced by a factor N. The principal advantage of alternate averaging is that due to the alternate addition and subtraction and successive ensemble elements, such inhomogenities tend to average out, which implies that the corresponding estimator becomes less biased. Instead of using the full ensemble for calculation of the alternate average and its corresponding spectrum, sub-ensemble averaging is preferred because the inhomgenities caused by trends, slow amplitude modulations of the signal or a slow changing character of the background etc. can be taken care.

The methods for separation of signal and noise spectra as discussed above are applicable when dealing with an ensemble in which each element is conceptually composed of an invariant signal and an additive stationary noise component, uncorrelated with this signal.

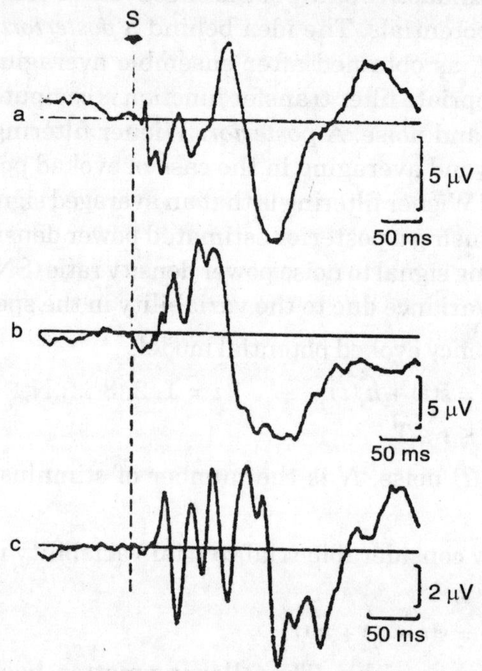

Fig. 14.16. Shows a typical examples of evoked potential from the human brain. (a) Somatosensory evoked potential (b) Visual evoked potential (c) brainstem auditory evoked potential.

SIGNAL PROCESSING IN HEART RATE VARIABILITY-LINEAR ANALYSIS

The heart rate variability (HRV) signal derives its significance from the facts that

(*i*) it provides a noninvasive window to study the autonomic nervous system (ANS),

(*ii*) it is altered in different disease states and

(*iii*) changes in ANS activity may be important indicators of patient outcome.

HRV analysis concerns with the systematic, quantitative study of the fluctuations in the heart rate.

The ECG is sampled at a sufficiently high rate (usually 500 Hz) to determine the time locations of the R waves at the accuracies needed for the analysis. The R waves are detected using a suitable algorithm, and the so-called normal-to-normal (NN) intervals (that is, all intervals between adjacent QRS complexes resulting from sinus node depolarizations) are determined. From this R-R interval series, several time domain descriptors of the variability are computed.

SPECTRAL DOMAIN ANALYSIS

However, a simple linear interpolation gives results as good. From this uniform interval HR series, the mean is then removed. Either non-parametric (FFT) or parametric (usually, Autoregressive) spectrum of this HRV signal is then obtained. Fig. 17 shows sample HRV spectra for supine and standing postures of a subject. By means of studies where the autonomic components were selectively blocked, they have identified that different frequency components in the HRV spectrum have been contributed by different aspects of the physiological system. Based on the results of these studies, the spectrum is divided into three distinct bands, namely, the very low frequency band (VLF, frequency range 0.01–0.04 Hz), the low frequency band (LF, 0.04–0.15 Hz) and high frequency band (HF, 0.15–0.40 Hz). Drugs such as atropine are selective parasympathetic blocking agents and by employing them on normal individuals, the HF peak has been identified to be correlated to the respiratory driven vagal (parasympathetic) efferent input to the sinus node. Similarly, propanolol is a strong sympathetic receptor blocker, with the help of which, the LF band (definitely during standing position) is known to represent the sympathetic vagal drive. The VLF band is supposed to be linked to the thermoregulatory system, though the evidences are inconclusive. Accordingly, the absolute power (in millisecond squared) in all the 3 frequency bands and ratios of HF and LF to total HRV power are calculated. A ratio of the energies in the LF and HF bands is currently being accepted as representing sympatho-vagal balance. LF norm and HF norm are the LF and HF powers in normalized units (i.e. LF or HF/(total power-VLF) * 100, where total power is defined as the power in the frequency band < 0.4 Hz. The representation of LF and HF in normalized units emphasizes the controlled and balanced behavior of the two branches of the ANS and also tends to minimize the effect of the changes in total power on the values of LF and HF components.

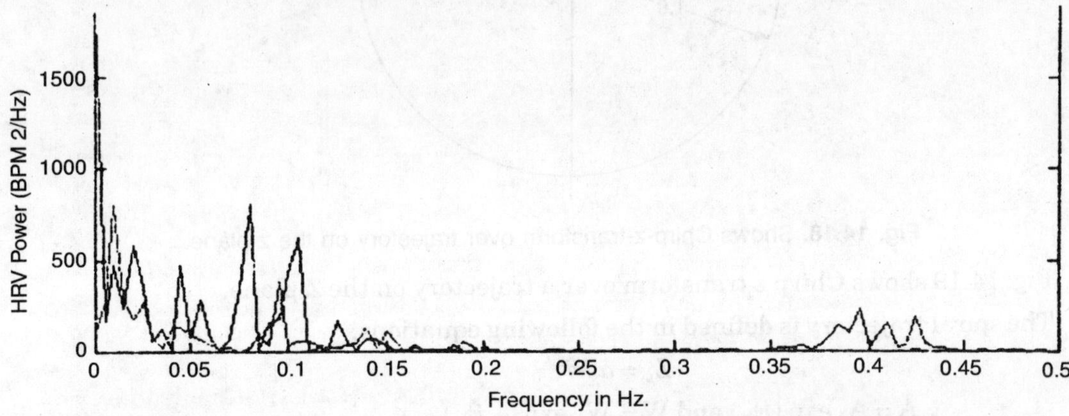

Fig. 14.17. Shows the power spectrum of HRV (I-Supine; II standing).

Though most studies have analyzed HRV samples, a few investigators [Murata] have directly obtained the power spectrum of the R-R interval series, ignoring the fact that the latter is a non-uniformly sampled data. These results are not always directly comparable to those obtained from the HRV series.

CLINICAL APPLICATIONS

The anatomic location of the autonomic nervous system (ANS) renders it inaccessible to direct physiological testing. The study of HRV Power Spectra is gaining acceptance as a non-invasive method for identifying the role of the ANS in regulating cardiac function. HRV decreases with age and this factor must be kept in mind while interpreting the results of any study. It may be possible to roughly normalize the data with respect to age. HRV analysis being a field of current research, the possible clinical applications are increasing. The following are some of the potential clinical uses already identified.

1. Decreased HRV is predictor and adverse outcome after a myocardial infarction. Low HRV for such patients means automatic unbalance which can be fatal.
2. Side effects of drugs in psychiatric patients causes HRV reduction. This is an extension of the Z-transform in sampled data (discrete) analysis of bio-signal.

CHIRP-z-TRANSFORM

Fig. 14.18 shows the Z-plane with a spiral trajectory drawn on it. The spiral trajectory is marked out at angular intervals ϕ corresponding to the M frequencies (values of ω) for which the z-transform has to be evaluated.

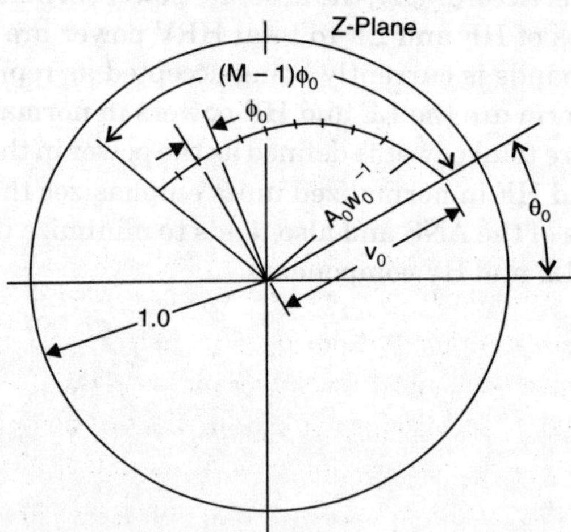

Fig. 14.18. Shows Chirp-z-transform over trajectory on the z-plane.

Fig. 14.19 shows Chirp z transform over a trajectory on the Z plane.

The spiral trajectory is defined in the following equations:

$$Z_k = a\, W^{-k}$$

$$A = A_0 \exp(j\phi_0) \text{ and } W = W_0 \exp(-j\phi_0),$$

$$k = 0, 1, 2, 3\ldots\ldots M-1$$

The chirp-z algorithm provides an efficient method for finding the transform $X(Z_k)$ given by

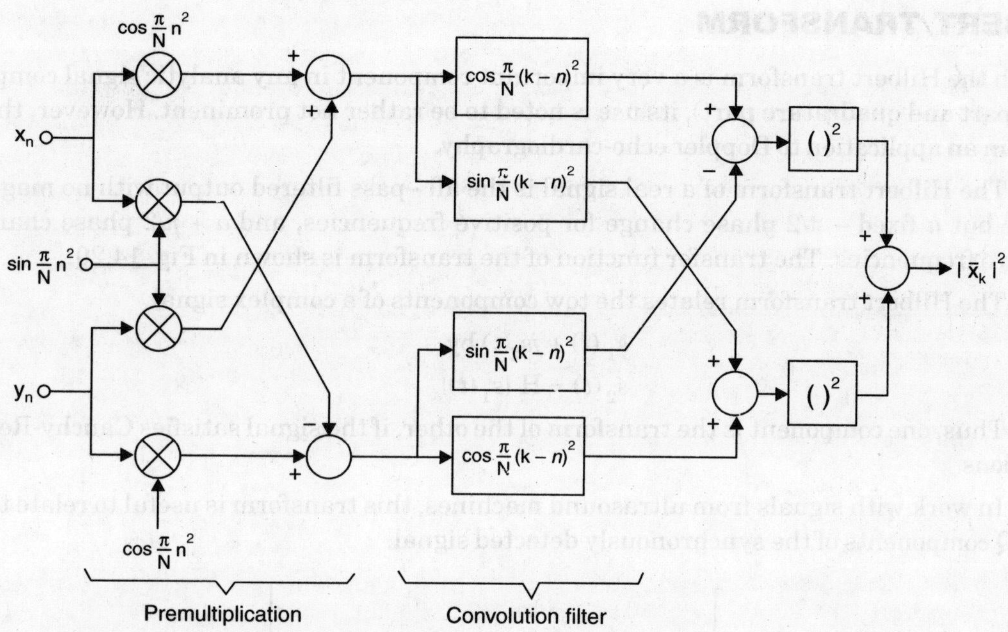

Fig. 14.19. Shows the phase quadrature scheme of doppler signal excitation.

$$X(z_k) = \Sigma\, x(n) z_k^{-n} = \Sigma\, x(n)\, A^{-n} W^{nk}$$

where the summations extend from 0 to M-1

Using the equation $2kn = k^2 + n^2 - (k - n)^2$, this expression is manipulated algebraically to give a convolution of two sequences with scaling as follows:

$$X(z_k) = W\, k^{n^2/2}\ \Sigma\, x(n)\, A^{-n}\, W^{n^2/2}\ W^{-(k-n)^2/2}$$

where $h(n) = W^{-n^2/2}$ and $g(n) = x(n)A^{-n}\, W^{n^2/2} = x(n)A^{-n}/h(n)$

This is the summation equivalent to $g(n)*h(n)$

Therefore $X(z_k) = [1/h(k)]\ \Sigma\, g(n)h(k - n)$

The summation is required convolution operation and the result $X(z_k)$ is a sequence, in principle of indefinite length which we truncate to give our required M output samples. It is interesting to note that h(n) is a complex exponential sequence with a linear increase in frequency.

$$h(n) = (W_0 \exp(-j\phi_0))^{n^2/2}$$

which may be rewritten as $h(n) = (W_0 \exp(-jn\ (\phi_0\ n/2))$

The brackets ($\phi 0\ n/2$) can be regarded as a frequency which steadily increases with time (n); such a signal is known as a chirp and it is from this that the operation gets its name. The convolution is carried out rapidly be means of an FFT routine and appropriate scaling is applied to the final result. The computations are as depicted in Fig.14.19.

The convolutions are performed using CCD ICs (R6502) in the ultrasound machines.

Fig. 14.19 shows chirp-z transform Computation of spectral power density.

HILBERT TRANSFORM

Though the Hilbert transform is a very important component in any analytic signal comprising a real part and quadrature part), its use is noted to be rather not prominent. However, this was useful in an application to Doppler echo-cardiography.

The Hilbert transform of a real signal is the all - pass filtered output with no magnitude change but *a* fixed $-\pi/2$ phase change for positive frequencies, and *a* $+\pi/2$ phase change for negative frequencies. The transfer function of the transform is shown in Fig. 14.20.

The Hilbert transform relates the tow components of a complex signal

$$s_1(t) + js_2(t) \text{ by}$$
$$s_2(t) = \mathrm{H}\{s_1(t)\}$$

Thus, one component is the transform of the other, if the signal satisfies Cauchy-Reimann conditions.

In work with signals from ultrasound machines, this transform is useful to relate the two I and Q components of the synchronously detected signal.

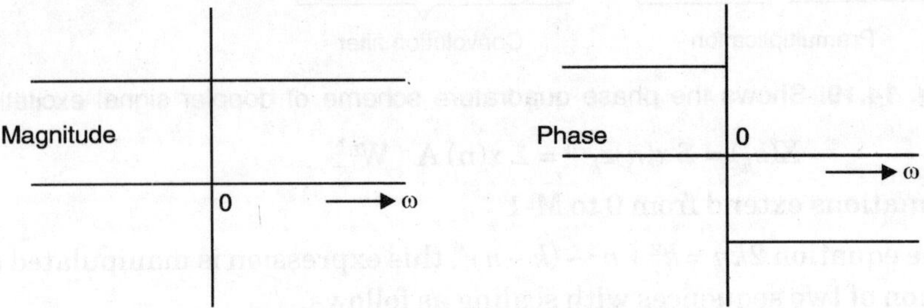

Fig. 14.20. Shows the Hilbert transform transfer function.

A program for quickly evaluating the Hilbert transform of a large set of data samples was written using a matrix formulation of relations. The Hilbert transform of a discrete sequence x_v is obtained by:

$$y_n = 2/\mathrm{N} \sum_{v=0}^{\mathrm{N}-1} x_v \sum_{k=1}^{\mathrm{L}} \sin(v-n)\, 2\pi k/\mathrm{N}$$

where L = (N/2) – 1 when N is even and (N – 1)/2 when N is odd.

The above Hilbert transformed sequence can be put in matrix notation as :

$$\mathrm{C}_{n,v} = (2/\mathrm{N})\, \Sigma \sin(v-n) \text{ and}$$

$$y_n = \Sigma x_y \mathrm{C}_{n,v}$$

or $\quad \mathrm{Y} = \mathrm{C}\ \mathrm{X}$ where $\mathrm{Y}^{\mathrm{T}} = |\ y_0, y_1 \ldots\ldots y_n\ |$

and $\quad \mathrm{X}^{\mathrm{T}} = |\ x_0, x_1 \ldots\ldots x_n$

Since the rows are circulant, by evaluating one row and keeping it stored, it was possible to generate the other rows by shift operations; the output vector is thus easily obtained as the product of sum. This operation can be the implemented very rapidly in DSP hardware and could show the waveforms as quickly as the machine shows the spectrogram.

ECG DATA COMPRESSION

AZTEC

The amplitude zone Epoch Coding (AZTEC) data-reduction algorithm has become an accepted from of data reduction for ECG monitors, and data bases recently. AZTEC takes raw ECG data and produces short lines and slopes. Fig. 14.21 shows how this is done.

Horizontal lines

As the monitor samples the ECG, the first sample is set equal to the initial conditions, one of Vmax and V_{min}. The next sample is compared to V_{max} and V_{min}. If the sample is greater than V_{max}, then V_{max} is made equal to the sample value. Conversely, if the sample is less than V_{min}, then V_{min} is made equal to the value of the sample. This process is repeated until either the difference between V_{max} and V_{min} is greater than a predetermined threshold, V_{thresh}, or more than 50 samples have been gathered. Either event produces a line. To store the line, first the number of samples examined minus one is saved at T_1 (time or length of line). Then the values of V_{max} and V_{min}, previous to the present sample, are averaged and set to V_1, which is saved (i.e., the value of the line, $V_1 = (V_{max} + V_{min})/2$ at time $(t-1)$. V_{max} and V_{min} are then set equal to the present sample and the process is continued. This is the first part of AZTEC algorithm and is called zero-order interpolation (ZOI). This ZOI produces lines of zero slope. The first value saved is the length of the line, while the second value is the amplitude of the line.

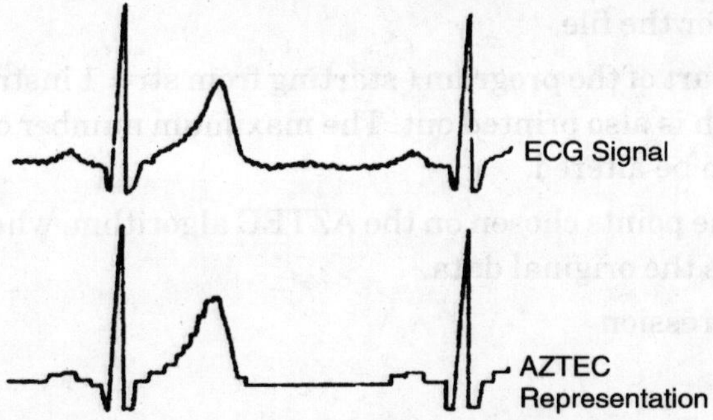

Fig. 14.21. Shows the original data and the output.

First, the value of the line is assigned to V_{slope1}. Second, the length of the line is assigned to Tslope1 (time or length of the slope1). This direction of the slope (+ or –) is also recorded. When the next line is produced, AZTEC determines whether or not the slope data should be updated or terminated. Then, the slope parameters are determined and saved. If the slope was terminated by a change in direction and / or the terminating line length is greater than 2, the amplitude of that line is saved, then the length of the line, and finally the amplitude of the lines are saved again.

AZTEC's data reduction is not constant. The reduction is frequently as great as 100/1000 or more, depending upon the nature of the signal itself and the value of the empirically determined threshold.

Although AZTEC produces a recognizable ECG signal, the step like quantization is unfamiliar to most nurses and physicians. Therefore, a curve smoothing algorithm to process the AZTEC data produces a more acceptable output for the nurses and physicians.

Parabolic fitting provides a smooth - curve approximation to each set of seven points in the original waveform.

$$P_0 = 1/2T\,(-\,2a_{k-3} + 3a_{k-2} + 6a_{k-1} + 7a_k + 6a_{k+1} + 3a_{k+2} - 2a_{k+3})$$

where P_0 is the new data point and

$a_{k\pm n}$ the original data points (AZTEC), and $k \pm n$ defines the time relationship.

For R wave detections, scanning through the data to look for a slope greater than 1/3 of the height of the normal QRS of the patient, is done. If no such R wave is found, the trial is done with a slope of 1/6 of the height. When no R wave is detected in a time of twice the R-R interval, a "missing beat" is indicated. If more than one R-wave is noted, the higher amplitude is taken as R wave, the other can be a P wave and R–R interval is used for calculating the sinus rhythm.

Therefore, we can take advantage of AZTEC's superior data compression while retaining the clinical information content of the ECG for diagnostic purposes.

AZTEC Program for ECG compression

The program (in Basic) given below is in 2 parts. First, for testing, it generates an ECG file of data points. Second, it compresses this file. The program also displays the two signals-the actual data plotted, and the points selected on the compression by AZTEC.

When using with data collected clinically, the first part of the program is removed; but the ECG clinical data must be available as a file {a: ecgfile}. It is possible to generate short ecg file from clinical data with a PC-based data acquisition card or via the printer port. The data for up to 5 or 6 ECGs are enough for the file.

Then, the second part of the program (starting from str = 1 instruction) is run to generate the compressed file, which is also printed out. The maximum number of compressed data in this program is 128, but it can be altered.

Please note how the points chosen on the AZTEC algorithm, when joined, give the ECG of almost the same shape as the original data.

```
rem ecg data compression
str=200
screen 12
dim azt(str)
open "a:ecgfile" for output as #1 ; rem generates sample ecg data file
for i=1 to 56*4
read e
write #1,e
line -(4+i*2,200-e*6)
next
close #1

data 1,1,1,2,2,3,4,5,6,6,6,5,4,3,2,1,1,1,2,1,2,1,1,1,0
data -1,-2,-3,-3,-2,-1,0,2,7,9,15,17,19,17,14,12,7,2,-2,-1,-1,0,1
data 1,1,2,2,2,1,1,1
```

```
data 1,1,1,2,2,3,4,5,6,7,8,8,7,7,7,6,5,4,3,2,1,0,1,1,1,1,1,1,1
data 1,1,1,2,2,3,4,5,6,6,6,5,4,3,2,1,1,1,2,1,2,1,1,1,0
data -1,-2,-3,-3,-2,-1,0,2,7,9,15,17,19,17,14,12,7,2,-2,-1,-1,0,1
data 1,1,2,2,2,1,1,1
data 1,1,1,2,2,3,4,5,6,7,8,8,7,7,7,6,5,4,3,2,1,0,1,1,1,1,1,1,1
data 1,1,1,2,2,3,4,5,6,6,6,5,4,3,2,1,1,1,2,1,2,1,1,1,0
data -1,-2,-3,-3,-2,-1,0,2,7,9,15,17,19,17,14,12,7,2,-2,-1,-1,0,1
data 1,1,2,2,2,1,1,1
data 1,1,1,2,2,3,4,5,6,6,6,5,4,3,2,1,1,1,2,1,2,1,1,1,0
data -1,-2,-3,-3,-2,-1,0,2,7,9,15,17,19,17,14,12,7,2,-2,-1,-1,0,1
data 1,1,2,2,2,1,1,1
data 1,1,1,2,2,3,4,5,6,7,8,8,7,7,7,6,5,4,3,2,1,0,1,1,1,1,1,1,1
data 1,1,1,2,2,3,4,5,6,6,6,5,4,3,2,1,1,1,2,1,2,1,1,1,0
data -1,-2,-3,-3,-2,-1,0,2,7,9,15,17,19,17,14,12,7,2,-2,-1,-1,0,1
data 1,1,2,2,2,1,1,1
data 1,1,1,2,2,3,4,5,6,7,8,8,7,7,7,6,5,4,3,2,1,0,1,1,1,1,1,1,1
data 1,1,1,2,2,3,4,5,6,6,6,5,4,3,2,1,1,1,2,1,2,1,1,1,0
data -1,-2,-3,-3,-2,-1,0,2,7,9,15,17,19,17,14,12,7,2,-2,-1,-1,0,1
data 1,1,2,2,2,1,1,1
rem program to read the ecgfile and compress it and write it
str=1
pset(1,200)
n= str
open "a:ecgfile" for input as #2
gosub ecg : vm1=e:vmn1=vm1
20 if str>57 then 200 else gosub ecg:

n=n+1
vmx=vm1
vmn=vmn1
v=e
locate 20,1
if n>10 then 100
if vmx < v then 60
      goto 70
60 vm1=v
70 if vmn > v then 80
      goto 90
80 vmn1=v
```

```
90 if (vm1 - vmn1) < 1 then 20
100 t1 = n-1
v1=( vmx+vmn)/2
if flag=1 then 140
if t1<=2 then 110
azt(str)=t1
105 print "t1=";t1;
print "v1="; v1;
azt(str+1)=v1
str=str+1
vm1 = v
vmn1 = v

n=1
tt=tt+t1
line-(2+tt*2,200-v1*6),15
rem 77 if inkey$="" then 77
goto 20
110 tsl=0
vsl=azt(str-1)
flag=1
sign=-1

if v1-vsl>=0 then sign=1
140 if t1>2 or (V1-Vsl)*sign<0 then 150
tsl=t1+tsl
vsl=v1
n=1
vm1=v
vmn1=v
goto 20
150 if str=128 then 200 :rem end
azt(str)= -tsl
? "tsl"; -tsl;
tt=tsl+tt : rem tt is total time
151 azt(str+1) = vsl
print "vsl=" ;vsl;
str=str+2
line-(2+tt*2,200-6*vsl)
flag=0
```

```
?"T1";t1
if t1< = 2 then 110
print "Extrav1-";v1;
azt(str-1) = v1
goto 105

data 1,1,1,2,2,3,4,5,6,6,6,5,4,3,2,1,1,1,2,1,2,1,1,1,0
data -1,-2,-3,-3,-2,-1,0,2,7,9,15,17,19,17,14,12,7,2,-2,-1,-1,0,1
data 1,1,2,2,2,1,1,1
data 1,1,1,2,2,3,4,5,6,7,8,8,7,7,7,6,5,4,3,2,1,0,1,1,1,1,1,1,1
ecg:
if eof(2) then 200
input #2,e
return
200 ? "printing data"
open "a:ecgcompr.dat" for output as #1: Rem data compressed saved
for str=1 to 128
? azt(str);
write #1,azt(str)
next
? "data points=";str]

close #2
close #1
end
```

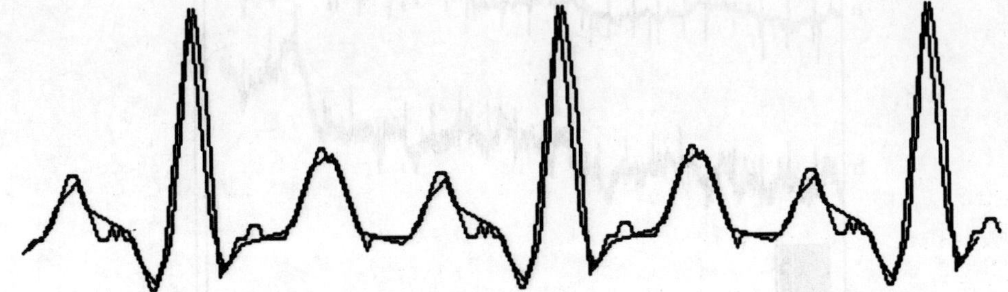

Figure above shows how the data of the compressed format merges almost with the actual data in the above AZTEC program.

The turning point algorithm

This is another algorithm. This reduces the sample points to half the original. Suppose 200 points were taken for one e.c.g. wave, it will become 100.

The first point sampled X_0, is called reference. The next two are X_1, X_2. Since among these three points, there can be only one of the following changes, the change that is relevant is shown and selected as the point for compressed data. Thus, if $X_0 - X_1 - X_2$ is a progressive rise, the X_2 point alone is selected.

The next 2 points are chosen, of which one is selected and so on goes the entire data compression.

Since, a program cannot recognize the figure shown here, the slopes of the point pair which are $X_2 - X_1$ and $X_1 - X_0$ are compared as positive or negative. The product is taken. X_1 is saved if it is negative, while X_2 is saved when it is positive or zero.

Thus

$$(X_2 - X_1)(X_1 - X_0) < 0 \text{ then Choose } X_1$$

$$(X_2 - X_1)(X_1 - X_0) >= 0 \text{ then Choose } X_2$$

A second application of the algorithm to the compressed data is sometimes done but it may not be good enough.

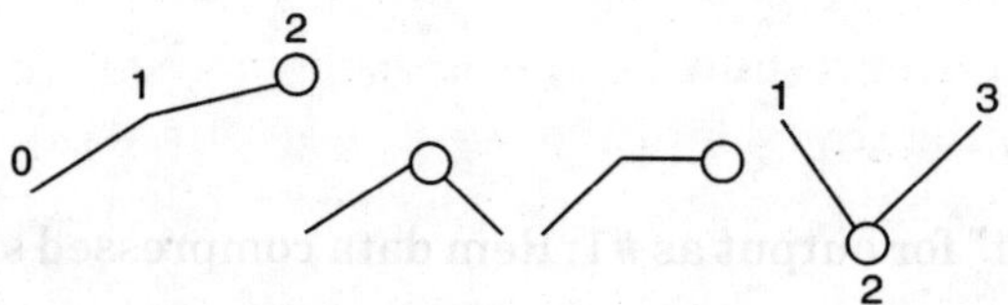

Showing method of choice of compressed point in Turning point algorithm.

ECG CLASSIFICATIONS

Fig. 14.22 shows how a computer classification of grade for an ECG would be (of course, all clinical ECGs are grade – 1 only).

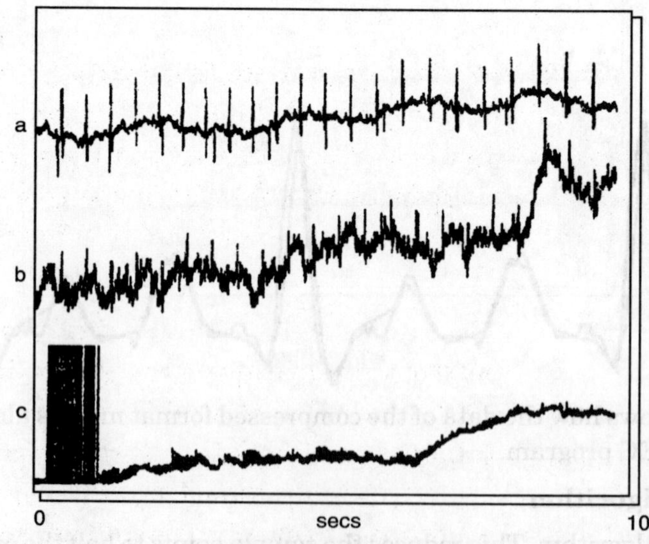

Fig. 14.22

An FIR or IIR bandpass digital filter may be used to pre- process the raw ECG before QRS detection. We prefer the use of FIR as an IIR filter of a high order, (for example eighth order); sometimes rings when excited by the narrow width QRS complexes which may complicate the precise location of the R wave. The filter specifications used in the study are as follows.

AZTEC	
Filter length	75
Sampling frequency	500 Hz
Stopbands	0–1Hz, 47–250 Hz
Passband	9 – 39
Pass band ripple	0.5 dB
Stopband attenuation	30 dB

Figs. 14.23 *a* to *c* show the filtered ECG data. Compared with the corresponding unfiltered raw data, figures a-c, the baselines shifts as well as the high frequency noise have been reduced in the filtered data (ignoring the transients and the initial transients in the filtered data). In the grade – 3 data, the ADC error appears as a burst which no doubt will confound most QRS detection algorithms.

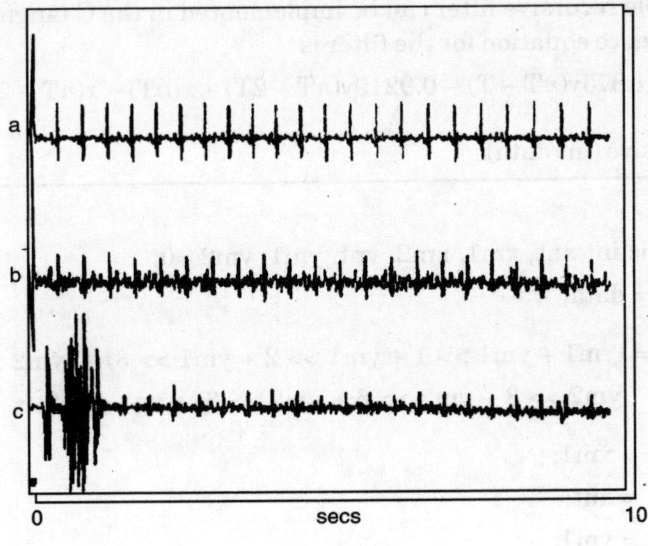

Fig. 14.23

Bandpass filtering on ECG

From the spectral analysis of the various signal components in the ECG signal, a filter can be designed which effectively selects the QRS complex from the ECG. Fig. 14.24 shows a plot of the signal-to-noise ratio (SNR) as a function of frequency. The study of the power spectra of the ECG signal, QRS complex, and other noises also revealed that a maximum SNR value is obtained for a bandpass filter with a center frequency of 17 Hz and a Q of 3.

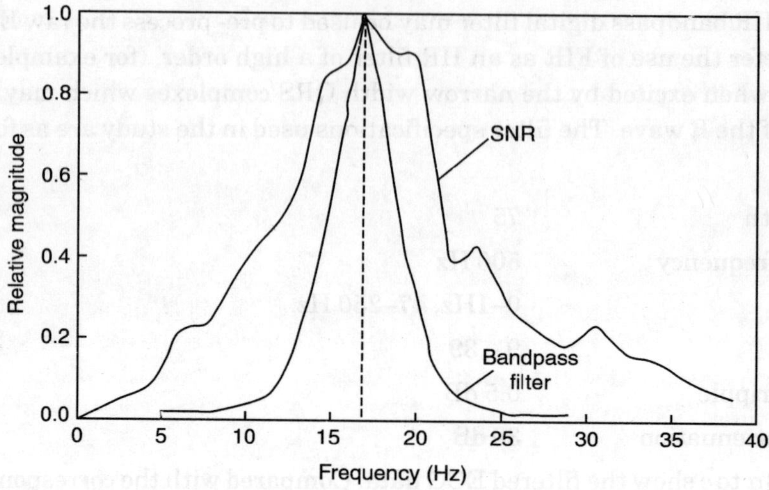

Fig. 14.24. Plots of the signal-to-noise ratio (SNR) of the QRS complex referenced to all other signal noise based on 3875 heart beats. The optional bandpass filter for a cardiotachometer maximizes the SNR.

Two Pole recursive filter

A simple two-pole recursive filter can be implemented in the C language to bandpass the ECG signal. The difference equation for the filter is

$$y(nT) = 1.875y(nT - T) - 0.9219y(nT - 2T) + x(nT) - x(nT - 2T)$$

Two Pole Recursive (int data)

```
{
        static int xnt, xm1, xm2, ynt, ym1, ym2 =0;
        xnt = data;

        ynt = (ym1 + ym1 >> 1 + ym1 >> 2 + ym1 >> 3) + (ym2 >> 1 + ym2 >>2 +
              ym2 >> 3 + ym2 >> 5 + ym2 >> 6) + xnt - xm2;

        xm2 = xm1;
        xm1 = xnt;
        xm2 = ym1;
        ym2 = ym1;
        ym1 = ynt;
        return(ynt);
}
```

This filter design assumes that the ECG signal is sampled at 500 samples/s.

It is to be noted that in this code, the coefficients 1.87635 and 0.9216 are calculated easily by

$$1.875 = 1 + ½ + ¼ + 1/8$$

and

$$0.9219 = ½ + ¼ + 1/8 + 1/32 + 1/64$$

so that right shift operations are useful.

INTEGER FILTER

QRS detectors for cardiotachometer applications frequently bandpass the ECG signal using a center frequency of 17Hz. The denominator of the general form of the transfer function allows for poles at 60°, 90° and 120°, and these correspond to center frequencies of a bandpass filter of T/6, T/4, and T/3 Hz, respectively. The desired center frequency can thus be obtained by choosing an appropriate sampling frequency.

A useful filter for QRS detection is based on the following transfer function:

$$H(z) = (1 - z^{-12})^2/(1 - z^{-1} + z^{-2})^2$$

This filter has 24 zeros at 12 different frequencies on the unit circle with poles at ±60°. The ECG signal is sampled at 200 sps, and then the turning point algorithm is used to reduce the sampling rate to 100 sps. The center frequency is at 16.67 Hz and the nominal bandwidth is ± 8.3 Hz.

The difference equation to implement this transfer function is

$$y(nT) = 2y(nT - T) - 3y(nT - 2T) + 2y(nT - 3T) - y(nT - 4T) + x(nT) - 2x(nT - 12T) + x(nT - 24T)$$

QRS Template

Most QRS detection methods rely on the availability of a representative QRS template against which the incoming ECG signal is compared. The template may be generated from raw ECG data by detecting and averaging several good QRS complexes. This may be done automatically or semi manually by visually examining a grade 1 ECG record and identifying good, unambiguous ECG complexes. The R waves are then synchronized and the QRS complexes averaged. A fixed QRS template may be used to detect *v* complexes or a new one may be generated at the start of each ECG record. An example of a QRS template obtained by averaging 69 QRS complexes in grade 1 data and then taking 31 samples (15 samples on either side of the R wave) of the averaged QRS complexes is shown in Fig. 14.25.

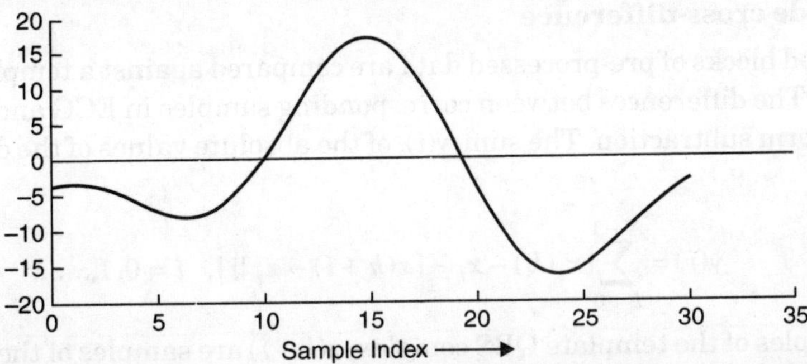

Fig. 14.25. An example of a QRS complex template. This is obtained by averaging over 69 QRS complexes in a grade 1 ECG, with the R-waves synchronized. The QRS complexes were detected with a threshold level of 13.

In a study, templates of various lengths were tried. Typically, the length of the template, N, is between 11 and 31 samples, that is a width of between about 20 ms and 60 ms at a sampling rate of 500 samples s^{-1}. Good results are obtained with two templates of lengths 11 and 31 samples.

QRS detection methods

A general block diagram of the QRS detection process is given in Fig. 14.26. The raw ECG data is first pre-processed to reduce the effects of noise. The pre-processed data samples are fed into a buffer one data point at a time. For each new data point fed into the buffer, the oldest data point is removed and the content of the buffer compared with a QRS template in the QRS detector. The output of the QRS detector is then thresholded. If this output exceeds the threshold value then a QRS is said to have occurred. Two conventional QRS detection methods are compared now, selected on the basis that they are either in practical use or potentially of practical use.

Many other QRS detection methods exist.

The methods are

1. average magnitude cross-difference(AMCD) (Lindecrantz) currently used in a new fetal monitor described in Lindecrantz and
2. matched filtering, which is a common QRS detection method and has been investigated by a number of workers (Azevedo and Longini).

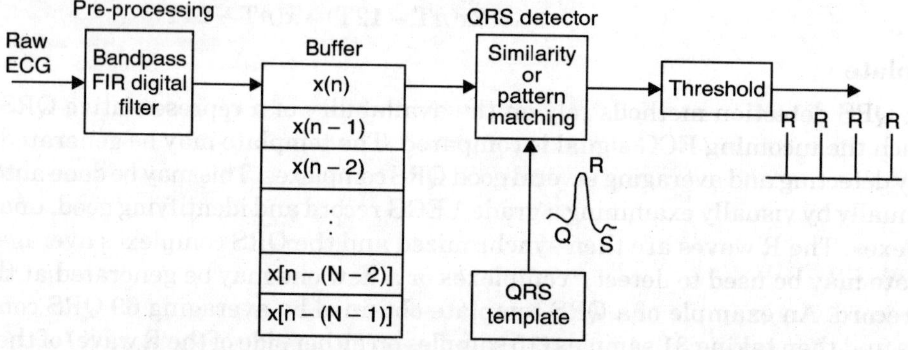

Fig. 14.26. Concepts of QRS complex detection from raw ECG.

Average magnitude cross-difference

In this method blocks of pre-processed data are compared against a template QRS complex as described above. The differences between corresponding samples in ECG and the template are computed by waveform subtraction. The sum, $y(i)$, of the absolute values of the differences is then computed:

$$y(i) = \sum_{k=0}^{N-1} | x_t(k) - x_t - [x(k+i) - x_i]\} |, \quad i = 0, 1, ...$$

where $x_t(k)$ are samples of the template QRS complex, $x(k + i)$ are samples of the ECG signal, N is the length of the template, and I is the time shift parameter. x_t is the mean value of the QRS template, and x_i the mean value of the ith data block for the ECG signal given by

$$x_t = (1/N) \sum_{k=0}^{N-1} x_t(i)$$

$$x_i = (1/N) \sum_{k=0}^{N-1} x(k+i)$$

When the ECG signal and QRS template are very similar in shape, that is in the neighbourhood of a QRS complex, the AMCD value, $y(i)$, becomes a minimum (theoretically zero).

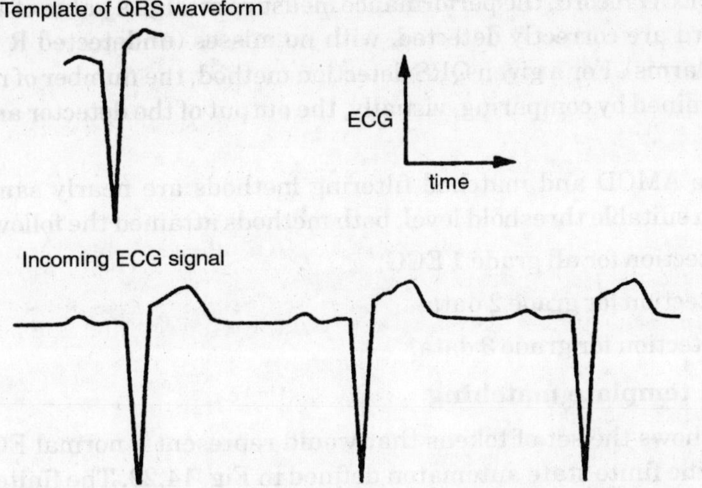

Fig. 14.27. In simple template matching, the incoming signal is subtracted, point by point, from the QRS template. If the two waveforms are perfectly aligned, the subtraction results in a zero value.

Fig. 14.27 shows the method used in simple template matching.

Digital matched filtering

Matched filtering is commonly used to detect time recurring signals buried in noise. The main underlying assumptions in this method are that the signal is time limited and has a known waveshape. The problem then is to determine its time of occurrence. The impulse response of a digital matched filter, $h(k)$, is the time-reversed replica of the signal to be detected. Thus in our case, if $x_t(k)$ is the QRS template then the coefficients of the matched filter are given by

$$h(k) = x_t(N - k - 1),\ k = 0, 1, \ldots, N - 1 \qquad \ldots(14.2)$$

The digital matched filter can be represented as an FIR filter with the usual transverse structure, with the output and the input of the filter related as

$$y(i) = \Sigma\, h(k)x(i-k)$$
$$= \Sigma\, x_t\,(N - k - 1)\, x\,(i-k)$$

where x(i) are the samples of the input ECG signal, $x_t(k)$ are the samples of the QRS template, N is the filter length, $h(k)$ are matched filter coefficients, and i is the time shift index. It is evident that when the template and the QRS complex coincide, the output of the matched filter will be a maximum. Thus by searching the output of the matched filter for a value above a threshold the occurrence of the QRS can be tested.

Performance measure for QRS detection

To evaluate and compare the algorithms requires a measure of performance. Following Azevedo and Longoni define the performance measure as

$$\frac{(\text{Total number of R waves} - \text{number of misses} - \text{number of false detections}) \times 100\%}{\text{Total number of actual R waves}}$$

For a given ECG record, the performance measure attains a value of 100% only if all the R waves in the record are correctly detected, with no misses (undetected R waves) and no false detections (false alarms). For a given QRS detection method, the number of misses or false detections can be determined by comparing, visually, the output of the detector and the pre-processed ECG.

Overall, the AMCD and matched filtering methods are nearly same in terms of their performance. With suitable threshold level, both methods attained the following performances:

- 100% detection for all grade 1 ECG;
- >90% detection for grade 2 data;
- > 60% detection for grade 3 data.

Automata-based template matching

Fig. 14.28 shows the set of tokens that would represent a normal ECG. Then this set of tokens is input to the finite state automaton defined in Fig. 14.29. The finite state automaton is essentially a state-transition diagram that can be implemented with IF...... THEN control statements available in most programming languages. The sequence of tokens is fed into the automaton. For example, a sequence of tokens such as zero, normpup, normdown, and normup would result in the automaton signaling a normal classification for the ECG.

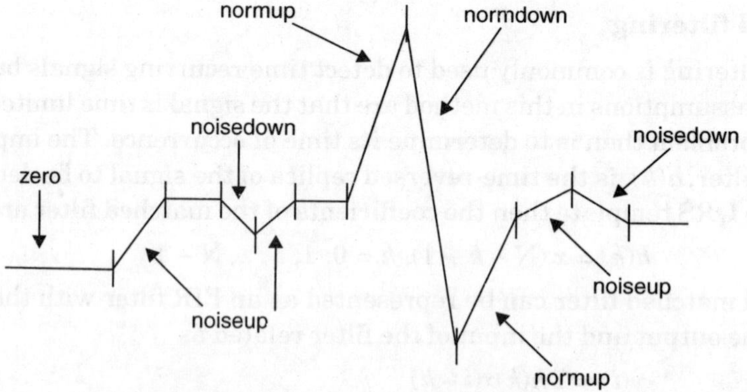

Fig. 14.28. Reduction of an ECG signal to tokens.

The sequence of tokens must be derived from the ECG signal data. This is done by forming a sequence of the differences of the input data.

This QRS detector first 'learns' about the R-wave, where the program approximately determines the peak magnitude of a normal QRS complex. Then the algorithm detects a normal QRS complex each time there is a deflection in the waveform with a magnitude greater than half of the previously determined peak. The algorithm now teaches the finite state automaton the sequence of tokens that make up a normal QRS complex. The number and sum values for a normal QRS complex are now set to a certain range of their respective values in the QRS complex detected.

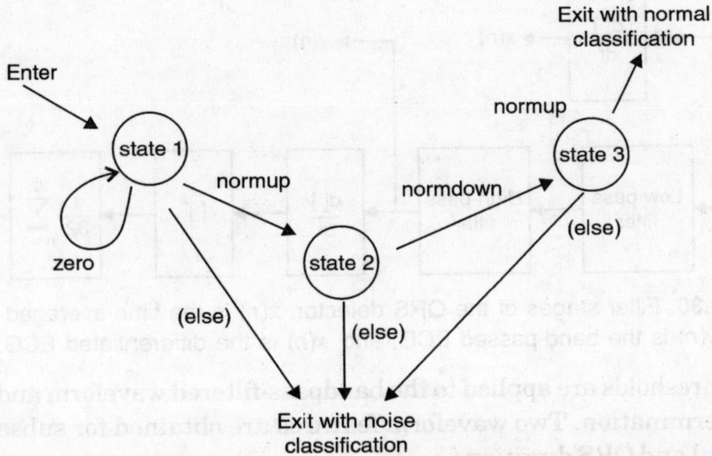

Fig. 14.29. State-transition diagram for a simple automaton detecting only normal QRS complexes and noise. The state transition (else) refers to any other token not labeled on a state transition leaving a particular false.

The program can now assign a waveform token to each of the groups formed previously, based on the values of the number and the sum in each group of differences. For example, if a particular group of differences has a sum and number value in the ranges (determined in the learning phase) of a QRS upward or downward deflection, then a normup or normdown token is generated for those group of differences. If the number and sum values do not fall in this range, then a noise-up or noise-down token is generated. A zero token is generated if the sum for a group of differences is zero. Thus, the algorithm reduces the ECG signal data into a sequence of tokens, which can be fed to the finite state automation for QRS detection.

Filter based QRS Detector

Fig. 14.30 shows the filter stages of the QRS detector. z(n) is the time-averaged signal y(n) is the band passed ECG, and x(n) is the derivative of the ECG.

A bandpass filter picks up the predominant QRS energy centered at 10Hz, attenuates the low frequencies characteristic of P, T waves and baseline drift, and also attenuates the higher frequencies. The next processing step is differentiation, a standard technique for finding the high slopes that normally distinguish the QRS complexes from other parts of ECG wave.

Next is a nonlinear transformation that consists of point-by-point squaring of the signal samples. This transformation serves to make all the data positive prior to subsequent integration, and also enhances the higher frequencies in the signal obtained from the differentiation process. These higher frequencies are normally characteristic of the QRS complex.

The squared waveform passes through a box-car moving window integrator. This integrator sums the area under the squared waveform over a 150 ms interval, advances one sample interval, and integrates on the new 150 ms window. The window's width has to be long enough to include the time duration of extended abnormal QRS complexes, but short enough so that it does not overlap both a QRS complex and a T wave.

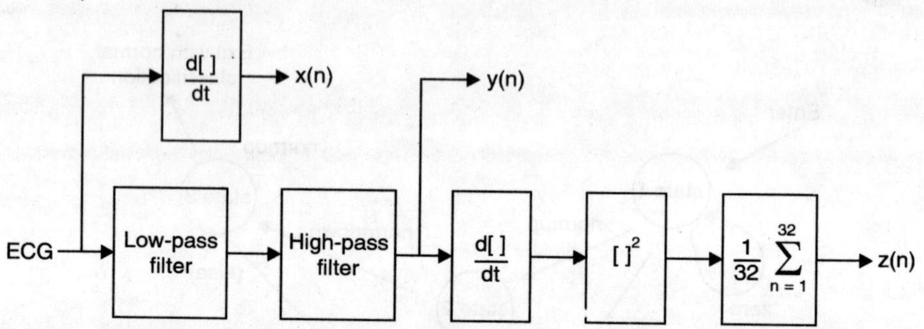

Fig. 14.30. Filter stages of the QRS detector, $z(n)$ is the time-averaged signal, $y(n)$ is the band-passed ECG, and $x(n)$ is the differentiated ECG.

Amplitude thresholds are applied to the bandpass-filtered waveform and decision processes make the final determination. Two waveform features are obtained for subsequent arrhythmia analysis-RR interval and QRS duration.

Chapter 15

Safety Measures in Bio-Medical Instruments

ARTIFACTS

The term artifact refers to the presence of an unwanted signal such as power line frequency interference or noise. When recording for example, the EEG, the presence of ECG or EMG information on the recording also constitutes artifacts. The most common source of artifact is power line interference; however, power line leakage is of paramount importance from a safety viewpoint and it is common from a safety consideration to seemingly contradict artifact - elimination considerations.

1. GROUNDING

If a subject were deliberately connected across a one-volt AC source, an AC current of perhaps a 100 μA would flow through the subject due to the finite impedance of our body (>10,000 ohms) and skin connections. Really, many instrumentation systems inadvertently produce a similar situation in the form of a ground loop.

If a 3-meter length of wire is connected between a patient's left arm and his right leg, a 60 Hz AC current will be induced through the patient as this wire acts as a transformer secondary, with current magnetically induced from adjacent power wiring and transformers. Although the magnetic coupling material involved is air and the amount of coupling therefore is extremely small, it is finite and an EMF will be induced into the loop which will in turn cause current to flow through the subject. This 3-meter length of wire may, in practice, be two separate grounding wires attached to a subject (Fig. 15.1).

As shown in Fig. 15.1, if either the ECG monitor or the "other monitoring equipment" is connected to the subject, a ground loop is not produced. However, if both instruments are simultaneously connected to the subject, the ground connections for each instrument form a ground loop. The ground loop shown produces a potential between the subject's right leg and left arm causing a current to flow through the patient's bulk body resistance. This current flow produces a voltage drop across different parts of the body which would appear as a 50 Hz artifact of the ECG monitor.

The ground loop produced by the configuration shown in Fig. 15.1 may simply be eliminated by removing one of the ground connections to the subject whenever both items of monitoring equipment are used simultaneously. If this is particularly inconvenient, the ground loop may be eliminated by adding a high impedance in series with one of these leads or the subject may be grounded at a single reference point so that any induced current does not flow through the subject's bulk body impedance. Both of these ground loop changes are shown in Fig. 15.1 and both changes

effectively eliminate the current flow through the subject, thus eliminating the mains frequency potential differences between various points on the subject.

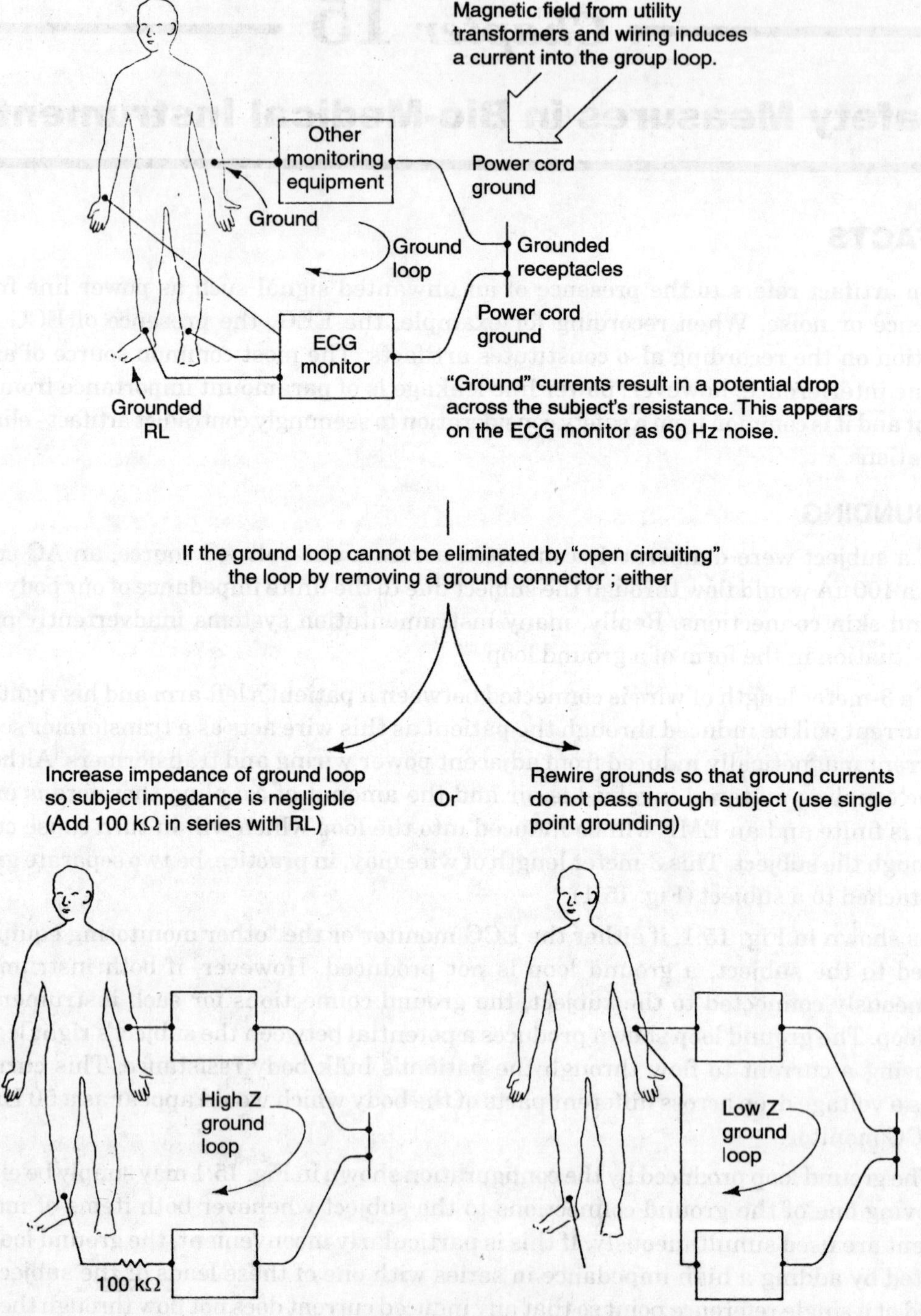

Fig. 15.1. Shows the induced ground current from a "ground loop".

2. INDUCED GROUND CURRENTS

A ground loop is an example of an induced ground current, the value of which can be reduced or eliminated by modifying the grounding configuration. Another form of induced ground current is illustrated in Fig. 15.2 where a current is induced into a ground wire via an instrument's power transformer. In this specific case, an induced 50Hz ground current is induced into the grounding circuit of an electrocautery unit. This ground current flows via the electrocautery ground plate, through the subject and to ground via a perspiration-damped bed sheet, a conductive rubber mat and the grounded operating table.

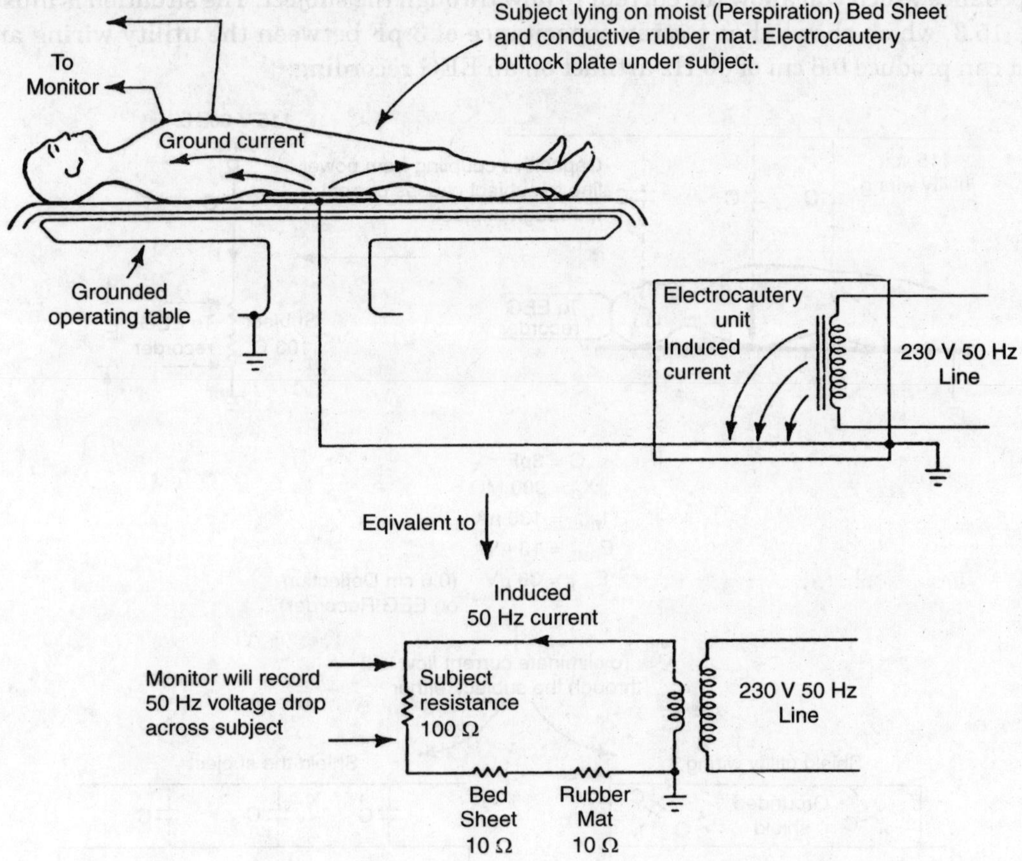

Fig. 15.2. Shows the induced ground current from electrocautery unit. An induced current of 350 nA will cause a 2 mm hum trace on the standard ECG Monitor.

The above type of induced ground current is particularly difficult to eliminate as safety considerations demand that the subject be grounded and that the electrocautery-unit buttock plate be well grounded to the electrocautery unit and to the subject to eliminate burns at electrode sites during electrocautery. This particular problem is often encountered when trying to monitor a subject's ECG in an operating room using an older style electrocautery unit. When these older units were designed, it was not expected that the ECG may be monitored while the electrocautery unit was connected to the line ready for use. Modern electrocautery units have more carefully designed internal-grounding configurations and incorporate shielding to prevent magnetically induced or capacitively induced current from entering the subject via the buttock plate. Perhaps the only solution that can be offered for an electrocautery unit of the older design is to discard the unit. The induced current produced by the electrocautery unit may be sufficient to cause death if grounded catheters are used on the subject.

3. ELECTROSTATICALLY INDUCED CURRENTS

Utility Wiring Capacitance

Capacitive coupling between the mains voltage (220 V/115) wiring and the subject constitutes an impedance which will allow the current to flow through the subject. The situation is illustrated in Fig. 15.3, which shows that a stray capacitance of 3 pF between the utility wiring and the subject can produce 0.6 cm of 50 Hz artifact on an EEG recording.

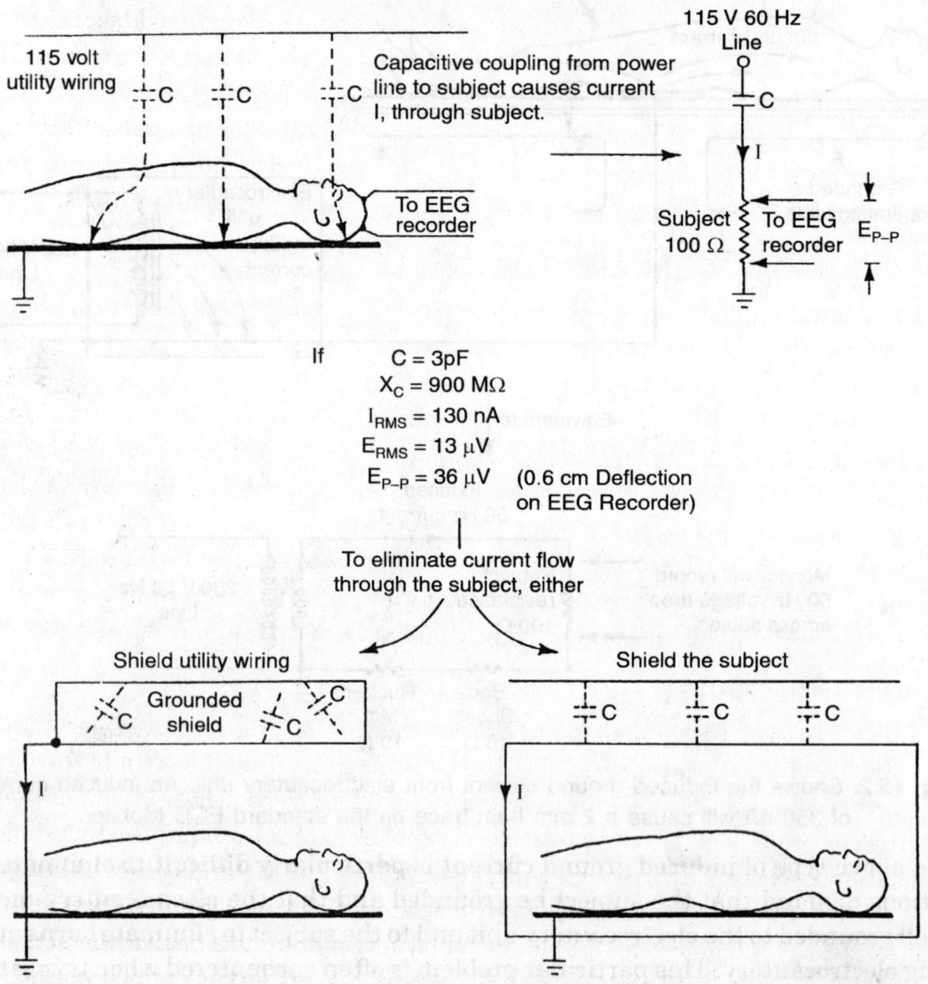

Fig. 15.3. Shows the electrostatic shielding.

Utility Wiring Shielding

To eliminate this electrostatically induced currents, it is necessary to provide an alternative path for this current to flow. This may be achieved by either shielding the mains supply wiring, in which case the current flows from this wiring to this shield. Alternatively, by placing the subject inside an electrostatic shield (Faraday cage), in which case the current flows to ground via the shield rather than via the subject. In either case, shielding is expensive and it may be preferable to locate a recording site in alternative part of the hospital or laboratory where electrostatically induced current is less bothersome. In the research environment, where high sensitive amplifiers are invariably employed, the subject and parts of the recording equipment should be enclosed in a screened room to effectively isolate the subject from capacitively induced currents from any source.

Recording Lead Shielding

Currents may be capacitively coupled to the leads connecting the subject to the recording equipment. Thus, these leads must be screened to effectively shield them. Care should be taken to ensure that these shields are, however, only grounded at one point. Otherwise, in attempting to eliminate interference by electrostatic shielding, one may inadvertently create 50 Hz interference by introducing ground loop. This interference may be produced by 50 Hz power wiring or it may be high frequency interference produced by radio and /or television transmitters.

4. ELECTRIC SHOCK CURRENT THRESHOLDS

When electric current is passed through the body, part of this current will pass through the heart and interfere with the normal function of the heart. Perhaps it can cause death. In cases of death by electrocution, almost all subjects are killed by the passage of electric current through the heart rather than by some related occurrences such as burns, or muscular paralysis of the muscles controlling breathing action. If a person receives a mains shock (110/220 V), it is not the voltage of the shock that is important but rather the current through the body. Thus, if a person receives a mains (220 V/115 V) shock standing in a dry environment insulated by normal clothing, the shock may hardly be felt, as a current may be well below 1 mA. If, however, a person receives a mains (220 V/115 V) shock while standing on back footed on a moist ground, the person would receive a severe shock and probably be killed as the current may exceed 100 mA.

Shock Current Thresholds

As shown in Fig. 15.4, experimental investigation on numerous subjects has indicated that up to 300 μA applied to the surface of the body, such as from one arm to the other, may be suggested as being reasonably safe for most subjects. It can be seen that 99.9 % of the population require 400 μA or more of 60 Hz current to perceive the current and that the threshold of perception or sensation increases as frequency increases above 100 Hz and below 10 Hz. At 10000 Hz and at DC, the threshold of sensation is approximately five times greater than at 50 Hz. While current above the threshold of sensation may not be detrimental to a healthy person, it may cause complications in a hospitalized person and will certainly create anxiety which would be detrimental to the patient's general well being.

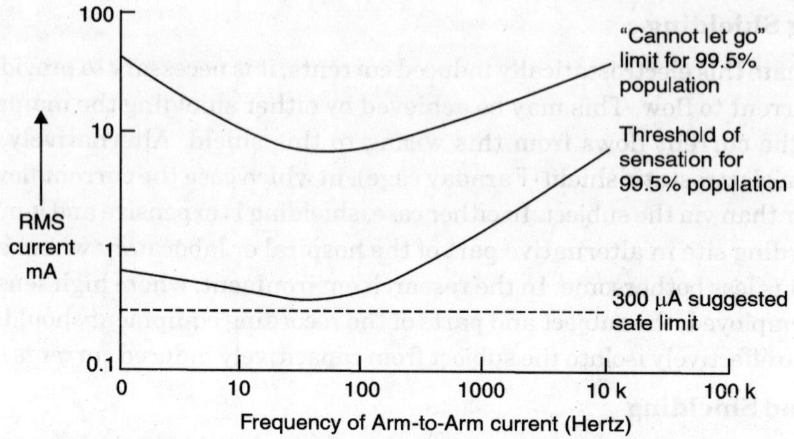

Fig. 15.4. Variation of current with frequency for "LET-go Current", "sensation current" etc. for humans.

'Let-go' current

The maximum current at which a person is capable of releasing a conductor by using muscles directly stimulated by that current is called the 'let-go' current.

From Fig. 15.4, it can also be seen that "can not Let go" current thresholds are one order of magnitude above sensation current threshold and that also increases for frequency below 10 Hz and above 100 Hz.

The muscular reactions caused by commercial—frequency alternating currents in the upper ranges of let-go current, typically 18-22 or more milliamperes, flowing across chest stopped breathing during the period the current flowed, and in several instances caused temporary paralysis of the middle finger. However, normal respiration resumed upon interruption of the current, and no advance after effects were produced as a result of not breathing for short periods.

Sinusoidal currents from 5 to 10000 Hz were used in these experiments. There is essentially no difference in the muscular reactions for frequencies between 50 and 60 Hz, which are the commercial frequencies used throughout the world.

Ventricular Fibrillation

Fig. 15.5, shows the physiological effects of 50 Hz arm-arm current and shows the threshold of sensation at 300 μA, a threshold of pain at 1mA, cannot let-go threshold at 10 mA and a ventricular fibrillation-induction threshold at 100 mA. 99.5 % of the population have thresholds above these values. Ventricular fibrillation refers to mal functioning of the ventricular musculature which will interfere with normal blood pumping action of the heart and eventually cause death.

"Vulnerable Period" in Cardiac Cycle

Ventricular fibrillation is produced by current directly through the heart during a specific portion of the cardiac cycle known as **"vulnerable period".** The vulnerable period occurs during the upstroke of the T wave and a single shock impulse lasting for less than 0.1 sec, could cause ventricular fibrillation if received during this vulnerable period.

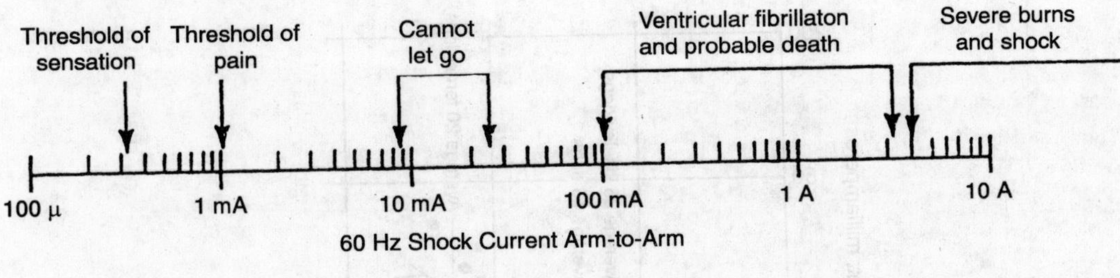

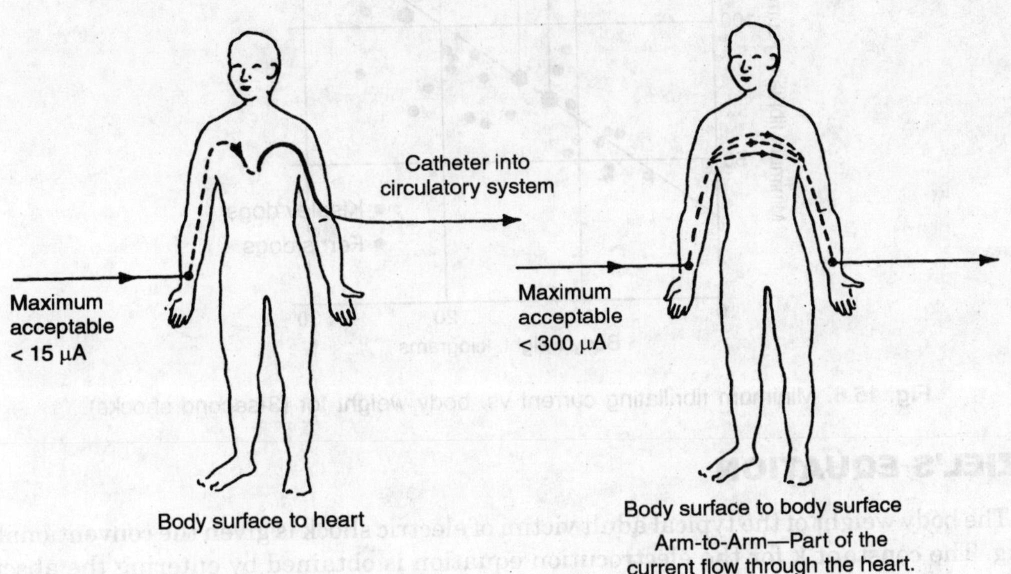

Fig. 15.5. Shows the physiological effects of 50 Hz electric current.

The 300 μA threshold refers to 60 Hz current applied from the arm to the other arm and is intended as a guide to acceptable leakage current levels. The acceptable level for any one subject may be somewhat above this value and will also depend on the size of the current contact. A very small point contact can undoubtedly be felt at 0.3 mA, but a current in excess of perhaps 1 mA may not produce sensation if the contacts are somewhat larger. Depending on size of contact, the threshold of pain may also be considerably above 1 mA, probably 10 mA, if the contacts are large enough. It is thus evident that current density is also important in the determining the physiological effects of electric current.

Relationship Between Fibrillating Current and Body Weight

Fig. 15.6 represents the relationship between minimum fibrillating current for 3 second shocks from the 35 Kiselev dogs and the ten Ferris dogs.(These are names of experimenters). The line of best fit, the regression line, was calculated by the method of least squares, using a standard statistical procedure. Although there is some scattering about this line, the trend to the response clearly shows that minimum current required to produce fibrillation is approximately proportional to the individual dog's body weight and the degree of association which is indicated by the correlation coefficient, is $r = 0.74$.

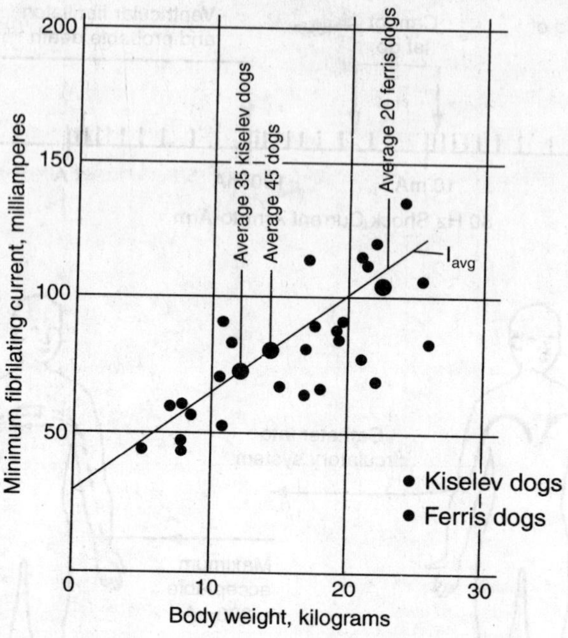

Fig. 15.6. Minimum fibrillating current vs. body weight for (3-second shocks).

DALZIEL'S EQUATION

The body weight of the typical adult victim of electric shock is given the conventional value of 50 kg. The constant k for the electrocution equation is obtained by entering the abscissa of Fig. 15.7 at a value of 50 kg and proceeding vertically to the two 0.5 percentile lines as follows :

0.5 percentile fibrillating current equation is 2.04 W + 5

0.5 percentile max. non-fibrillating current equation is 1.15 W + 10

Put W = 50. Then,

$$I = k / \sqrt{T}$$

$$k = \sqrt{T} \,.\, I$$

$$k = \sqrt{3} \times 107 = 185 \text{ maximum}$$

$$= \sqrt{3} \times 67 = 116 \text{ minimum}$$

$$I = 116 - 185/\sqrt{T} \Big|_{0.3\text{ sec}}^{5\text{ sec}} \quad \text{mA (rms)}$$

Unfortunately there is no direct evidence available regarding threshold fibrillating currents for children. A value of $53 - 69/\sqrt{T}$ is suggested by Dalziel.

The shortest time for which data are available represents a half wave of 50 Hz AC, and the majority of shorter shocks might be classified as impulse shocks. There is little information about the effects of shocks of longer duration than 5 seconds.

At higher currents, fibrillation does not occur, and very strong shocks will stop a fibrillating heart. This is the basis for defibrillating techniques—now standard hospital operating room routine for stopping fibrillation, which frequently results from several causes in addition to electric shock.

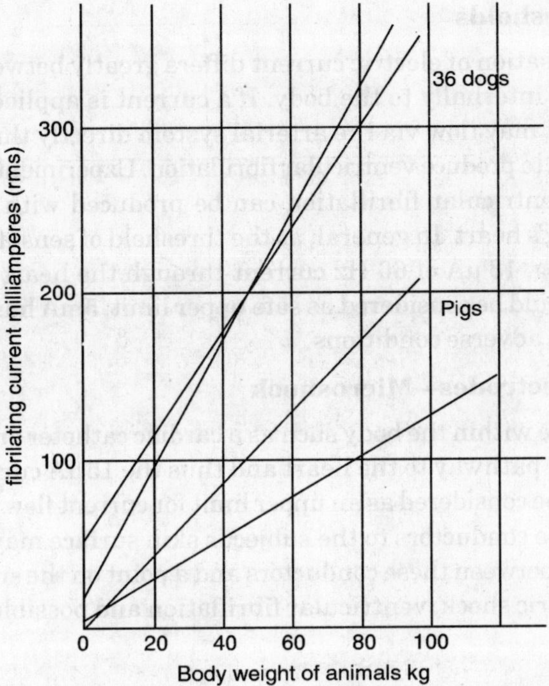

Fig. 15.8. Fibrillating current vs body weight for some animal speicies.

Lethal Effects of Electric Shock

1. A long continued current in excess of one's let -go current, passing through the chest, may produce collapse, unconsciousness, asphyxia, and death.
2. Ventricular fibrillation is probably the most common cause of death in electric shock cases, and may be produced by moderately small currents that cause derangement of coordination within the heart rather than physical damage to that organ. When fibrillation takes place, the rhythmic pumping action of the heart ceases and death rapidly follows.
3. Shocks administered to hundreds of animals indicate that the minimum commercial—frequency electric current causing ventricular fibrillation is proportional to body weight and inversely proportional to the square root of the shock duration. For a current pathway between major extremities in 50 kg mammals, the relationship is approximately 116 to $185/\sqrt{T}$ milliamperes. It is believed that ventricular fibrillation in a normal adult worker is unlikely if the shock intensity is less than $116/\sqrt{T}$ milliamperes, where T is in seconds.
4. Currents flowing through the nerve centers controlling breathing may produce respiratory inhibition, which may last for a considerable period even after interruption of the current.
5. Cardiac arrest may be caused by relatively high currents flowing in the region of heart.
6. Relatively high currents may produce fatal damage to the central nervous system.
7. Electric currents may produce deep burns, and currents sufficient to raise body temperature substantially produce immediate death.
8. Delayed death may be due to serious burns or other complications.

Internal Current Thresholds

A threshold of sensation of electric current differs greatly between currents applied arm-arm and current applied internally to the body. If a current is applied internally, a far greater percentage of the current may flow via the arterial system directly through the heart, thus less overall current is required to produce ventricular fibrillation. Experiments with dogs have indicated that, in some animals ventricular fibrillation can be produced with current as low as 17 μA applied directly to the dog's heart. In general, as the threshold of sensation of the man may not be much higher than the dog, 13 μA of 60 Hz current through the heart may produce ventricular fibrillation. And 15 μA would be considered as safe upper limit; 5mA has been postulated as a safe upper limit under certain adverse conditions.

Internal Probe and Electrodes—Microshock

A probe or electrode within the body such as a cardiac catheter or pacemaker electrode will provide a direct electrical pathway to the heart and thus the 15 μA current limit proposed in the above paragraph, should be considered as an upper limit for current flow through these conductors. The impedance from these conductors to the subject's skin surface may typically be 1000 ohms ; thus a potential of 30 mV between these conductors and a point on the surface of the subject's body is sufficient to cause electric shock, ventricular fibrillation and possible death.

High Accident Rate

It has been proposed that the introduction of the internal electrode has been the leading factor in the present high incidence of accidents in hospital patient care areas and operating rooms. Cardiac catheterization for diagnostic or therapeutic purposes has become common in recent years. Sensing catheters may have electrodes or transducers at their tips for ECG recording, blood pressure measurements and other diagnostic procedures. Fluid filled catheters are also in common use and, although they are not normally considered to be a probe or electrode within the body, the fluid in these catheters may be conductive; thus they also may provide an electrical pathway to the heart.

Electric Shock Hazards in Hospitals

Microshock

More serious – 5 μV – 50 μA, by wired in catheters causes ventricular fibrillation.

Macro shock ; This is due to contacts at exterior body surfaces

Table I

Shock level	Remarks
1 mA (1 sec)	Perception
5 mA	Accepts as maximum harmless (Resistance of body with well prepared electrodes 1–1.6 K)
10–20 mA	"Let-go"
50 mA	Pain, fainting, exhaustion, injury heart and respiration continues.

100–300	Ventricular fibrillation will start but respiratory. center alright
> 300	Involuntarily jerked away from contact
6000	Sustained myocardial contraction followed by normal rhythm, burns Temporary respiration failure
	Current required for fibrillation—smallest at 50 Hz

Isolated Input Circuits

No conductance path, using h.f. transformers. Patient is completely isolated from the mains supply (right leg not grounded). (Fig. 15.8 a)

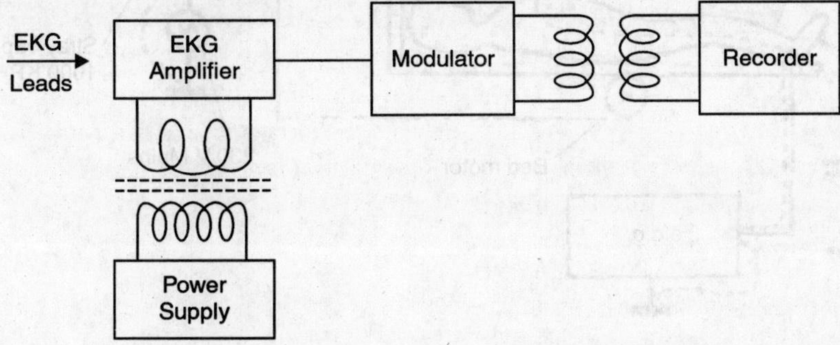

Fig. 15.8a & b. Shows the isolated—input circuit.

Power Isolation Transformers

The current through the body of heart with implanted electrodes not to exceed 10 μA. So allowable voltage is **5 mV only.**

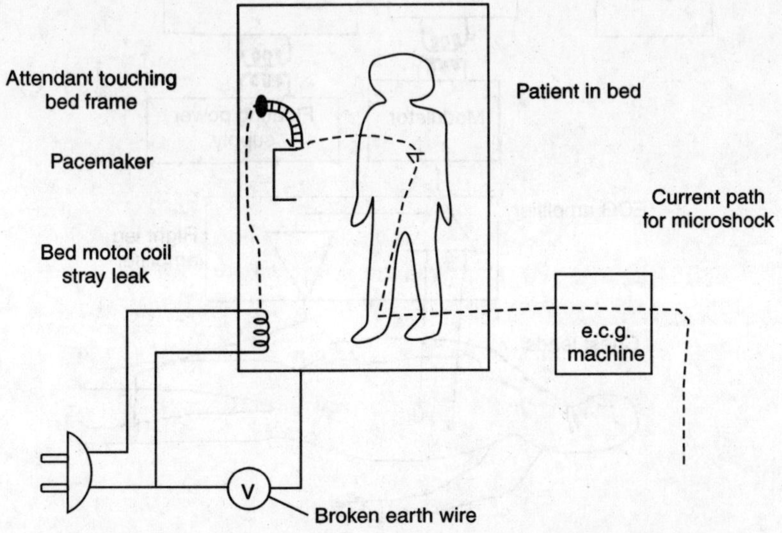

Fig. 15.9. Micro-shock Accident in a broken earth lead case.

Suppose an internal live-ground occurs; the fault current is several amperes.

The patient in a typical intensive care unit (ICU) and cardiac output (CCU) is being exposed to the danger of microshock because of increasing practice of using internal conductive electrodes or saline filled catheters in the vicinity of the heart (Fig. 15.9).

Fig. 15.9 shows the microshock accident in a bed in ICU due to bed motor leak and attendant touching bed and pacemaker adjustment made, causing leakage current to flow as per dotted line via heart.

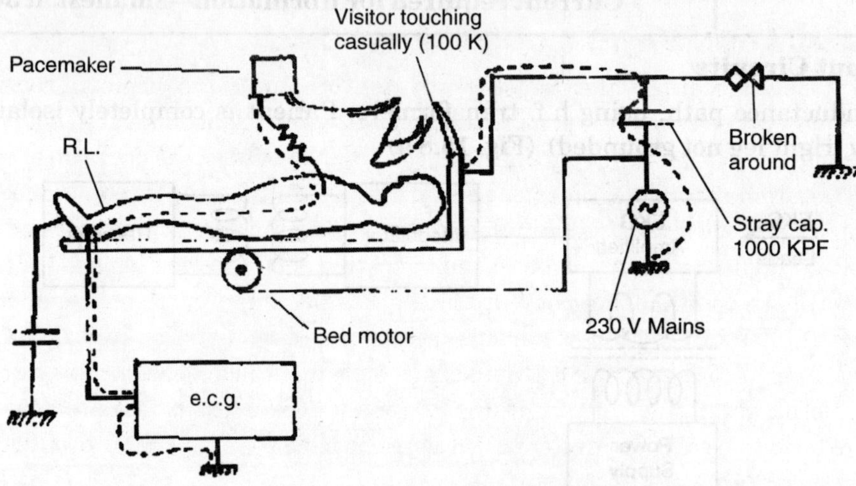

Fig. 15.10. Shows the another microschock scene in a bed.

As observed from Fig. 15.9, the shock is due to the bed-frame. Arrow indicates leakage current path supplied by attendant.

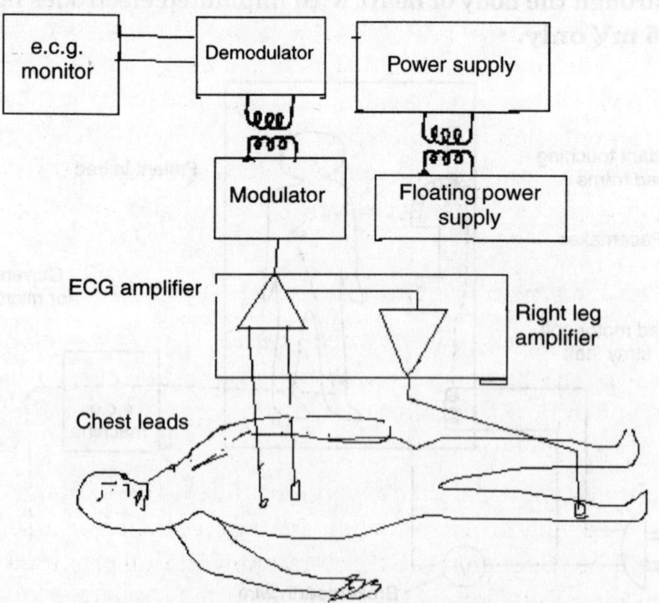

Fig. 15.11. Use on isolated input circuit for ECG machine.

Fig. 15.11 indicates the Isolated ECG amplifier circuitry. Arterial and venous pressure measurement can be designed so that the saline column in the catheter is not connected to the chassis of the pressure monitor through shield in transducer cable.

Fig. 15.11 Use of isolated input circuit for ECG machine.

Other ICU probes used are the temperature probes, Heart sound mikes and the respiration transducers.

5. INSTRUMENTATION SAFETY CONSIDERATIONS

Earlier the electrocautery unit was the only item of electronic equipment routinely used in the operating room. Any electrical shock hazard associated with this instrument was far outshadowed by the risk of explosion from flammable anesthetic gases. Nowadays, the operating room is packed with electronic equipment, all of which is necessary for the fulfillment of today's modern surgical procedures, and the risk of explosion from flammable anesthetic agents is considered of secondary importance. All of the instruments used in the operating room may be used alone with relative impunity however, in combination they produce an unprecedented electrical shock hazard of giant proportions. The interaction of various units connected to the subject demand a system approach which may be foreign to the training of medical staff and may also not be fully understood by the manufacturers of the various items of instrumentation. Some medical instrument manufacturers tend to be oblivious to this problem and tend to regard their product as an entity within itself rather than a part of an over-all system.

Power Transformer Leakage Currents

The major source of potentially lethal currents in any instrument is leakage current from mains power transformer primary. This leakage current is largely due to capacitive coupling from the power transformer primary to other parts of the transformer or other parts of the instrument. Instruments are usually designed so this leakage current flows to the instrument case and then to ground via the three-wire power cord provided with the instrument. Most modern general-purpose instrumentation may be expected to produce up to 500 μA of leakage current; however instrumentation designed for use in the medical environment should preferably have a leakage below 100 μA. By special design techniques, it is possible to decrease this leakage to well below 10 μA.

Shock Currents from Ungrounded Instruments :

Fig. 15.12 Shows microshock accident when Vacuum cleaner on electric line (top) is switched on, causing difference of 80 mV between the two earths of the two monitoring equipment, causing more than 50 μA current to flow through heart, although this may not always be practical although this may not always be practical.

As long as the instrument is adequately grounded, the leakage current will not flow through the subject. A problem arises when instrumentation is used in an ungrounded configuration, as would be the case if the three-pin power plug provided with the instrument was replaced by a two-pin plug to allow the instrument to be used with the older style two-pin power receptacles. Under these conditions the ground leakage current may flow through the subject

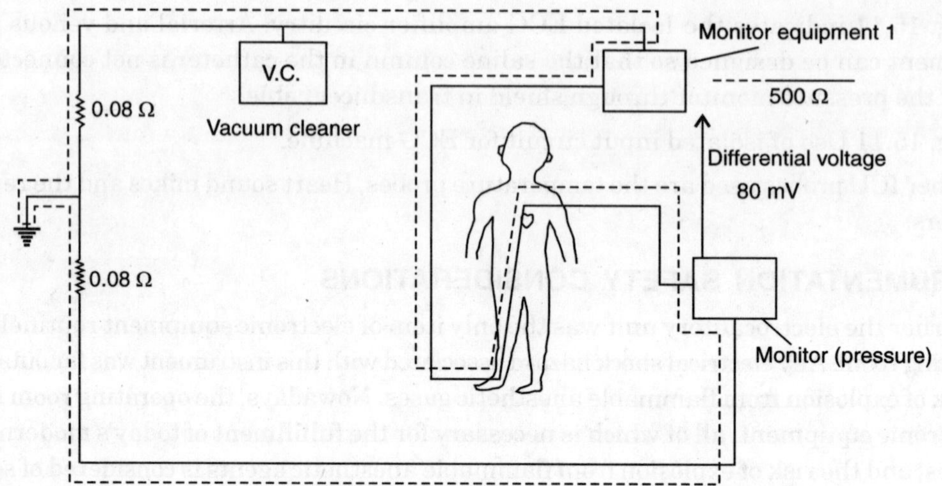

Fig. 15.12. Shows microshock accident when Vacuum cleaner (drawing/Amp.) on electric line (top) is switched on, causing difference of 80 mV between the two earths of the two monitoring equipment, causing more than 50 uA current to flow through heart.

as shown in Fig. 15.13, and if one of the conductor is an internal electrode, such as a catheter, death will almost certainly result.

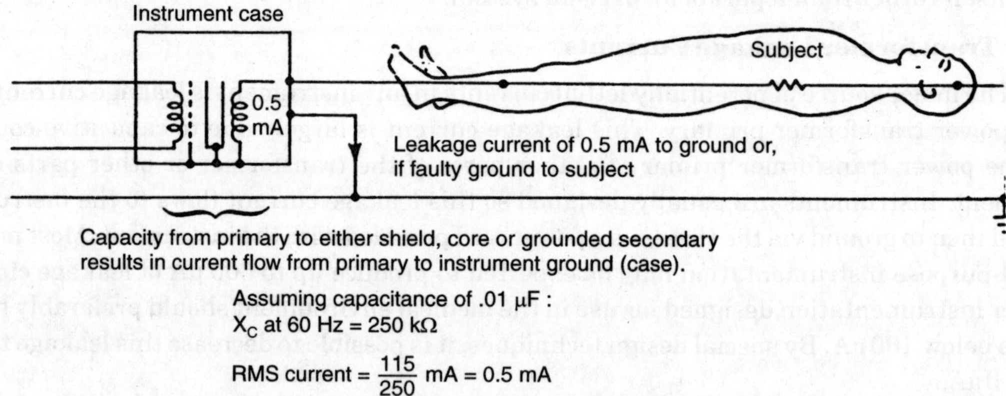

Fig. 15.13. Shows the transformer capacitive leakage currents.

Shock Currents to Isolated Subjects

It is apparent that if the subject were 'floating' or isolated , then a path to ground would not be provided for the leakage current mentioned in the previous para, and no current would flow through the subject. In practice, however, this does not reduce the risk as fault currents could still flow between various items of equipment without involving 'ground' in the current circuit; also, if a subject inadvertently touched a grounded item, such as a bed frame or water pipe, then the isolation would be nullified and electrocution may result. It is, therefore, apparent that protection systems must be organized on a grounded system concept.

Second order shock protection

The various hazards mentioned so far in this chapter primarily refer to current flowing through the subject if a fault occurs or if something abnormal happens. As in any situation, faults do occur and abnormalities do happen, thus, it is desirable to offer some second order protection to the subject.

Current limiting

Under normal operation of, for example, an ECG unit, only a small signal current should flow in any of the active electrodes or the right-leg ground electrode. Under abnormal or fault conditions, however, current may flow through any one of these paths and second order protection can be offered by incorporating some form of current limiting, The simplest from of current limiting, and a form adequate for use with the 'right-leg' ground electrode, is to use a large value resistor in series with the electrode. Series resistance current limiting is not, however, always possible. In any amplification equipment, such as an ECG monitor, series resistance will degrade the common-mode rejection-ratio (CMRR) specifications of the instrument to a point where mains frequency interference may be intolerable. It is often required to use a more sophisticated form of current limiting.

Most of the physiological monitors (such as Tektronix-type 410) are specifically designed for operating room use and incorporating series resistance current limiting in the right-leg ground electrode and more sophisticated current limiting in series with the active electrodes. This current limiting utilizes field effect diodes, the impedance of which is approximately 1000 ohms, when the current is less than 1 μA. However, the diodes limit fault currents to a maximum of 300 μA as their impedance increases as the current attempts to exceed the 300 μA level. It is thus apparent that current limiting within the physiological monitor provides adequate second order subject protection for **'arm-to-arm'** fault currents delivered by surface electrodes. It does not provide adequate protection to allow the monitors to be used with **intracardiac-catheter** electrodes.

Current Limiting Adapters

Many oscilloscopes and other electronic instrumentation produced by various manufacturers are used in the operating rooms and in intensive-care room(ICUs) on live human subjects. While designing all the instruments related to medical laboratories, operating rooms and other ISC's equipments, the secondary protection should be incorporated. This is necessary to avoid the risk involved with the human subject/patient lives. Electrical shock protector may be used in series with the mains supply. This is called alternatively as GFI or Ground Fault Interrupter.

6. ELECTRICAL SERVICE GROUNDING

As discussed earlier in this chapter, a potential of only 30 mV between two supposedly grounded conductors may allow enough current to flow through a subject as a microshock current to cause death by electrocution. If multiple ground points are available in an operating or intensive care room, there is no guarantee that all of these are at the same potential and a voltage may exist between, for example, a grounded wall outlet and a nearby water pipe. These subtle ground potential differences are difficult to detect, but they may be fatal if left undetected. It is not uncommon to find two electrical power services available in older hospitals; the second service having been provided to handle increased power demand since the hospital was constructed. This second service may come from a different part of the hospital and the potential at its ground conductor may differ from the potential of the ground conductor of the older service by a volt or more. If subtle differences in ground potential are detected, they can usually be almost completely eliminated by interconnecting each ground point with heavy gauge copper grounding bus. As currents of several amperes may flow in this interconnecting grounding bus, the copper wire used should be at least a ¼ inch in diameter. Such subtle ground difference can be detected with a differential AC voltmeter.

Remote fault Currents

As given in Fig. 15.14, it is apparent that two ground points from the same power service may show a potential gradient due to a fault current in equipment connected elsewhere in the power service. Although the fault current of 1 A shown in Fig. 14 is sufficient to trip a circuit breaker in the active line of the power service, it is sufficient to produce a voltage drop of 50 mV across 20 feet standard service ground wire. Once again this 50 mV may be enough to cause a fatality by microshock. To avoid this difficulty, the service outlets should be grouped together to provide a **single point ground.**

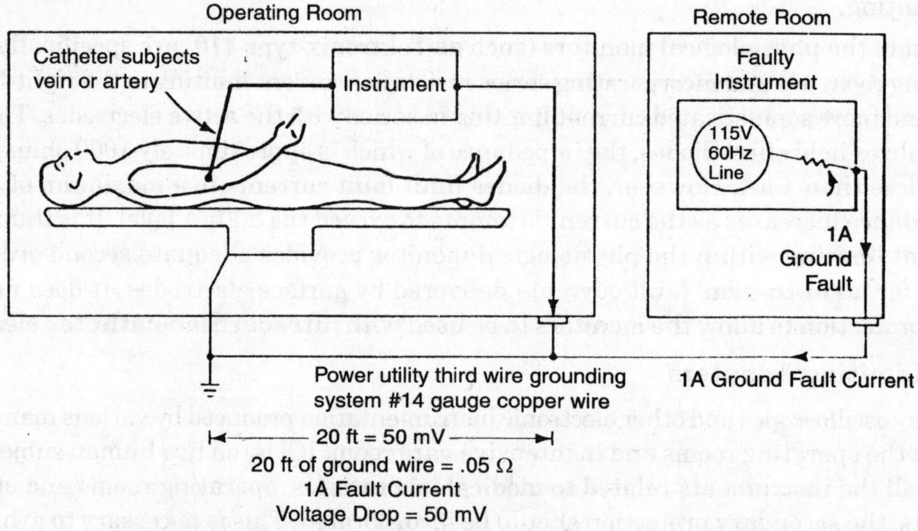

Fig. 15.14. Shows the subject injury caused by a "remote" electrical fault.

Response time of protection devices :

A catastrophic remote electrical fault may produce a fault current of perhaps 50 A which will cause the primary circuit breaker to trip. This circuit breaker may, however, take several hundred milliseconds to disconnect the service after the fault has occurred, thus the fault current may flow for more than 100 ms. As discussed earlier, if this fault current occurred during the 'vulnerable period' of a subject's cardiac cycle, any potential produced between different ground points attached to the subject may be enough to cause death.

7. OPERATING ROOM ISOLATION

Static Charge Prevention

In an effort to reduce the risk of flammable anesthetic ignition in an operating theatre, conductive ground flooring is used, the subject is connected to a grounded operating table by a conductive rubber mat and moist bed sheet and the operating personnel wear conductive clothing. These precautions prevent the build-up of static electricity and the subsequent spark caused by the discharge of this static electricity.

Fault Current Monitors

Due to the presence of this extensive grounding in the operating room, the electrical service to operating rooms normally has both conductors isolated from ground; so, if a fault develops between one conductor and ground, no fault current can flow. The integrity of this isolation is monitored continuously by ground fault detectors installed between either side of the service and ground. These detectors normally signal when it finds any ground fault causing to flow in excess of 1 mA. Unfortunately, there is no worse item of electrical equipment in the operating room than the ground fault monitor; if the monitor alarm sounds, the operating room personnel often suspect the monitor rather than heed its warning. It should also be noted that 1mA level at which the ground-fault monitor alarm sounds may be low enough to protect the subjects against currents flowing from surface contacts to his body but it is not low enough to protect the subject from shock from internal electrodes or catheters (microshocks).

8. ELETROCAUTERY AND DEFIBRILLATION

The diathermy unit which is often called as electrocautery unit is extensively used in operating rooms. As discussed in another chapter, it is used to provide a source of high frequency

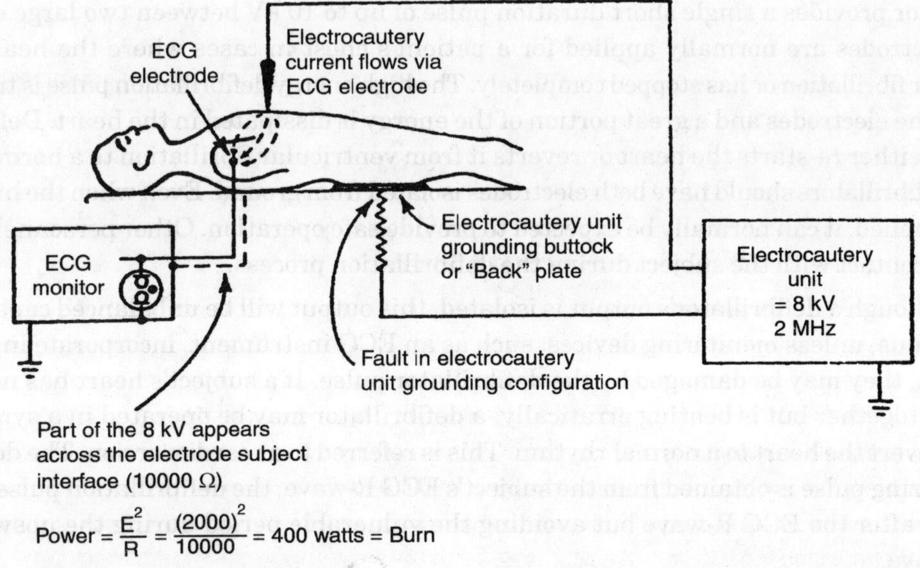

$$\text{Power} = \frac{E^2}{R} = \frac{(2000)^2}{10000} = 400 \text{ watts} = \text{Burn}$$

Fig. 15.15. Shows how the electrocautery diathermy unit causes burns at electrode site.

RF current for either cutting tissue or welding tissue together. The electrocautery probe provides a high frequency source of 2 MHz and up to 15 kV with respect to ground. When this probe is applied to the subject during surgery, current flows between this probe and ground. This unit is always used in conjunction with a large buttock plate underneath the subject in such a way as to provide a large surface. An electrocautery current of several amperes will thus flow between the electrocautery probe and the buttock plate. However, the energy dissipated will cause appreciable heating and burning only in the region of the probe as the current density flowing in the region of the large surface area buttock plate will be quite low.

Electrode Burns During Elecrocautery

If the electrocautery unit does not provide an excellent ground to the subject, either due to poor application or due to a fault within the buttock plate grounding circuit, then the electrocautery current will be diverted to other grounded points on the subject. It is not common for ECG electrodes to provide this alternative grounding point as all ECG monitoring equipment essentially provide a low impedance for the path to this high voltage, high frequency current. Unfortunately, the ECG electrode does not behave in the same manner as the buttock plate, as the contact area involved is smaller by a factor of at least 100, perhaps 1000. The current density is thus increased by a corresponding factor and will almost certainly cause heating and burns at the ECG sites. The high frequency current used in electrocautery is at higher frequency and will not cause ventricular fibrillation. In practice, if a surgeon suspects that the electrocautery unit "is not cutting too well" he should be suspicious of the electrocautery ground circuitry and should have the electrocautery unit adequately checked before continuing to use it.

Defibrillation

The defibrillator is another high voltage device commonly used in patient care units. The defibrillator provides a single short duration pulse of up to 10 kV between two large electrodes. These electrodes are normally applied for a patient's chest in cases where the heart got into ventricular fibrillation or has stopped completely. The high energy defibrillation pulse is transmitted between the electrodes and a great portion of the energy is dissipated in the heart. Defibrillation hopefully either re-starts the heart or reverts it from ventricular fibrillation to a normal beating action. Defibrillators should have both electrodes isolated from ground. Even when the high voltage pulse is applied, it can normally be expected to provide safe operation. Other personnel are not to have any contact with the subject during the defibrillation process.

Although a defibrillator's output is isolated, this output will be unbalanced capacitively to ground. Thus, unless monitoring devices, such as an ECG instrument, incorporate input circuit protection, they may be damaged by the defibrillator pulse. If a subject's heart has not stopped beating altogether but is beating erratically, a defibrillator may be operated in a synchronized mode to revert the heart to a normal rhythm. This is referred to as cardioversion. The defibrillator synchronizing pulse is obtained from the subject's ECG R-wave, the defibrillation pulse occurring sometime after the ECG R-wave but avoiding the vulnerable period during the upswing of the ECG T-wave.

CONCLUSION

In this Chapter, the essential requirements for operating and intensive care room safety considerations with respect to electric shock hazards were outlined with relevant examples as reported thus far. This does not mean that it is an exhaustive description. It is likely that with the newer and modern electronic equipment coming into use, new types of hazards are also more likely. Hence, the principles enunciated in this Chapter will have to be used in making safety assessments in any such room and persons should be trained in this aspect to make such assessment before handing over the room equipment to the care of medical personnel.

Chapter 16

Electro Chemical Instruments

The survival of a living cell and of a whole organism depends entirely on the existence of chemical reactions. These reactions are ordered and controlled by biological catalysts called enzymes. To understand the processes which characterize life, it is necessary to measure the molecular and ionic concentrations of the materials which participate in these reactions. Accordingly, the measurements of pH, pCO_2 and pO_2 are the main parameters in understanding the chemical energy exchanges which are called metabolism. This chapter deals with the methods to study the above parameters, and to study the methods of transduction of these quantities, as they appear in solution, into an electrical signal. The detection of other important ions, such as sodium, calcium and potassium are also done often clinically.

Electrode potential

The electrode potential measurement gives the concentration of ions in solution. Electrode potential is the potential developed at the interface between two material phases. For example, in the case of a metal—solution interface, an electrode potential results from the difference in rates between two opposing processes.

1. Passage of ions from the metal into the solution
2. The combination of metallic ions in solution with electrons in the metal to form atom of metal.

When equilibrium is reached, a layer of charge is formed in proximity to the electrode; that next to the electrode is of one sign, that in the solution is of the opposite. The charge distribution is called the electrical double layer. Although diffuse, the layer in its simplest form was considered by Helmholtz to be a uniform layer of charge. The double layer of charge constitutes a capacitance which is of importance in determining the electrical impedance of the interface. The potential appearing across the metal electrolyte interface at equilibrium is electrode potential. Table–1 gives the various ion- to metal potentials.

Table 1. Gives the Half cell potentials for various metals

Name of the metal	Potential (volts)
$Aluminum^{+++}$/aluminum	– 1.66
$Iron^{++}$/Iron	– 0.44
$Nickel^{++}$/nickel	– 0.250
$Lead^{++}$/lead	– 0.126

Hydrogen$^+$/hydrogen	0.0 (Reference)
Copper^{++}/copper	+ 0.337
Copper$^+$/copper	+ 0.521
Silver$^+$/silver	+ 0.799
Platinum^{++}/platinum	+ 1.2
Gold$^+$/gold	+ 1.68
Gold^{+++}/gold	+ 1.50

(Hand book of Chemistry and Physics)

(**Note.** the potentials are listed in the reference as oxidation potentials and accordingly carry a sign opposite to that shown here.)

An electrode potential is also developed if an interface is created by imposing a semipermeable barrier or membrane between two liquid phases so that the membrane allows irreversible transfer of a particular ion.

PHOTOELECTRIC TRANSDUCERS

In the measurement of physiological events in living subjects photoelectric transducers are employed in two ways;

1. As a detector to detect the intensity of light of a given wavelength
2. As a detector to detect intensity of light where the wavelength is relatively unimportant.

There are three types of photoelectric transducers. They are:

1. The photoemissive (phototube) transducers
2. The Photoconductive type
3. The Photo-electric type.

ELECTROCHEMICAL MEASUREMENT

As discussed earlier, a chemical sensor produces an electric signal which will be proportional to the concentration of the biochemical analytes. These sensors use chemical as well as physical principles in their operation.

A human body consists of several living cells. These cells are essentially a large number of chemical cells. The input to these cells is from metabolic food and the output from these cells is waste product. These are referred to as the building blocks for the organ system in the body. The functional status of an organ system is obtained by measuring the chemical input and output analysis of the cells. Generally, the majority of tests made in the hospital or the medical doctors deal with analyzing the chemistry of the body, before start of the clinical treatment for the patient if required or if he suspects for any uncommon symptom in the patient.

The important critical care analysis are :

The blood levels of pH, PO_2, PCO_2, hemotocrit, total hemoglobin, O_2 saturation, electrolytes including sodium, potassium calcium and chloride, and various metabolism such as Glucose, lactae, urea etc. Table-1 gives the normal ranges in blood for the above variables.

Table 2. Shows the Analysis of chemicals in the blood

Sl. No.	Blood gases and related parameter	Typical values	Electrolytes	Metabolites
1.	PO_2	80-104 mm Hg	Na^+ 135-155 m mol/l	Glucose 70-110 mg/100 ml
2.	PCO_2	33-48 mm Hg	K^+ 3.6-5.5 M mol/l	Lactate 3-7 mg/100 ml
3.	Ph	7.31-7.45	Ca^{2+} 1.14-1.31 Mmol/l	Creatinine 0.9-1.4 mg/100 ml
4.	Hematocrit	40-54%	Cl-98-109 m mol/l	Urea 8-26 mg/100 ml
5.	Total Hemoglobin	13-18 g/100 ml		
6.	O_2	95-100%		

The above parameters are normally analysed in a central clinical chemistry laboratory.

Measurement of pH

The measurement of pH is done by utilizing a glass electrode that generates an electric potential when solutions of differing pH are placed on the two sides of membrane. Since it is not possible to use the standard hydrogen electrode to determines pH here, the glass electrode is ordinarily employed. The schematic diagram of the pH electrode is shown in Fig. 16.1. The glass electrode is a belonging to the member of the class of ion–specific electrodes that react to any extent only with a particular ion.

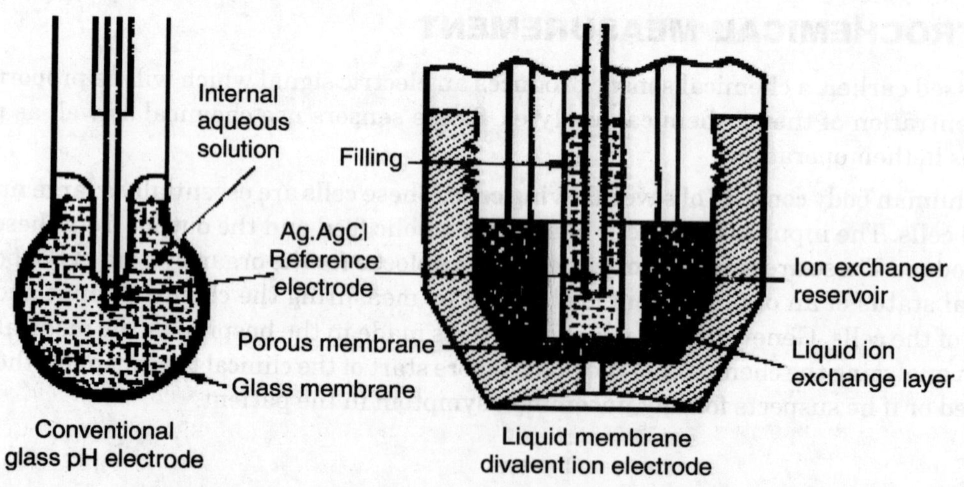

Fig. 16.1. (a) The Glass composite electrode for pH (b) Same.

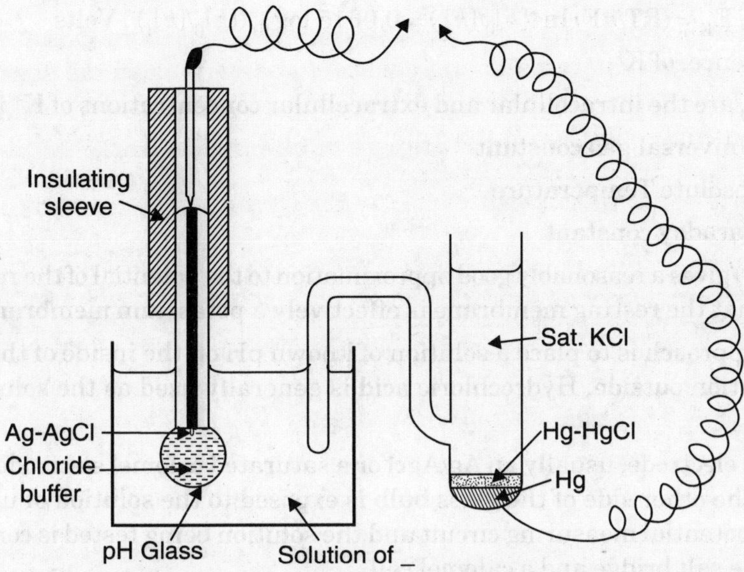

Fig. 16.1. (c) The Glass electrode used with the separate calomel reference electrode for pH measurement.

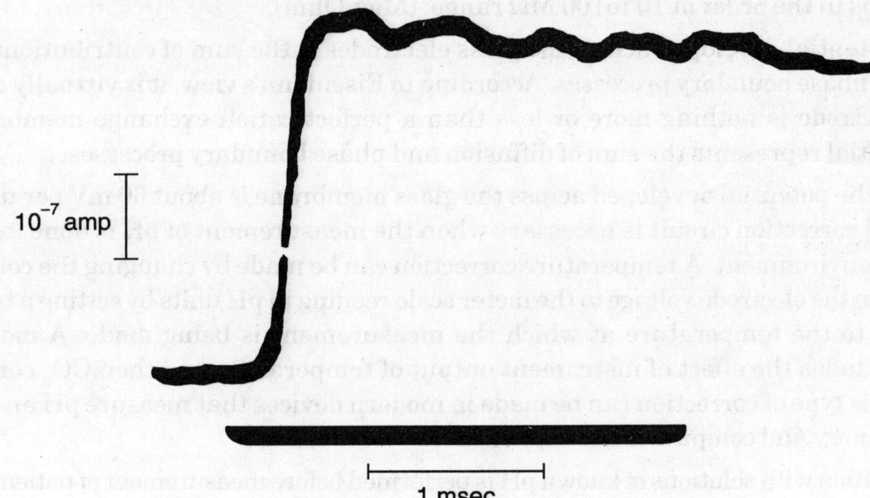

Fig. 16.1. (d) Response time of an open type PO_{2e} Electrode.

The glass electrode consists of a thin glass membrane which permits the passage of only hydrogen ions. (in the form of (H_3O^+). The usual configuration consists of a spherical bulb of 6 mm diameter. On the inside of the pH-responsive glass bulb is placed a buffer solution usually of pH = 1 which is immersed in an Ag-AgCl nonpolarizable electrode.

The approach of a hydrogen ion to outside of the membrane causes the silicate structure of the glass to conduct positive charge (hole) into the ionic solution inside the electrode. As per Nernst equation (1) given below, the voltage developed across the membrane changes by 60 mV/ pH unit. The Physiological change of pH is only 0.06 units, the pH meter must be able to measure accurately the change in pH value in the order of only 0.01 mV.

$$E_K = (RT/nF) \ln ([k]_0/[k]_i) = 0.0615 \log_{10} ([k]_0/[k]_I) \text{ . Volts} \quad \dots (1)$$

where n is the valence, of K^+,

$[k]_i$ and $[k]_0$ are the intracellular and extracellular concentrations of K^+ in one liter

R = Universal gas constant

T = absolute Temperature

F = Faraday constant

Equation (1) gives a reasonably good approximation to the potential of the resting membrane, which indicates that the resting membrane is effectively a potassium membrane.

The basic approach is to place a solution of known pH on the inside of the membrane and the unknown solution outside. Hydrochloric acid is generally used as the solution with known pH.

A reference electrode, usually an Ag/Agcl or a saturated calomel electrode, is placed in this solution. That is the other side of the glass bulb is exposed to the solution of unknown pH. The connection of the potential measuring circuit and the solution being tested is completed though a potassium chloride salt bridge and a calomel cell.

The potential developed across the membrane of the glass electrode is read on the meter provided which will generally have a high input impedance because the internal impedance of the pH electrode is in the order of 10 to100 MΩ range. (Meg-Ohm).

The potential developed across the glass electrodes is the sum of contributions from both diffusion and phase boundary processes. According to Eisemann's view, it is virtually certain that the glass electrode is nothing more or less than a perfect cation exchange membrane whose electric potential represents the sum of diffusion and phase boundary processes.

Thus, the potential developed across the glass membrane is about 60 mV per unit of pH at 30°C. A small correction circuit is necessary when the measurement of pH is done in a different temperature environment. A temperature correction can be made by changing the constant used to convert from the electrode voltage to the meter scale reading in pH units by setting a temperature control knob to the temperature at which the measurement is being made. A more complex correction includes the effect of instrument output of temperature and then CO_2 content of the specimen. This type of correction can be made in modern devices that measure pH and PCO_2 and also have memory and computational capabilities.

Calibration with solutions of known pH is performed before measurement of patient specimens are made.

The glass electrode made the determination of pH in the laboratory as a simple and routine procedure. Bull (1943) listed the following advantages of the glass electrode.

1. The glass electrode is independent of oxidation reduction potentials.
2. It is not required to pass a gas through the solution or to add any material to it.
3. It is possible to use a vary small quantities of solution sample.
4. It is possible to use this electrode for coloured or for turbid solutions.
5. The electrode gives accurate values in unbuffered solution.
6. Equilibrium is reached rapidly.

Of course, the electrode has some of the disadvantages. They are :

1. The range of measurement is restricted unless a Special glass is used for the electrode. (for example, some error often exists in both highly acidic solutions (near pH = 0) and alkaline solutions (above pH = 9).

Because the pH is determined by measuring the potential developed across the pH glass electrode, it is important that the magnitude of the potential be accurately measured. A simple meter using an LCD display panel meter module is shown below, using front end high input impedance Operational amplifier.

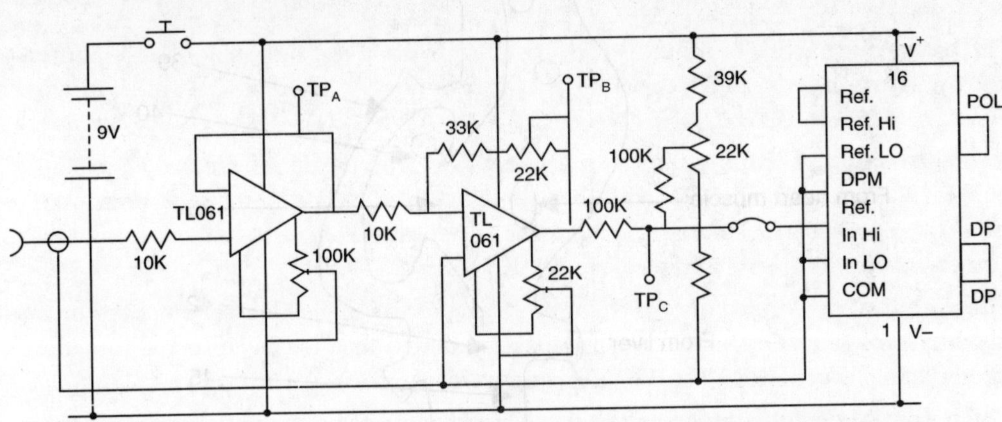

Fig. 16.2. The circuit for a simple pH meter using OPA TL 061 and LCD panel meter.

MEASUREMENT OF PO_2

The term PO_2 (oxygen tension) P = partial pressure

Fig. 16.3 shows PO_2 of blood at various places in the inferior vena cava and right of heart. The liver and heart are big consumers of O_2; kidneys do not, nor the muscles (at rest).

DALTON'S LAW

The pressure exerted by a gas in a mixture of gases is equal to the pressure the same quantity of gas would exert in isolation. For example, dry atmosphere exerts 760mm Hg pressure. Oxygen which makes up to 20.96% of atmosphere thus accounts for 20.96% × 760 = 157.2 mm. If we bubbled air through a sample of blood, the air and blood would rapidly come into equilibrium such that the blood could take up no more oxygen. The blood PO_2 would then be 15.2 mm Hg. The air in the alveoli of the lungs contains 14.2% of oxygen and water vapor equivalent to 45 mm Hg. Because PO_2 is always expressed in terms of dry air, we must subtract the 45 mm from 760 to get the partial pressure of alveolar oxygen: 14.2 % of (760-45) = 101.53 mm Hg.

The average PO_2 of venous blood is 40mm Hg, that of arterial blood is 100 mm Hg. In other words, blood comes into perfect equilibrium with the alveolar air during its passage through the lungs (in as little as 0.3 sec).

All photometric methods for determining the PO_2 of the blood depend on the different light reflection characteristics of Hemoglobin (Hb) and HbO_2. Note that at wavelength 6.1×10^{-7} meters (orange part of the spectrum), the difference between the two is at the maximum ; HbO_2 absorbs much less orange than Hemoglobin–hence its bright red appearance . But at wavelength of 8×10^{-7} m (800 nm) (in the infra red) Hemoglobin and HbO_2 absorb identical amounts of light. Here, then, is the basis for measurement: one wavelength at which the two substances behave identically, another at which their difference is maximum. NB : visible light – 3600 – 7700°A.

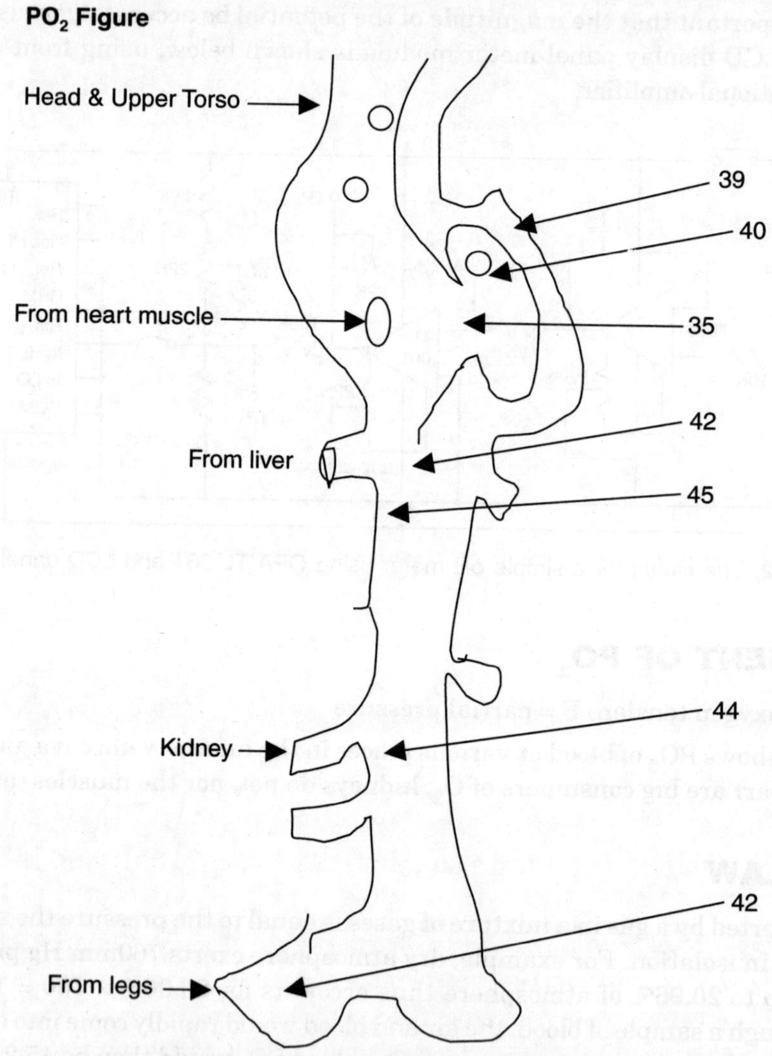

Fig.16.3. Shows PO_2 Oxygen Tension.

Basic design of reflection photometer is outlined. Two photocells are set back to back and wired in opposition to each other. To set up the light is shone into a cuvette filled with Indian ink. The signal from the compensating cell is adjusted , through the variable compensating resistance, giving zero deflection. This eliminates the effect of light reflected from cuvette glass. The next reading is taken with a standard dye and the "sensitivity "control adjusted to give a standard deflection. A blood–filled cuvette is then exposed to light filtered at 610 and then at 800 millimicrons and the two readings can be interpreted in terms of blood PO_2.

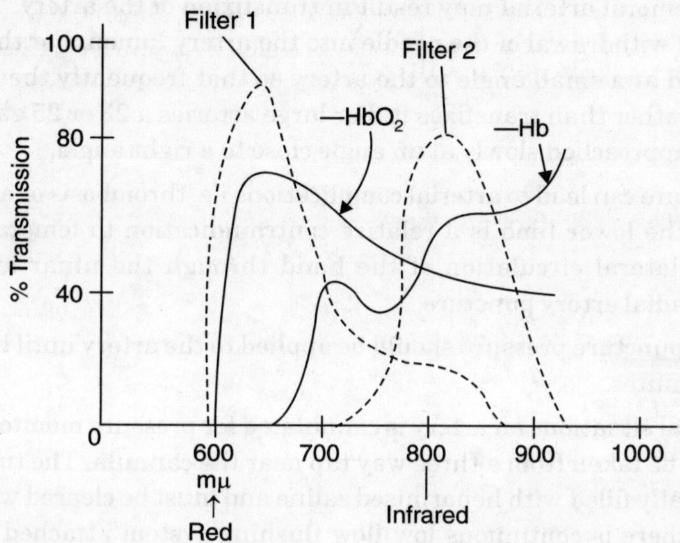

Fig. 16.4. Shows the Isobestic curve and schematic of measurement.

Errors: to Anemia (less Hb conc.)

To Hemoglobin (destroyal of red cells and Hb in plasma)

Formaldehyde vapor in pathology lab.

Dyes in blood (patient underwent Dye solution test).

PRESENT TECHNIQUES FOR MEASURING pH STATUS

pH electrode, Blood sampling

Having seen pH measurement in general, it is enough to say that pH of biological fluids is measured likewise using a glass electrode. A simple description of the glass electrode for pH was given above.

A blood sample for measuring pH parameters is collected in a glass syringe which is lubricated and heparinised. Heparin solution 1000 units/ml is used to wet the inside of the syringe and the excess emptied out leaving the dead space filled with solution. When as is usual now a plastic syringe is used to take blood samples for assessment of pH status the material of the syringe should not allow the diffusion of gas. Some commercially available blood gas syringes allow gas diffusion.

Arterial puncture is performed and the blood should fill the syringe under its own pressure. Verification that the blood sample is from an artery is important. Movement of the plunger of the syringe with the pulse is a necessary condition.

The common sites for arterial puncture are the radial, femoral or brachial arteries. Less common sites are the superficial temporal or dorsalis pedis arteries. The technique for puncture of the brachial and femoral arterial may result in transfixion of the artery. The sample is then obtained during slow withdrawal of the needle into the artery lumen. For the radial artery the needle should be held at a small angle to the artery so that frequently the needle goes up the lumen of the artery rather than transfixes it. For large arteries a 23 or 25 gauge needle may be used and the artery approached slowly at an angle close to a right angle.

Arterial puncture can lead to arterial complications i.e. thrombosis or embolus. Peripheral vascular disease in the lower limb is a relative contraindication to femoral artery puncture. Absence of good collateral circulation of the hand through the ulnar artery is a relative contraindication to radial artery puncture.

After arterial puncture pressure should be applied to the artery until bleeding stops. This usually takes five minutes.

In many clinical situations an artery is cannulated for pressure monitoring. In these cases arterial samples can be taken from a three way tap near the cannula. The tube between the tap and the artery is usually filled with heparinised saline and must be cleared with blood before the sample is taken. If there is continuous low flow flushing system attached this should not be reconnected between the flushing of the system with blood and the attachment of the syringe to collect the blood sample. That is the 3 way tap should be turned to 45° between clearing of the line and the taking of the sample.

Any air in the syringe should be removed and then the syringe capped and labelled. If analysis cannot be done immediately the syringe should be cooled in a container containing ice and water and sent to the laboratory.

Use of some plastic syringes, excessive amount of heparin and the presence of small bubbles of air in the blood may lead to errors in the results, but these will usually not be critical in the clinical situation in adults and large children. There are micro-techniques available for use in small children and neonates. When these are used the technique of collection of the blood samples is critical.

The Astrup Method

This requires three measurements to be made:

(*i*) pH of arterial blood collected anaerobically (actual pH),

(*ii*) and (*iii*) pH of two samples of the same blood after equilibration with two standard gases containing known partial pressures of CO_2. The Siggaard-Andersen nomogram is a log PCO_2-pH graph.

(*ii*) and (*iii*) are plotted on it and a straight line drawn through the points. On this plot the PCO2-pH line is approximately straight. From the log PCO_2-pH line can be read

(*a*) PCO_2 at pH of the anaerobically collected arterial blood, *i.e.*, $PaCO_2$.

(*b*) pH at $PaCO_2$ = 40mmHg, *i.e.*, non-respiratory pH.

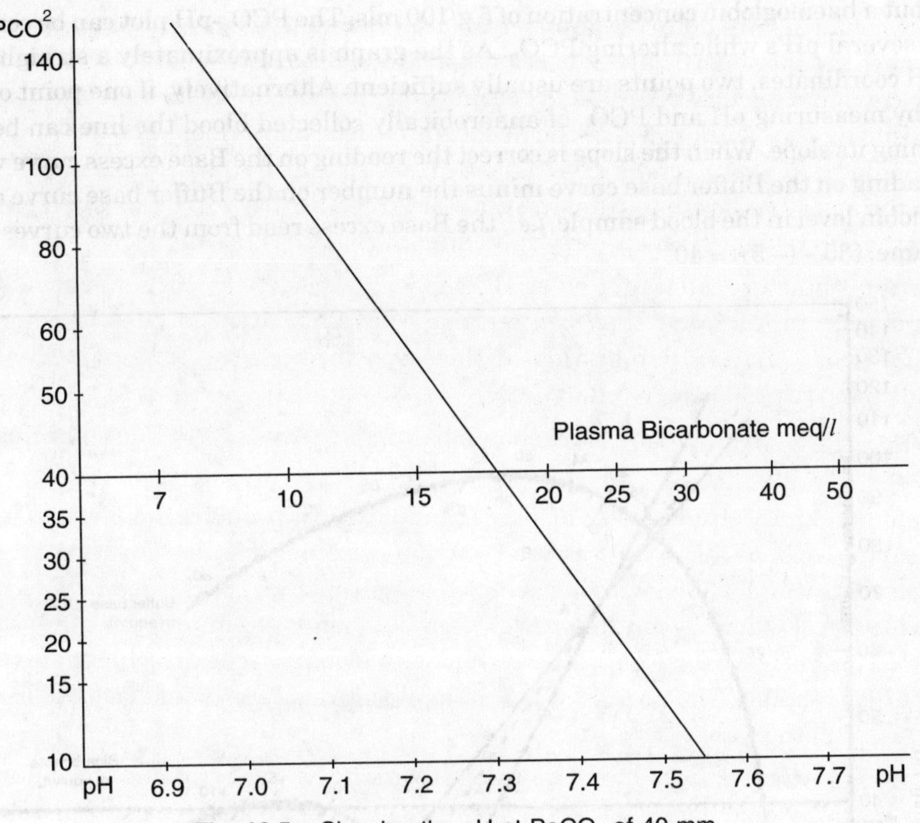

Fig. 16.5a. Showing the pH at $PaCO_2$ of 40 mm.

pH and PCO_2 Electrode Systems

A PCO_2 electrode is a pH electrode surrounded by a layer of electrolyte solution and calibrated for PCO_2. With this and a pH electrode actual pH and actual $PaCO_2$ can be measured. Other acid-base parameters can be calculated or derived from Siggaard-Andersen nomogram using pH, $PaCO_2$ and haemoglobin. The pH and PCO_2 set one point on the plot and the haemoglobin determines the slope.

Either of the methods will give:

(*i*) pH (actual in patient).

(*ii*) $PaCO_2$ (actual in patient).

(*iii*) Non-respiratory pH (pH at PCO_2 = 40 mmHg).

The actual pH, the $PaCO_2$ (or $[H_2CO_3]$) and non-respiratory pH are derived by measuring the blood pH and constructing the pH/PCO_2 titration curve. This curve is approximately a straight line on pH/log PCO_2 coordinates. It is called a "buffer" line although "pH/log PCO_2" line is a better description. The $PaCO_2$ is read off at the point where the pH/log PCO_2 line crosses the actual pH value :

This is a PCO_2-pH plot. I and II represent PCO_2-pH plots for two samples with pH 7.08 and PCO_2 70 mmHg. I is plasma. II is whole blood. III represents a similar plot for a fluid containing plasma but a haemoglobin concentration of 5 g/100 mls. The PCO_2-pH plot can be constructed by plotting several pH's while altering PCO_2. As the graph is approximately a straight line on log PCO_2-pH coordinates, two points are usually sufficient. Alternatively, if one point on the plot is defined by measuring pH and PCO_2 of anaerobically collected blood the line can be defined by determining its slope. When the slope is correct the reading on the Base excess curve will be equal to the reading on the Buffer base curve minus the number on the Buffer base curve opposite the Haemoglobin level in the blood sample, *i.e.*, the Base excess read from the two curves will have to be the same. (35 – (– 5)) = 40.

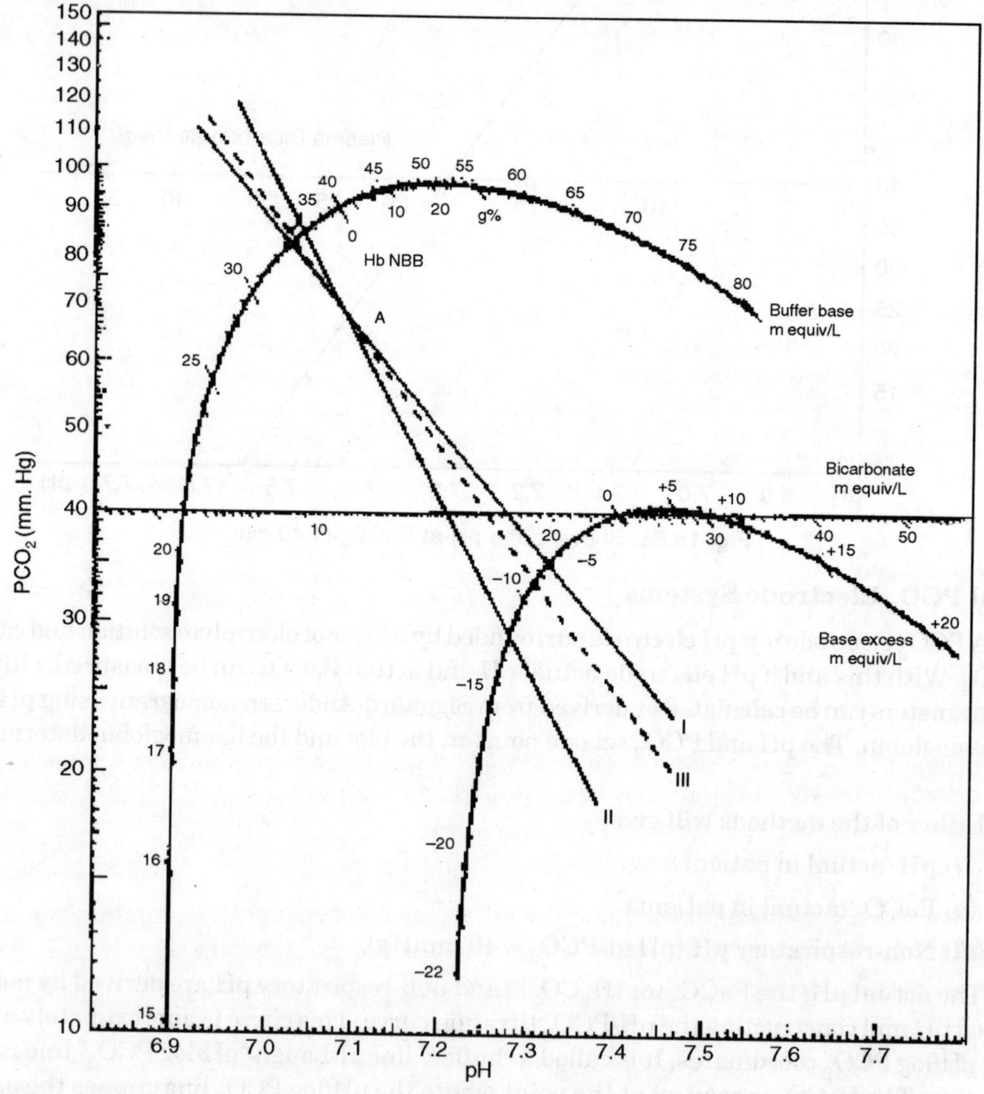

Fig. 16.5b. The nomogram method for finding PCO_2.-Siggaard-Andersen Nomogram.

Figure copied from O.Siggaard-Andersen. Therapeutic Aspects of Acid-Base Balance from Modern Trends in Anaesthesia, 3rd Ed. F.T. Evans and T.C. Gray. Pub. Butterworths, 1967, p.102.

The non-respiratory pH is read off at the point where the line crosses the isobar $PCO_2 = 40$ mmHg-see Figures below:

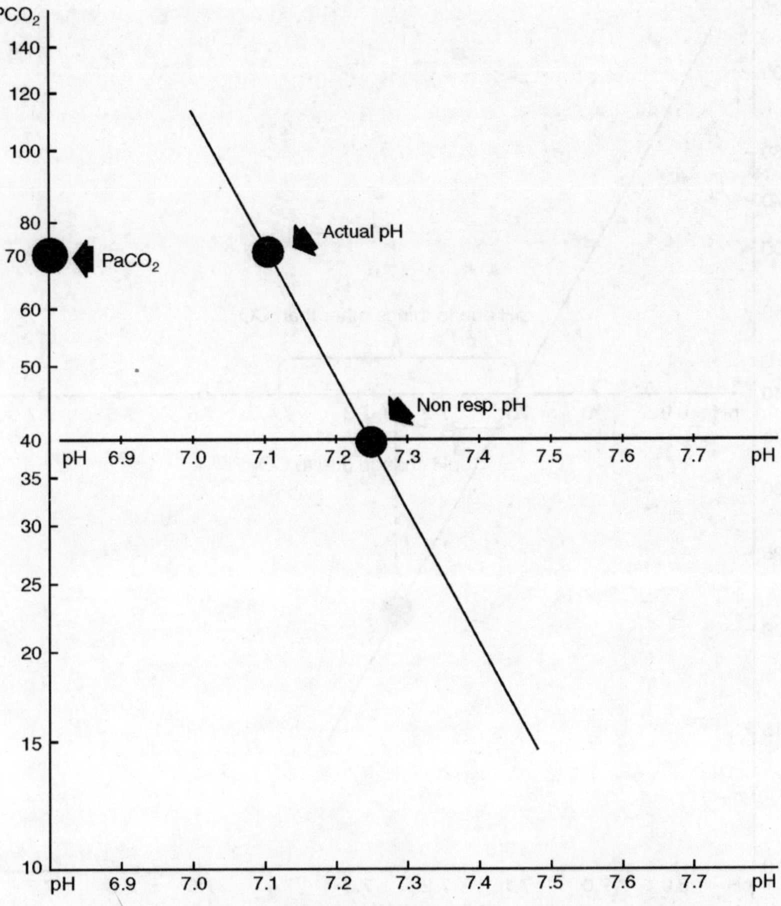

Fig. 16.6. Method showing the pH change due to CO_2.

Non-respiratory pH. A Siggaard-Andersen Nomogram on which a pH/PCO_2 line has been plotted and the actual pH marked. Non-respiratory pH is where the pH/PCO_2 line crosses the $PCO_2 = 40$ mmHg line. In this case it is 7.1 (actual pH).

Non-respiratory pH plotted as in Fig. 16.6. In this case non-respiratory pH is 7.23 (approx).

7.4 minus non-respiratory pH equals the fall in pH due to acids other than carbonic or to bases (change in pH due to non-respiratory acids or bases). Non-respiratory pH minus actual pH equals the fall in pH due to carbonic acid (change in pH due to respiratory (carbonic) acid). Negative results equal rises.

Separation of pH changes due to CO_2 from those due to other acids or bases. This plot is the same as in Figure 16.7. pH change due to CO_2 is + 0.14 units. pH change to other acids and bases is – 0.3 units.

Separation of pH changes due to CO_2 from those due to other acids or bases. This plot is the same as in Figure c. pH change due to CO_2 is – 1.3 units. pH change due to other acids or bases is – 1.7 units.

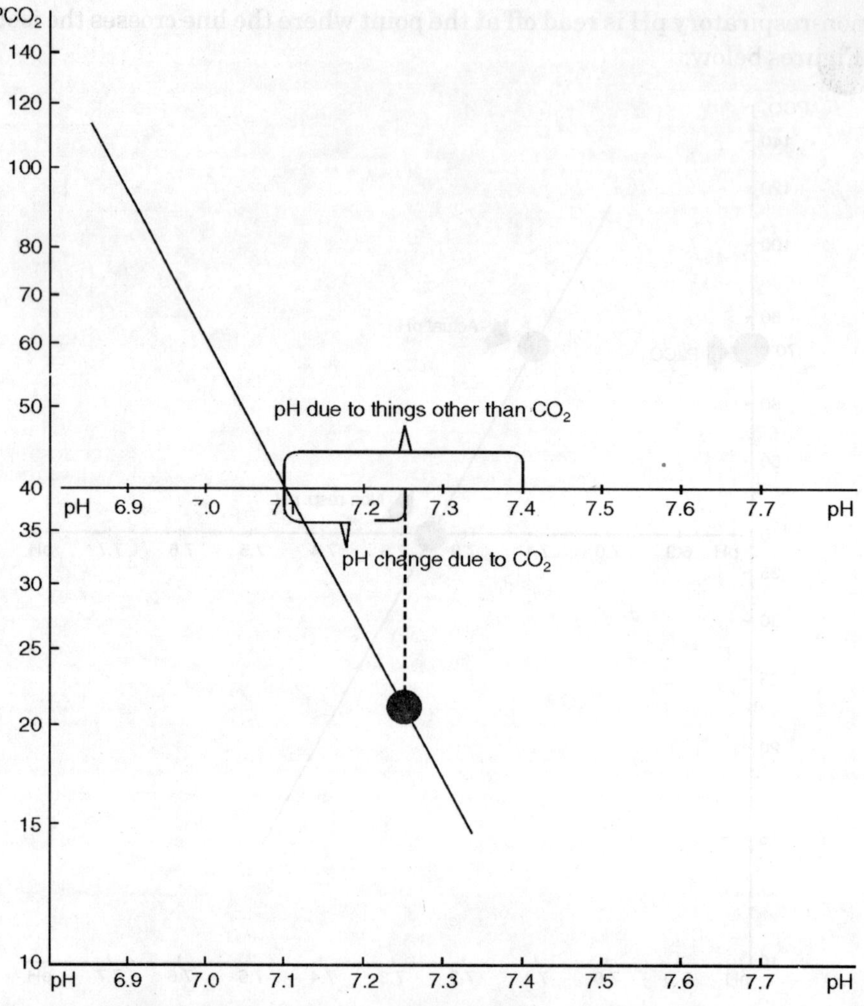

Fig. 16.7. Method showing the pH change due to CO_2.

SUMMARY

A. Actual pH of the blood may be changed by changes.

1. In carbonic acid, and/or

2. In acids other than carbonic, or in bases.

B. If the PCO_2 is corrected to normal (40 mm Hg) the resulting pH deviation from 7.4 (7.4 minus non-respiratory pH) is due to acids other than carbonic or to bases.

C. Any other deviation in pH (non-respiratory pH minus actual pH) is due to carbonic acid changes.

D. The primary disurbance usually produces the greater change in pH.

TABLE 2. Showing possible combinations of actual pH, $PaCO_2$ and non-respiratory pH. To show compatibility between this system and the base excess/standard bicarbonate system (Section 4.3), these parameters are also noted.

Actual pH	$PaCO_2$	Non-resp. pH	Base excess	Status
N	N	N	0	Normal
□	□	N	0	Acute resp. alkalosis (a)
□	□	□	Negative	Chronic resp. alkalosis with renal compensation
□	□	□	Negative	Chronic resp. alkalosis
□	□	□	Positive	Non-resp. alkalosis with respiratory compensation
□	□	N	0	Acute resp. acidosis(a) without compensation
□	□	□	Positive	Chronic CO_2 retention with compensation(b)
□	N	□	Negative	Non-resp. acidosis without respiratory compensation
N	□	□	Negative	Complete compensation or
N	□	□	Positive	Mixed disturbance
□	□	□	Negative	Mixed respiratory and non-respiratory acidosis
□	□	□	Positive	Mixed respiratory and non-respiratory alkalosis

Measuring Acidosis or alkalosis

Acidity and alkalinity of blood and urine are of great diagnostic value.

Depends upon hydrogen ion concentration (H^+)

A strong alkali has 10^{-14} gm of H^+ per liter.

A strong acid has 10^{0}(*i.e.*, 1 gm) of H^+ per litre.

Take log scale, we get 0 to + 14.

By conversion, $pH = -\log (H^+)$

The mid point is 7, the pH of pure water.

Acids 0 to 7 **Akalines 7–14.**

Uses a glass electrode–tubular membrane of special glass (5.0 mm dia, 0.4 mm thick)

Blood volume needed is 1 cc.

In healthy blood , pH never stays for long outside 7.37 to 7.45. (*i.e.*, alkaline even though the end products of metabolism are acidity).

Metabolic process

↓

Initial 'Lactate' chain

↓

Glycogen converted to Lactic acid

80% of this acid are constructed to glycogen. Remaining parts together with proteins and fats goes through a complex cycle reaction called 'Krebs cycle' whose end products are CO_2 and water.

$$CO_2 + H_2O \rightleftharpoons H_2CO_3$$

Most of the steps in this process yield energy.

The acidic end products tend to increase the blood H^+ concentration. This is defended by

1. Buffers that mop up H^+ ions. Alkaline hemoglobin (kHb) in the red cell tends to mop up H^+ ions and fixes them temporarily as acid Hb (HHb). The product of this reaction is HCO_3 which diffuses into the plasma and further depletes H^+ ions by

$$H^+ + HCO_3 \longrightarrow H_2CO_3$$

2. At the lung there is a sharp change in the partial pressures of CO_2 and O_2 (compared with the tissues). The blood with PCO_2 of 46 meets the lung ($PCO_2 = 40$) surface and the reaction.

$$H^+ + HCO_3 \longrightarrow CO_2 + H_2O$$

is driven forward, reducing the H^+ ions in the blood.

The kidneys quite simply have the ability to pull H^+ ions out of the blood (urine pH is 5–6). Strong acids produced by metabolism drive the equilibrium in such a way that the weakly acidic bicarbonate is produced in their stead.

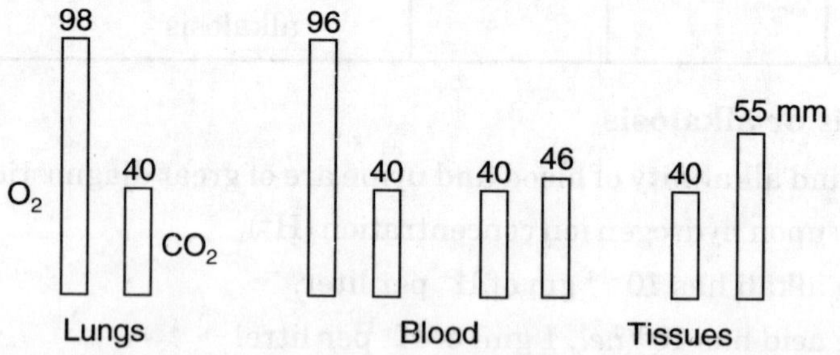

Fig. 16.8. Partial pressures of O_2 and CO_2 in lungs, blood + tissues.

TABLE. Partial pressures of O_2 + CO_2 in lungs, blood + tissues

The kidneys provide the coarse adjustment of pH. The lungs finely adjust it.

If a patient has poor lungs, the CO_2 will not be removed very efficiently leading to a fall in blood pH. The kidneys then step up their export of H^+ and retain HCO_3 above the normal level (24 mg/l).

On the other hand, if the patient's kidneys were poor or has circulation restricted, there will be a rise in blood activity and his lungs will vent more CO_2 to compensate.

Fall in blood pH is called 'acidosis'—can be due to

1. Rise in PCO_2^+ because of faulty lungs.
2. Fall on HCO_3^- because of faults in kidneys, circulation, Blood pressure (BP) and metabolism. 'Alkalosis' (rise in pH) may be due to fall in PCO_2 due to hysterical overbreathing or to a rise in HCO_3^{+-} through some other organic failure. If the PCO_2 alone changes it is called **'respiratory acidosis or alkalosis'**. If the HCO_3^- alone changes it is called **'metabolic acidosis'**. The distinction localizes the seat of failure.

By measuring the pH, PCO_2 and HCO_3^- concentrations in the blood plasma , we can tell to within fine limits about the patient. The patient's blood is sampled into three parts. One part is measured for pH. The other is shaken in an atmosphere with CO_2 well below the normal level and the third with an atmosphere well above normal CO_2 (54 and 27 mm Hg respectively). (4% CO_2 in O_2 + 8% CO_2 in O_2).

By measuring the pH of these samples, we can plot an upper and lower point on the graph and connect them with a line on which patient's actual pH must lie. Reading across this line, we can tell this actual PCO_2.

The four lines radiating from the normal point define pure states of respiratory and metabolic acidosis or alkalosis.

The PCO_2 Electrodes and Measurement by Electrode Method

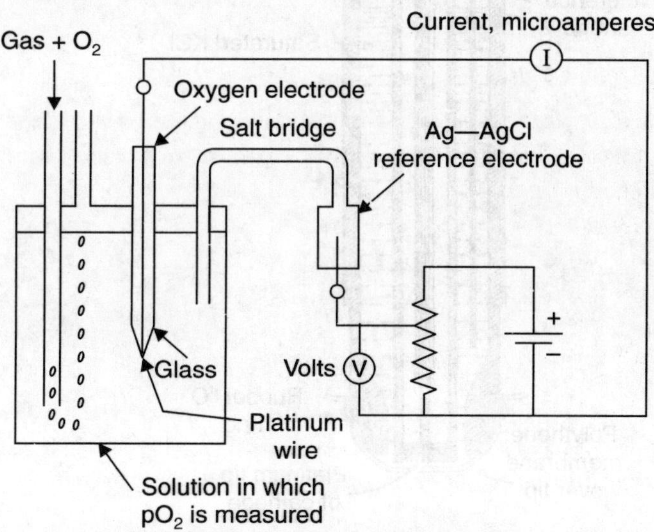

Fig. 16.8. The PO_2 Electrode.

It consists of a standard pH electrode covered with a rubber membrane permeable to CO_2. Between the glass surface and the membrane was a thin film of water. The solution under test, which contained dissolved CO_2, was presented to the outer surface of the rubber membrane. The film of water equilibrated with the CO_2 solution under test by diffusion of CO_2 across the membrane. After equilibration, the pH of the aqueous film was measured by the glass electrode and interpreted in terms of pCO_2 on the basis of the linear relationship between log pCO_2 and pH (as described by the Henderson-Hasselbalch equations).

The Stow pCO_2 electrode was improved by Severinghaus and Bradely (1958), who showed both analytically and experimentally that the sensitivity of the electrode could be doubled by including bicarbonate ion in the aqueous medium between the rubber membrane and the glass electrode. These investigators have found the wet Teflon backed with a layer of cellophane 0.002 inch thick was superior membrane. The optimum aqueous solution consisted of 0.01 M $NaHCO_3$ and 0.1 *M* NaCl in which the cellophane had been soaked for several hours. In addition to these modifications of 'Stow's electrode, Severinghaus and Bradely added NaCl to the solution surrounding the silver reference electrode, thus increasing the conductivity of this solution and stabilizing the reference electrode. The resulting modified CO_2 electrode was twice as sensitive and drifted much less than before. The response time was as such that equilibrium was reached in about 2 minutes after a fourfold rise in CO_2 and in about 4 minutes after fourfold fall in CO_2.

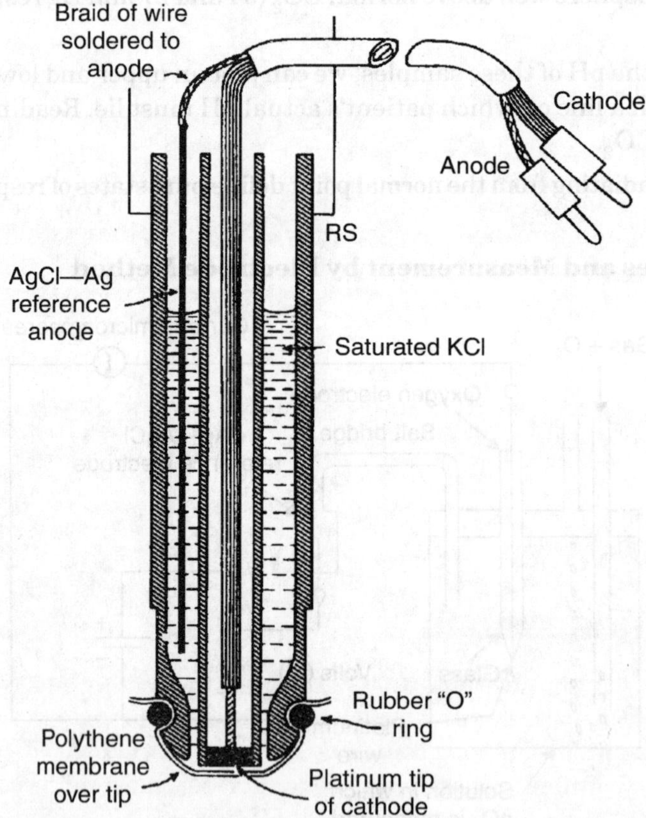

Fig. 16.10. The Clark-type pO_2 electrode. [From B.J. Sproule et al., J. Appl. Physiol. 11:365—370 (1957). By permission.]

OXYGEN SATURATION MEASUREMENT BY MEMBRANE METHOD

The choice of the semi-permeable membrane is based on the trade off between consumption of O_2 and the time required for the PO_2 values in the specimen and measurement chambers to equilibrate.

The more permeable the membrane to O_2, the higher the consumption of O_2 and the faster the response. Polypropylene is less permeable than Teflon and is preferable in most applications. Polypropylene is also quite durable, and it maintains its position over the electrode more reliably than other membrane materials.

The membrane thickness and composition determine the O_2 diffusion rate; thicker membranes extend the sensor time response by significantly increasing the diffusion time and produce smaller currents.

Because the electrode consumes O_2, it partially depletes the oxygen in the immediate vicinity of the membrane. If movement of the sample takes place, undepleted solution brought to the membrane causes a higher instrument reading—the "stirring" artifact. This is avoided by waiting for a stagnant equilibrium to occur.

The reaction is very sensitive to temperature. To maintain a linear relationship between PO_2 and current, the temperature of the electrode must be controlled to ± 0.1°C. This has been traditionally accomplished by using a water jacket. However, new blood-gas analyzers are now available that use precision electronic heat sources. The current through the meter is approximately 10 nA/mm Hg (75 nA/kPa) O_2 at 37°C, so the instruments must be designed to be accurate at very low current levels.

The system is calibrated by using two gases of known O_2 concentration. One gas with no O_2 (typically a CO_2—N_2 mixture) and a second with a known O_2 content (usually an O_2—CO_2—N_2 mixture) are used. The specimen chamber is filled with water, and the calibrating gas containing no O_2 is bubbled through it. The PO_2 meter output is set to zero after equilibrium of O_2 content is achieved-usually in about 90 s. Next the second calibrating gas is used to determine the second point on the PO_2-versus-electrode-current calibration scale, which is electrically set in the machine. Then the value of the specimen PO_2 can be measured. Note that the time required to reach equilibrium is a function of the PO_2 of the specimen. It may take as long as 360 s for a specimen with a PO_2 of 430 mm Hg (57 kPa) to reach equilibrium (Moran et al., 1966). Dragerwerk Aktiengesellschaft, Lubeck, Germany, manufactures a gas O_2 sensor with 2-s response in which gas diffuse into a PO_2 electrode.

CHEMICAL FIBROSENSORS

Rapid advances in the communications industry have provided appropriate small optical fibers, high-energy sources such as lasers, and wavelength detectors. The fiber-optic sensors that were developed were called optodes, a term coined by Lubbers and Opitz (1975). Which implies that optical sensors are very similar to electrodes. As we shall see, however, the properties and operating principles for optical fibrosensors are quite different from those for electrodes. The term optrode, with an r, is currently used.

Chemical fibrosensors offer several desirable features.

1. They can be made small in size.
2. Multiple sensors can be introduced together, through a catheter, for intracranial or intravascular measurements.
3. Because optical measurements are being made, there are not electric hazards to the patient.

4. The measurements are immune to external electric interference, provided that the electronic instrumentation is properly shielded.
5. No reference electrode is necessary.

In addition, fibro-sensors have a high degree of flexibility and good thermal Stability, and low-cost manufacturing and disposable usage are possible. In reversible sensors, the reagent phase is not consumed by its reaction with the analyte. In nonreversible sensors, the reagent phase is consumed. The consumption of the reagent phase for nonreversible sensors must be small or there must be a way to replenish the reagent.

Optical-fiber sensors have several limitations when compared with electrode sensors. Optical sensors are sensitive to ambient light, so they must be used in a dark environment or must be optically shielded via opaque materials. The optical signal may also have to be modulated in order to code it and make it distinguishable from the ambient light. The dynamic response of optical sensors is normally limited compared with that of electrodes. Reversible indicator sensors are based on an equilibrium measurement rather than a diffusion-dependent one, so they are less susceptible to changes in flow concentration at the sensor (Seitz, 1988).

Long-term stability for optical sensors may be a problem for reagent based systems. However, this can be compensated for by the use of multiple wavelength detection and by the ease of changing reagent phases. In addition, because the reagent and the analyte are in different phases, a mass-transfer step is necessary before constant response is achieved (Seitz, 1988). This limits the temporal response of an optical sensor. Another consideration with optical sensors is that for several types of optical sensor, the response is proportional to the amount of reagent phase. For small amounts of reagent, an increased response can be achieved by increasing the intensity of the source. An increased response, however, results in an increase in the photo-degradation process of the reagent. Designers of optical sensors, then, must consider amount of the reagent phase, intensity of the light source, and system stability (Seitz, 1984).

These limitations can be alleviated by an appropriate design of the optical sensor and instrumentation system (Wise, 1990). The systems described in the following paragraphs incorporate many features specifically for this purpose.

INTRAVASCULAR MEASUREMENTS OF OXYGEN SATURATION

Blood oxygen can be monitored by means of an intravascular fiber-optic catheter. These catheters are used to monitor mixed venous oxygen saturation during cardiac surgery and in the intensive-care unit. A Swan-Ganz catheter is used, in which a flow-directed fiber-optic catheter is placed into the right jugular vein. The catheter is advanced until its distal tip is in the right atrium, at which time the balloon is inflated. The rapid flow of blood carries the catheter into the pulmonary artery.

Measurements of mixed venous oxygen saturation give an indication of the effectiveness of a cardiopulmonary system. Measurements of high oxygen saturation in the right side of the heart may indicate congenital abnormalities of the heart and major vessels or the inability of tissue to metabolize oxygen. Low saturation readings on the left side of the heart may indicate a reduced ability of the lungs to oxygenate the blood or of the cardiopulmonary system to deliver oxygen from the lungs. Low saturation readings in the arterial system indicate a compromised cardiac output or reduced oxygen-carrying capacity of the blood.

Fig. 16.10 shows the optical-absorption spectra for oxyhemoglobin, carboxyhemoglobin, hemoglobin, and methemoglobin. Measurements in the red region are possible because the absorption coefficient of blood at these wavelengths is sufficiently low so that light can be transmitted through whole blood over a distance such that feasible measurements can be made with fiber-optic catheters. Note that the 805-nm wavelength provides a measurement independent of the degree of oxygenation. This isosbestic wavelength is used to compensate for the scattering properties of the whole blood and to normalize the measurement signal with any changes in hemoglobin from patient.

Oxygen saturation is measured by taking the ratio of the diffusely backscattered light intensities at two wavelengths. The first wavelength is in the red region (660 nm); the second is in the infrared region (805 nm); which is known as the isosbestic point for Hb and HbO_2, Oxygen saturation considers the optical density of the blood-the light transmitted through the blood-according to Beer's law. For hemolyzed blood (blood with red cells ruptured), Beer's law holds, and the absorbance (optical density) at any wavelength is.

$$A(\lambda) = WL\,[a_o(\lambda)C_o + a_r(\lambda)\,C_r]$$

where W = weight of hemoglobin per unit volume

L = optical path length

a_o and a_r = absorptivities of HbO_2 and Hb

C_o and C_r = relative concentrations of HbO_2 and Hb

$(C_o + C_r = 1.0)$

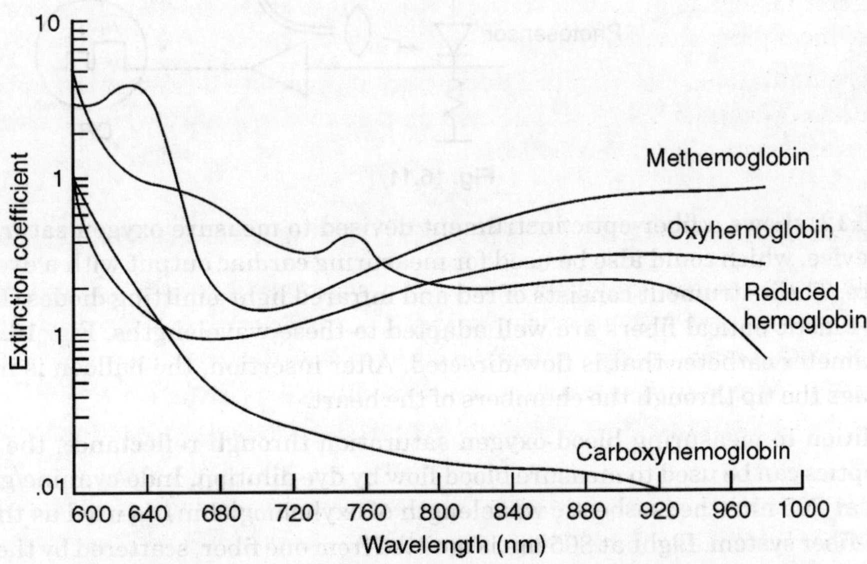

Fig. 16.10 shows that a_o and a_r are equal at 805 nm, called the isosbestic wavelength. If this wavelength is λ_2, then

$$WL = \frac{A(\lambda_2)}{a(\lambda_2)}$$

where $a(\lambda_2) = a_o(\lambda_2) = a_r(\lambda_2)$ as (λ_2 is isobestic) and $C_o + C_r = 1$.

Therefore $$A(\lambda) = \frac{A(\lambda_2)}{a(\lambda_2)} [a_o(\lambda)C_o + a_r(\lambda)C_r]$$

When absorbance is measured at a second wavelength λ_1, the oxygen saturation is given by

$$C_o = x + \frac{yA(\lambda_1)}{A(\lambda_2)}$$

Where x and y are constants that depend only on the optical characteristics of blood. In practice, λ_1 is chosen to be that wavelength at which the difference between a_o and a_r is a maximum, which occurs at 660 nm. (Fig. 16.11).

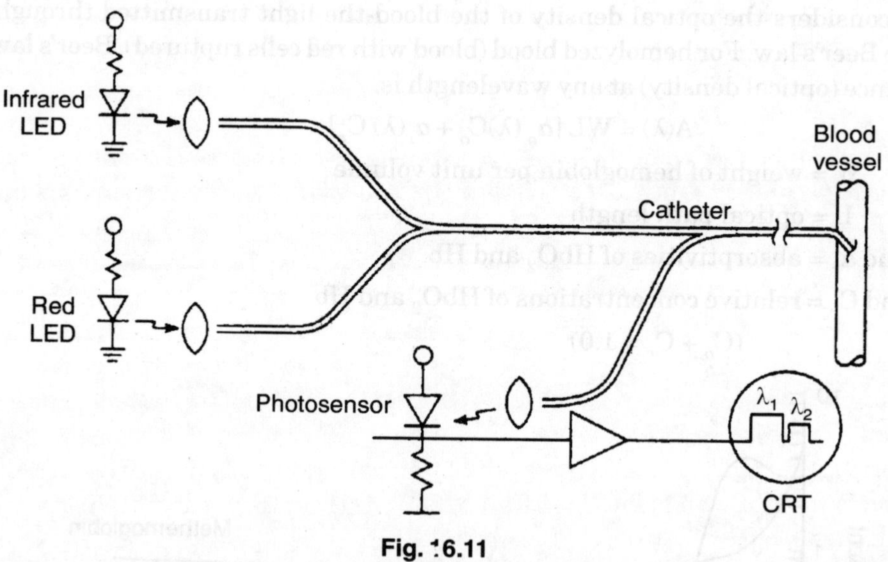

Fig. 16.11

Fig. 16.12. shows a fiber-optic instrument devised to measure oxygen saturation in the blood. This device, which could also be used for measuring cardiac output with a dye injected, is described here. The instrument consists of red and infrared light-emitting diodes (LEDs) and a photosensor. Plastic optical fibers are well adapted to these wavelengths. Fig. 16.12. shows a fiber-optic oximeter catheter that is flow-directed. After insertion, the balloon is inflated, and blood flow drags the tip through the chambers of the heart.

In addition to measuring blood-oxygen saturation through reflectance, the same dual-wavelength optics can be used to measure blood flow by dye dilution. Indo/cyanine/green, which absorbs light at 805 nm (the isosbestic wavelength of oxyhemoglobin), is used as the indicator. This is a dual-fiber system. Light at 805 nm is emitted from one fiber, scattered by the blood cells, attenuated by the dye in the blood, and partially collected by the other fiber for measurement. The second wavelength, above 900 nm, is used as a reference; this is the region where the light is absorbed by the dye. It is used to compare the effect of flow-rate light scattering. In effect, a dual-beam ratiometric system is developed for dye-dilution measurement of blood flow. Cardiac output is determined via the dye-dilution method described earlier.

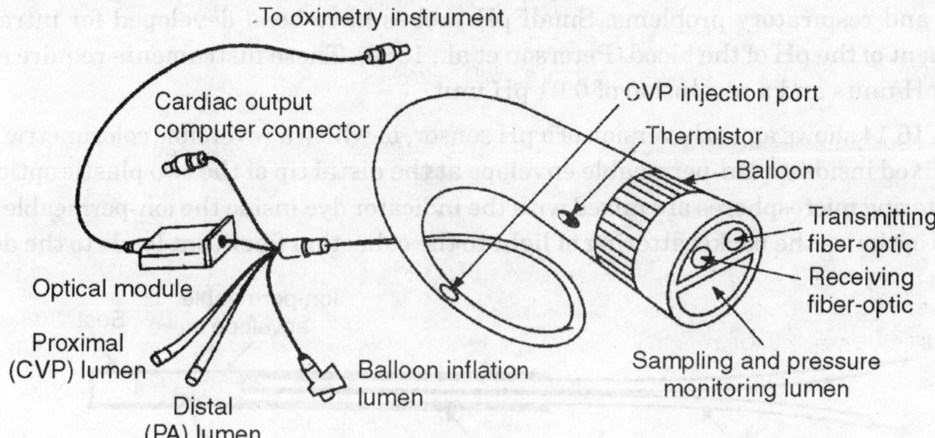

Fig. 16.12

A significant difference exists between two-wavelength oximetry systems and the Abbott three-wavelength Oximetry Opticath® System. In two-wave-length systems an important limitation, in the vivo measurement of oxygen saturation below 80%, is the dependence of the reflected light's intensity on the patient's hematocrit. Hematocrit varies from subject to subject, and within one subject it varies for different physiological conditions. Catheter tip oximeters require frequent updates of a patient's hematocrit. Various correction techniques have been devised to correct the oxygen-saturation measurements for errors due to hematrocrit variations. (This limitations is eliminated in the three-wavelength Abbott Opticath Oximetry System.) False readings occur in situations in which hemoglobin combines with another substance besides oxygen, such as carbon monoxide. Hemoglobin has a strong affinity for carbon monoxide , so oxygen is displaced. The optical spectra for HbO_2 and HbCO overlap at 660 nm (Fig. 16.8), causing an error in SO_2 if CO is present in the blood.

A three-fiber intravascular fiber-optic catheter that measures mixed venous oxygen saturation and hematocrit simultaneously has been developed and tested (Mendelson et al., 1990). The system consists of a catheter with a single light source in two equally spaced, near and far detecting fibers. The ratio of backscattered-light intensities measured at the isosbestic wavelength (805 nm) by the two detecting fibers (IR near/IR far) serves a correction factor that reduces the dependence of oxygen-saturation measurements on hematocrit.

This approach also provides a means for determining hematocrit independently. The principle of the measurement is based on the fact that variations in blood pH and osmolarity affect the shape and volume of the red blood cells. The IR near/IR far ratio is affected by variations in red blood cell volume and thus in hematocrit. The reflected-light intensities, measured by the two detecting fibers, are due to the higher-order multiple scattering. The intensity of the reflected light becomes more pronounced as source-to-detector separation distance increases. Details concerning the transcutaneous measurement of arterial oxygen saturation via pulse oximetry are given earlier.

REVERSIBLE-DYE OPTICAL MEASUREMENT OF pH

The continuous monitoring of blood pH is essential for the proper treatment of patients who have metabolic and respiratory problems. Small pH probes have been developed for intravascular measurement of the pH of the blood (Peterson et al., 1980). These instruments require a range of 7.0 to 7.6 pH units and a resolution of 0.01 pH unit.

Fig. 16.14 shows an early version of a pH sensor, in which a reversible colorimetric indicator system is fixed inside an ion-permeable envelope at the distal tip of the two plastic optical fibers. Light-scattering microspheres are mixed with the indicator dye inside the ion-permeable envelope in order to optimize the backscattering of light to the collection fiber that leads to the detector.

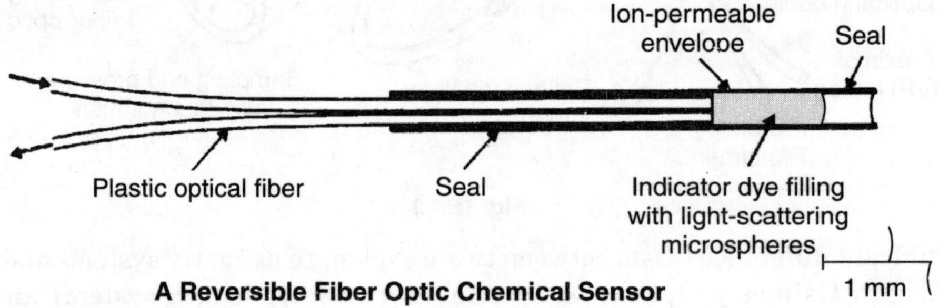

Fig. 16.14.

The reversible indicator dye, phenol red, is a typical pH-sensitive dye. The dye exists in two tautomeric (having different isomers) forms, depending on whether it is in an acidic or a basic solution. The two forms have different optical spectra. If the absorbance is plotted against wavelength for phenol red for the base form of the dye, it is indicating that the optical-absorbance peak increases with increasing pH. The ratio of green to red light transmitted through the dye is (Peterson, 1988)

$$R = k^* \, 10^{[-C(10^{-\Delta} + 1)]}$$

where Δ = Difference between pH and pK of the dye

R = I (green)/I(red) = measured ratio of light intensities

K = I_o (green)/I_o(red) = a constant (I_o = initial light intensity)

C = a constant determined by (1) the probe geometry, (2) the total dye concentration, and (3) the absorption coefficient of the dye's basic tautomer

BLOOD-GLUCOSE SENSORS

Accurate measurement of blood glucose is essential in the diagnosis and long term management of diabetes. This section reviews the use of biosensors for continuous measurement of glucose levels in blood and other body fluids.

Glucose is the main circulating carbohydrate in the body. In normal, fasting individuals, the concentration of glucose in blood is very tightly regulated-usually between 80 and 90 mg/100 ml, during the first hour or so following a meal. The hormone insulin, which is normally produced by beta cells in the pancreas, promote glucose transport into skeletal muscle and adipose tissue. In those suffering from diabetes mellitus, insulin-regulated uptake is compromised, and blood glucose can reach concentrations ranging from 300 to 700 mg/100 ml (hyperglycemia).

Accurate determination of glucose levels in body fluids, such as blood, urine, and cerebrospinal fluid, is a major aid in diagnosing diabetes and improving the treatment of this disease. Blood glucose levels rise and fall several times a day, so it is difficult to maintain normoglycemia by means of an "open loop" insulin delivery approach. One solution to this problem would be to "close the loop" by using a self-adapting insulin infusion device with a glucose controlled biosensor that could continuously sense the need for insulin and dispense it at the correct rate and time. Unfortunately, present-day glucose sensors cannot meet this stringent requirement (Peura and Mendelson, 1984).

Electro enzymatic Approach. Electroenzymatic sensors based on polarographic principles utilize the phenomenon of glucose oxidation with a glucose oxidase enzyme (Clark and Lyons, 1962). The chemical reaction of glucose with oxygen is catalyzed in the presence of glucose oxidase. This causes a decrease in the partial pressure of oxygen (PO_2), an increase in pH, and the production of hydrogen peroxide by the oxidation of glucose to gluconic acid according to the following reaction:

$$\text{Glucose} + O_2 \xrightarrow[\text{Oxidase}]{\text{Glucose}} \text{Gluconic acid} + H_2O_2$$

Investigation is done to measure changes in all of these chemical components in order to determine the concentratin of glucose. The basic glucose enzyme electrode utilizes a glucose oxidase enzyme immobilized on the membrane or a gel matrix, and an oxygen-sensitive polarographic electrode. Changes in oxygen concentration at the electrode, which are due to the catalytic reaction of glucose and oxygen, can be measured either amperometrically or potentiometrically.

Because a single-electrode technique is sensitive both to glucose and to the amount of oxygen present in the solution, a modification to remove the oxygen response by using two polarographic oxygen electrodes has been suggested (Updike and Hicks, 1967). Figure16.15. illustrates both the principle of the enzyme electrode and the dual-cathode enzyme electrode. An active enzyme is placed over the glucose electrode, which senses glucose and oxygen. The other electrode senses only oxygen. The amount of glucose is determined as a function of the difference between the readings of these two electrodes. More recently, development of hydrophobic membranes that are more permeable to oxygen than to glucose has been described (Updike et al., 1982).

The major problem with enzymatic glucose sensors is the instability of the immobilized enzyme and the fouling of the membrane surface under physiological conditions. Most glucose sensors operate effectively only for short periods of time. In order to improve the present sensor technologies, more highly selective membranes must be developed. The features that must be taken into account in designing and fabricating these membranes include the diffusion rate of both oxygen and glucose from the external medium to the surface of the membrane, diffusion and concentration gradients within the membrane, immobilization of the enzyme, and the stability of the enzymatic reaction (Jaffari and Turner, 1995).

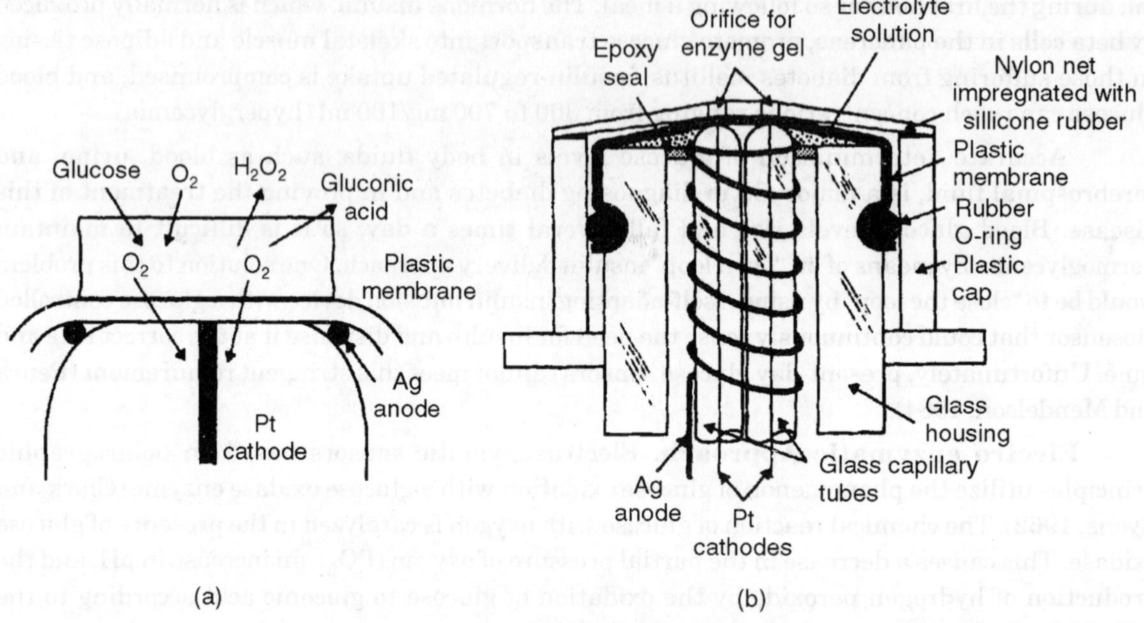

Fig. 16.15. Enzyme electrode and dual cathode electrode.

Optical Approach

A number of innovative glucose sensors, based on different optical techniques, has been developed in recent years. A new fluorescence-based affinity sensor has been designed for monitoring various metabolites, especially glucose in the blood plasma. The method is similar in principle to that used in radioimmunoassay. It is based on the immobilized competitive binding of a particular metabolite and fluorescein-labeled indicator with receptor sites specific for the measured metabolite and the labeled ligand (the molecule that binds).

Fig. 16.16 shows an affinity sensor in which the immobilized reagent is coated on the inner wall of a glucose-permeable hollow fiber fastened to the end of an optical fiber. The fiber-optic

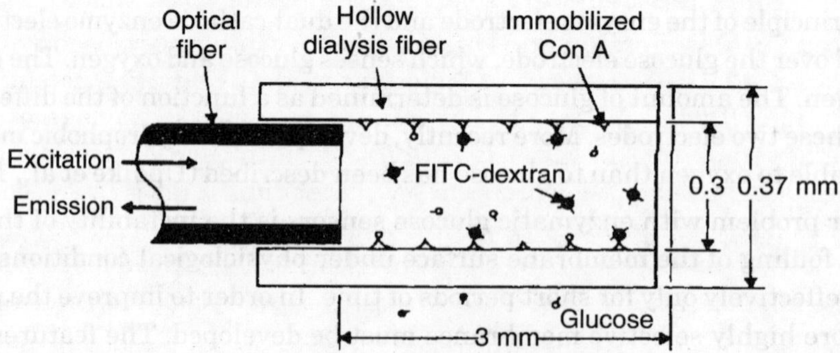

Fig. 16.16. An affinity sensor.

catheter is used to detect changes in fluorescent light intensity, which is related to the concentration of glucose. The feasibility of its miniaturization, has lead to an implantable glucose sensor. Fig. 16.17 is a schematic diagram of the optical system for the affinity sensor. The advantage of this is implantation through a needle. In addition, as with other fiber-optic approaches, no electric connections to the body are necessary.

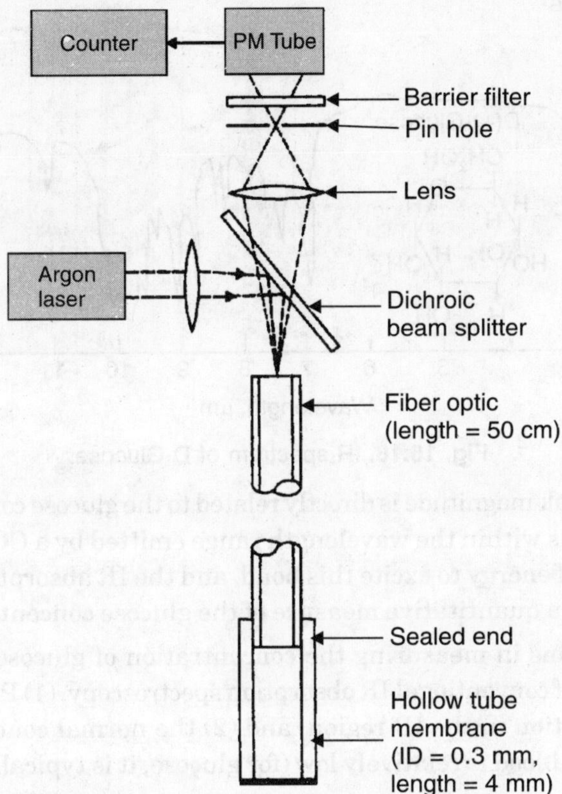

Fig. 16.17. Optical system for the affinity sensor.

The major problems with the approach are the lack of long-term stability of the reagent, the slow response time of the sensor, and the dependence of the measured light intensity on the amount of reagent, which is usually very small and may change over time.

Attenuated Total Reflection and Infrared Absorption Spectroscopy. The application of multiple infrared ATR spectroscopy to biological media is another potentially attractive noninvasive technique. By this means, the infrared spectra of blood can be recorded from tissue independently of the sample thickness, whereas other optical-transmission techniques are strongly dependent on the optical-transmission properties of the medium. Furthermore, employing a laser light source makes possible considerable improvement of the measuring sensitivity. This is of particular interest when one is measuring the transmission of light in aqueous solutions, because it counteracts the intrinsic attenuation of water, which is high in most wavelength ranges.

Absorption spectroscopy in the infrared (IR) region is an important technique for the identification of unknown biological substances in aqueous solutions. Because of vibrational and rotational oscillations of the molecule, each molecule has specific resonance absorption peaks, which are known as fingerprints. These spectra are not uniquely identified; rather, the IR absorption peaks of biological molecules often overlap. An example of such a spectrum is shown in Fig. 16.18, which is the characteristic IR spectrum of anhydrous D-glucose in the wavelength region 2.5-10 μm. The strongest absorption peak, around 9.7 μm, is due to the carbon-oxygen-carbon bond in the molecule's pyran ring.

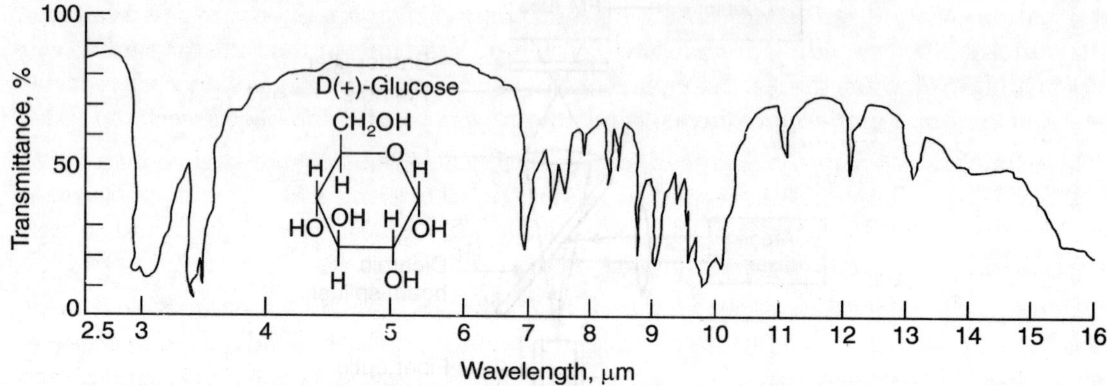

Fig. 16.18. IR spectrum of D-Glucose.

The absorption-peak magnitude is directly related to the glucose concentration in the sample, and its spectral position is within the wavelength range emitted by a CO_2 laser. Thus a CO_2 laser can be used as a source of energy to excite this bond, and the IR absorption intensity at this peak provides, via Beer's law, a quantitative measure of the glucose concentration in a sample.

There are problems in measuring the concentration of glucose in an aqueous solution, such as blood, by means of conventional IR absorption spectroscopy. (1) Pure water has an intrinsic high background absorption in the IR region, and (2) the normal concentration of glucose and other analytes in human blood is relatively low (for glucose, it is typically 90-120 mg/dl, or mg%).

Significant improvements in measuring physiological concentrations of glucose and other blood analytes by conventional IR spectrometers have resulted from the use of high-power sources of light energy at specific active wavelengths. In the case of glucose, the CO_2 laser serves as an appropriate IR source.

SUMMARY

Many biosensors produce signals that are correlated with the concentration of glucose in body fluids. These small sensors are fit for implantation. Nevertheless, further progress must be made before these sensors can be used reliably for long-term monitoring of glucose in the body. The problems that have yet to be solved involve operating implanted sensors in the chemically harsh environment of the body, where they are subject to continuous degradation by blood and tissue components. The device must be biocompatible, properly encapsulated, and well protected against elevated temperature and saline conditions. Furthermore, it should be possible to calibrate the sensor in situ.

NONINVASIVE BLOOD-GAS MONITORING

Blood-gas determination can provide valuable information about the efficiency of pulmonary gas exchange, the adequacy of alveolar ventilation, blood-gas transport, and tissue oxygenation. Although taking the blood to determine arterial blood gases is still widely practiced in many clinical situations, simple, real-time, continuous, and noninvasive techniques are now available. Also, intermittent blood sampling provides historical data valid only at the time the sample was drawn. Delays between when the blood sample is drawn and when the blood-gas values are reported average about 30 min. Furthermore, invasive techniques are painful and have associated risks.

These limitations are particularly serious in critically ill patients for whom close monitoring of arterial blood gases is essential. Continuous noninvasive monitoring of blood gases, on the other hand, makes it possible to recognize changes in tissue oxygenation immediately and to take corrective action before irreversible cell damage occurs.

Various noninvasive techniques for monitoring arterial O_2 and CO_2 have been developed. This section describes the basic sensor principles, instrumentation, and clinical applications of the noninvasive monitoring of arterial oxygen saturation (SO_2), oxygen tension (PO_2), and carbon dioxide tension (PCO_2).

TRANSCUTAVEOUS ARTERIAL OXYGEN SATURATION MONITORING (PULSE OXIMETRY)

The two-wavelengths approach was discussed, is successful for intravascular oximetry applications, but to the transilluminated ear or fingertip resulted in unacceptable errors due to light attenuation by tissue and blood absorption, refraction, and multiple scattering. And because of differences in the properties of skin and tissue, variation from individual to individual in attenuation of light require frequent calibration. Oximeters can be used to measure SO_2 noninvasively by passing light through the pinna of the ear. Because of the complications caused by the light-absorbing characteristics of skin pigment and other absorbers, measurements are made at eight wavelengths and are computer-processed. The ear is warmed to 41°C to stimulate arterial blood flow.

A two-wavelength transmission noninvasive pulse oximeter was introduced by Yoshiya in 1980. This instrument determines SO_2 by analyzing the time-varying, or ac component of the light transmitted through the skin during the systolic phase of the blood flow in the tissue (Fig. 16.19). This approach achieves measurement of the arterial oxygen content with only two wavelengths (660 and 940 nm, for instance). The dc component of the transmitted light, which represents light absorption by the skin pigments and other tissues, is used to normalize the ac signals.

A transcutaneous reflectance oximeter based on a similar photoplethysmographic technique has been developed by Mendelson in 1983. The advantage of the reflectance oximeter is that it can monitor SO_2 transcutaneously at various locations on the body surface, including more central locations (such as the chest, forehead, and limbs) that are not accessible via conventional transmission oximetry.

Because of these and other significant improvements in the instruments, measurements of ear, toe, and fingertip oximetry are used. Noninvasive measurements of SO_2, can be made with a 2.5% accuracy for saturation values from 50 to 100%.

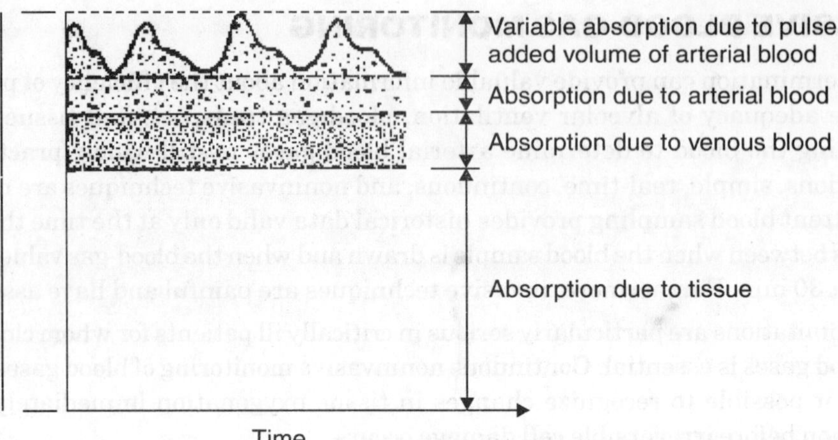

Fig. 16.19. Variation in absorption with time during pulse.

Transcutaneous SO_2 Sensor. The basic transcutaneous SO_2 sensor, for both the transmission and the reflective mode, make use of a light source and a photodiode. In the transmission mode, the two face each other and a segment of the body is interposed; in the reflection mode, the light source and photodiode are mounted adjacent to each other on the surface of the body.

Fig. 16.20 shows an example of a transcutaneous transmission SO_2 sensor and monitor. These transmission sensors are placed on the fingertips, toes, ear lobes, or nose. A pair of red and infrared light-emitting diodes are used for the light source, with peak emission wavelengths of 660 nm (red) and 940 nm (infrared). These detected signals are processed, in the form of transmission photoplethysmograms, by the oximeter, which determines the SO_2.

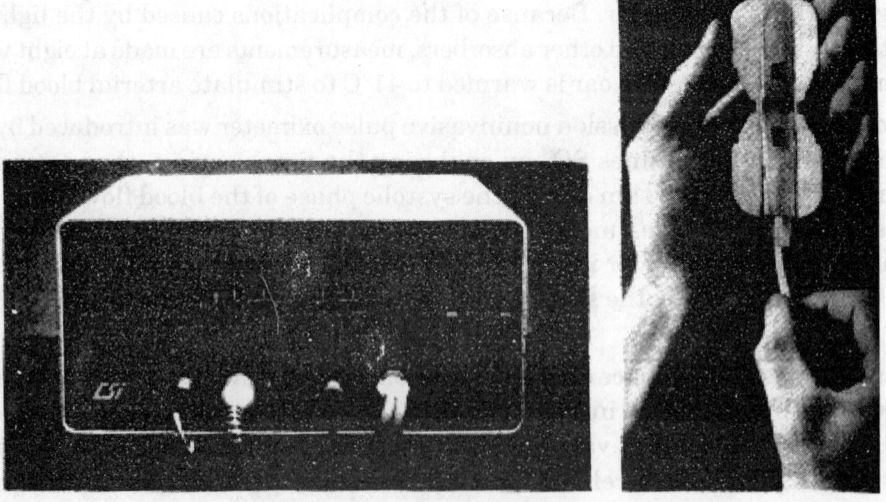

Fig. 16.20. (a) Noninvasive patient monitor capable of measuring ECG, noninvasive blood pressure (using automatic oscillometry), respiration (using impedance pneumography), transmission pulse oximetry, and temperature. (From Criticare Systems, Inc. Used by permission) (b) Disposable transmission SO_2 sensor in open position. Note the light sources and detector.

Applications of SO_2 Monitoring. As we have noted, the applications of noninvasive So_2 monitoring by direst assessment of the adequacy of tissue oxygenation can be made Oximetry is applied during the administration of anesthesia, pulmonary function tests, bronchoscopy, intensive care, and oral surgery, in neonatal monitoring, in sleep apnea studies, and in aviation medicine.

Noninvasive oximetry is also used in the home for monitoring self-administered oxygen therapy. Noninvasive oximetry provides time-averaged blood oxygenation values and can be used to determine when immediate therapeutic intervention is necessary. A lightweight (less than 3 g) and a small (20 mm diameter) optical sensor makes this transcutaneous reflectance sensor appropriate for monitoring newborns, ambulatory patients, and patients in whom a digit or ear lobe is not accessible. Problems with both transmission and reflectance oximetry include poor signal with shock, interference from lights in the environment and from the presence of carboxyhemoglobin, and poor trending of transients.

AUTO ANALYZER

(Vickers make) Multi-channel 300 m/c) ; Takes a new sample every 12 seconds. Each takes 10 minute to analyse for 14 blood constituents. Flame photometer and calorimeter is used. (reactions change colour, whose density is measured). At any moment 50 samples are undergoing analysis (300/ hour). Vials are labeled and results printed.

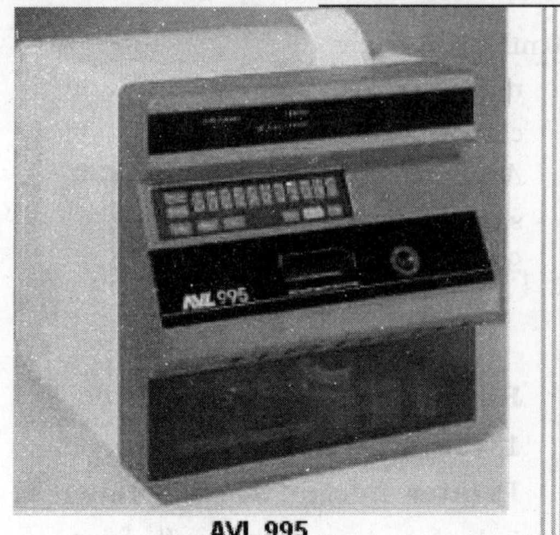

AVL 995

AVL Blood Gas Analyser model 995

- Blood Gas Analyzer
- pO_2, pCO_2, pH
- 30 samples/hour
- 18 × 16 × 22 in (46 × 41 × 56 cm), 65 lbs (29 kg)

AVL 995 Hb

— pH, pcO_2, pO_2, tHb

Call for specifics: 763-497-0172 or email to: **richard@gmi-inc.com** or via our **Contact Page**

Fig. 16.20. The Auto analyzer model AVL 995 Hb.

Current designs of instruments providing blood gas and electrolyte results make them suitable for use in a point of care (POCT) setting. Such instruments may be sited away from the main laboratory in accident and emergency departments, intensive care, coronary care and special baby care units.

The AVL 995-Hb measures carbon dioxide partial pressure, oxygen partial pressure, hydrogen ion concentration expressed as pH and hemoglobin in whole blood. The AVL 995-Hb also measures gas partial pressures in expired gas. The AVL 984-S determines sodium, potassium and ionized calcium in whole blood, serum, dialysate fluids and urine. The two instruments work independently of each other and require individual sample input. However they can be interfaced electronically so that patient results from the 984-S are transmitted to the 995-Hb for printing on a combined blood gas and electrolyte report. Hydrogen ion concentration, electrolytes and blood gas partial pressures are measured using electrode technology. Hemoglobin is quantified by measurement of the absorbance of a haemolysate at 546 nm. Thirteen other parameters are derived mathematically from the measured parameters.

The measurement of all the available analytes was evaluated. Whole blood samples were used for blood gas, pH and hemoglobin assessment and whole blood and plasma samples for sodium and potassium; calcium measurement was assessed using quality control material only. The evaluation included assessment of the analytical performance, carryover, ease of use, safety and reliability of the analyzer.

Adjustments can be made to the instrument's calibration to enable satisfactory correlation with other instrumentation. Instrument maintenance was straightforward.

Main features of both analysers, quoted by the manufacturer

Analytes measured: 995-Hb: Carbon dioxide and oxygen partial pressures, hydrogen ion concentration reported as pH, hemoglobin 984-S: Sodium, potassium and ionized calcium

Analytical system: Flow through, separate sample for each analyzer, electrolyte measurement by ion-selective electrode.

Operator interface: 995-Hb: 2 row display, touch sensitive membrane keyboard 984-S: Dot-matrix LED display, 'Yes' and 'No' buttons

Sample: 995-Hb: 95 μL whole blood or 50-100 mL expired air

984-S: 120 μL whole blood, serum, dialysate fluid or diluted urine

Sample collection: Anaerobic for blood gas analysis; heparin anticoagulant

Calibration of blood gases: Integral gas mixer produces mixtures from compressed air and carbon dioxide

Analysis rate: 995-Hb: Up to 30 samples/hour

984-S: Up to 40 samples/hour

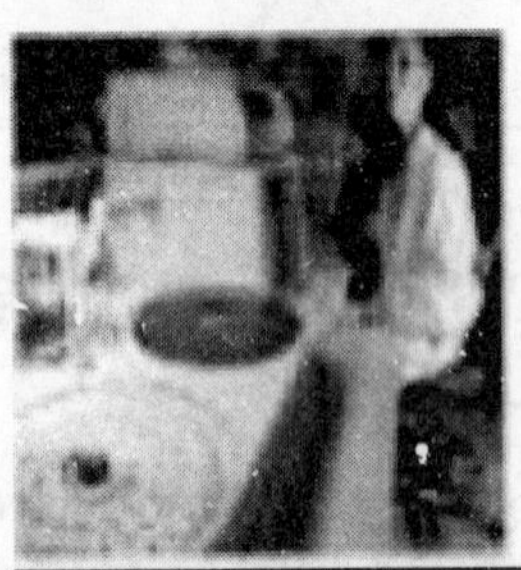

Results: 7 measured parameters and 13 calculated parameters

Printer: Integral thermal printers in both instruments, results from 984-S can be automatically transferred to the 995-Hb.

Result recall: Last sample, can be recalculated using revised patient data

Interface ports: 995-Hb: several; 984-S: RS 232 C

Analyzer dimensions: 995-Hb: 400 mm W × 450 mm H × 557 mm D 984-S: 300 mm W × 345 mm H × 270 mm D

Analyzer weight: 995-Hb: 35·5 Kg; 984-S: 11 Kg.

Chapter 17

Patient Monitoring System and Bio-Telemetry

PATIENT MONITORING SYSTEM

Most diseases of the heart and of the circulatory system, referred to as cardiovascular diseases, strike without warning and prompt treatment is required if death is to be averted. Such treatment is best provided in a specialized area of hospital referred to as "intensive care unit."(ICU). These specialized hospital units provide constant observation of the subject, constant monitoring of the subject's physiological condition and provide immediate emergency treatment whenever it is required. There are three important intensive care units which are given below.

1. Coronary intensive care units
2. Stroke intensive care Units
3. Pulmonary intensive care units

1. Coronary Intensive Care Units

Coronary intensive care units are used for treatment of diseases of the heart such as the Myocardial infarction or "heart attacks".

2. Stroke Intensive Care Units

Stroke intensive care Units are used for treatment of diseases of the circulatory system such as stroke.

3. Pulmonary Intensive Care Units

Pulmonary intensive care unit s are used for treatment of respiratory diseases. An intensive care unit may consist of one or more subject-monitoring sites, referred to as "beds" as each site, is in fact, a bed. Electronic instrumentation at each subject—monitoring site monitors various physiological signals from one subject and activates alarms should these physiological signals go above or below predetermined limits. The complete intensive care unit consists of not only the necessary monitoring equipment but also the necessary trained personnel and emergency equipment to allow immediate treatment of cardiac malfunctions.

Intensive care units (ICUs) are usually constructed to suit a particular hospital's requirements. Widely varying approaches are taken to the physiological functions to be monitored and the type of monitoring equipment required. In general, no two intensive care units are alike. Intensive care instrumentation is continuously being developed to accomplish more advanced physiological monitoring techniques. The following discussion on intensive care concepts is intended to present some of the physiological functions that may be monitored and some of the typical instrumentation that may be used to monitor these functions. The discussion is conceptual in nature and in no way attempts to survey all current intensive care applications and instrumentation.

PHYSIOLOGICAL FUNCTIONS TO BE MONITORED DURING INTENSIVE CARE

Since, subjects in coronary intensive care units are suffering from cardiovascular diseases, all physiological functions associated with the heart and circulatory system should be monitored.

The following are the important physiological signals to be monitored in intensive care unit is given below:

1. ECG Monitoring
2. Blood pressure Monitoring
3. Respiration and
4. Body temperature

1. ECG Monitoring

The principal physiological signal monitored in an intensive care unit is often the electrocardiogram. The electrocardiogram is usually monitored in the lead-II configuration with two active electrodes. These two electrodes are placed approximately 12 inches apart along the maximum potential axis of the subject's heart. A third electrode (ground) should be located elsewhere on the chest. This electrocardiogram monitoring configuration is referred to as three-lead chest cluster. Tektronix produces a patient cable for use with their type 410 physiological monitor that is specifically intended for monitoring during intensive care.

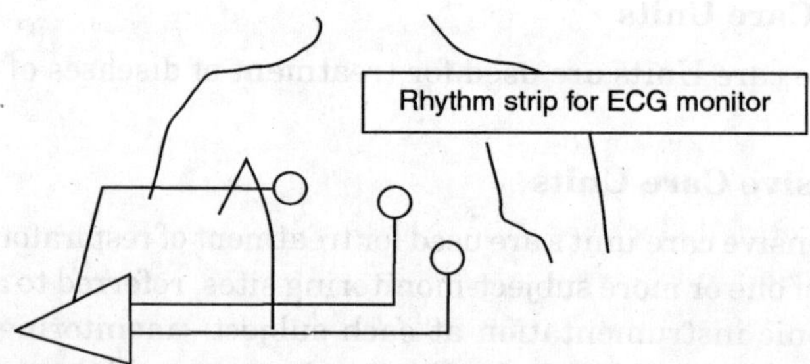

Fig. 17.1a. Showing the Rhythm strip for Intensive care ECG monitoring.

The electrodes used for ECG monitoring during intensive care must be suited for long term monitoring applications. The Tektronix silver / silver-chloride electrode system provided with a physiological monitor is ideally suited for this application as the electrode paste supplied produces no subject discomfort or skin irritation. A relatively large amount of paste is required between the subject and the electrode which prevents the paste from drying out due to evaporation and skin absorption.

The set of leads used for monitoring purpose is called 'rhythm' strip and its purpose is just to note the heart beat and not for analyzing it. Intensive care units have monitors built with either a long persistence monitor C.R.O. or with digital Raster scan display based non-fading displays.

The bedside non fading display type ECG monitor for use in such ICUs can use either the TV type raster scan display with microprocessor board and memory or else use a graphics LCD display. Such a unit is shown in Fig.17.1*b*.

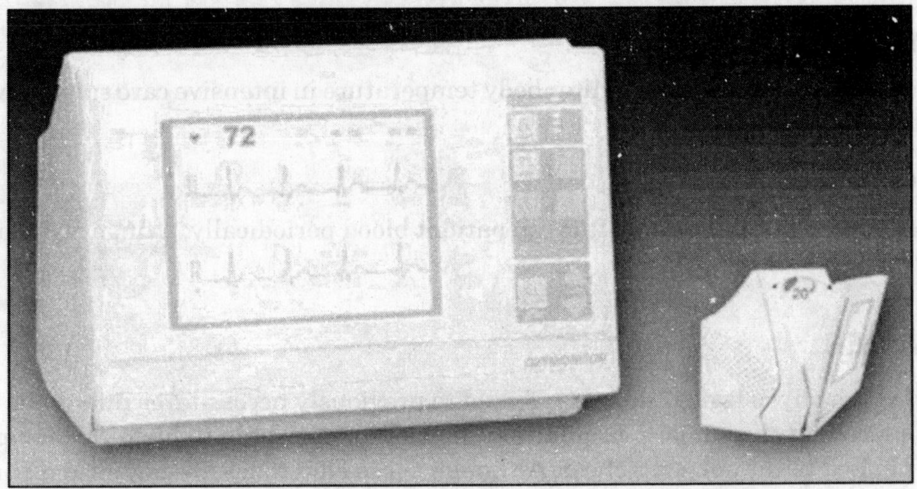

Fig. 17.1b. A nonfading LCD display monitor for ICU use.

2. Blood Pressure Monitoring

The second physiological parameter often of prime importance in intensive care monitoring is blood pressure. Blood pressure can be and often is monitored using intra - arterial catheter and transducer; however, the catheter results in considerable subject discomfort and many intensive care units prefer to monitor blood pressure by some alternative method only.

Korotkoff system-Riva-Rocci Method

Blood pressure can be monitored using the automatic cuff pump and Korotkoff microphone blood- pressure measurement system given in chapter-3. Although, this system is occasionally used in intensive care units. , it also possesses the disadvantage of being somewhat uncomfortable to the subject (bruises), and more importantly, being a sampling technique, it does not provide a continuous record of the subject's blood pressure. Thus, if for some reason the subjects blood pressure were to suddenly drop, this system may take some minutes or so to detect this pressure drop.

Plethysmograph

Blood pressure monitoring with plethysmograph offers the least discomfort to the subject; however, it provides only a relative indication of the well being of the circulatory system rather than providing absolute values for diastolic and systolic pressure.

Digital blood pressure monitors are now-a-days often used in many intensive care units. Any intensive care unit may employ one or more of these techniques and indeed all three may be available if required. Although diastolic and systolic arterial pressure are commonly monitored, mean arterial pressure and venous pressure are also be monitored in some instances.

3. Respiration Monitoring

It is often desirable to monitor the subject's respiratory activity during intensive care ; this may be accomplished with a thermistor pneumograph placed in the subject's nostril.

4. Body Temperature

It is often also desirable to monitor body temperature in intensive care subjects via a rectal or armpit thermistor probe.

5. Blood Chemistry PO_2

In order to measure and monitor the patient blood periodically, a finger type oximeter is also required.

PACEMAKER

Monitoring of the physiological signals referred to previously necessitates numerous electrodes etc., being placed on the subject. In addition, it is often desirable to have cardiac pacemaker electrodes applied to the subject's chest. Although these electrodes are not used during routine intensive care, they should be connected to a cardiac pacemaker for immediate emergency use if required.

INSTRUMENTATION REQUIREMENTS FOR INTENSIVE CARE UNITS

A conceivable intensive care instrumentation system is shown in Figs. 17.1, 17.2 and 17.3. Fig. 17.1 shows the instrumentation in an intensive care unit for four beds. Each of the four beds includes separate subject-monitoring instrumentation. This provides an indication of the subject's physiological condition as shown in Fig. 17.2. Signals from each of these four instrumentation modules are also connected to a central nurse on duty, to allow selective recording of the ECG, and to allow the ECG signal and or audio/visual information to be transmitted throughout the hospital via a closed circuit television link. The television camera and closed circuit link may be regarded as "luxury items", most other features shovn are essential.

PLETHYSMOGRAPH

Referring to the patient monitoring instrumentation located beside each intensive care bed as shown in Fig. 17.2, the following four parameters are monitored .

1. Relative arterial blood pressure
2. Respiration activity
3. The electrocardiogram
4. Body temperature

Relative arterial blood pressure is monitored by using a plethysmograph on either the subject's forehead, his nasal septum or the lobe of his ear. Finger plethysmographs are rarely used in intensive care units due to their susceptibility to subject movement. The instrumentation associated with the plethysmograph may provide an alarm signal should the cardiac rate go over or below preset limits or should the amplitude of signal produced by the plethysmograph fall below the predetermined level which indicates the loss in blood pressure or blood flow.

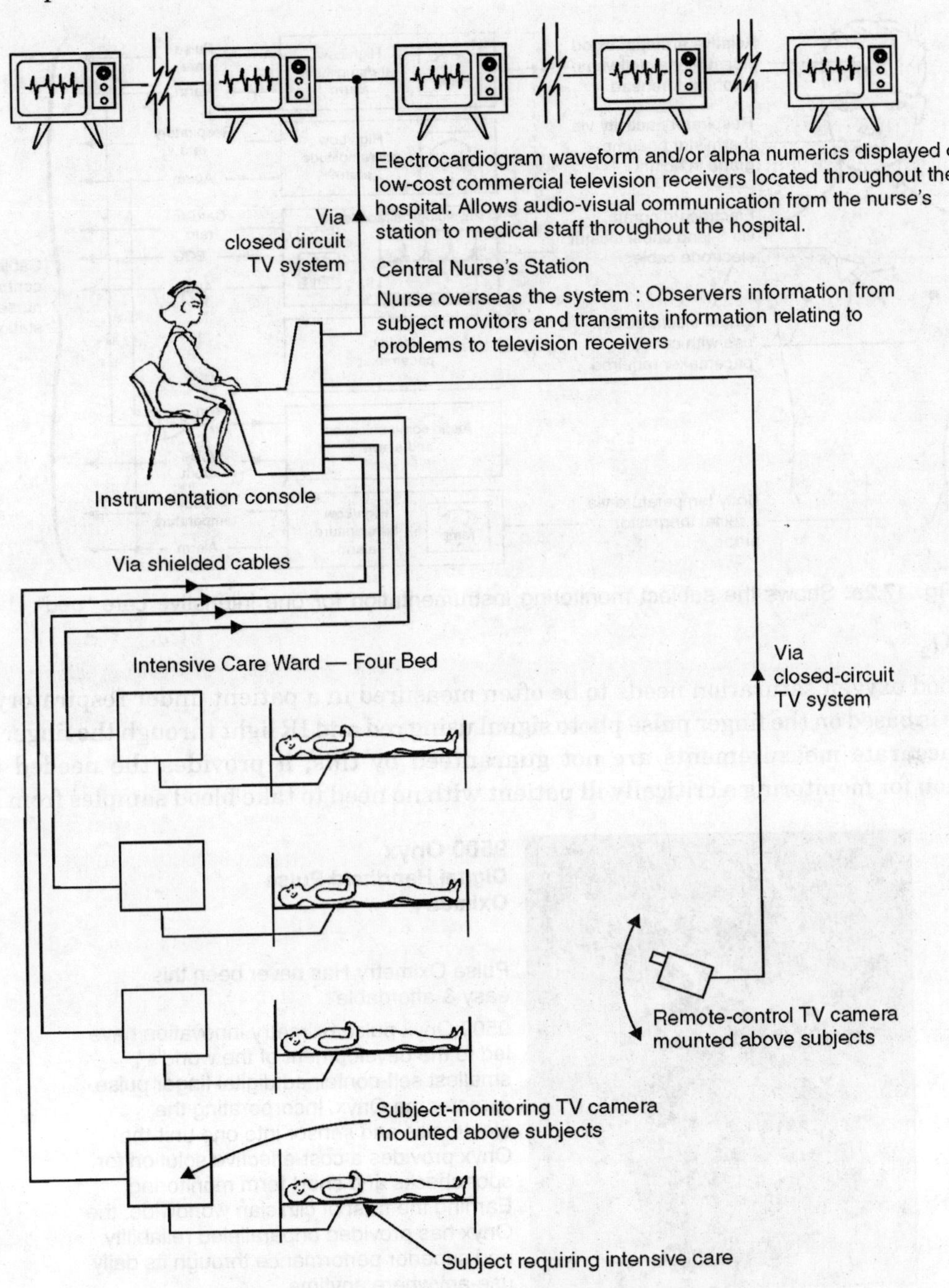

Fig. 17.1. Shows the instrumentation in an intensive care unit.

Respiratory activity is monitored via a thermistor pneumograph in the nostril with the associated instrumentation providing an indication of respiratory rate as well as providing an alarm if this rate falls outside the predetermined limits or if the signal level produced by the thermistor pneumograph is reduced below some predetermined amplitude. This indicates the loss of respiratory activity.

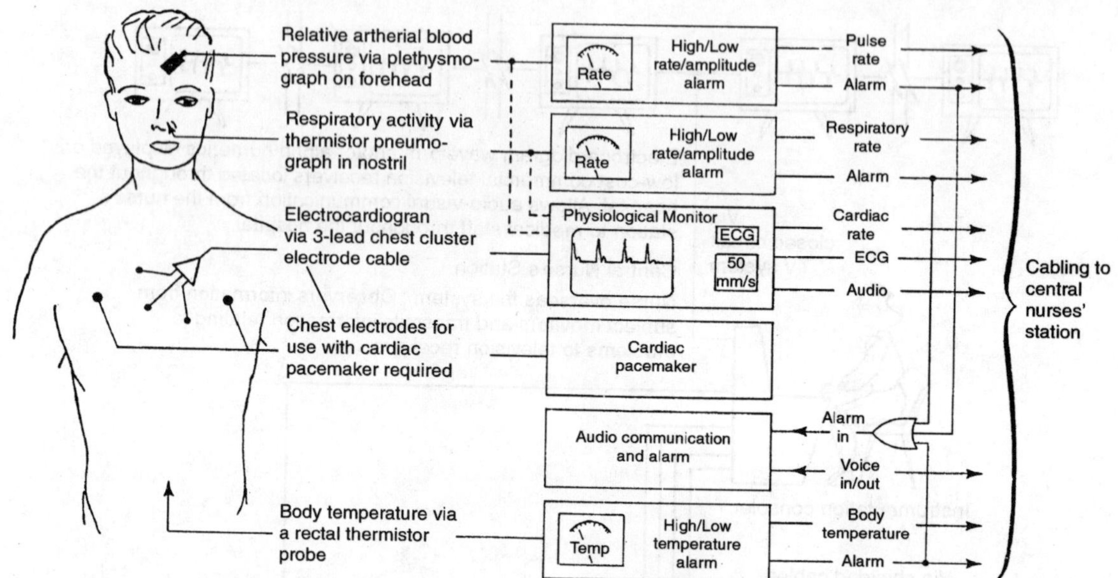

Fig. 17.2a. Shows the subject monitoring instrumentation for one intestive care "bed".

Blood PO_2

Blood oxygen saturation needs to be often measured in a patient under respiratory care unit. This is based on the finger pulse photo signal using red and IR light through the finger pulp. Though accurate measurements are not guaranteed by this, it provides the needed trend information for monitoring a critically ill patient with no need to take blood samples from him.

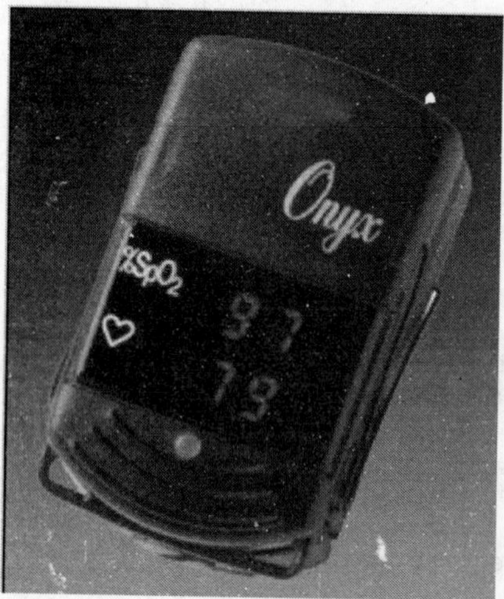

9500 Onyx
Digital Handheld Pulse
Oximetry

Pulse Oximetry Has never been this easy & affordable

9500 Onyx pulse oximetry innovation have led to the development of the world's smallest self-contained digital finger pulse oxmeter the Onyx. Incorporating the electronics and sensor into one unit-the Onyx provides a cost-effective solution for spot-checks and short term monitoring. Earning the trust of clinician worldwide, the Onyx has provided unparalleled reliability and superior performance through its daily use-anywhere anytime.

Fig. 17.2b

The Fig. 17.2*b*, *c* shows a unit of such a type which is handy and portable. It uses bright LED display for clear visibility.

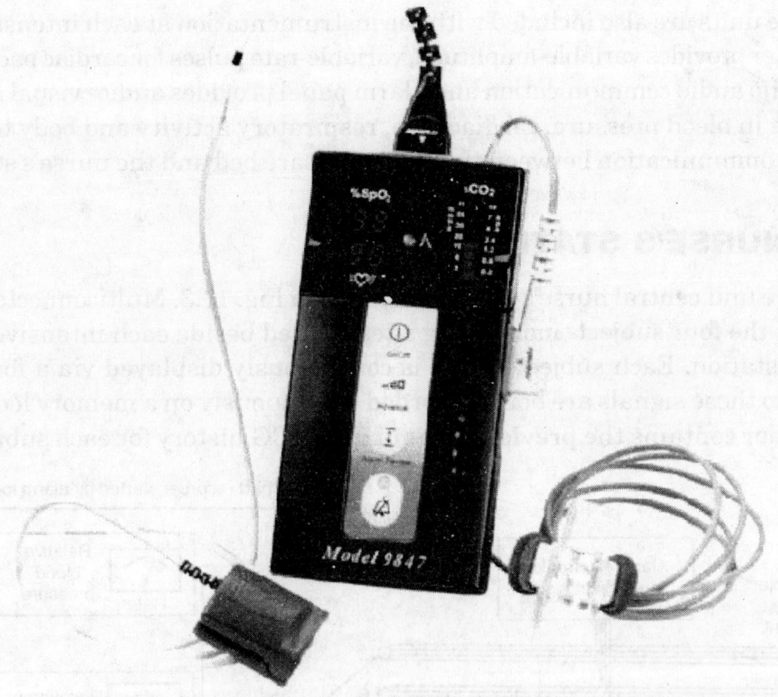

Fig. 17.2c

The electrocardiogram is monitored by the rhythm string having three chest leads. The physiological monitor provides an ECG output with a low audibility to indicate the cardiac rate or to indicate a loss of cardiac activity.

Thermistor probe

Body temperature is monitored by using a rectal thermistor probe. The associated instrumentation indicating body temperature may also contain an alarm system. It will be activated if the body temperature falls outside predetermined limits

Television Monitoring

Instrumentation located bedside each intensive care bed, should preferably be away from the subject's range of vision as its presence can be somewhat disturbing the subjects. The intensive care ward may also contain a closed - circuit television system to allow one or more subjects to be viewed via a television camera. This television camera may continuously scan the subjects in the intensive care ward or its position may be controlled from the central nurse's station.

OTHER EQUIPMENTS

In addition to physiological and visual monitoring of the subject, the following modules are required along with the instrumentation in intensive care unit. They are:

1. A cardiac pacemaker module and a defibrillator unit for emergency
2. Audio communication module and
3. Alarm module.

The above units are also included with the instrumentation at each intensive care bed. The cardiac pacemaker provides variable-amplitude, variable-rate pulses for cardiac pace-making should it be required. The audio communication and alarm panel provides audio- visual alarm indication of abnormalities in blood pressure, cardiac rate, respiratory activity and body temperature and provides audio communication between the intensive care bed and the nurse's station.

CENTRAL NURSE'S STATION

An intensive care unit central nurse's station is shown in Fig. 17.3. Multiconnector cable connects the output form the four subject- monitoring sites located beside each intensive care bed to the central nurse's station. Each subject's ECG is continuously displayed via a four channel CRT display. And also these signals are being recorded continuously on a memory loop tape recorder. This tape recorder contains the previous one-minute ECG history for each subject by recording

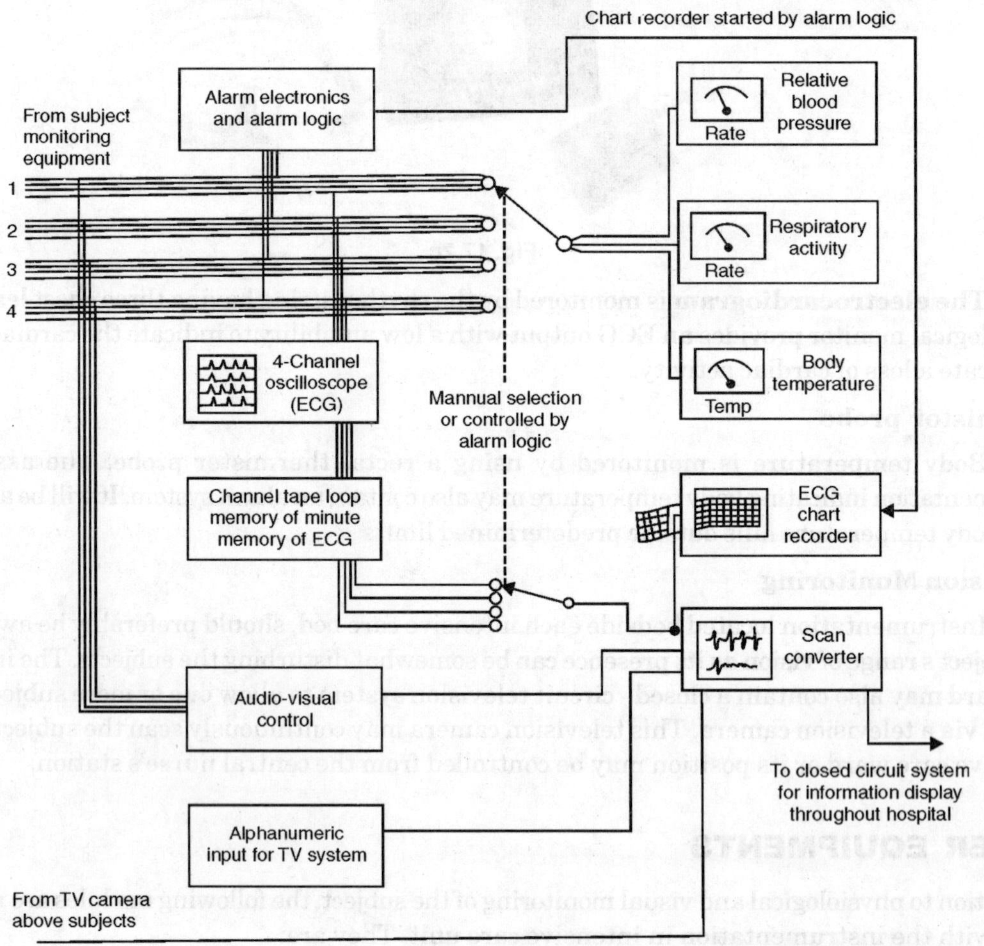

Fig. 17.3. Shows the central monitoring station for ICU beds.

the ECG on a tape loop "one minute" in length. Some central stations duplicate physiological indicators for relative blood pressure, respiratory activity and body temperature. These indicators can be manually switched between the four beds or the switching may be activated by the alarm system with the monitors being automatically switched to the bed providing the alarm signal. When an alarm is received at the central nurse's station, it may also be used to connect the appropriate ECG signal to a scan converter and ECG chart recorder and to start the chart recorder. In this way, a permanent record is achieved on the chart recorder beginning one minute prior to the alarm being sounded and information is displayed on the scan converter for transmission via the hospital closed circuit TV system to other medical personnel involved. The scan converter and closed-circuit TV system may also incorporate alphanumeric input to allow alphanumeric data relating to the intensive care subject to be displayed on television receivers located throughout the hospital.

COMPUTERS IN INTENSIVE CARE UNITS

Increasing use is being made of digital computers in intensive care units. These computers provide storage of the subject's physiological data and can continuously interrogate this data to determine if it is within the predetermined limits. The computer can perform multivarient analysis of the subject's ECG and can compare his ECG with previous records to indicate changes in the ECG which may be clinically significant. The advent of the time shared computer system allows one computer to simultaneously perform many tasks throughout a hospital, thus making the computer economically feasible for many hospitals.

MICROPROCESSOR BASED NON FADING DISPLAY PATIENT MONITOR

As discussed earlier, the three important parameters in any intensive care unit of small hospitals are ECG, pulse and respiration rate. Manually observing these by a physician is possible periodically, but during night time, for critically ill patients, it is necessary to have an electronic unit for automatically monitoring and displaying the ECG, preferably the other two parameters as well. This design involves a simple microprocessor circuit and its necessary interfacing circuitry and it is less expensive than the commercial machines. In each small hospitals in rural areas this may installed.

The environment around the patient is simple. A rhythm strip of three electrodes (two on chests and one on right leg) generates the ECG voltage. The finger pulse pick up generates the sphygmo or pulse waveform. The bead thermistor in the oxygen mask funnel gets the respiration rate signal (Fig. 17.4). The waveforms (or just the ECG only if required) are displayed on a 30 cm TV screen as a non-fading trace, using memory. Additionally, an alarm output sounds for fast pulse rates or low values. These are present in the unit and can be changed if required. The system works from mains power only and is compact enough for the bedside and simple to maintain.

ANALOG CIRCUITRY

The power supply for the analog circuitry is obtained from a mains transformer of special insulation resistance with an inter-winding shield. A dual stabilized DC of + and – 6V is obtained for all analog circuitry and + 5V for the microprocessor and the digital logic devices. Alternatively, a + 12V accumulator battery can be employed which can also power the TV unit. The ECG signal is

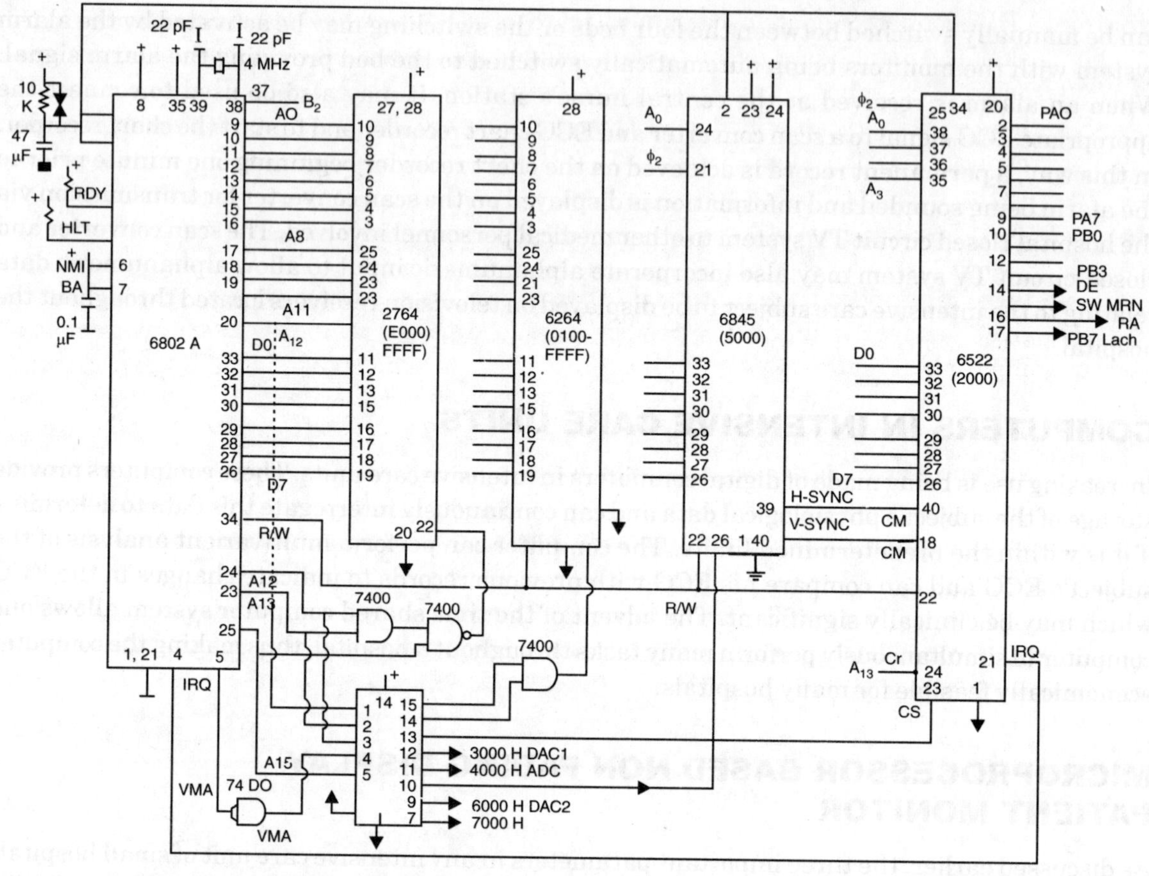

Fig. 17.4. The microprocessor part of the patient monitor unit on a CRT display. Note the 6845 CRT Controller and the VIA 6522.

fed to the pre-amplifier comprising of one dual FET which alone provides maximum hum rejection and superior performance. The input impedance is very high but is limited by the pair of 10 MΩ resistors at the input lead end. The gain is around 15dB. The common mode rejection is over 60 dB easily.

The post amplification of the ECG signal is done in a second FET input operational amplifier. This signal is directly used by the video signal forming circuitry described later. For use by the microprocessor, this signal is converted into a TTL pulse relating to the QRS complex by using a time constant filter and a TTL Schmitt trigger monostable. This TTL ECG pulse is read by the microprocessor and used for determining rate, which is displayed on the 3 digit LED 7-segment display on the microprocessor board. It is used by the software programs to check for the upper and lower limits and issue alarms as well.

The pulse pick up employs a light dependent resistor (LDR) of high resistance and of size 0.5 cm which is kept just opposite to a high brightness miniature LED and the unit is worn on the thumb of the patient whereby the reflected signal of light from the blood flowing in the capillaries causes the pulse signal to be generated. In some hand worne units is enclosed the required high gain pre-amplifier using a small transistor. A two core shielded cable connects this pick up to the unit from a DIN connector on its back panel. The respiration pick up can be incorporated in the oxygen mask of the patient and in that case, a micro-miniature glass coated bead thermistor is used. Alternatively, chest band elastic resistive pick-up can also be employed. A few tens of millivolt signal got there from this is amplified in a DC amplifier using a BI-FET operational amplifier and a ± 2V for respiration is obtained.

GENERATION OF VIDEO PULSES FOR ANALOG SIGNALS

There are three high speed comparators which are employed one for each analog input signal. These are given to negative input. The positive input of all three comparators are given a signal which is ramp wave of range + 5V to – 5V, generated by horizontal sync. signal by an integrating amplifier (Fig. 17.5). Therefore, when a ramp wave crosses the level of the input signal, the comparator gives an output. This is used to trigger the dot generating monostable, again one for each comparator, using TTL gates, for a time period of about 350 ns. This gives a resolution of about ten dots to a centimeter on the screen. These dot pulses are combined in a OR gate, so that the dot pattern for all the three signals are available together on each horizontal line of the raster.

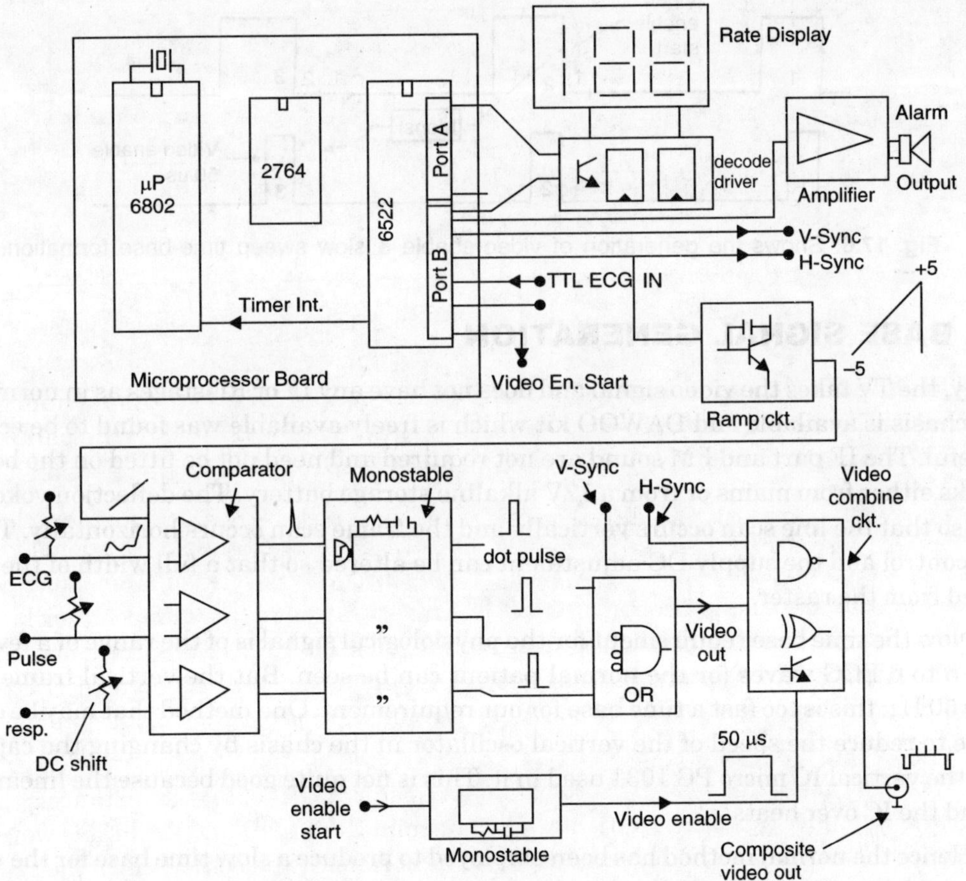

Fig. 17.5. Shows a analog to video signal generation, Microprocessor control and display.

DC shift signals can be added at each comparator from three variable presets so that the three waves appear shifted from each other much like an oscilloscope. These combined dots constitute the video signal. The same is combined with a microprocessor generated H-sync and V-sync pulses in an EXCLUSIVE OR gate and a transistor so that a final composite video signal to be given to the TV unit is obtained.

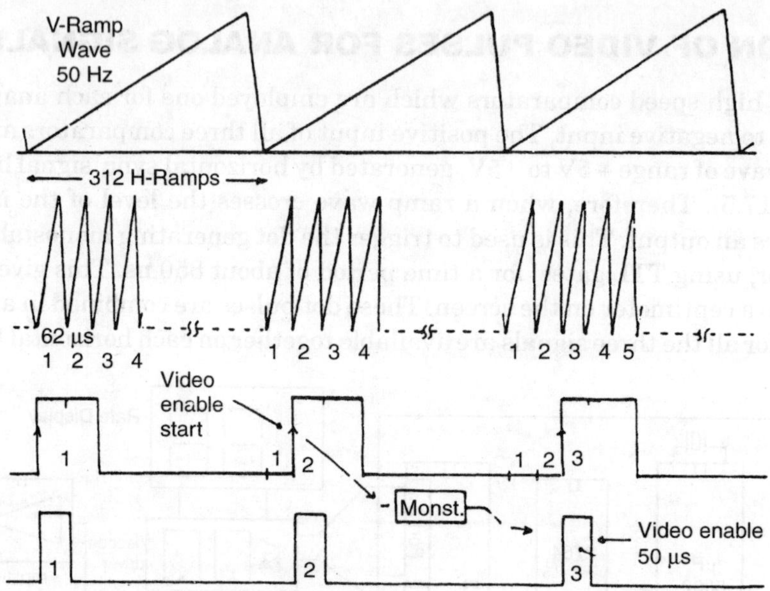

Fig. 17.6. Shows the generation of video-enable & slow sweep time-base formation.

TIME BASE SIGNAL GENERATION

Actually, the TV takes the video signal and does not have any IF or RF stages as in normal set. 35 cm TV chasis is available and DAWOO kit which is freely available was found to be economical and useful. The IF part and FM sound are not required and need not be fitted on the board. The kit works either from mains or from a 12V alkaline storage battery. The deflection yoke is tuned by 90°, so that the line scan occurs vertically and the frame scan occurs horizontally. The frame height control and the supply DC adjustment can be altered so that a full width of the screen is obtained from the raster.

Now the time base requirement for the physiological signal is of the range of a few seconds so that 5 to 6 ECG waves for the normal patient can be seen. But the vertical frame signal is usually 50 Hz; this is too fast a time base for our requirement. One method that may be employed could be to reduce the speed of the vertical oscillator in the chasis by changing the capacitor at pin7 of the vertical IC micro PC 1031 used in it. This is not quite good because the linearity is not good and the IC over heats.

Hence the normal method has been employed to produce a slow time base for the view. Fig. 17.6 explains the principle employed in a quick glance. The top wave is the vertical ramp waveform which generates the frame movement of the cathode ray beam on the tube. This is at usual at 50

Hz frame rate. The second wave that is shown in Fig. 17.6 is the line ramp. There are 312 such ramps in the time of 1 frame ramp. The third signal that is shown is the video enable signal which comprises of the pulses, each of one line duration occurring only once on each frame and displaced by one line count for each frame until the 312 are covered, whereupon the pulse starts on the first line again. Such a pulse waveform can of course be generated by a microprocessor ! Each pulse is of an exact line duration being generated by a hardware monostable only timed for 15 μs. But the short trigger is generated by a bit on the microprocessor PIA. The same is programmed to count the H-sync pulses which it generates by the PIA's timer and time the video enable signal. The principle is that of a sampling oscilloscope. In each frame only the line which is enabled by this pulse will be visible. Thus, in the first frame, one sees the first line. On the second frame, the 2nd line and so on till the end of the raster at the last 312th line. Thus, for the view, the apparent frame speed is just 50 lines a second and therefore the total screen is moving in a time of 312/50 or about 6 sec. This is the time-base.

MICROPROCESSOR AND ITS FUNCTIONS

The microprocessor board employs a 6802 Motorola 8-bit processor with on chip clock and RAM. An EPROM 2764 holds all the software needed. There is only one other chip, a PIA 6522, which is versatile enough for the requirement. The same contained two programmable ports, programmable bit wise; it has a pair of 16-bit timer counter. It supports interrupt logic for these 6802.

One port of 8-bit is used for outputting the two BCD digits up to 99 for the heart rate. Another bit from the second port lights up the 100th place if it occurs. External BCD to seven segment decoder-driver Integrated circuits (ICs) are required for the 10th and unit LEDs while a transistor is used for the MSB-LED digit. Two bits of the second port are employed for generating alarm logic high output which drive external alarm sounder piezo unit. The PB_7 bit is programmed to generate the line rate signal at 1/625 Hz. The same also is programmed to interrupt its 6802 which then counts the lines and outputs the video enable signal approximately as per Fig. 17.6 on another B-port bit. Two other bits generate its clock start pulses for the H-sync and V-sync while external monostable times the actual Hsync and Vsync outputs for standard width. One other bit is used as an input bit to receive the ECG TTL pulse (Fig. 17.4).

The microprocessor board and the several monostables, one for H and another V-sync generation, the third for video enable signal are mounted on the PCB. A second analog board receives the transducer signal and does the amplification, dot pulse generation, video formation and composite video output. The power supply is separately mounted. The analog ground and digital ground lines in the boards are kept separate.

TYPICAL COMMERCIAL ELECRONIC-PATIENT MONOTORING UNIT

Specifications of a Commercial Patient Monitoring Unit (Electronic) is given below.

I. BLOOD PRESSURE CHANNEL

Measuring Principle	Sensing by arterial puncture; carrier frequency method with inductive transducer

Measuring ranges – 1 torr to +10 torr (mm Hg)

- 2 torr to + 20 torr (mm Hg)
- 5 torr to + 50 torr (mm Hg)
- 10 torr to + 100 torr (mm Hg)
- 20 torr to + 200 torr (mm Hg)
- 30 torr to +300 torr (mm Hg)

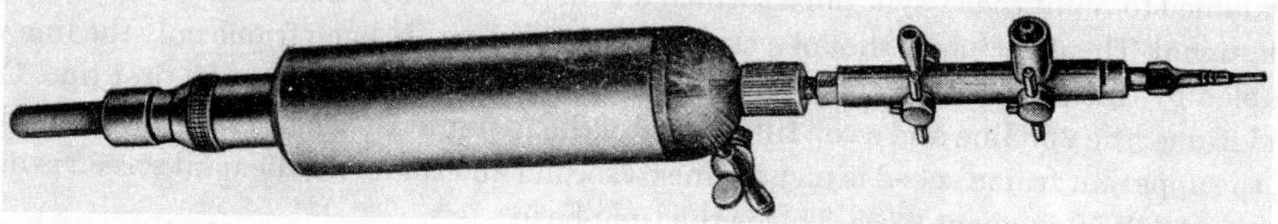

Kind of measurement

(Attenuation)	(1) Without Filter limit >100 Hz (2) With filter limit = 10 Hz (3) With filter (integrated value $t = 1$ sec.)
Signal Outputs	Output sockets for display units and recording Instruments.
Weight of Transducer	400 g approximately.
Dimensions of Transducer	35 mm dia, 130 mm length.

II. TEMPERATURE CHANNEL

Measuring Principle	Carrier frequency bridge with platinum resistor
Types of Temperature Probes	(1) Oesophageal (2) Rectal and vaginal
Measuring Ranges	0° C to 12°C 10°C to 22°C 20°C to 32°C 30°C to 42°C
Signal Output	Conjunction with low-speed recorder and threshold monitor

III. PLUG-IN HEART RATE METER

Measuring Principle	Averaging over about 5 sec
Measuring Range	40–250 pulses/min.
Response voltage	≥ 500 mV

Physiological quantities usable for evaluation	ECG, waveform signals of blood pressure, pulse rate, etc.
Signal Outputs	Conjunction to low speed Recorder and threshold monitor

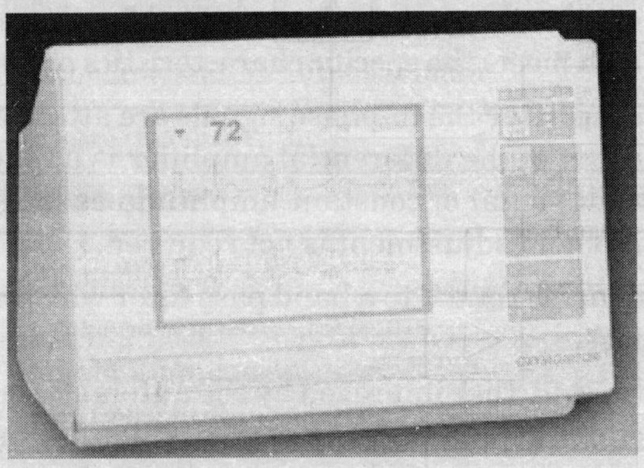

Fig. 17.7a. Shows a typical Patient monitoring unit in an intensive care ward.

Fig. 17.7*b*. shows the Defibrillator for ICU use.

Fig. 17.7*c*. shows the block schematic of the patient monitoring unit.

The functional schematic unit for bedside set-up is given in Fig. 17.7(*b*).

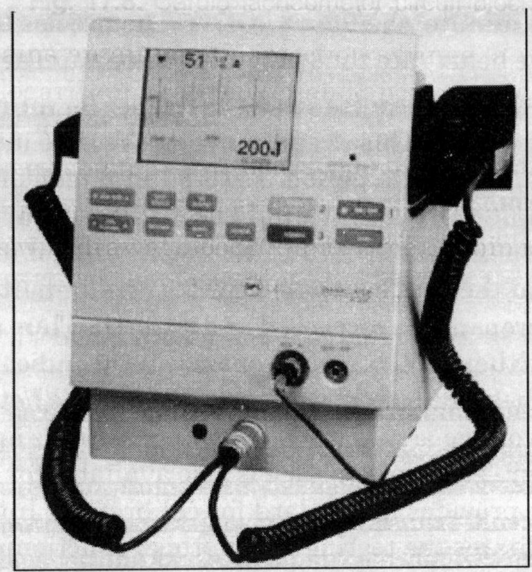

- < 5 Second to charge to 360 J with Battery
- Charge upto 360 J in AC without battery
- <100 charge discharge cycles with fully charged battery
- LCD for sharp bright non fade display
- Visual and auto alerts

Fig. 17.7b. Showing the Cardiac Defibrillator in an ICU.

CARDIOTACHEOMETER

The use of a tacheometer for cardiac rate in small rural intensive care units at an economical cost is felt worthy of design and such units have been in use since long.

The circuit of the 104 cardio tachometer is shown schematically (Fig. 17.8). Each signal that is picked up by the electrodes is successively examined for phase, amplitude, frequency and time and only that signal which meets the specific characteristics of the QRS complex is measured.

In the **differential amplifier** the in-phase signals are attenuated with respect to the out-of-phase ECG signal the output of the differential amplifier is applied to the AGC circuit. This essentially provides an output signal of constant amplitude as long as the input is within the specified limits. Hence a threshold adjustment is not required.

The now regulated signal is routed to a band pass filter which allows the 15Hz fundamental of the QRS complex to pass.

Signal to artifact ratio is further improved by the automatic dead time switch. The signal derived from the band pass filter will, to a certain degree, still contain artifact elements. Now the simplest approach to eliminate these would be to short circuit the amplifier, the moment a pulse has passed and to keep it in that state until the next pulse occur. A 99% elimination could thus be obtained. However, since the heart rate is subject to continuous variations, a 99% elimination is evidently impracticable since, after a sudden one-period change of heart rate, the nest pulse would occur within the dead time and consequently would not be registered. On the basis of studies the dead time at a heart rate of 80 beats/min was fixed at 35% of the time interval between successive heart beats. For 180 beats per minute, the figure is 67%. The precise length of the dead time is automatically controlled by the heart rate thus providing maximum artifact elimination.

The leading edge of the dead time pulse serves as trigger for **monostable multivibrator** which in turn triggers a timing circuit. This circuit converts the time interval between beats into a proportional voltage, which during one period is stored in a memory capacitor. The voltage across this capacitor as a result will vary in proportion to any heart rate change. Since the efficiency of the storage at the next beat is C.75%, the meter will not follow the rate increase or decrease for the full 100% but at the next beat will lag C.25% behind. At the second beat after the variation 75% of this 25% discrepancy is recovered and so forth. Thus at a high jump of for e.g., 12 beats per min in one period, there will be a discrepancy in the indication of 3 beats/min at the next beat and of less than one beat/min after two beats. It should be noted that a high jump is an extreme case. Finally the d-c voltage across the memory capacitor is applied to the panel meter via an isolation power amplifier. The same voltage is also available for operation of an auxiliary recorder. A built-in calibrator provides a standard for calibration. Internally connected to the input, this calibrator also facilitates the testing of the proper fnnctioning of the instrument.

The actual no. of heart beats can be registered by an electro mechanical counter which emits a click sound with each registered heart beat.

Applications

Occupation physiology sports, cardiology, As hospital monitor.

Tracerlab, 277 chaussee d'Arvers malinies, Belgium

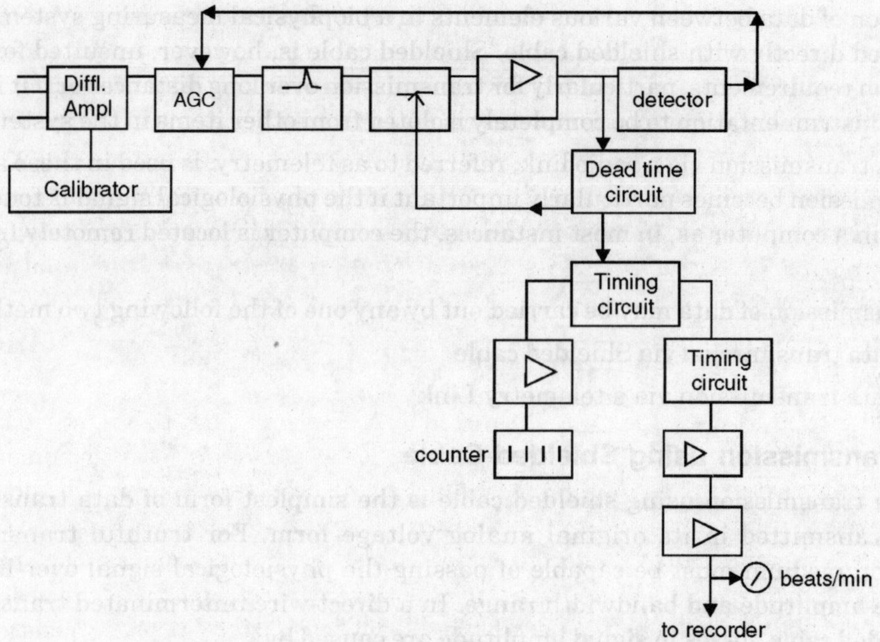

Fig. 17.8. Cardio tacheometer circuit block diagram.

Hematron contains an automatic injection syringe, a withdrawal pump, a scintillation detector, a linear and logarithmic rate meter and an x-y recorder.

After injection and withdrawal, needless have been connected to the desired arteries of the patient, the automatic sequence is started by pressing the 'inject' button. This causes 1cc of I^{125} serum albumin to be injected into patient. At the same time, the x-y recorder makes a graph of the radioactivity of the withdrawal blood, (x-axis-time), 3 min is total x-travel.

Graph used

- Cardiac output
- Total femoral artery outflow
- flow after vasodilation
- blood volume
- circulation time
- Limb blood volume

I^{125} prefered (longer half-life). Lower background with minimum shielding.

Hematocrit measuring equipments

Based on the electrically insulating characteristics of red blood cells. Essentially the conductivity of a carefully controlled blood volume is measured and the results read from a meter directly calibrated in hematocrit percentage units.

Designed to eliminate the need for a centrifuge. Draw up blood into cell, adjust printer, place cell on contacts, push betton, read value.

BIO-TELEMETRY FOR GENERAL USE

Transmission of data between various elements in a biophysical measuring system is normally accomplished directly with shielded cable. Shielded cable is, however, unsuited for many data transmission requirements, particularly for transmission over long distances or if it is desired for one item of instrumentation to be completely isolated from other items in the system.

Data transmission via a radio link, referred to as telemetry, is used in these applications. Data transmission becomes particularly important if the physiological signal is to undergo data processing in a computer as, in most instances, the computer is located remotely from the data source.

Transmission of data may be carried out by any one of the following two methods;

1. Data transmission via Shielded cable
2. Data transmission via a telemetry Link

1. Data Transmission using Shielded Cable

Data transmission using shielded cable is the simplest form of data transmission; the signal is transmitted in its original analog voltage form. For truthful transmission, the transmission medium must be capable of passing the physiological signal over its maximum conceivable amplitude and bandwidth range. In a direct-wire unterminated transmission link using shielded cable, losses in signal amplitude are caused by;

1. Cable reactance and
2. Length, to which it is in direct proportion.

For most physiological data transmission applications, cable reactance imposes a practical maximum cable length of about 1000 feet when the cable is driven by normal Instrumentation providing signals form an output impedance of perhaps 100 ohms. Within the bandwidth of interest in biophysical measurements (DC to 30,000 Hz) , the capacitance from the shielded cable inner conductor to the shield is the most important single factor limiting the high frequency performance of the transmission system. The bandwidth of the shielded cable transmission system, when driven from a voltage source, is given by:

$$f_{3dB} = 0.16 \times 10^{12}/\text{RCL} \quad \text{...(1)}$$

where R = the output resistance of the driving source in ohms

C = the nominal capacitance of the shielded cable in pico-farads/m.

L = is the length of the cable in metres.

Instrumentation providing an output signal via a voltage follower circuit provides a typical driving source impedance of < 1000 ohms; Instrumentation providing an output signal via a transistor emitter follower circuit provides a typical driving source impedance of < 100 ohms. Most shielded cable has a capacitance of between 60 to 120 pF/ meter; the common of 0.6 cm diameter shielded cable used in many physiological applications and in laboratories exhibits a typical capacitance of 90 pF/meter. Relating this information to the previous formula (eqn.1), a 30 m length of 90 pF/meter shielded cable, when driven from a source impedance of 100 ohms, provides transmission system bandwidth of 50 kHz. Practically, the system bandwidth will be somewhat less than this as the driving amplifier does not "see" only the capacitance of the line, but its inductance and resistance components as well. At 50 kHz, a 300 metre line, allowing for propagation velocity in the cable, is a significant fraction of a wavelength long.

Although, unterminated direct wire transmission links using a shielded cable can be used to about 300 m, it is recommended that terminated systems can be used for analog data transmission in excess of 15m. Terminated systems require the shielded cable to be driven from a source of its own characteristic impedance. And also this should be terminated with the same value of the characteristic impedance. To avoid ground loops, it is customary, and usually essential, to transmit from a single ended driver having the line characteristic impedance. This is received by a differential amplifier between line and shield having a high common mode impedance, and a differential input impedance equal to the characteristic impedance of the line.

The overall bandwidth of a bio-physical measurement system is given by,

$$f = \frac{1}{\sqrt{1/f_1^2 + 1/f_2^2 + 1/f_3^2 + \ldots \text{etc.}}} \quad \ldots(2)$$

where f_1, f_2, f_3 etc., are the bandwidths (upper-3 dB frequency limits) of the individual components in the system including the transmission components between individual instruments.

2. Amplitude Modulation Techniques

Wire transmission can be done over very long distances by employing an amplitude modulated carrier frequency with the information to be transmitted being used to amplitude modulate a carrier frequency. This carrier frequency must be higher than the highest frequency component in the modulating signal by a factor at least five, to allow low distortion demodulation at the receiver end. Any amplitude modulated transmission system, is only as good as the ability of the system to faithfully reproduce amplitude variations. Four important parameters are to be taken care when we transmit any physiological signals. They are:

1. System attenuation
2. System amplitude noise
3. System non-linearity and or
4. Interference from other sources

The above parameters produce errors in the information transmitted. For this reason, amplitude modulated data transmission techniques are limited to wire transmission rather than to radio link transmission.

DATA TRANSMISSION VIA A TELEMETRY LINK

Telemetry links used in biophysical measurement range from the short range systems used in behavioral studies laboratories to the extremely long range systems used in aerospace industry.

The major difference between the short range and long range systems is the power output capability of the transmitter and the sensitivity of the receiver.

SHORT RANGE TELEMETRY SYSTEMS

Short range telemetry systems are used in behavioral studies to completely isolate a subject or laboratory animal from a recording system. A small telemetry transmitter may be attached to the subject to transmit, for example, the subject's ECG; a telemetry receiver may be located only a few feet away to allow this ECG signal to be processed by a physiological measurement system. This allows complete subject freedom of movement and thus allows for more natural subject behavior. As a telemetry transmitter is normally a completely isolated battery operated device, telemetry offers a degree of safety unattainable with conventional instrumentation due to the complete elimination of direct electrical connections between the subject and the instrumentation.

FREQUENCY MODULATION TECHNIQUES IN TELEMETRY LINK

Short range telemetry systems usually use FM (Frequency Modulation) Techniques and may transmit in the FM broadcast band (88 to 108 MHz). They may be simple systems providing only one data channel or more complex systems providing multi channel capability by using sub carrier modulation. A typical single channel telemetry link is shown in Fig. 17.9 The single channel battery powered FM transmitter shown would normally be one cubic inch or so in volume, providing several hundred hours of operation from one or two miniature mercury batteries. The receiver must provide DC coupling from the discriminator to give the system a DC signal transmission capability, and, to avoid DC drift, both transmitter and receiver should be crystal controlled.

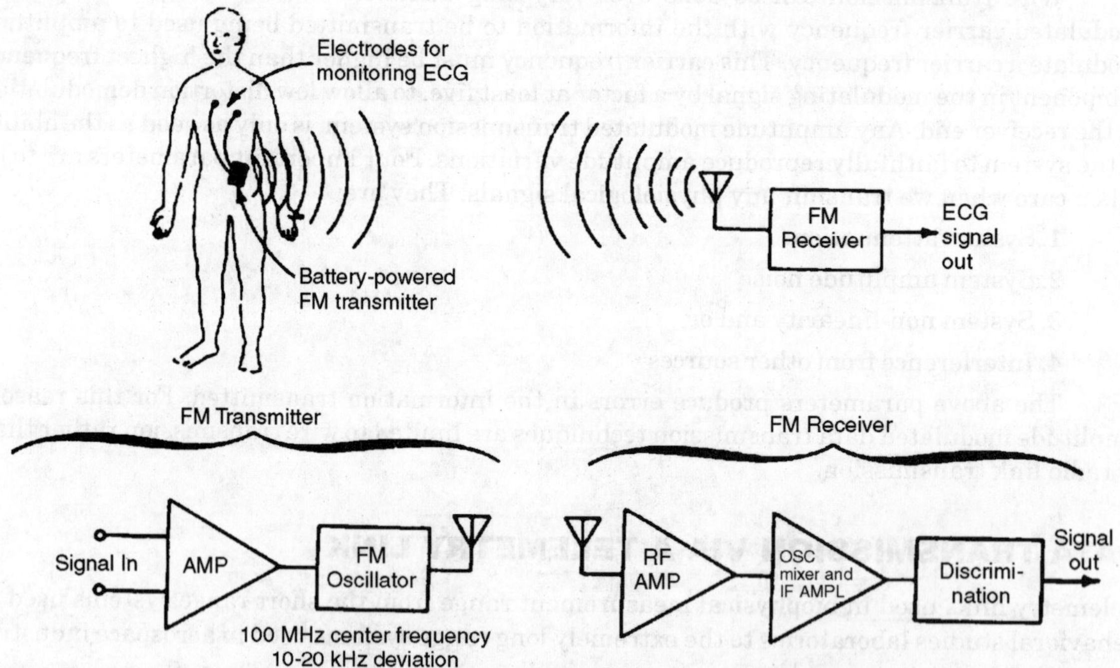

Fig. 17.9. Shows a typical single-channel telemetry link.

A typical multi channel telemetry link is shown is Fig. 17.9*b*. The input signal is used to frequency modulate sub carrier oscillators operating below 100 kHz; the frequency modulated outputs from these three sub carrier oscillators are mixed and used to frequency modulate a higher frequency oscillator. This system is referred to as FM/FM system as both the sub carrier oscillators and the main oscillator are frequency modulated. A list of IRIG FM/FM sub carrier frequency bands is shown in Fig. 17.9. The maximum signal that can be transmitted via the telemetry is known as the nominal intelligence frequency . This nominal intelligence frequency is directly proportional to the bandwidth of the sub carrier channel used. It can be seen from Fig. 17.9, that at a sub channel bandwidth of 24.75 kHz, the nominal intelligence frequency is only 2.5 kHz. Many multi channel telemetry systems use wider channel bandwidths and thus require correspondingly greater channel separations. Sub carrier bands 1 through 21 shown in Fig. 17.9 have relatively narrow bandwidth; however, sub carrier bands A through H have wider bandwidths to allow higher frequency component of information to be transmitted.

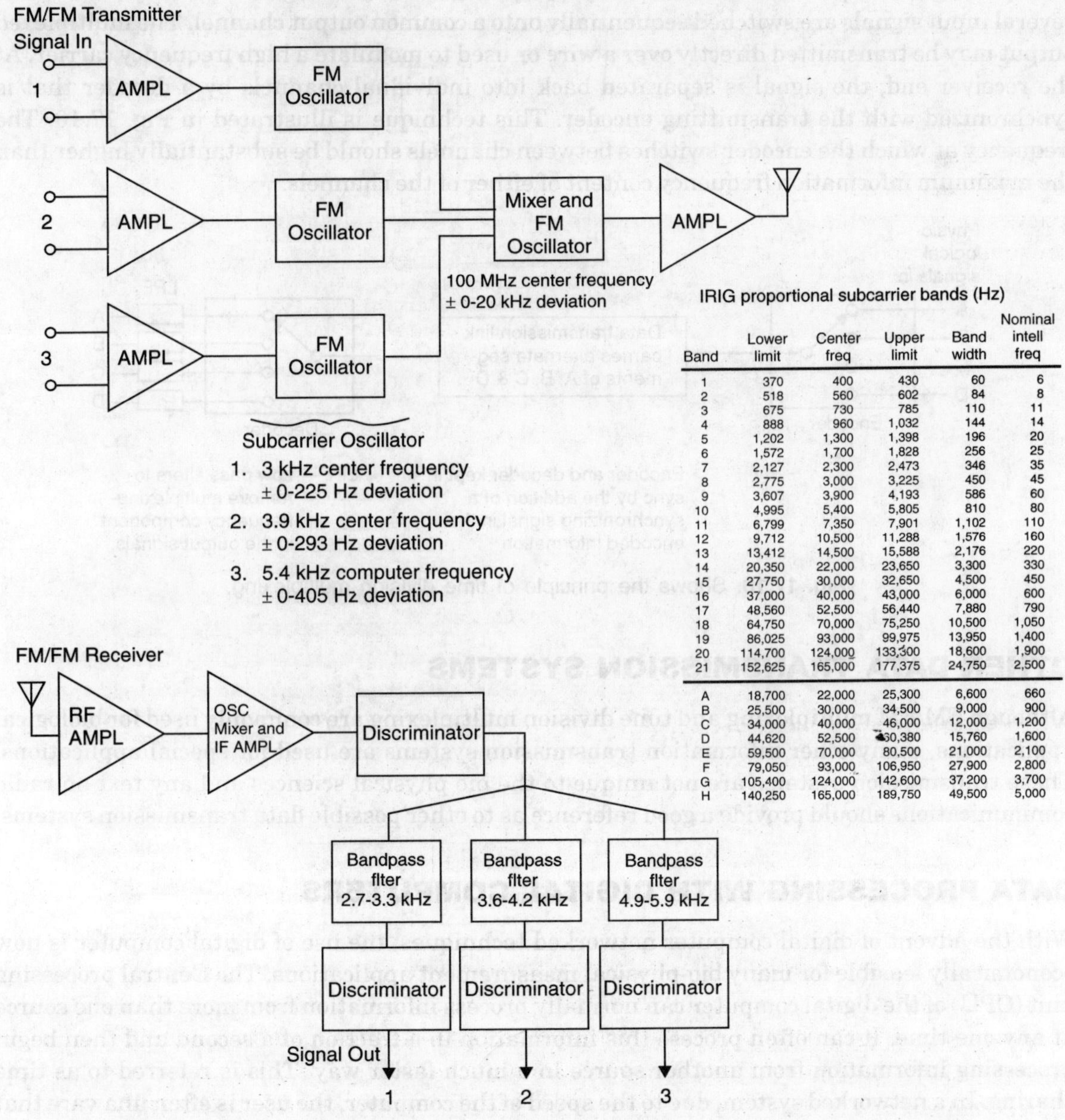

IRIG proportional subcarrier bands (Hz)

Band	Lower limit	Center freq	Upper limit	Band width	Nominal intell freq
1	370	400	430	60	6
2	518	560	602	84	8
3	675	730	785	110	11
4	888	960	1,032	144	14
5	1,202	1,300	1,398	196	20
6	1,572	1,700	1,828	256	25
7	2,127	2,300	2,473	346	35
8	2,775	3,000	3,225	450	45
9	3,607	3,900	4,193	586	60
10	4,995	5,400	5,805	810	80
11	6,799	7,350	7,901	1,102	110
12	9,712	10,500	11,288	1,576	160
13	13,412	14,500	15,588	2,176	220
14	20,350	22,000	23,650	3,300	330
15	27,750	30,000	32,650	4,500	450
16	37,000	40,000	43,000	6,000	600
17	48,560	52,500	56,440	7,880	790
18	64,750	70,000	75,250	10,500	1,050
19	86,025	93,000	99,975	13,950	1,400
20	114,700	124,000	133,300	18,600	1,900
21	152,625	165,000	177,375	24,750	2,500
A	18,700	22,000	25,300	6,600	660
B	25,500	30,000	34,500	9,000	900
C	34,000	40,000	46,000	12,000	1,200
D	44,620	52,500	60,380	15,760	1,600
E	59,500	70,000	80,500	21,000	2,100
F	79,050	93,000	106,950	27,900	2,800
G	105,400	124,000	142,600	37,200	3,700
H	140,250	165,000	189,750	49,500	5,000

Fig. 17.9. Shows a typical multichannel telemetry link-frequency division multiplexed.

TIME DIVISION MULTIPLEXING

Multiplexing refers to the combining of several channels of information to allow this information to be transmitted via one data transmission link. The FM/FM telemetry system discussed previously is an example of frequency division multiplexing. By using the FM/FM technique, all the signals are transmitted simultaneously by using various frequency bands to separate the signals. Whereas frequency division multiplexing is true simultaneous transmission of separate channels of data, time division multiplexing consists of sequential transmission of separate channels of data. This multiplexing technique is best illustrated by the operation of a rotating commutator in which the several input signals are switched sequentially onto a common output channel. The multiplexed output may be transmitted directly over a wire or used to modulate a high frequency carrier. At the receiver end, the signal is separated back into individual channels by a decoder that is synchronized with the transmitting encoder. This technique is illustrated in Fig. 17.10. The frequency at which the encoder switches between channels should be substantially higher than the maximum information frequency content of either of the channels.

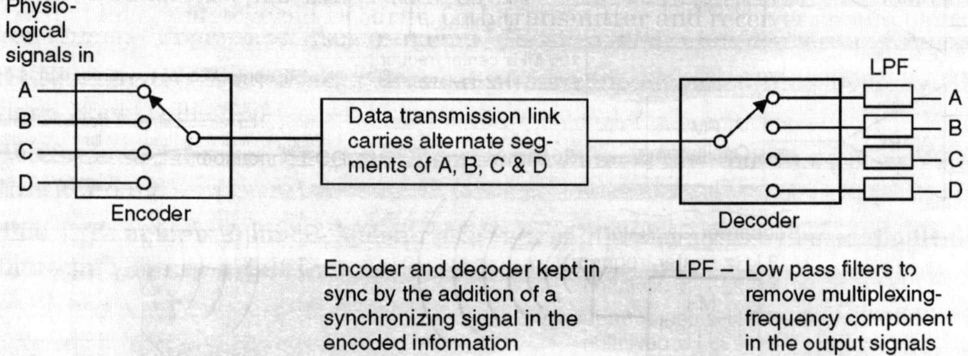

Fig. 17.10. Shows the principle of time division multiplexing.

OTHER DATA TRANSMISSION SYSTEMS

Although FM/FM multiplexing and time division multiplexing are commonly used for biological applications, many other information transmission systems are used for special applications. These transmission systems are not unique to the bio physical sciences and any text on radio communications should provide a good reference as to other possible data transmission systems.

DATA PROCESSING WITH DIGITAL COMPUTERS

With the advent of digital computer networked techniques, the use of digital computer is now economically feasible for many bio-physical measurement applications. The Central processing unit (CPU) of the digital computer can normally process information from more than one source at any one time. It can often process this information in a fraction of a second and then begin processing information from another source in a much faster way. This is referred to as time sharing. In a networked system, due to the speed of the computer, the user is often unaware that the central processing unit is sharing its time between him and many other users.

It is customary to process the data to the digital computers in digital form. That is, data must be presented to, and is received from, a digital computer in a digital format. If analog data is to be processed with a digital computer, it must, therefore, be converted to digital form using analog to digital converting techniques. This conversion of analog signal into digital format can be done using different techniques. Some important analog to digital conversion techniques are:

1. Successive approximation technique using a Digital to Analog Converter (DAC).
2. Counter type analog to digital converters
3. Dual slope integration method and
4. Flash type analog to digital converters (high speed).

By using any one of the above techniques, the analog data can be converted into digital form and the same can be given to the digital computer for processing. Each method has its own merits and demerits, but depending on the application one will have choice of using any one method mentioned above.

If a computer is remotely located, from the analog data gathering site, then it is preferable to transmit and receive data in analog form. If the data is digitized on site, it must be either transmitted in parallel to the computer (one cable per bit), which is very expensive, or serially, which is also possible with present day technological improvement in the field of communication, in a much faster and less expensive way. It is quite feasible for ECG or EEG data, but impractical for direct brain recording of action potentials.

REAL TIME PROCESSING

Since the time scale of analog data is usually important, this time scale must be maintained when processing analog data via a digital computer. It is thus necessary that the computer process this data in real time as shown in Fig. 17.11*a*. This precludes the direct use of a time shared computing system unless the priorities in the time shared system are arranged so that processing of this analog information takes absolute priority over any other processing. In this case, the time shared computer system would process this data in real time. For this reason, many self contained small computers are used in this application.

The time scale of analog data is usually important and must be maintained during a data processing procedure; but it is possible for a time shared computer system to indirectly process this data in other than real time and then reconstruct the data in real time after a finite delay through the use of storage devices. Referring to Fig. 17.11*b*, analog data is converted to digital data using an analog to digital converter; this digital data is then stored in a digital storage device. The time shared computing system then accepts data from the digital storage device on time shared basis with transfer being controlled by the computer. Digital data from the computer will then be produced in segments as the computing system finds time to process stored data. These segments of digital data can then be converted to analog data and shown or they may be stored in a digital storage device before converting. All of the analog data can then be withdrawn from the storage device to preserve the time scale of the data.

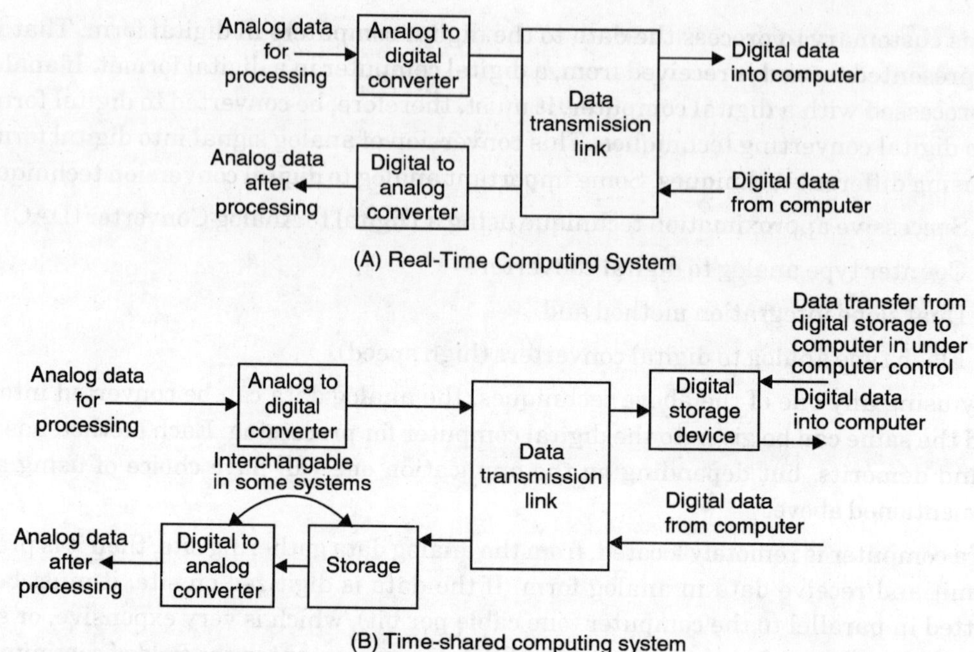

Fig. 17.11. Shows a analog data to and from a digital computer.

A graphic computer terminal shown in Fig. 17.12, when interfaced wit a custom analog input module, is was used to analog input data processing with a time shared hospital computing system. The terminal when used in conjunction with "modem" (modulator / demodulator) and data communication service provides necessary electronics to implement the time shared computing system discussed in the previous paragraph. The storage function is achieved by using memory cards/sticks (removable). The communication lie provided by the data communication service should have sufficient bandwidth (baudrate capability) to allow data transmission in real time. The ECG signal typically requires only a 400 baud rate.

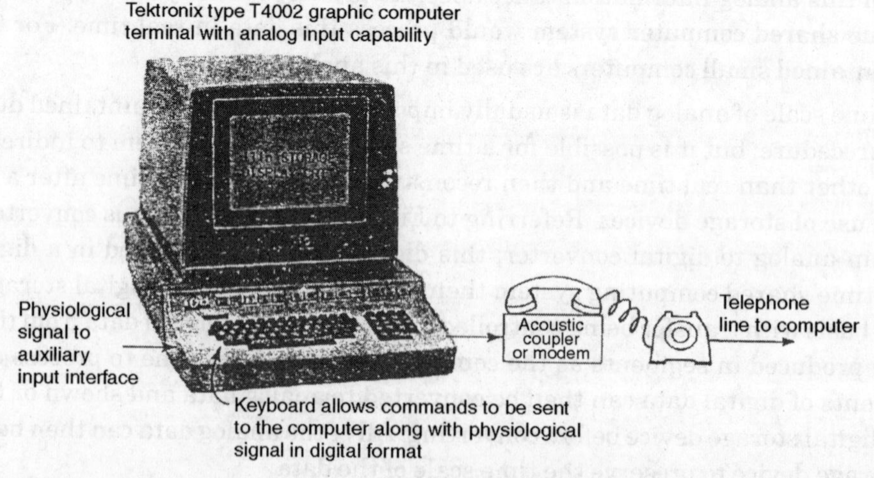

Fig. 17.12. Shows a computer terminal used for physiological signal analysis and processing via a remote computer. A modern card is in-built in the motherboard in PCs today.

DATA PROCESSING APPLICATIONS AND DEVELOPMENTS IN SOFTWARE

Data processing applications in biophysical measurements require application software (computer programs) to control the computer in performing specific tasks. This software is continuously being developed by computer manufacturers, computer users and many other companies and they have "library" of software programs available to their customers.

The digital computer is particularly suited to signal averaging. Any computer that also permits prestimulus averaging and computation of statistical information such as standard deviation and trends is useful. The digital storage display unit with an analog to digital converter serves as a complete signal averaging instrument.

ECG ANALYSIS USING COMPUTERS

Computers are now extensively used for analysis of ECG waveforms. The information storage and waveform comparison capability of the computer allow it to compare an ECG signal with other ECG signals is within its acceptable statistical limits. Long back in the 80's the Control Data Corporation provided software for electrocardiogram analysis to use with their model 1704 computer; the complete package of computer software and peripheral equipment is designated the "1700 computer electrocardiogram analysis system". This system identified, measured and analysed waveforms of 12-lead electrocardiograms by performing a pattern recognition analysis on the electrocardiogram and provided a printout of the results for diagnostic use.

Today, computers are ideally suited to simulation of physiological systems; thus, in many cases, they allow an analysis of physiological systems within a computer rather than performing physiological measurements.

Computer based medical simulators, with realistic visuals and touch sensations, enables one to hone their skills. The mist VR system (Muse Tech., ltd., Albuquerque, NN) is used to train on Laperoscopic surgery. The colour monitor displays shapes, not body parts. An interface device has the handles of Tools for surgery on gall bladder etc.

TELEMETRY IN OPERATING ROOM

The use of telemetry in operating rooms is to perform a higher degree of patient safety such as electric shocks etc. And also for elimination of the hanging interconnection of leads from the patient which are required in direct - wired equipment.

Generally several parameters are monitored in surgical patient monitoring. Most common being are:

1. ECG
2. Blood pressure
3. Peripheral pulse and
4. EEG

The above are the four parameters observed generally.

A 4-channel telemetry system is ideally suited for this application. Basically the signal recording is based upon frequency modulation of four sub carriers centered around 2.2, 3.5 , 5 and 7.5 kHz respectively. The Bandwidth of a typical system is of the order of 100 Hz at the 3 dB point and the discriminator provides 1v dc output for a 10% shift in the subcarrier associated with each of the four channels. For ECG signals, 2 V peak to peak (0.05 to 100Hz), 100 μV of EEG signal (1 to 40 Hz), 100 mmHg of arterial blood pressure (dc to 40Hz) and 400 μV peak to peak for the values of peripheral pulse (0.1 to 40 Hz). The four sub-carriers are summed and used to frequency modulate a radio frequency carrier oscillator which is tuned in such a way that the frequency is within the FM band. The transmitter signals are then tuned by a FM tuner whose output is fed to a 4th channel discriminator. This separates the sub-carriers through filter circuits and demodulation is done by using phase -locked loop (PLL). The demodulated signals are displayed on the monitor.

SPORTS PHYSIOLOGY STUDIES THROUGH TELEMETRY

Monitoring of pulmonary ventilation, heart rate and respiration rate are required for the study of energy expenditure during physical work especially for sports such as squash, handball, tennis and track etc. A radio telemetry system is used for the above measurements on human subjects during vigorous exercise. The transmitter uses pulse duration modulation. In this technique, each channel is sampled sequentially and a pulse is generated. The width of the pulse is proportional to the amplitude of the corresponding signal. At each end of the frame, a synchronization gap is inserted to ensure that the receiving system locks correctly on to the signal.

Each channel is sampled 200 times a second. With each clock pulse, a counter advances one step making the gates to open sequentially. At the starting of a particular gate, the corresponding physiological signal is obtained and it is given to the comparator. The comparator compares with the ramp signal and finds out where the signal exactly lies on the ramp. When the ramp voltage exceeds the signal voltage, the comparator changes state. Thus, the time required for the comparator to change state depends upon the amplitude of the signal. The counter and gate serve as multiplexer.

The pulse train at the output of the comparator is used to frequency modulate the RF oscillator in 88–108 MHz band. The transmitter is designed to work in a range of 100 m, which can be extended using whip antenna. Such telemetry transmitter dissipates approximately 60 mW and the batteries give continuous service for 125 hours. Single ended amplification was found to be quite enough to readable ECG recordings. The electrode thermistor were placed at the sternum. The pulmonary ventilation and respiration rate were derived from the thermistor transducer.

At the receiving end, the system contains a FM tuner and a circuitry which converts the pulse width changes into analog voltages and a multichannel pen recorder to display the physiological signals. Fig. 17.13 shows a three channel telemetry system for monitoring the physiological data of a sprinter.

Monitoring of breathing pressures inside the face mask in exercising subjects, mobile and stationery is another interesting application of radio-telemetry. (Fig. 17.14)

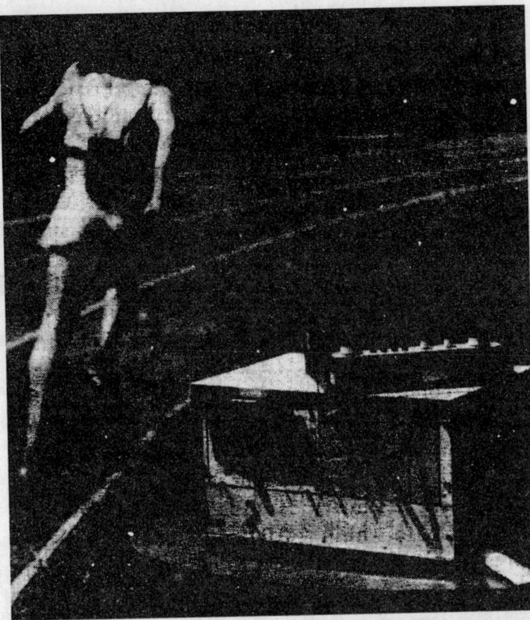

Fig. 17.13. Shows a three channel telemetry system to monitor the physiological data of a sprinter (Courtesy Hellige, W. Germany).

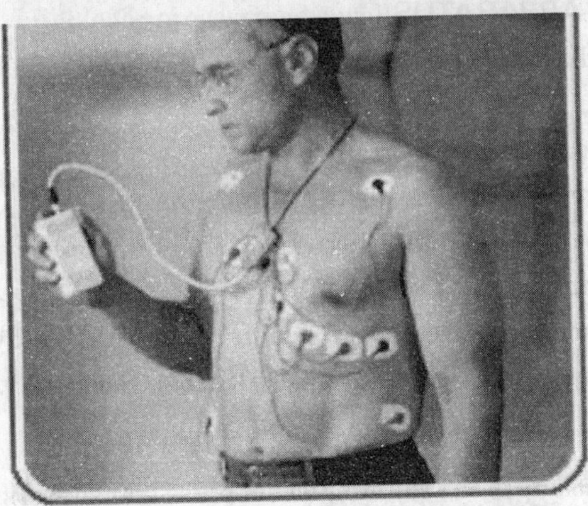

Fig. 17.14. 12 Lead Recorder/Transmitter (ECG).

- Uses a 10-wire patient cable for 12 lead lead ECG recording.
- Simultaneously records 2.5 seconds per lead and 10 seconds of lead II as rhythm lead.
- Sequentially transmits 12 lead ECG separated by 1 mV calibration signal via telephone.
- Direct transmission of ECG via RS232 to PC computer (optional).
- Pocket-sized. Weighs 110 grams without battery.
- Frequency response : 0.05–150 Hz.

Chapter 18

Practical Electronic Medical Laboratory Experiments

I. PERPHERAL PULSE MEASUREMENT

EXPERIMENT

To prepare a transducer for pulse (arterial) measurement and

1. To record the pulse waveform
2. To determine the heart rate.

Additional experiments might involve the design of a suitable active 50 Hz active notch filter for the signal picked up from the photo detector.

LIST OF PARTS AND APPARATUS

1. LDR CdS 1cm dia with dark resistance of 100K ohms -1 or
2. Photo transistor IPL33 -1
3. Circuit components as per diagram given.
4. An electrical wiring PVC Conduit T of 1 inch dia.
5. A filament bulb of 3 V 45 mA as found in mini hand torches
6. A 5 V power supply, ripple free.(10 mV)
7. A long persistance oscilloscope 5mV sensitivity, 1 MHz bandwidth enough.
   or a digital storage oscilloscope such as TDS2024 (Scientific).

PROCEDURE

The finger pulse pick up is one the simplest of pulse transducers to know the arterial blood flow and also to determine the heart rate. The same signal can also be used to determine the Diastolic pressure in the indirect blood pressure measurement (see Expt.2).

The ***T*** tube of PVC is ideal for inserting the thumb of the left finger into the vertical hole and then the two sides of the T are for housing the lamp on the one side and the photo detector circuit board on the other.

A circuit for the same using the LDR was given in the Chapter on Circulation measurements. It is given again here.

The circuit provides the output of 100-200mV at the collector of the transistor. This can be directly observed on a long persistence CRO or the Digital storage oscilloscope. The reason why general purpose oscilloscopes are not useful is that here, the time base is to be set as 2 seconds per sweep and the signal is coming so slowly that the trace fades away before permitting one to view the complete sphygmogram.

In a (crange phosphor) long persistence tube CRO, this is visible. In a Digital storage oscilloscope, since only the stored data is repeatedly presented, the trace is visible, even though the effective sweep is 2 second.

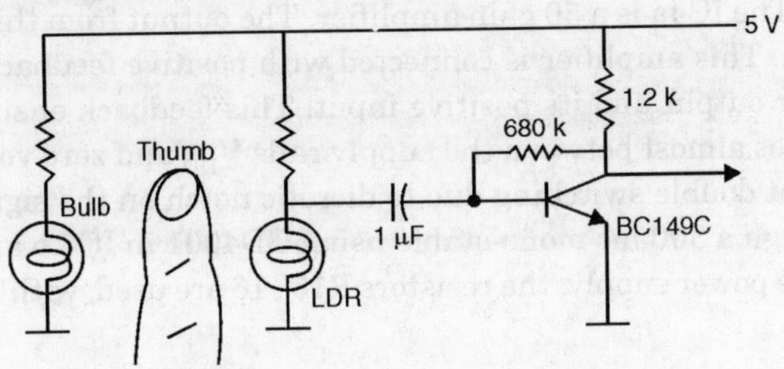

Fig. 18.1. Pulse pick up circuit.

In DSOs, there is provision to send the waveform data, after "freezing" it to a PC through the interface provided on the scope. Usually RS232 interface is simple, and the copy can be printed on the PC printer.

The data file is available for processing as well.

Fig. 18.2 below shows another circuit for the pick up.

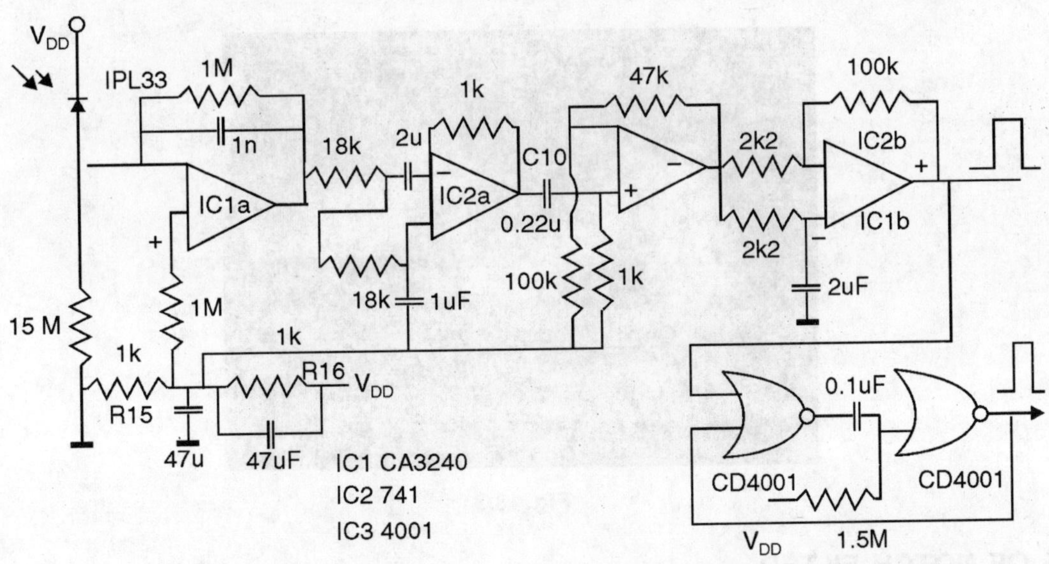

Fig. 18.2. Showing the circuit of the pick up amplifier and the pulse shaper.

The use of the photodiode can be similarly made as the LDR, but the current through the diode is operated at a much less value since the diode is actually worked in reverse mode. So, a high input operational amplifier is useful for picking up the signal. A dual IC OPAMP (CA3240) is chosen for the initial amplification because of its relatively low noise and high impedance FET input. The reverse leakage current as affected by the light passing through the finger pulp is amplified.

The second amplifier is connected as a second order low pass filter with a cut off frequency of 15 Hz.

The sphygmo signal is available at the capacitor C10. Further to this, two more stages of OPAMPs are shown. The IC4a is a 50 gain amplifier. The output from this is connected to IC1b, via resistors 2 K each. This amplifier is connected with positive feedback by connecting 100 K between the amplifier output and its positive input. This feedback ensures that the amplifier output voltage switches almost between the supply rails V_{DD} and zero volts. It is like a Schmitt trigger. To ensure that double switching due to dicrotic notch on the signal does not occur, the signal is passed through a 300 ms mono-stable using CD4001 in IC3 b and a. To get the center voltage from the single power supply, the resistors R15 , 16 are used, with decoupling by 47 micro Farad capacitors.

The power supply for this circuit would be 9V from a regulated supply, using a 7809. The bulb is series connected with a current limiting resistor which absorbs the balance voltage. For *e.g.*, if a 3.6 V bulb is used, then the 4.4 V divided by the current of 50 mA in the bulb will need a resistor of 91 ohms, 1/2 W.

EXPERIMENT

Record the waveform of the finger pulse for several subjects and compare between them through amplitude,Frequency and wave shape. (Fig. 18.3)

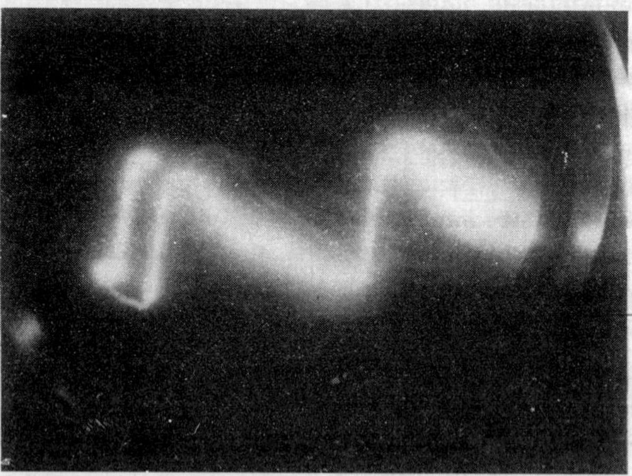

Fig. 18.3

USE OF NOTCH FILTER

The signal might be picking up 50 Hz hum due to improper filtering of the power supply to the bulb, causing the hum through the light source. For this purpose, a filter of high Q using active op-amp can be used.

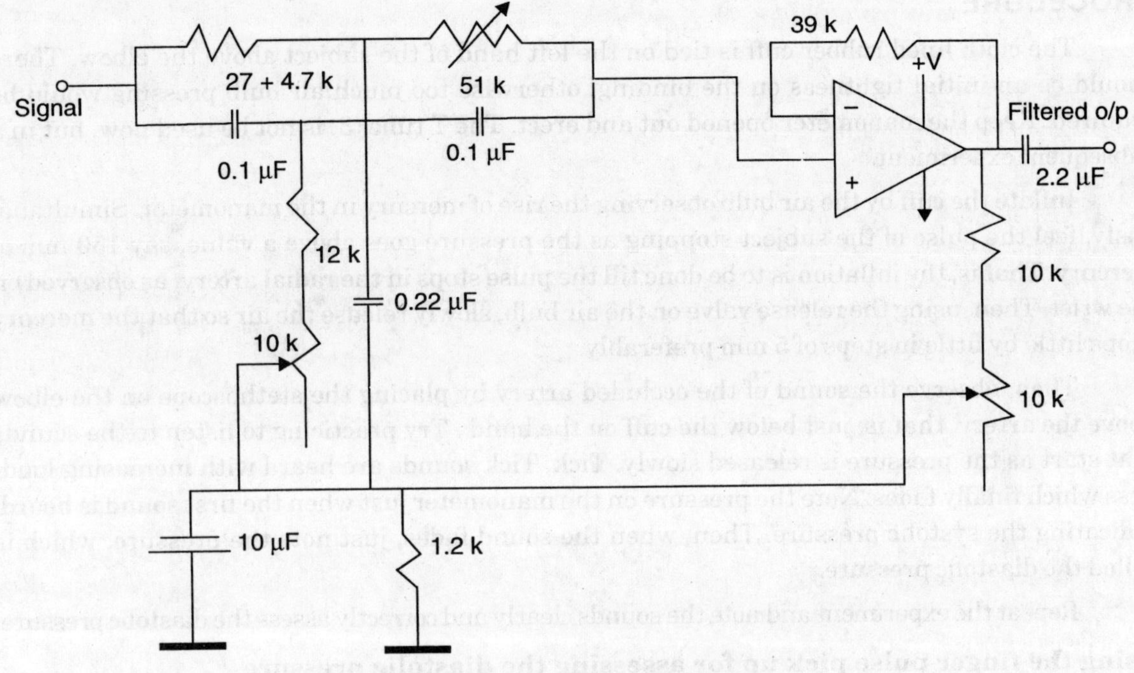

Fig. 18.4. Active Notch Filter Circuit.

By adjusting the 51 K and the 10 K resistor at the left, the frequency is tuned to 50 Hz for rejection, using an audio frequency generator. Then, the Q of the filter is adjusted by the right 10 K resistor for best notch effect as observed on the signal of interest, the sphygmo signal.

II. BLOOD PRESSURE MEASUREMENT WITH THE SPHYGMOMANOMETER

EXPERIMENT

To learn to measure the Blood pressure of a subject properly, using the Riva-Rocci method. Also, to investigate the alternatives in measuring the diastolic pressure.

APPARATUS

1. The mercury well sphygmomanometer with inflating cuff and a stethoscope.
2. Alternatively the CH-403C Citizen make B.P. automatic measurement apparatus. (available here)
3. A glass T tube of size to fit on the rubber tubing used in the above units.

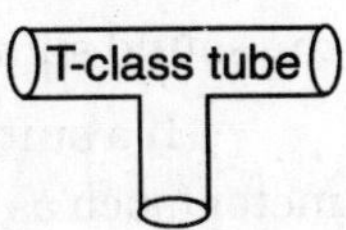

4. The finger pulse pick up with a storage oscilloscope for viewing the signal, or else a long persistence amber screen scope.

PROCEDURE

The cloth lined rubber cuff is tied on the left hand of the subject above the elbow. There should be an initial tightness on the binding, otherwise too much air bulb pressing would be required. Keep the manometer opened out and erect. The T tube (3) is not be used now, but in a subsequent experiment.

Inflate the cuff by the air bulb observing the rise of mercury in the manometer. Simultaneously, feel the pulse of the subject stopping as the pressure goes above a value, say 150 mm of mercury. That is, the inflation is to be done till the pulse stops in the radial artery, as observed on the wrist. Then, using the release valve on the air bulb, slowly release the air so that the mercury drops little by little in steps of 5 mm preferably.

Then, observe the sound of the occluded artery by placing the stethoscope on the elbow above the artery, that is, just below the cuff on the hand . Try practicing to listen to the sounds that start as the pressure is released slowly. Tick, Tick sounds are heard with increasing loudness which finally fades. Note the pressure on the manometer just when the first sound is heard, indicating the systolic pressure. Then, when the sound fades, just note the pressure, which is called the diastolic pressure.

Repeat the experiment and note the sounds clearly and correctly assess the diastolic pressure.

Using the finger pulse pick up for assessing the diastolic pressure

If the finger pulse pick up is also used with the subject, then it is possible to measure the diastolic pressure by noting when the signal increases and reaches a maximum and falls. The signal will rise as the cuff pressure is released below systolic pressure. Then, when it reaches the lower diastolic pressure value, the artery fully admits blood flow and hence the signal increases. This signal increase can be observed on the scope, by using a slow time base as in Fig. 18.3. Then, when the rise is maximum and then it falls, note the pressure, which is the diastolic pressure.

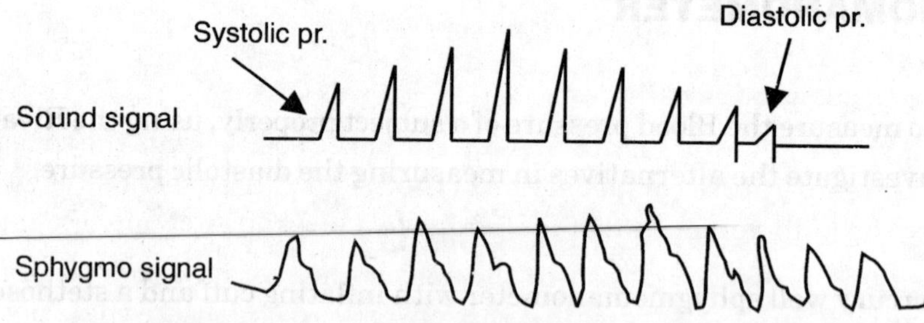

Fig. 18.4

After reaching maximum value, the pulse signal remains constant as it should be, whereas the sound signal is absent after diastolic pressure.

If a suitable meter is provided on the output of the finger pulse signal, using a 500 uA mini meter (such as the one available as VU-meter for audio parts shops for Rs. 30/-), then the observation of the peak of the signal would be easier.

A good electronics enthusiast could relate this maximum rise point to switch on to the pressure channel to show the diastolic pressure accordingly on a display.

USE OF SENSYM PRESSURE SENSOR

Instead of measuring the pressure by a manometer, as the unit CH403 (Citizen make) does, one can use a pressure transducer for measuring the pressure and use the signal output from it for a digital read out.

APPARATUS

1. Sensym pressure transducer 0 to 30 psia (SX30AN)
2. Circuit for getting the analog value of the pressure from the sensor

The Sensym products are of USA origin but they are available locally. The pressure transducer is small size unit like a matchbox and has a tube connection for connecting to the pressure line. That is why, the T tube is used to connect the pressure tube to this inlet in addition.

The Sensym pressure transducer is a bridge of semiconductor strain gauge mounted on the flexing diaphragm under pressure applied. The signal is generated by passing a constant current to the Wheatstone bridge like configuration inside the unit. The output signal is to be amplified by an OPAMP.

There are four pins on the small unit for connecting to the internal bridge.

The transducer is sensitive, fast in response and fairly accurate, after calibration of the signal.

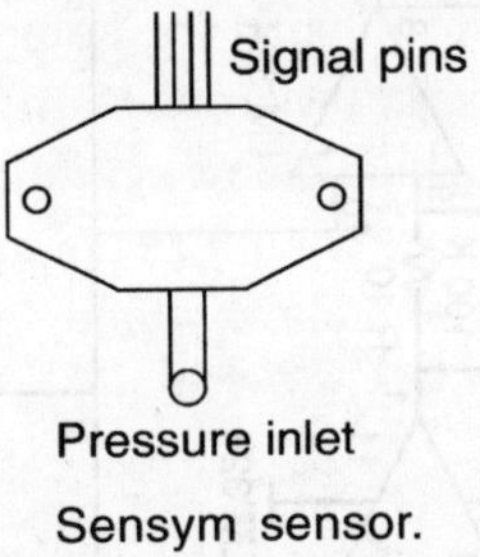

Sensym sensor.

Schematic of the pressure transducer

The circuit is shown below in Fig. 18.5. A 5 V stabilized source feeds the sensor bridge. The Diodes D1-D4 are for temperature compensation of the bridge. Three sections of LM324 OPAMP are used to amplify the milli-volt output of the bridge to a level for A/D conversion.

When there is no pressure applied to the sensor the voltage between pins 2,4 is zero. However, there may be a small voltage, called zero offset. To compensate that , pot R16 allows a small DC volts to be fed to the amplifier that would negate the offset voltage.

When the sensor is exposed to 30 psi, corresponding to about 760 mm of mercury on a manometer, the bridge will generate about 35 mV. This is only a rough figure, that might vary from one sensor to another. R6 adjusts amplifier gain.

The ICL 7106 is an A/D converter together with the LCD display. The voltage between pins 7 and 8 is the output which is fed to the IC. The reference voltage is between pins 35 and 36. This is set by R2-R4 to be 240 mV.

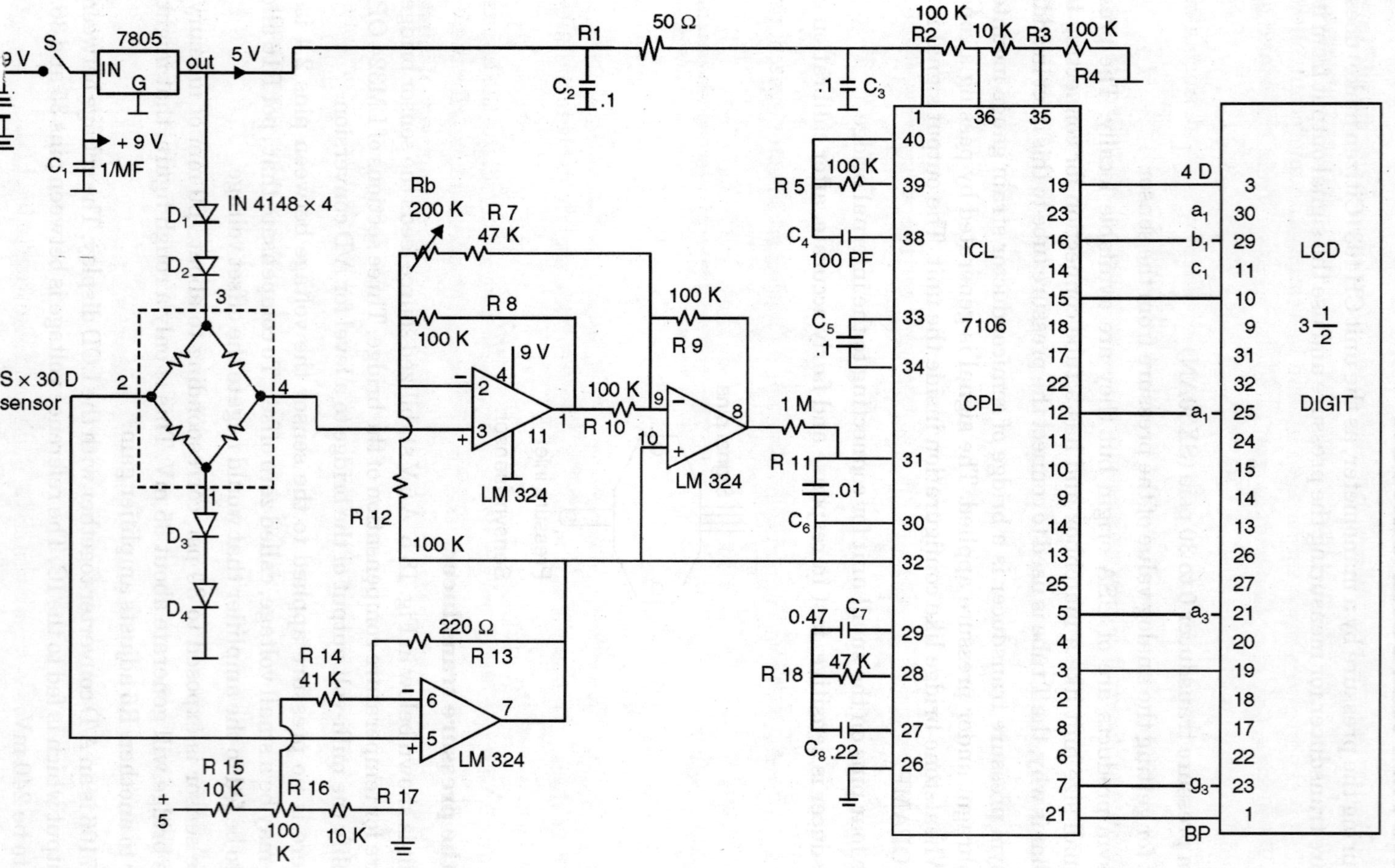

Fig. 18.5. Circuit of Sensym Sensor based Blood Pressure Meter.

If this circuit board is made and kept ready, then the experiment can be performed easily.

A microcontroller based circuit board can also made to order and the output from the bridge can be analog digital converted and used by the microcontroller to display the value. Also, the sound signal as picked from a mike under the cuff can be read by the microcontroller. The logic can be programmed to display the systolic and diastolic pressure from the sound signal sensing through a software on the unit.

A typical microcontroller board with LCD alphanumeric display is ideal. Such a circuit can be referred to from Electronics for You Magazine, Jan.2003 issue.

Fig. 18.5 showing the circuit of Sensym pressure transducer and LCD display 7106.

III. STUDY AND MEASUREMENTS ON THE COMMERCIAL MEDICAL ECG RECORDER

EXPERIMENT

To study the use of the ECG recorder on a subject and get the waveforms of the ECG correctly without any artifacts.

APPARATUS

1. A hot stylus recorder based portable ECG machine with lead selector switch, patient cable
2. Chart paper, jelly tube, electrode clips for limbs and suction cup electrodes for chest.
3. Signal output to CRO

PROCEDURE

Note the markings of the colour on the leads and connect the patient cable to the subject in lying position, with chest open.

The colours of the leads I to III are used to connect the patient electrodes to the hands, feet. The chest lead is either taken one by one, or in some machines, they keep all cups for the V leads at the same time. This solves the problem of smearing of jelly on the chest causing signal interaction among the V leads.

The subject must be lying on a wooden table. There may not be any jewels or ornaments of metal on the person.

Jelly is applied in small dots at the places of contact on the limbs and chest positions V1 to V6, as shown in the Chapter on ECG.

1. First the Machine is switched on. Then, the calibrate button is pressed, so that the chart paper moves and shows the 1 mV pulse standard. Note that is consitently the same amplitude.
2. Then take the lead selector switch to Lead I position and the ECG should be moving on the paper.
3. Take two or three waves and switch to lead II and likewise to lead III.
4. Then switch to the recording of the auxiliary leads aVR, aVL, aVF.

5. Then connect to the V leads and obtain the six records.
6. Finally, for Lead II, take a Ecg after asking the subject to take and hold a deep breath for ½ min and record 3 cycles of ECG.

Do not waste chart paper unnecessarily.

Now, switch off the machine, clean the subject free of jelly and then look at the records.

Technical aspects

1. Is the record in all cases free from base line shift?
2. Is the record showing 50 Hz hum in any one or more leads?
3. Is the record showing adequate amplitude as a normal subject ?

Medical aspects

4. Draw the cardiac vector on the Einthoven triangle and measure the angle. Is there any deviation from normal?
5. Observe all V leads and find their uniform change from V1 to V6. The T waves must all be upright.
6. Observe the ST segment and note that it is iso-electric.
7. Observe the QRS complex at each of the 12 leads and see if there is a proper QRS with no broadening or Q-wave indication or notched QRS.
8. Since the subject you will be using is not likely to have any abnormalities, the waveforms should be showing normal ECG only.
9. In order to observe and study pathological conditions, it would be necessary to take to a hospital.

EXPERIMENT

To study the frequency response and transient response of the ECG recorder.

APPARATUS

Same as per the above experiment, but no need for jelly or patient electrode clips. An audio oscillator with calibrated output (or with meter)

PROCEDURE

1. Frequency Response

This is to be determined for the ECG machine from externally applied signals from a variable frequency oscillator. We are going to use only upto 150 Hz.

How to connect the oscillator output to the ECG machine?

Since the signal from an audio oscillator is likely to be in the Volts range and since we have to feed only millivolts to the machine, the signal output from the oscillator is to be attenuated by resistor divider.

Further, the signal has to be applied in differential mode, i.e., between any two leads with earth lead being the ground of the oscillator.

One way to give this is shown in figure below.

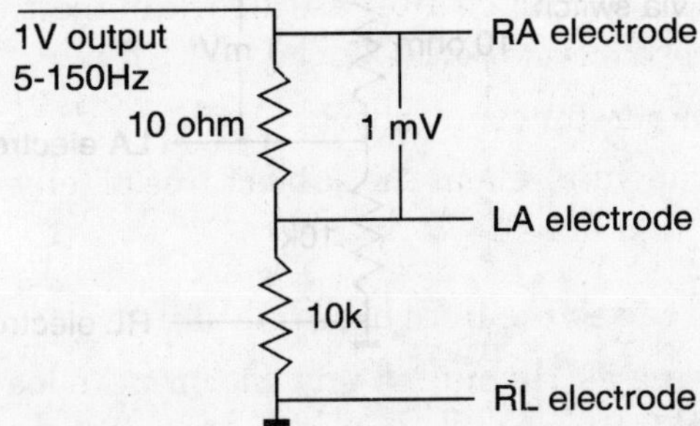

Measure the voltage as above to be 1 mV on a digital 4.5 digit LCD meter on the AC scale.

Then connect the lead wires to this resistor network as shown and switch to LEAD 1 position.

Then, apply the signal from oscillator little by little varying the frequency and noting the record response.

The chart paper should not be wasted and just enough movement for each spot frequency is to be taken.

Tabulate the results indicating amplitude and frequency.

Plot the response on a graph paper.

One can use computer software for drawing the graph using a graph program such as EXCEL.

Precaution is that it is necessary to maintain the voltage at 1 mV in all frequencies.

The response curve should match the standard given by AHA.

Observations

1. Is there is any notch or peak in the frequency region at any frequency?
2. Did you find there is a dip at 50 Hz? If so, the filter select must be deselected.
3. Is there any response above 100 Hz?
4. What will be the shape of the normal ECG if the instrument's response was peaking at 2 Hz.

For example? How will it affect the QRS and T waves?

Transient response

In order to record the transient response, it is necessary to apply a step input of 1 mV. For this, a DC voltage of 1 V is applied to the network. But the recorder is kept on before switching the DC voltage on.

The response curve should indicate the fast rise over a division of one or 2 mm and there may be a slight overshoot.

The response of course includes the amplifier part and the recorder part put together.

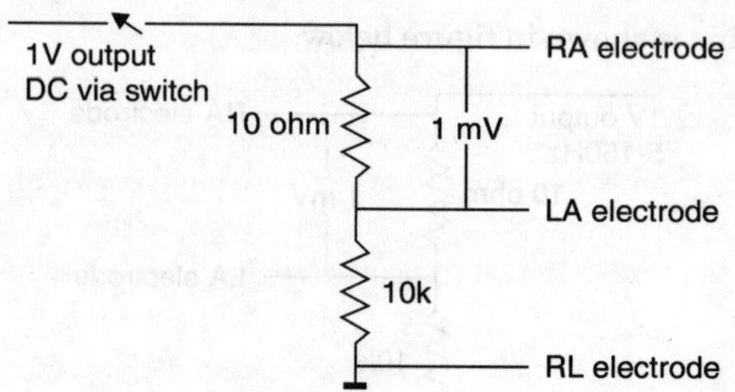

IV. BIOLOGICAL AMPLIFIER-E.E.G SIGNAL RECORDING

EXPERIMENT

To use the Biological amplifier in the EEG-mode and record scalp EEG signals.

A strip chart recorder for fast recording. Dedicated hot stylus or pen motor type recorders are not available. This can be a PC based recording on printer if the signal is coupled through a serial port to the computer and a software on the same outputs the record to the printer (dot matrix) with continuous feed paper.

Or

Use a multi-channel EEG machine to record EEG signals.

PRINCIPLE

The use of biological amplifier in the most sensitive EEG mode is made use of in order to record EEG signals. However, with this, only a sample EEG signal can be noted. This is not meant for studies relating to signals from the brain, since that would need a large number of signals from several sets of electrodes.

Just recording a single signal from any one set of electrodes on the brain is only for the purpose of detecting brain activity such as during the progress of anesthesia administration. It is also useful for simple evoked potential experiments from flash light signals by signal processing.

However, for a full EEG signal recording, the use of an EEG machine is necessary, but since the same is expensive, a biological amplifier which has got provision for ECG, EEG or filtered signal outputs is sufficient.

A description of the Devices Inc., make Biological amplifier is given at the end of this experiment.

Accessories

Electrode for scalp-1 pair

Head belt with holes for fixing the electrode

Indifferent electrode-1 no.

Flashing source of light with a pulse output at the moment of the flash. Argon flash bulb based units are available.

PROCEDURE

1. The use of a shielded cage for the subject is essential for this experiment. The table or bench on which the subject lies is enclosed with a cage of copper or brass wire mesh and the shielded cable from the electrodes reach the amplifier which is outside the cage. The cage can be a size of 1.5 m × 2.5 m × 2 m in $l \times b \times w$ dimensions. The mesh must be connected to ground connection of the power outlet or to separate ground pipe laid for the laboratory.
2. The amplifier can be either battery operated with built in storage battery as it is now-a-days available. In that case, the hum pick up will be minimal.
3. After fixing two electrodes on the occipital lobe position O1 and O2, and the common ground electrode somewhere outside the head, near the ear or chin, the subject is asked to lie down and react to the signals applied to him through light flash.
4. The amplifier output is recorded on a strip chart recorder. The record can take quite a bit of time, even up to 30 minutes.
5. During the record, the flash light is made to blink which the subject watches for a minute. The record is taken note on the paper when the flash appears. The blink rate can be 1 or 2 seconds.
6. It is dangerous to apply these flash light signals to persons who are sensitive and prone to epileptic attack.

After completing the records, the waveform is looked up and analysed. If the data is fed to the computer, the analysis can be done through ensemble averaging by separating the records to several groups of 1 minute duration each and then averaging the signals. Each such group should begin with the instant of the flash correctly, which can be also fed to the computer through a signal available from the flashing light.

The records show the evoked response of the photic stimulation. This should be within limits on the records.

If the EEG machine itself is used, the same is provided with the flash source and the records can be observed on the length of chart paper. Even here, the signal averaging requires communication of the signal to a computer and then average processing is done there.

RESULTS

The results of the EEG recording would be the observation of the standard alpha to theta rhythm of the brain which, when there is evoked response, does not show easily on the record, but only with extensive recording and averaging the signal samples.

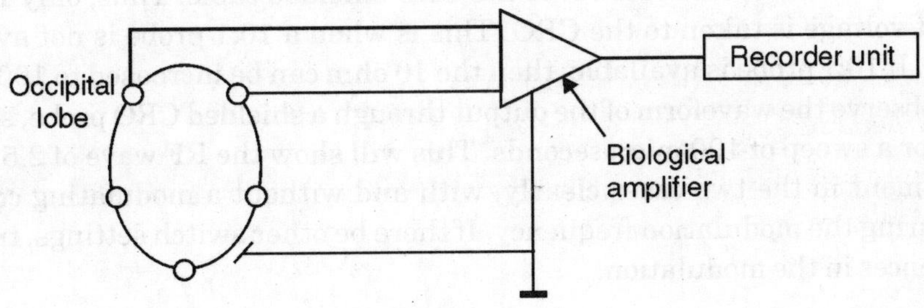

V. DIATHERMY MACHINE FOR SURGERY

EXPERIMENT

To study the details of the surgical diathermy apparatus and to use it for mock cutting and examine the safety aspects of using the instrument. Observation of variations in waveform for cutting and coagulating modes.

Apparatus

Surgical Diathermy apparatus 500 W or 1 KW S.W. (Short wave)

Electrodes for cutting and coagulating.

The back plate for patient.

Wire wound resistors of value 1 K, 10 ohms, 200 ohms at 10 W and 200 ohms 22 W.

Any 10MHz bandwidth C.R.O., with shielded probe. (10:1 probe)

PRINCIPLE

The Short wave diathermy apparatus is of two types - either the spark gap discharge based or generator based. The latter is predominantly in use today.

The short wave power is delivered at a level which can be adjusted.

The cutting action uses a burst of the R.F. power while for coagulating, it modulates the waveform with a lower frequency.

The use of the apparatus is by means of a foot switch for controlling the on and off by the surgeon.

The indifferent electrode is a large stainless steel plate which is kept under the back of the patient undergoing surgery. This must make the best contact with his body.. If there is a small contact resistance there, then the current, being large, when passing through that resistance, will heat the skin sufficiently high and cause burns on the back.

This is one of the problems in using this apparatus.

Further, there are problems of burns happening at other points of the body also, where too, a contact with the earthed bed might be there.

EXPERIMENTS

1. **Waveform observation.** Switch the instrument on and wait for a time of 1 minute. Then apply the patient switch after setting the control to cutting/coagulating. Connect a 1 K 10 W resistor to the electrode in series with a 10ohm 10 W. Then take wires from the 10 ohm resistor and connect to the CRO shielded cable. Thus, only 1/100 the of the output voltage is taken to the CRO. This is when a 10:1 probe is not available for the C.R.O. If 10:1 probe is available, then the 10 ohm can be increased to 100 ohms. In each case, observe the waveform of the output through a shielded CRO probe, setting the time base for a sweep of 100 microseconds. This will show the RF wave of 2.5 MHz from the instrument in the two cases clearly, with and without a modulating component. Try measuring the modulation frequency. If there be other switch settings, try and note the differences in the modulation.

2. Connect a high wattage 200 ohm 22 W resistor to the output and then switch on. Now observe the effect of applying the power. There will be instant heating up of the resistor and it may be burnt off. This shows that adequate power output is available.
3. Use the electrodes for seeing the effect. But this is very dangerous without using a hand glove of rubber. Use some heavy vegetable item such as a melon and keeping it on the back plate, try using the cutting electrode with lowest power output. As the electrode is just brought near, a spark will occur and then by dragging the electrode, the matter is cut. The voltage is high enough to start an arc at the cutting point. When trying in the coagulate switch position, the power level is less and the effect will be noted to be different. In actual surgery, coagulation seals up the blood vessels and prevents excessive bleeding after a cut has been made.
4. The safety aspect at the indifferent electrode: Some units try to measure the contact resistance of the back plate. If there is provision for it, then there will be an additional resistance measuring electrode on the patient's skin fixed near to the plate location. For the experiment, then, that plate will have to be brought into contact with the big plate for the unit to work. Try connecting a resistance of wire wound 10 ohms between the small sensing electrode plate and the main plate. See if the unit works or gives a warning light. Because even a small resistance of contact can cause undue heating of the skin, the unit needs to monitor the same.

For units not having this feature, the user must take the adequate precautions to see that the contact resistance is minimal and by keeping the patient well in contact with the plate. (He will any way be under anesthesia).

VI. E.M.G. APPARATUS EXPERIMENTS

EXPERIMENTS

To understand the principles of Electro myographic measurements with simple equipment and understand the problems of accurate recording of muscle potentials and diagnosing muscular problems and related nerve conduction problems.

Apparatus

1. A C.R.O. preferably of long persistence or else a Digital storage type with high sensitivity of at least 2 mV/cm.
2. An EMG differential amplifier
3. Electrodes of several types for observation only. Needle, concentric needle, small plate and circular metal (chlorided silver) types.
4. External stimulator for stimulus based experiments.

PRINCIPLES

The possibilities of conducting EMG experiments have already been outlined fully in the chapter on EMG.

Here, the simple and basic experiment on voluntary muscle contraction and associated action potential complex can be measured. The conduction velocity of nerve can be an additional experiment.

PROCEDURE

Two surface pick up electrodes are fixed to the thumb at the extremities and the ground plate is held tied to the wrist. The ground electrode is a conducting strip and is often a saline soaked strap wrapped around the patient's limb, i.e., above the wrist.

The differential amplifier output is connected to the CRO.

The differential amplifier is set for a gain of 1000 fixed. It must be having a CMRR of over 10,000.

The subject then makes contractions of his hand muscle and the observations are noted on the CRO at a gain setting of 2 mV per cm. The time base will be 100 or 200 ms sweep.

The potential waveforms are of the order of a few milliseconds and the amplitude will be within 5 mV. Thus only weak signals can be noted with the set up.

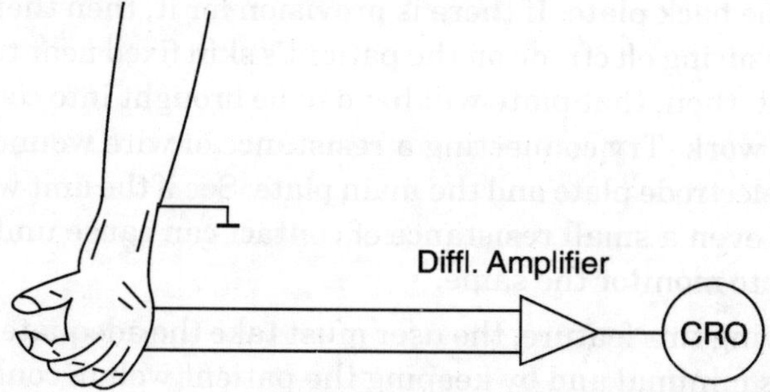

Fig. 18.6. Showing the set up for the voluntary muscle action potential measurement.

Propagation velocity of nerve impulse on a motor nerve

The details of the above were given in the Chapter on EMG.

The stimulus is to be applied to the stimulus electrodes and the signal applied is a 30–40 V pulse stimulus, single pulse, biphasic. A stimulator set up for this purpose must be first tested for its function and the level of voltage must be kept adjusted properly before the same is applied to the leg. If a stimulator is not available, a capacitor of 100 microfarad 63 V is kept charged to 50 V from a DC supply and then discharges through a switch into a small 50 mA 220 V/6 V mains transformer through the secondary. Then the primary winding is connected in series with a 2K resistor to the stimulus point for stimulation.

From the measurements made of the delay obtained from the trigger point and the peak of the action signal, the velocity of the nerve conduction can be estimated.

VII. STUDY OF PACEMAKER AND DEFIBRILLATOR

EXPERIMENT

To study the external demand pacemaker unit and to examine its functions

To study the defibrillator unit and learn to maintain it.

Apparatus

Pacemaker unit - external use model.

D.C. defibrillator unit with external pad electrodes.

PRINCIPLE

The pacemaker is an adjunct to an intensive care bed for cardiac patients. The catheter based pacing is meant for external pacing.

The Demand pacemaker uses the QRS complex to time the pulse only after the vulnerable period.

The unit has to be studied side by side with its circuit diagram, opening out the parts for visibility.

A typical unit may comprise of three sub systems.

1. Timing functions along with the rate indicating meter, the pulse output circuit
2. This senses the input ECG signal, if one is applied. This identifies the QRS complex if present and inhibits system 1 for a duration determined by the rate chosen.
3. This part is the power supply, the circuit including the microcontroller that operates the several sections.

The section 2 is the most important part of the unit. The ECG strip signal from the patient is processed by amplification and filtering. Then, a programmed refractory period is waited for, and signals arriving outside this period reset the timing control circuit. A hysterisis period is also programmable in some units.

The purpose of hysterisis is to stop the output from the pulse generator if the heart produces ECG even at a rate slightly below the programmed pacing rate. Hysterisis timings can be from 0, 100, 200 to 375 ms.

PROCEDURE

1. Set up for a rate of 72 beats per minute on the pacemaker front control.
2. Observe the nature of the waveform at the output pins. The pulse need not be a pure rectangle. Observe the leading and trailing edge values.

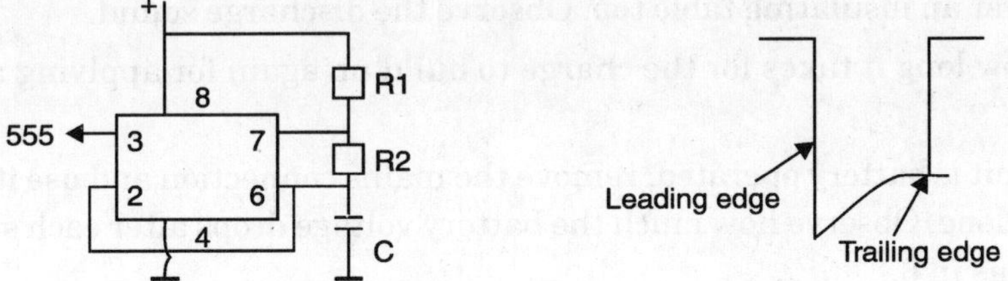

Fig. 18.7. Test circuit for testing demand pacing.

Measure the width of the pulse

3. Vary the rate to 120 and observe the same, noting if the width decreases. It must not.
4. In order to generate and ECG and examine demand pacing action, set up a short pulse generator using a 555 timer, which times at a rate of 0.8 second per pulse and make the pulse width very narrow, about 50 ms. Try R1 = 100K + 470 K variable, R2 = 10 K and C = 4.7 uF.

5. Apply this pulse to the ECG input socket of the pacemaker at a low amplitude, about 0.1 V through a potentiometer.
6. Observe if inhibition takes place at the output when the rate is set at 72.
7. Vary the rate and observe the inhibitive effect.
8. Measure the output voltage for various loading resistors, from 50 to 500 ohm.

Keep the output level setting at a fixed point.

Other features

There are pacemakers which are programmable by external programming feature.

The same may be a magnetic card or any other type. The programming information can be fed in the command code to tell the rate, width, amplitude and mode of operation.

VIII. D.C. DEFIBRILLATOR

Study the portable defibrillator unit

1. Is it provided with the ECG monitor?
2. Is it a synchronized type? In the synchronized type, the application of the shock pulse of defibrillation is avoided for 25-30 ms after the R wave, if exists.
3. Note if there is an energy level indicator for the charged capacitor.
4. Is the unit mains powered or only uses it for charging its internal batteries?
5. When the Defib button is pressed, note what relay inside operates. Is it a glass vacuum relay?
6. Examine the output sockets how high level of insulation is provided for the contacts and also the patient cable.
7. Is there a push switch on the paddles?
8. Now, charge the unit and press the electrodes on conducting foam pad kept on a metal plate over an insulating table top. Observe the discharge sound.
9. Note how long it takes for the charge to build up again for applying a second shock, if need be.
10. If the unit is battery operated, remove the mains connection and use it from the battery power alone. Observe how much the battery voltage drops after each shock delivered by testing as in 8.
11. Note how long it takes for the battery to get its full charge with mains input given. This figure might increase with age of the battery and hence a record of this will indicate the condition of the batteries.

IX. MICRO SHOCK DEMONSTRATION EXPERIMENTS

EXPERIMENT

To demonstrate on a phantom how microshock currents flow through a patient in an I.C.U. or surgery unit.

APPARATUS

A mock ECG recording with display unit

A mock Defibrillator

A mock pressure transducer for arterial puncture catheter based measurement

A mock patient motorized bed

A toy patient positioned on the bed.

PRINCIPLES

It is commonly learnt that possibilities of small currents of a.c. supply of the order of 500 A and above pass through the heart itself, which will instantly set the heart into a fibrillating state.

These small currents through the heart of a patient are produced unknowingly through fault or leakage currents diverted through the catheter and electrodes inserted into the body of the patient during surgical or intensive care operations.

Therefore, the equipment connected to a patient through internal or even well contacted surface electrodes must be free from faults and all conditions that might lead to such a current flow through the heart should be not only well known to everyone and be averted.

Since it is not possible to actually see such a condition in any I.C.U., in order to understand how and why such a microshock could happen totally in an unexpected manner, this experimental schedule is built using mock components and is meant to demonstrate the same under several possible conditions.

All apparatus applied to a patient must have earthed power supply with the metal case well earthed. Then, when two equipment are employed with a patient, one of which takes a lead into the patient through a catheter, such as for arterial pressure measurement, then, any differential voltage that can exist between the two equipment earths will send a current through the patient's internal organs, almost through his heart.

Suppose there is a 2 V differential voltage between such earth electrodes, which can occur possibly due a leak in one of the circuitry of the units, then the current that might flow in the patient would be limited only by the contact resistance which may be 1000 ohms or less. This will send 2 mA current, which is dangerous.

PROCEDURE

The mock ECG unit is just built using a simple microcontroller to generate pulses like the heart rate at about 80 per minute, which will cause a display on its LCD to show a mock ECG.

The other unit is a mock pressure transducer which shows the pulse on the LCD in a mock way, having just a lead connected into the catheter transducer attached through the toy patient kept on the mock bed.

The earth of the second unit can be made to have a potential difference with respect to the first (ECG) mock unit, by a resistor connected from the internal power supply to the case and leaving the earth connection open for it, as a means of showing a fault.

A resistor fault is introduced in the second unit by connecting a resistor between the hot lead and the earth, raising the earth potential of the unit by a certain 2-5 V. Then, a current will flow through the patient, which can be metered.

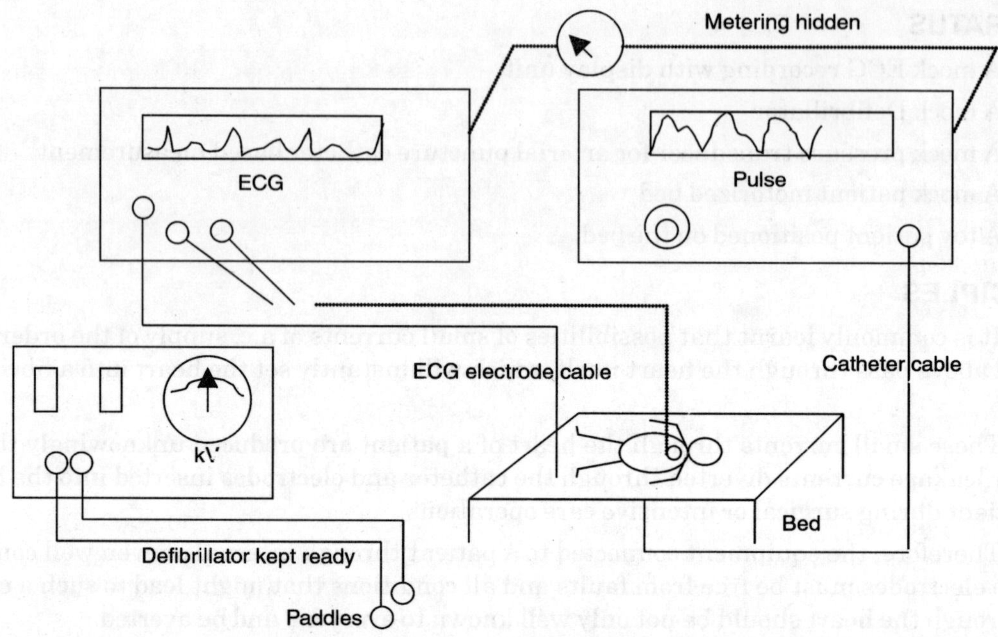

Fig. 18.8. Mock Microshock Demo experiment (*Courtesy* : V.I. Microsystems, Chennai-96).

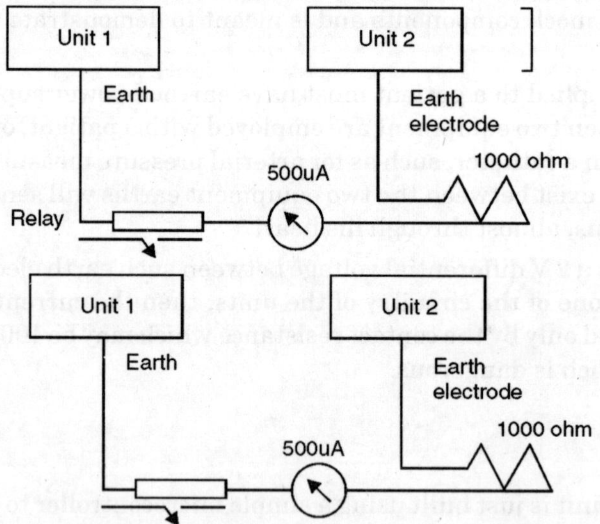

Fig. 18.9. Shows meter for earth difference current measurement and use of read relay.

This current will be made to flow when the fault is introduced at the unit 2 by connecting the resistor as already described. Then, this current flowing through the earth leads will cause a reed relay to close. These meter and relay are kept only for the view of the experiment.

This is sensed by the unit on Unit 1 through a connection hidden within the ECG lead cable itself and makes the microcontroller to sense the same and change the ECG pattern on the LCD screen to a mock fibrillating waveform.

An alarm also sounds with a blinking light on the unit1.

Then, the hospital assistant rushes and places the paddle defibrillator electrodes on the chest of the patient (mock).

This action of pressing the button on the paddle is also sensed by unit 1 microcontroller through another port bit. This then reverts the display back to ECG normal and the alarm ends. Then unit 2 is suddenly removed from mains and the catheter also removed from patient to prevent a repeating of the fault.

This session is totally arranged for a mock demonstration of how a microshock can ensue and how it is averted by timely action.

APPENDIX

A circuit for mock ecg and pulse display with microshock alarm.

The circuit is programmed to show the mock ECG or pulse waveform in the units 1 and 2 and this is possible by using the CG RAM feature of the LCD module. The ECG and pulse are split into three patterns which, together, show the ECG and pulse. These three characters are output one by one in the LCD with shift mode, so that a continuous display is visible. Then, the reed switch closes when a current of more than the micro-shock limit flows through the mock patient. Then, the same is sensed and the waveform changes to a random fibrillating signal on the LCD, simultaneously eliciting the sound from buzzer.

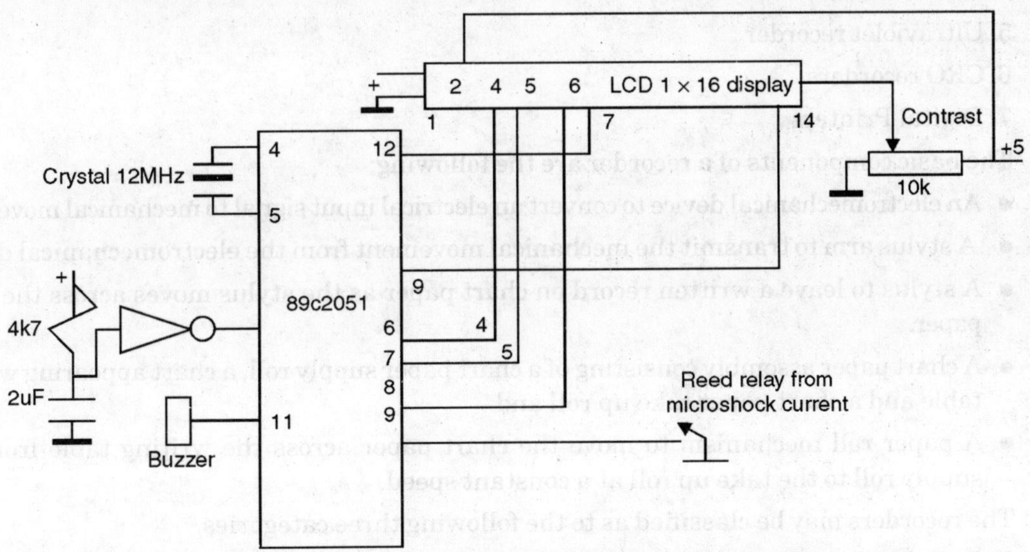

Fig. 18.10. Microcontroller with LCD Display Unit for 18.8.

Then, when the paddle switch of the defibrillator is pressed, that causes the reed relay to open and then the alarm stops, the wave reverts back to ECG from fibrillation.

Thus, an otherwise difficult event to demonstrate is made possible for mock demonstration with this microcontroller unit and LCD display, (two of which are needed) which act like mock ECG and Pulse transducer units.

Chapter 19

Recorders in Medical Instruments

A continuous visual record of physiological data versus time may either be obtained with a graphic recorder or with a digital storage oscilloscope along with a computer interface. Continuous motion CRT photography, while offering almost unlimited bandwidth and extremely fast recording rates, does not provide an immediate record of the recorded data. A graphic recorder, while inherently possessing limited high frequency response characteristics, does provide an immediate record of the recorded data for observation. Graphic recorders are often referred to as strip chart recorders, oscillographic recorders or chart recorders.

The recorders may be classified as follows:

1. Galvanometric recorders
2. Potentiometric recorders
3. EM recorder
4. Jet recorders
5. Ultraviolet recorder
6. CRO recorders
7. Digital Printers

The basic components of a recorder are the following:

- An electromechanical device to convert an electrical input signal to mechanical movement.
- A stylus arm to transmit the mechanical movement from the electromechanical device.
- A stylus to leave a written record on chart paper as the stylus moves across the chart paper.
- A chart paper assembly consisting of a chart paper supply roll, a chart appearing writing table and a chart paper take up roll and
- A paper roll mechanism to move the chart paper across the writing table from the supply roll to the take up roll at a constant speed.

The recorders may be classified as to the following three categories.

1. Basic Mechanism which converts an input current or voltage into mechanical movement of the recording stylus ; may use either a galvanometric or a potentiometric principle.

Recording Format in which the geometrical relationship between stylus movement and the chart paper will either result in a curved line or a straight line being transcribed on the chart paper when the stylus is abruptly moved to a new position.

Writing principle. A written record is transcribed on the chart paper with either an ink-pen stylus, a heated stylus or a rounded-point stylus.

Basic Recorder Mechanism

An input current or voltage is converted to mechanical movement of the stylus by either a galvanometric or a potentiometric principle.

Galvanometric recorders utilize a moving coil and magnet assembly with a stylus arm attached to the moving coil. This assembly is somewhat similar to the common d'Arsonval galvanometer assembly used in most conventional panel meters; however, the assembly used in a graphic recorder must develop sufficient torque than assembly used in the panel meter to overcome forces associated with stylus pressure and to provide good transient damping. The various recorder types shown in Fig. 19.1, all use galvanometric recorder mechanisms. These mechanisms are normally constructed so that angular deflection of the stylus arm is proportional to the magnitude of input current, that is, the relationship between input current and angular deflection is linear.

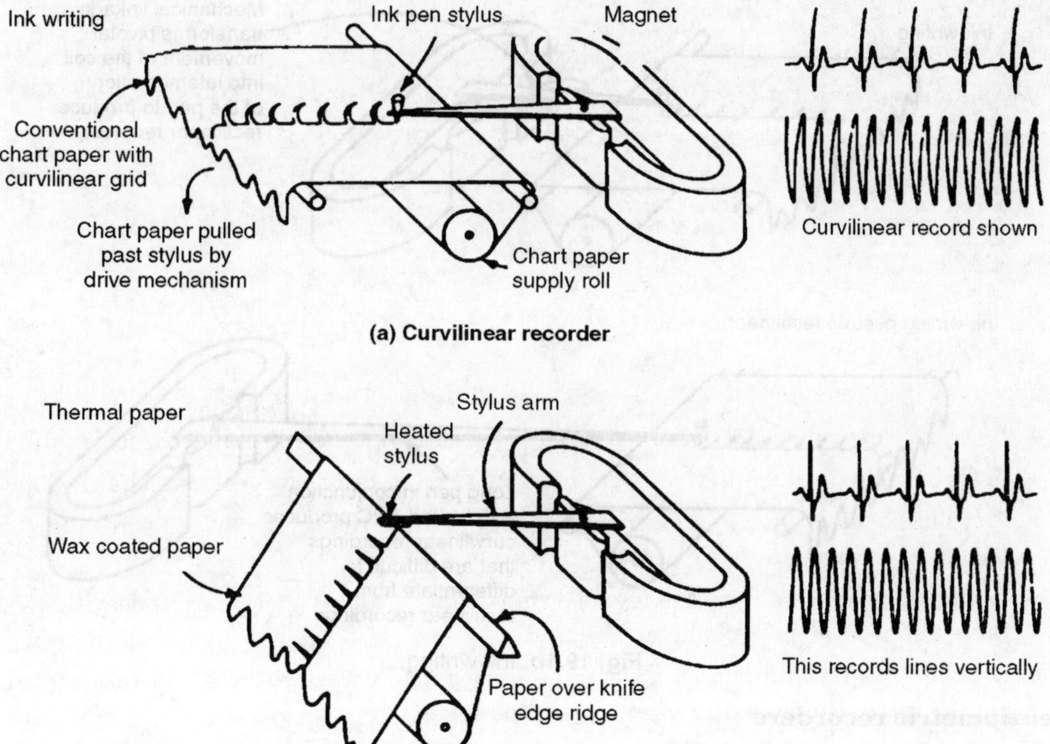

Fig. 19.1a. Shows the two forms of the galvanometric recorder (stylus short).

Damping is particularly important in a galvanometric recorder. If the moving-coil mechanism is at rest and a current is suddenly applied to the coil, the coil, the stylus arm and stylus will commence to move to a new position. The stylus and arm will gain momentum during this movement and when the new equilibrium position is reached this momentum will cause them to overshoot this position. The process is then reversed with the stylus and arm oscillating about the equilibrium position for some time until finally coming to rest. Damping must be added to a galvanometric recorder mechanism to overcome these oscillations, the mechanism being referred to as critically damped when the stylus and arm assume an equilibrium position as quickly as possible without overshooting the position. A slight overshoot is better because then it settles quicker. It is most important that pen- to paper friction constitutes only a very small part of the pen system damping, which should be supplied electrically, otherwise the damping will be unreliable over a period of time, and will tend to vary from one side of the chart to the other.

Frequency response. Due to finite force developed by a galvanometric recorder mechanism and the finite mass associated with a stylus and arm, the maximum angular acceleration of the system is defined and thus the frequency response of the system is defined. Most of the galvanometric recorder mechanisms offer a maximum frequency response of less than 200 Hz, this being directly proportional to the force developed by the galvanometric mechanism and inversely proportional to the moment of inertia of the coil, stylus arm and stylus assembly.

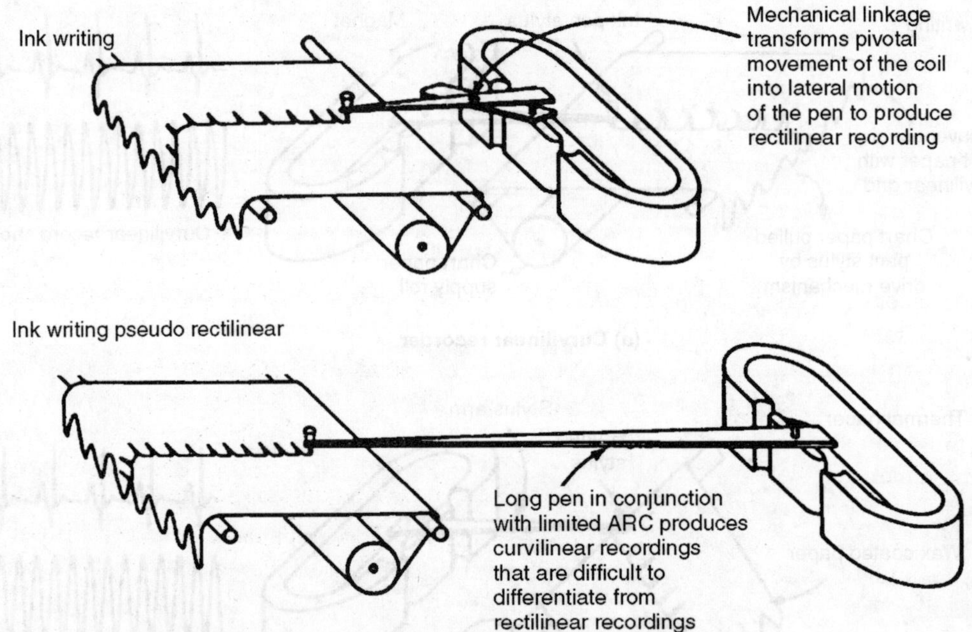

Fig. 19.1b. Ink writing.

Potentiometric recorders

Potentiometric recorders operate on a servo principle with the position of the stylus arm being detected via a contact mechanism attached to the arm and in contact with a fixed slide-wire as shown in Fig. 19.2. The servo system will move the stylus arm and stylus until the potential between the slide-wire contact and the input voltage is zero. The linearity and accuracy of the potentiometric recorder mechanism is dependant only on the characteristics of the slide wire and the associated electronics. The relationship between input voltage and the position of the contact on the slide wire is to be linear. Potentiometric recorder mechanism in general provides higher accuracy and better linearity than galvanometric mechanism. But the response is slower.

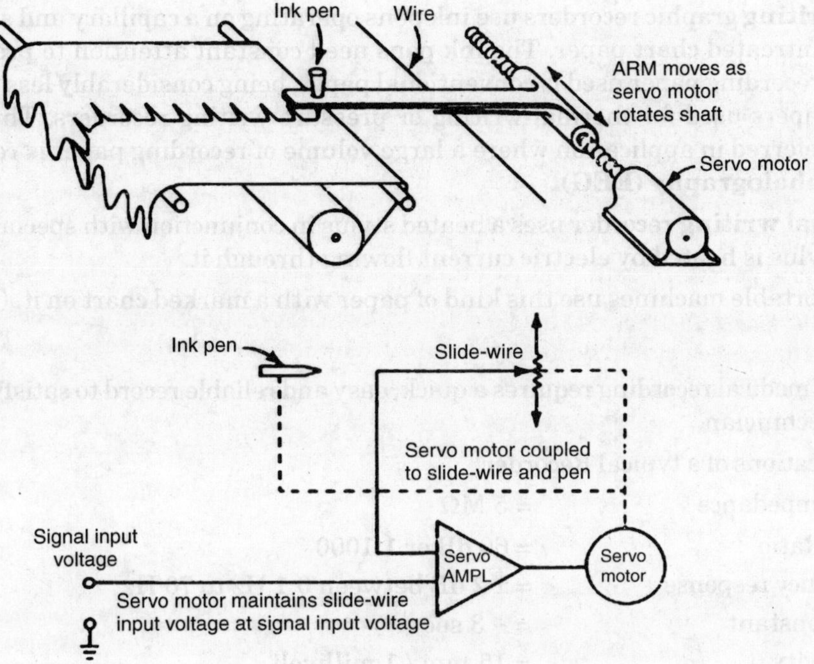

Fig. 19.2. Potentiometric servo type Recorder mechanism. Note that the wire is a potentiometer.

Recording Formats

The geometrical relationship between stylus movement and the chart paper is either referred to as curvilinear and rectilinear.

Curvilinear recording. The pivoted stylus arm will transcribe an arc at its tip if the arm is caused to rotate about its pivot point. A stylus at the tip of the arm will, therefore, transcribe a curved line on stationery chart paper located beneath the stylus. Since the line is curved, the recording format is referred to as curvilinear recording.(Fig. 19.1*a*). The basic galvanometer shown in Fig. 19.1*a* produces curvilinear recording. A typical **ECG** and sine wave recorded are shown with a curvilinear recorder. These recorders are less expensive than rectilinear recorders and are extensively used, particularly for less critical application such as may be encountered in a laboratory.

Rectilinear Recording. Movement of a stylus in a straight line perpendicular to the direction of movement of the chart paper would transcribe a straight line on stationary chart paper located beneath the stylus. Since the line is straight, the recording format is referred to as rectilinear recording. The potentiometric mechanism shown in Fig. 18.2 produces rectilinear recording. This recording may also be achieved with the galvanometric recorder mechanisms shown in Fig. 18.1*b*.

Writing Principles

The stylus in a graphic recorder must cause a written record to appear on the chart paper as the stylus moves across the surface of the paper. This written record may be achieved with a pen attached to the stylus arm, or with a rounded point attached to the stylus arm. The writing techniques are referred to as ink writing, thermal writing and pressure writing, respectively.

Ink Writing graphic recorders use ink pens operating on a capillary and siphon principle to record on untreated chart paper. The ink pens need constant attention to prevent blockage; however, the recording paper used is conventional paper, being considerably less expensive than the treated papers used for thermal writing or pressure writing recorders. Thus, ink writing recorder is preferred in application where a large volume of recording paper is required such as **electroencephalography (EEG).**

Thermal writing recorder uses a heated stylus in conjunction with specially coated chart paper. The stylus is heated by electric current flowing through it.

ECG portable machines use this kind of paper with a marked chart on it. (Chapter ECG).

Recorders

Electro medical recording requires a quick, easy and reliable record to satisfy every demand of a medical technician.

Specifications of a typical Recorder:

Input Impedance	= 5 MΩ
Discr. Ratio	= 60 dB or 1:1000
Frequency response	= ± 2 dB between 0.1 Hz to 70 Hz
Time constant	= ~ 3 sec
Sensitivity	= 15 mm / 1 millivolt
Linearity	= < 10% at ± 15 mm
Stability	= ± 10V fluctuation in mains voltage does not influence base line
Recording method	= Heater stylus, 50 mm recording paper
Speeds	= 25 mm/sec, 50 mm/sec
Standardization	= 1.3 V mercury cell
Power (KVA)	= 40 VA
Temperature of working	= 10–50°C

Recording Systems

Potentiometric Recorders

Pen or stylus is driven across the chart by a servomotor which simultaneously drives the slider of a potentiometer. The servomotor is controlled by an amplifier, the input to which is the difference between the signal and the slider potential. When the slider potential equals that of the signal, the motor stops and restarts in the appropriate direction when the signal changes. There is generally a finite minimum signal change needed to restart the motor; so the pen moves in a series of small steps, the value of each step is 0.1% of full scale deflection (f.s.d) usually.

The range is determined by the voltage applied to slide wire (1V). Recorders of 1mV full scale deflection are also available. Here, signal is compared with a small fraction (1/1000)th of the slider voltage and a high gain amplifier used to control the servomotor. Inertia of moving system limits speed.

Full Scale Deflection Times-0.1 sec to 1 sec. for various makes.

This is one limitation, but accuracy is good. (0.1%). Chart is large and clear, more reliable and running cost is very less.

For slowly varying variables : Oxygen tension, CO_2 tension, pH and pressure

Pen Motor (EM) recorders (EEG etc.)

1. Moving coil measurement or (Fig. 19.4)
2. Moving coil loud speaker movement (type 2) (Fig. 19.5)

In both the above, highest magnetic field is required.

Amplifiers. To drive 1 mm on paper/μV, anti-microphonic construction needed. Discrimination > 5000 : 1.

Should be maintaining this for long periods.

Noise level. 2 μV pp or less at the input grids of the unit with recorder in use (at frequencies up to 70 Hz).

Drift free during normal operation. That is not more than 1 mm per hour.

Facility for equalization of deflection for a common input calibrated signal is also required.

High frequency (H.F) controls must give varying degrees of attenuation for example, 15% less at 15, 25, 72 Hz.

Time constant – 0.03, 0.1, 0.3, 1 sec.

Amplifiers must have individual step gain controls at 6 dB each (totally 8). Master gain control to override the individual gain control.

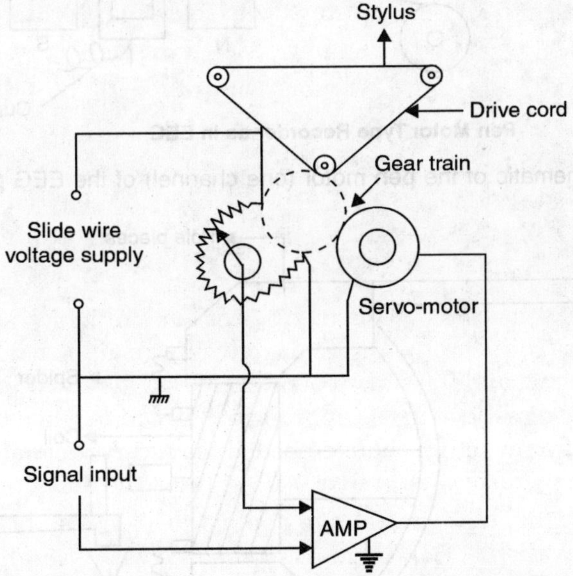

Fig. 19.3. Gear drive based servomotor in potentiometric recorder.

Amplifier must drive the recorder and provide adequate damping, without excessive overshoot. Power supply must be well stabilized.

Pen Recorder-Frequency response – 0–80 Hz.

It should be critically damped without any large resonance or phase distortion.

Pen arm length less than 10 cm (to reduce arc distortion) and a maximum deflection of 2 cm/sec.

Calibrator–5, 10, 20, 50, 100, 200, 500 mV or 1 mV. These signals are to be injected in amplifier with respect to earth.

Also with respect to earth differentially between the grids to adjust discrimination.

Inter-channel coupling < 2 %.

Paper Speeds–1, 5, 3 and 6 cm/sec ± 2%.

A minimum of 1 meter length of paper to be visible from the pen tips.

Earlier units used two valves at the front end, V1 and V2. These are critically selected for low noise as well as the anode resistors. Today's units employ dual FETs with matched performance.

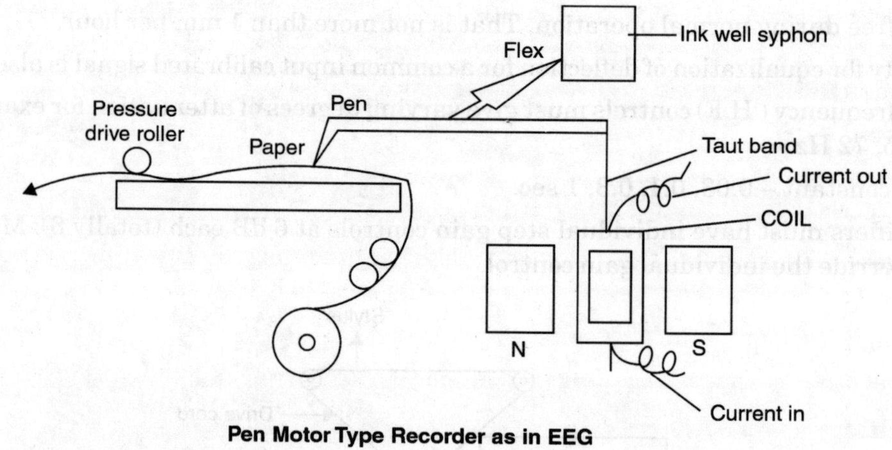

Fig. 19.4. A schematic of the pen motor (one channel) of the EEG paper recorder.

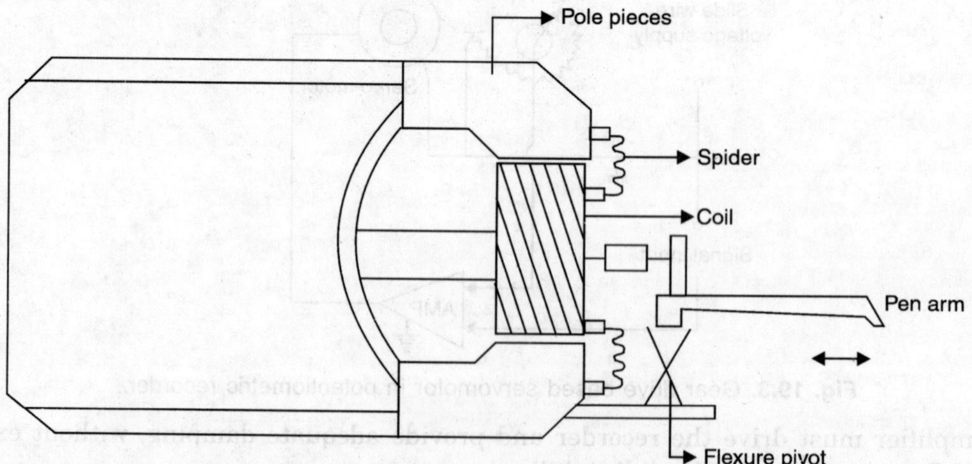

Fig. 19.5. Recorders of the moving coil-Pen Motor (types 1 and 2).

JET RECODERS

No pens are used. Fine jet ink emitted from a nozzle is directed by the movement of the coil.

Frequency response—500 Hz, even, up to 1000 Hz.

Disadvantages

Poor trace definition, ink drops at low speed, poor or faint trace at high frequencies.

Advantages

Best response. The whole width of the paper can be used for each trace in a multiple-trace unit, unlike stylus recorders, where the pen arms must not cross.

Ultraviolet recorder

Photographic paper is available which produces a visible trace without any chemical processing, after a few seconds exposure to ordinary room lighting.

Mirror galvo is used – 'Pencil type' which is derived from the high speed resistive galvanometer originally developed by Hill and Downing.

Various interchangeable galvos are available .

1 μA/cm (20 Hz natural frequency)

50 mA/cm (5000 Hz ,, ,,)

Biological transducers can directly actuate them. (5μ – 10 mA / cm types).

As a general purpose recorder, it is unequalled in performance. Linearity 1% , no hysterisis. Immediately available records, but high running cost, expensive paper.

The high pressure lamp (UV source) has a short life only.

One recorder now available uses iodine - quartz lamp (cheaper and long lasting).

Photographic recording galvos

These use ordinary white light and ordinary photo paper is needed which is anyhow wet processed. Light source needed is light and small (even dry batteries would do).

This has better resolution-can use even lower speeds of photo paper, for same resolution.

CRO Recorders

Linearity ± 1%

Beam switching-more traces

High input impedance

Voltage sensitivity is however not high , typically .2 to 2mm / m volt only.

Lab scopes – 10 mV/cm (DC to 15 MHz)

1 mV / cm (DC to 100 KHz)

Higher sensitivities available only in a.c.

Long persistence scope is needed for all biological recording , except EMG.

Non Graphic recording

For example, when we need to obtain a record of the variation in heart-rate over say 24 hour or a plot of frequency distribution, we need a non-graphic record.

Then we use a tape recorder and a timing and counting equipment.

Playback allows the same data to be processed in a number of different ways.

Playback can be faster or slower than the original recording.

Speech and music recorders have only a 30 – 10000 Hz response, which is unsuitable in biological work (lower frequencies needed).

Recording by carrier frequency modulation, amplitude modulation or pulse modulation can all be used. But these are costly.

Digital Printers

These add automation to the traditional experimental scientist with his pencil and note book but restricted to slowly changing signals. The accuracy is high, however.

The recorder is only a standard digital voltmeter (0.01%) coupled to electronic typewriter.

A Standard single channel high speed recorder by Devices Inc.

Uses interchangeable plug-in pıeamplifier units.

For example, the R2 system makes use of a special transistor chopper technique. It offers complete strain gauge amplifier and pen recorder facilities with power supplies-mains or battery operated in a single portable unit.

The pen writer provides a linear deflection of 50 mm, has frequency a response which is relatively flat from 0 – 50 Hz (3 dB down 75 Hz).

Recording methods for such standard Recorder

1. Hot stylus on heat sensitive paper-dense black trace writes in rectilinear co -ordinates.
2. Ink pen on untreated paper writes in curvilinear co-ordinates. An ink reservoir is supplied.
3. Paper drive is servo controlled to 2%. Accuracy and six speeds 1, 2.5, 5, 10, 25, 50 mm/sec are provided.
4. Either mains powered 250 V or by 12 V accumulator, with a current rating of 2.5 A.

Figure shows the Schwazer recorder. A stylus of special shape presses the recording paper running past in the direction of the arrow against 'writing edge' fixed at the right angles to the plane of travel. The carbon paper moving in the opposite direction, passes over the same writing edge and makes contact with the recording paper at the point of pressure of the recording stylus. Since the recording paper is moving in the opposite direction slight mutual friction is set up at the point of contact. So, a major proportion of the effort required to draw the trace comes from the paper feed mechanism and only a few grams of stylus pressure are needed to make an impression. The stylus can thus be made feather light and its minute moving mass combined with the small amount of friction and the small dimensions give a good frequency response. Very fine trace (0.15 mm) is got. The speeds of the recording and carbon paper feed are in a 2.5 : 1 ratio, even if paper speed is changed. The stylus is illuminated from below. Separate plastic gear wheels are used for paper speed adjustment.

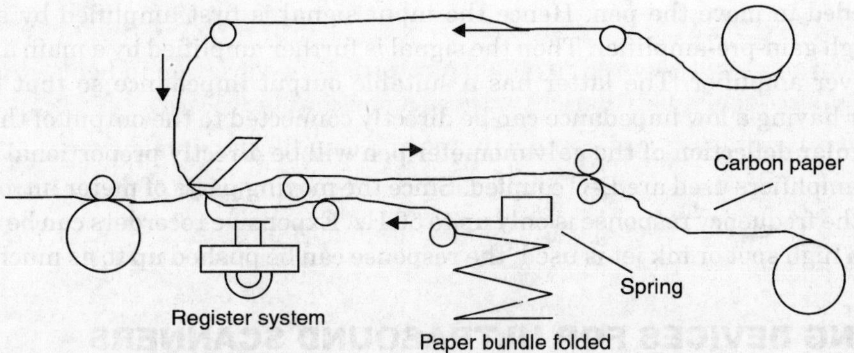

Fig. 19.6. Schwazer carbon paper + paper recorder.

Applications

Application	Pre Amplifiers	Transducers-electrode leads etc.
Blood Pressure	Uses a special tr. Chopper technique-1 kHz. 20 μV/cm DC input impedance or 3 kΩ or 200 μV/cm DC input impedance 30 kΩ, push pull zero drift 2 μV/°C. 10V DC isolated bridge supply with maximum current loading of 35 mA. Frequency response – 3 dB at 50 Hz. 10 step range switch either 0.1 mV – 100 mV or 10 – 500mm Hg for pressure measurements. **Sub unit.** Coarse and fine balance controls for external bridge (min. res. 100 Ω). Test button injects bridge calibrating resistor.	**Devices–Make Blood pressure transducer**
ECG	0.5mV /cm A.C., time constant 2 seconds Input impedance 1 MΩ Push pull HF response 3 dB down at 1.5 KHz. Control 'mute', × 1, ÷ 2. 'Fine gain' 'balance', filter for suppression of high frequencies. Lead selector, Std. I, II, III, AVR, AVL, AVF, V, CRCLCF, Std. Injects 1mV DC	ECG Electrodes–straps and patient cable.

For EEG and EKG, galvanometer type recorders are used. The galvo type recorder produces a permanent record on a strip of paper which during recording process moves at a pre determined rate. Since the pen of the galvanometer presses against the paper, there are frictional forces opposing the movement of the pen. In addition, the pen and the coil have inertia. So, considerable torque is needed to move the pen. Hence the input signal is first amplified by a high input impedance high gain-pre-amplifier. Then the signal is further amplified by a main amplifier and then to a driver amplifier. The latter has a suitable output impedance so that the coil of a galvanometer having a low impedance can be directly connected to the output of this amplifier. Then the angular deflection of the galvanometer pen will be directly proportional to the input voltage. The amplifiers used are D-C coupled. Since the moving parts of meter introduce inertia and friction, the frequency response is only up to 50 Hz. Expensive recorders can be available up to 200 Hz. If a high spot or ink jet is used, the response can be pushed up to as much as 3.5 kHz.

RECORDING DEVICES FOR ULTRASOUND SCANNERS

Recording devices recording the ultrasound image on a hard copy is essential. This helps us to review the scans and compare it while following up a patient. In the West, recording is compulsory from a legal stand. Recording devices are of various types.

1. **A Polaroid camera** is used for instantaneous photographic pictures, but this is too expensive to use ordinarily.
2. **35 mm camera** is simple to use and also cost-effective. Good reproduction of the image can be obtained. The negatives can be stored for future reference. This needs a photographic dark room back up and processing.
3. **Multi format cameras.** Two types are available, automatic and manual. These cameras use standard 10 × 8 inch special imaging films which is single side coated. In the automatic camera, the movement of the camera is automatic. In the manual type, the film has to be moved by the operator. This can result in double exposure if one is not careful. However, this costs only 50 % less than the automatic variety. 4 and 6 image formats on a single film are available.
4. **Strip Chart recorder.** In this type, silver paper is mechanically moved and the image is recorded. These have fallen into disuse due to unreliability of the equipment and also due to excessive running costs.
5. **Video Printers.** This is a new system, wherein inexpensive heat - sensitive paper is used for recording. This is the one used today for ultrasound machines. Unfortunately, the images recorded are not permanent.
6. **Video Recording.** This modality is useful for recording live images and Doppler audio signals. Storage of images facilitates reviewing and off-line analysis. Colour images can also be stored. Video recordings are useful for teaching programs.

Chapter 20

Computers and Medical Data Base Management Including Web

ACQUISITION OF BIOMEDICAL SIGNALS DATABASES

As biomedical signal databases are used for scientific and reference purposes, one specific aim is to obtain the best signal quality possible. Therefore, quality assurance during data acquisition is a very important task.

The International Classification of sleep Disorders (ICSD), which was developed in 1990 and revised in 1997, defines 88 sleep disorders based on symptoms and findings from sleep recordings. In order to objectify a diagnosis, a sleep recording must be done in a sleep laboratory. Biosignals reflecting neurophysiological, respiratory, and cardiac activities are recorded for eight to ten hours during the night. During the recording, the signals are also monitored.

Table 1. Minimal and optimal requirements for digital polysomnography as a basis for automatic sleep scoring. The digital amplitude resolution is chosen according to the measurement precision of the underlying instrument (n.a. = non-applicable).

Function	Signal	Minimum Sampling Rate	Optimal Sampling Rate	Digital Resolution
Neurophysiology	Electroencephalogram	100 Hz	200 Hz	0.5μV/bit
	Electro-oculogram	100 Hz	200 Hz	0.5μV/bit
	Electromyogram	100 Hz	200 Hz	0.2 μV/bit
Respiration	Oro-Nasal Airflow	16 Hz	25 Hz	n.a
	Respiratory Movements	16 Hz	25 Hz	n.a
	Oesophageal pressure	16 Hz	100 Hz	0.5 mmHg/Bit
	Capnography	16 Hz	25 Hz	0.1% / bit
	Oxygen saturation	0.5 Hz	1 Hz	1%/ bit
	Transcutaneous pO_2, pCO_2	0.5 Hz	1 Hz	0.1 mmHg/Bit
	Breathing Sounds	1 Hz	5000 Hz	n.a

Cardiovascular	ECG	100 Hz	250 Hz	10 µV/bit
	Heart Rate	1 Hz	4 Hz	1 bpm
	Blood Pressure	50 Hz	100 Hz	1 mmHg/Bit
Auxiliary	Body Temperature	0.1 Hz	1 Hz	0.1 Celsius /Bit
	Body position	0.1 Hz	1 Hz	n.a.

The SIESTA project, an Europeon work, was developed as an enhanced computer-based system for analyzing polysomnographies in a reliable, reproducible way. It serves as an example of medical database creation and management.

SIGNAL ACQUISITION CONDITIONS

As different signals in channels are interpreted together, the inter-signal synchronization is also important and must be thought of when selecting the recording equipment.

Sampling rates must be chosen in such a way that the requirements of subsequent analysis are covered. The different biomedical device modules needed for polysomnography are depicted in Fig. 20.1. Processing of the signals using the different sampling rate was done using two approaches. For many analysis methods applied, resampling of the raw signals was performed to come up with the agreed minimum sampling rate of 100 Hz. In the case of QRS detection in the ECG, the original sampling rate was preserved and the analysis was adapted to the conversion rates 100 Hz, 128 Hz, 200 Hz, 250 Hz, 256 Hz, and 400 Hz, respectively.

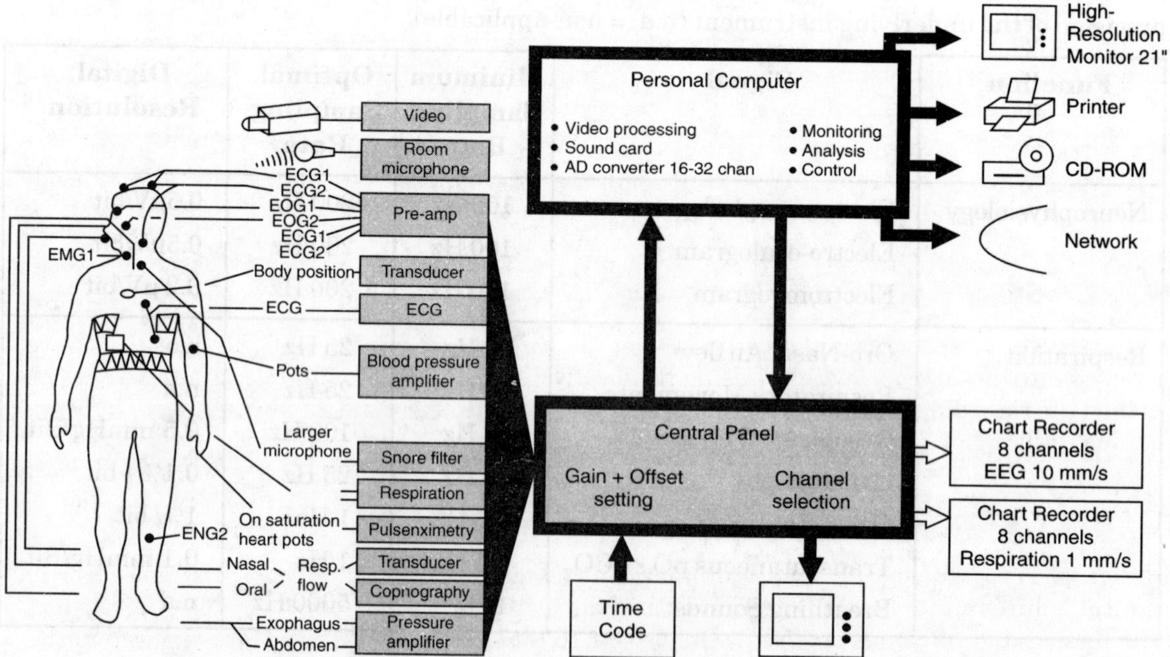

Fig. 20.1. The modules required for cardiopulmonary polysomnographic database creation, with personal computer and accessories.

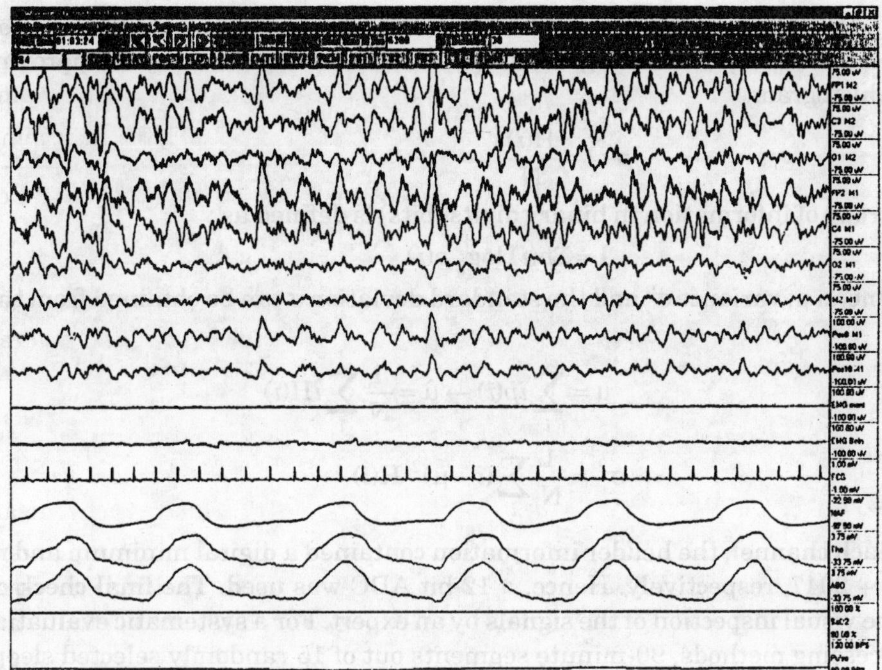

Fig. 20.2. Showing the Visual evaluation of biosignals of a sleep recording is performed using segments of 30 s. Sleep stages are based on the patterns, and then one of the buttons (each corresponding to a sleep stages) is activated. Here a signal data view is presented.

For respiratory movement recording, piezo transducers of different kinds, pneumatic belts, and inductive plethysmography were used. The resulting waveforms had different signal characteristics, so that no uniform analysis of respiration could be implemented. For respiratory flow, different kinds of thermistors and thermocouples were used. The differences between the resulting waveforms were smaller than the differences found in respiratory movement signals.

For oxygen saturation, pulse oximetry devices from different manufacturers were used. The devices were modules partially integrated in the equipment itself.

DATABASE STRUCTURES

All signals were either directly recorded using the European Data Format (EDF) or they were converted into the EDF format after using the locally available equipment. Filename conventions specified the recording site, the running number of the subject, and the number of the night being recorded (either 1 or 2). The order of the signals in the file was also specified.

QUALITY CONTROL AND RECORDED SIGNALS

The digitized recordings were tested automatically using a histogram analysis in order to identify technical failures and artifacts. The bin-width of the histograms was chosen to be the quantization of the analog-digital converter (ADC). In case of 16 bit signed integer numbers, as used in the EDF format, the histogram H(i) has bins in the range – 32768 = i = 32767.

When the total number of samples N goes to infinity, the normalized histogram is the probability distribution $p(i)$. For large N, the probability distribution may be approximated by the normalized histogram.

$$p(\hat{i}) = \frac{H(i)}{N} \quad ...(1)$$

and the entropy of information in binary digits (bits) is defined as :

$$I = \Sigma p(i) \log_2 p(i) \quad .(2)$$

The mean μ, variance σ^2 and the standard deviation σ can be obtained from the histogram H(i) :

$$\mu = \sum_i ip(i) \rightarrow \hat{\mu} = \frac{1}{N} \sum_i iH(i) \quad ...(3)$$

$$\sigma^2 = \frac{1}{N} \sum_i (i - \hat{\mu})^2 H(i) \quad ...(4)$$

For each channel, the header information contained a digital minimum and maximum of – 2048 and + 2047, respectively. Hence, a 12-bit ADC was used. The final check of the signal quality is the visual inspection of the signals by an expert. For a systematic evaluation of various artifact processing methods, 90-minute segments out of 15 randomly selected sleep recordings were visually analyzed and annotated. Nine types of artifacts (EOG, ECG, muscle, movement, failing electrode, sweat, 50 Hz, breathing, pulse) were visually identified, resulting in a total of 563192 1-s epochs.

Different artifact detection methods (least mean squares algorithm, regression analysis, independent component and principal component analysis, etc), which are able to remove technical and signal artifacts, were tested on the selected set of recordings with the annotated artifacts (Table 20.2). After validating different artifact processing algorithms, adaptive FIR filtering, regression analysis, and template removal were recommended to minimize the ECG interference, 50-Hz notch filtering for muscle and movement detection, and combined overflow and flat line detector for failing electrode artifacts.

ARCHIVING CONSIDERATIONS

A recordable CD-ROM can hold four recordings of this size. Sleep recordings require two consecutive nights with recording of all signals.

Table 20.2. Gives possible artifacts in the EEG signal

The methods to detect and remove these and the solution chosen within the SIESTA Project. (ICA= independent component analysis, PCA= principal component analysis)

Artifact	Detection and Removing	Solution Chosen
EOG	Regression Analysis, PCA, ICA,	Minimizing
ECG	Regression Analysis, PCA, ICA, Template Removal	Minimizing

Muscle Activity	Adaptive Inverse Filtering	Detect and Mark Data
Movement	Adaptive inverse filtering, overflow check	Detect and Mark Data
Failing Electrodes	Detect Typical Step Function with Exponential Decay, Combined Overflow and flat line Detector	Detect and Mark Data
Sweating	High-Pass filtering	None
50 Hz interference	Notch filter	Off-Line Filter
Breathing	Not Important for EEG	No Action
Pulse	Cross Correlation in Time, (did not appear in the SIESTA artifact database)	

When setting up a study design for the acquisition of a signal database, this has to be done on the basis of defined hypotheses with a fixed protocol. On the basis of a calculation on the number of subjects needed, the decision has to be made as to whether a multi-centre study is in need. For large signal databases this is usually the case.

CHOOSING THE PROPER DATA FORMAT FOR BIOSIGNAL EXCHANGE AND ARCHIVING

Floating point vs fixed point format

Signals are hardly ever sampled as floating point numbers, and the lack of support for this data type is not a serious flaw to a storage format. Sometimes there may, however, arise a need to store intermediate analysis results (e.g., autoregressive model parameters of an EEG signal segment) along with the original signals, and in that case the use of the floating point data type is necessary.

Digital Video

Digital video is becoming more and more commonplace in the intensive monitoring laboratories of epilepsy. A mechanism to link the video and the signals together in time is necessary to analyze the origin of the symptoms seen on the video. Voice annotations are not that hard to imagine to accompany biosignal recordings in some circumstances. Sometimes a simple image of, for example, the electrode positions on the head in a special EEG recording may come in useful. It is easy to foresee that the biosignal format could also provide some mechanisms to either embed these multimedia data into the biosignal file or to have links to point to those data in other files.

SOME FORMAT SPECIFICATIONS

One standard data format has been established as European prestandard CEN ENV 1064, and it is widely available for ECG recordings. This prestandard is also known as the SCP-ECG standard.

At this instance the handling of images is also mentioned in the SCP-ECG specification. Data compression is possible within format, SCP-ECG is supported by many manufacturers of ECG equipment and details are available on the WWW. Therefore, it is a recommendable alternative for ECG databases.

ASTM 1467 SPECIFICATION

The only standard for neurophysiology thus far that is supported by an official standardization body is the ASTM E-1467-94.

In addition to digitized biosignal waveforms of multiple channels, the primary data includes channel identifications, sensitivities, filter settings and sampling frequencies etc. The ASTM-1467 message consist of a sequential series of segments, with each segment conveying one aspect of a message. There are header segments, segments that contain the order of an investigation, and segments of the result. Segments consist of fields that define one attribute of the segment. A field may also be a hierarchical structure containing subfields. ASTM-1467 defines a number of data types.

The Mayo foundation (Rochester, Minnesota, USA) has provided software support to the ASTM-1467 user group including format conversions.

EDF SPECIFICATION

EDF (European Data Format) is a simple format for exchange and archiving. An EDF file has an ASCII header containing mainly patient and time identification, the number of signals, and the technical characteristics.

All information about EDF including its full specification, list of EDF-supporting companies, many links to downloads of software and data, the floating-point scheme, and a FAQ list including the annotations scheme is available on the Internet (www. hsr.nl./edf).

ALTERNATIVE SPECIFICATIONS

The Extensible Biosignal Format (EBS) was designed by the epilepsy research group of the University of Erlangen.

The SIGIF format was designed with neurophysiological biosignal exchanges in mind at the University of Aveiro, Portugal. In addition to the above, other format specifications have been published as well (MIT arrhythmia database format, IFFPHYS from Australia, etc.).

The EDF Format and Use

In most cases, the biomedical signals are sampled by a single device and their dynamic range can be covered by 16-bit (or less) integer values. In those cases, the EDF has proven its usefulness. The specification of this format takes only one page, and it is simple and many companies and researchers are already exchanging data using EDF. The format specification does not give defined signal labels, nor sampling rates nor other restrictions. Thus, the format can be used for many signals using free signal definitions without violation. This is avoided in the more complex ASTM 1467-94 and CEN / FEF formats. The general issue in designing data formats is the balance between free handling of the data format and giving as few definitions as possible. EDF is good example) and on the other extreme define codes that have to be filled in each single place in the file (ASTM and SCP - ECG being examples). The first extreme is the ideal format for developers because their acquisition software will almost every time work right due to the few restrictions. As labor costs form the majority of costs in health care, the trend is toward fully interoperable automatic systems (with extensive coding schemes) that do not require human intervention.

THE INTERNET AN IDEAL TOOL FOR BIOMEDICAL SIGNAL DATA ACQUISITION

Biomedical data can be collected using a variety of hardware interface methods including data acquisition cards inserted into the PC bus, hardwired interfaces (RS232, USB etc), or wireless connections to the PC. Data can also be generated within the computer in the form of questionnaire responses.

WIN-ECG

An example of web-enabled data acquisition of biomedical signals is the Win-ECG. These controls are compiled software components based on Microsoft's Component Object Model (COM) technology. The ActiveX controls in Win-ECG are simple button controls, which are embedded in the Web pages. Similar techniques may be used to acquire data from any biomedical signal source in the laboratory, clinic or from remote and unattended locations.

STORAGE AND ANALYSIS

The choice of a database management system (DBMS) is an important design consideration. DBMSs are either shared-file-based databases or client/server data-bases. Shared-file databases are usually stored and accessed on a local computer, thus making access to data by multiple remote users difficult.

The main drawbacks of client/server systems when applied to the remote acquisition and storage of biomedical signals are a requirement for an online network connection, the added cost of run-time software licenses, and the complexity of installation of the run-time engines on the remote client computer.

Data processing can be performed on either the client computer or the database server. However, data processing on the client server makes system upgrades difficult as changes must propagate to all clients. This problem can be overcome by shifting processing to the data base server; system changes are then automatically accessible by all simple client applications. However, this approach places more load on the data base server, as it is responsible for processing all client requests.

Multi-tiered systems can be used to solve these problems of client, and server-side processing. A multilayered system comprises a simple client data processing server and a data base server. By having a separate server or unit dedicated to data processing and brokering, the load on the database server can be reduced. The separate data processing server will process requests from clients and retrieve data from the data base server. After the data is retrieved, it is processed and presented to the client.

SYNCHRONIZATION

In the case of local database replicas, the client stores a subset of the server database and periodically inserts new records as they are collected. These database changes are flagged and on connection to the server, are transmitted to the server for updating or insertion. Similarly, changes in the server database specific to the client are replicated at the client side. Both client and server are able to track changes and synchronize their data using technologies such as Microsoft's ActiveX Data Objects (ADO), Inprise MIDAS, and CORBA. This store-and-forward method of updating the database also allows the utilization of flexible, low-cost, off-peak communication links. Periodic synchronization of the database with the server provides sufficient updates.

SECURITY FACTORS

Data encryption should be considered mandatory for any transmission of identified patient data, including physiological records. RSA public-key encryption technology is commonly used. User authentication is another important security issue. The SIESTA project considered only catering to password authentication. However, the ability to embed ActiveX controls within the web page that link to external hardware devices would allow more sophisticated user authentication paradigms.

RETRIEVAL AND QUERY ENGINES

For example, in a home tele-care application, the client may wish to query his /her own longitudinal data records or these data may need to be automatically analyzed and reformulated for transmission to the client's primary care physician.

ACTIVE X DATA OBJECTS (ADO)

ActiveX Data Object was designed by Microsoft to be a single application programming interface (API) that allows access to a wide variety of data sources. Simply, it is a wrapper object for OLEDB (see below) and open database connectivity (ODBC) data sources that encapsulates a simplified set of properties and methods for accessing these data sources. ADO is built as a general-purpose COM-based object model. This property allows ADO to be optimized or customized for accessing different data base types, while preserving a constant object model. Since ADO uses a language - neutral API, it can be used in a variety of languages such as C++, Visual Basic, or Delphi.

The ADO model consists of three main objects; Connection, Record-set, and Command. To use ADO, a Connection object is created that specifies the ODBC provider or OLE DB driver. The ODBC provider acts as an interface between the ODBC driver and the ADO object, exposing methods and properties for accessing the data. Data can then be retrieved or stored from the database by creating a Record Set object. In addition, database-specific commands and SQL can be sent to the database using a Command object.

OLE DB

OLE DB is a COM based API that allows access to any data independent of its data type. This eliminates the need to convert non-SQL data such as a spread sheet data into an equivalent ANSI SQL database format before it can be accessed using ODBC. OLE DB architecture is composed of the Data Consumer, Data Provider, and Service Provider components. These can be customized using a variety of exposed interfaces using the object model to maintain communication with each other. Through these various interfaces, OLE DB can represent all types of data in a standard tabular form, thus allowing them to be easily accessed and manipulated.

For example, if an application or Data Consumer requires data from a spreadsheet program, it calls the Data Provider. By using various interfaces, the provider exposes the underlying spreadsheet data as a table. This table can then be accessed and processed by the Data Consumer using SQL. The Service Provider encompasses both the Data Consumer and Data provider components. This component performs complex operations such as table joins and query processing. Examples of a service Provider are a query processor or cursor library.

SYSTEM DESIGN

Data acquisition and storage in a multi-tier information system begins with the patient or user acquiring biomedical signals data on a personal computer running the client application as shown in Fig. 20.3.

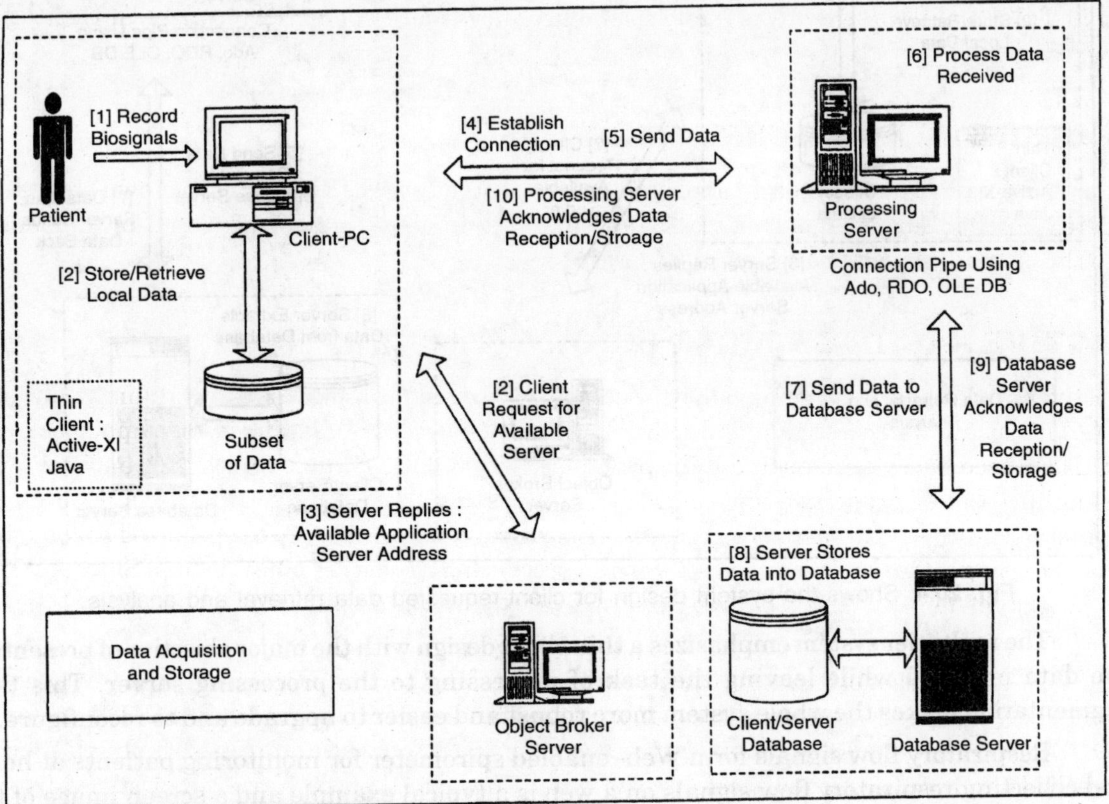

Fig. 20.3. Shows the System design for data acquisition and storage of biomedical signals.

DATA RETRIEVAL AND ANALYSIS

In a multi-tier information system, the process of data retrieval begins by the client requesting a specific piece of information (Fig. 20.4). The client then connects to the object broker requesting an available processing server address. Upon receiving the address, the client connects to the processing server and sends the request. The processing server processes the request by retrieving the appropriate data from the database server and transforming it into information. Generally, data transformation is performed through a client-defined command or a pre-specified set of rules residing on the server. The design allows automated server-side processing of the acquired data using an intelligent agent. These processing tasks can be triggered by database updates and insertions or by client-side requests. The information retrieved is exposed to the client through a database table. The client can then access this data and format it appropriately for presentation to the user.

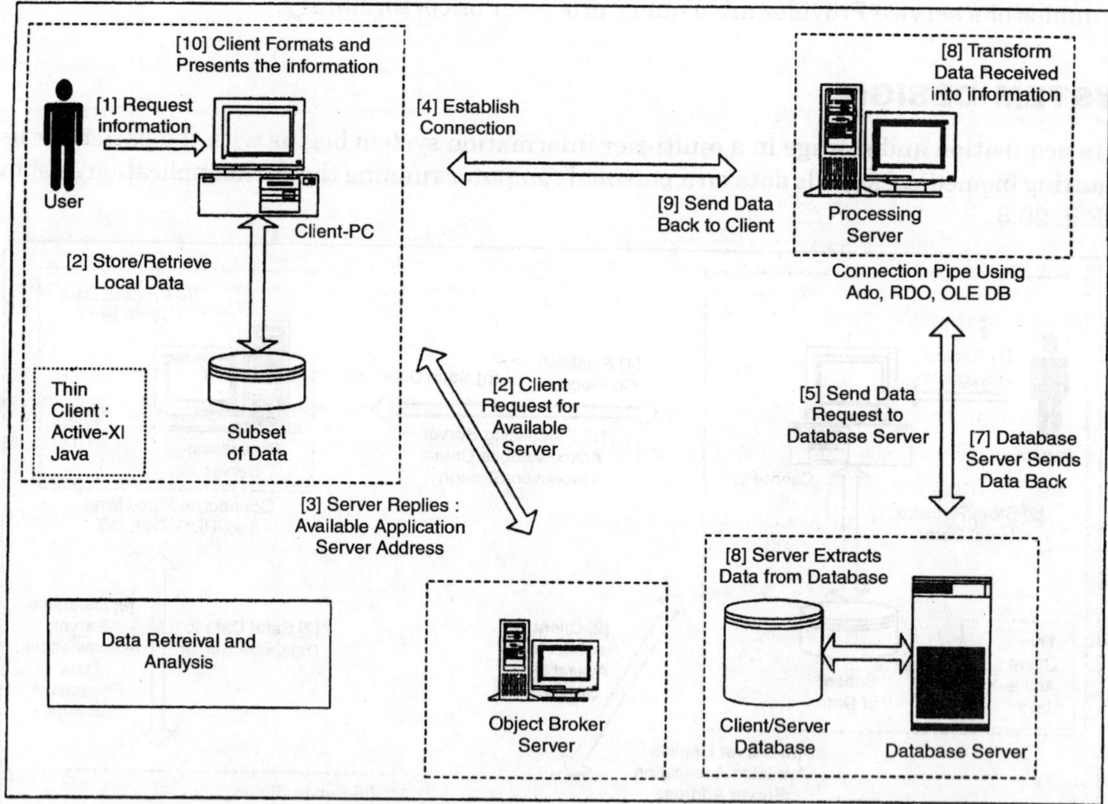

Fig. 20.4. Shows the system design for client-requested data retrieval and analysis.

The multi-tier system emphasizes a thin client design with the major objective of presenting the data provided while leaving the task of processing to the processing server. This task segmentation makes the whole system more robust and easier to upgrade and to reconfigure.

Respiratory flow signals form Web- enabled spirometer for monitoring patients at home and collecting respiratory flow signals on a web is a typical example and a screen image of the lung measurement software (Fig. 20.5).

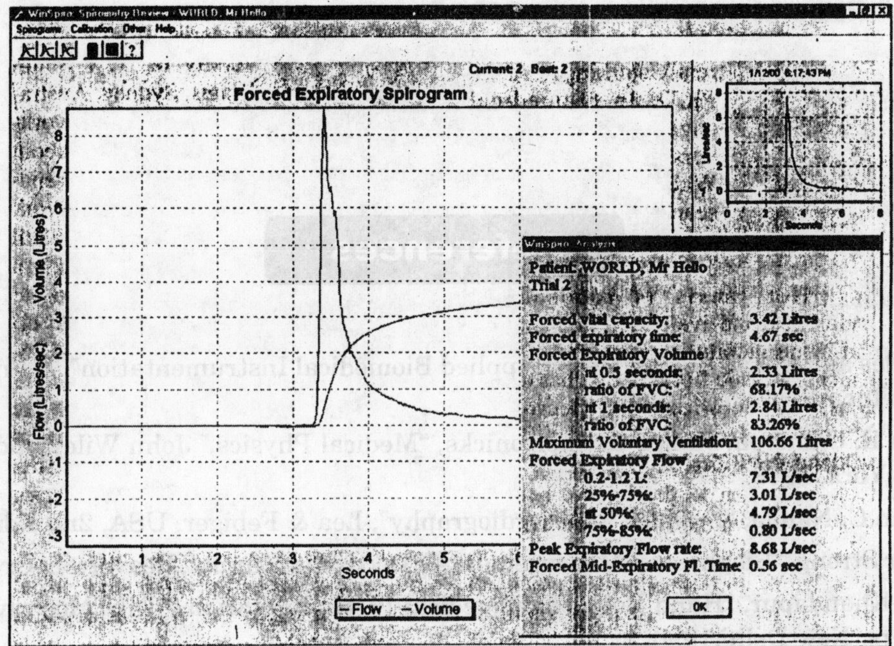

Fig. 20.5. Shows a screen image of the lung measurement software.

CONCLUSION

The advantages associated with a WEB interface include familiarity with browser design and navigation (for the user), as well as the ability to rapidly customize interfaces for particular requirements (for the programmer). Naturally, signals collected from particular target populations, (for example, lung function measurement associated with asthma in young children as opposed to chronic obstructive pulmonary disease assessment in the elderly) require different user interfaces.

References

1. Geddes and Bakar, "Principles of Applied Biomedical Instrumentation", John Wiley and Sons Inc., New York, 1968.
2. John R. Cameron, James G. Skofronicks, "Medical Physics," John Wiley and Sons Inc., New York, 1978.
3. Navin.C. Nanda, "Doppler Echocardiography", Lea & Febiger, USA, 2nd Edition, 1993.
4. Peter Strong, "Biophysical Measurements", Tektronix Manual, Beaverton, Oregon, 1970.
5. R.S. Khandapur, "Hand Book of Biomedical Instrumentation," Tata McGraw Hill Publishers, New Delhi,1990.
6. T.W. Graham Soloman, "Organic Chemistry", John Wiley and Sons, New York, 1996 (Sixth Edition).
7. Willis. J. Tompkins, John G. Webster, "Design of Microcomputer Based Medical Instrumentation", Prentice Hall International Inc, London, 1981.

Index

C

D

E

O

P

Q

R

S

T

U

V

W

X

Z